Coding Companion for OB/GYN

A comprehensive illustrated guide to coding and reimbursement

2013

Publisher's Notice

Coding Companion for OB/GYN is designed to be an authoritative source of information about coding and reimbursement issues affecting obstetrics and gynecological procedures. Every effort has been made to verify accuracy and all information is believed reliable at the time of publication. Absolute accuracy cannot be guaranteed, however. This publication is made available with the understanding that the publisher is not engaged in rendering legal or other services that require a professional license. If you identify a correction or wish to share information, please email the Optum customer service department at customerservice@optum.com or fax us at 801.982.4033.

American Medical Association Notice

Our Commitment to Accuracy

Optum is committed to producing accurate and reliable materials.

To report corrections, please visit www.optumcoding.com/accuracy or email accuracy@optum.com. You can also reach customer service by calling 1.800.464.3649, option 1.

Copyright

Acknowledgments

Kelly Armstrong, *Product Manager*
Karen Schmidt, BSN, *Technical Director*
Stacy Perry, *Manager, Desktop Publishing*
Lisa Singley, *Project Manager*
Debbie Hall, *Clinical/Technical Editor*
Jillian Harrington, MHA, CPC, CPC-P, CPC-I, CCS-P, MHP, *Clinical/Technical Editor*
Karen M. Prescott Adkins, CPC, CPC-I, CCS-P, *Clinical/Technical Editor*
Tracy Betzler, *Senior Desktop Publishing Specialist*
Hope M. Dunn, *Senior Desktop Publishing Specialist*
Katie Russell, *Desktop Publishing Specialist*
Kimberli Turner, *Editor*

Technical Editors

Deborah C. Hall

Ms. Hall is a new product subject matter expert for Optum. She has more than 25 years of experience in the health care field. Ms. Hall's experience includes 10 years as practice administrator for large multi-specialty medical practices. She has written several multi-specialty newsletters and coding and reimbursement manuals, and served as a health care consultant. She has taught seminars on CPT/HCPCS and ICD-9-CM coding and physician fee schedules.

Jillian Harrington, MHA, CPC, CPC-P, CPC-I, CCS-P, MHP

Ms. Harrington has more than 19 years of experience in the health care profession. She recently served as President and CEO of ComplyCode, a health care compliance consulting firm based in Binghamton, NY. She is the former Chief Compliance Officer and Chief Privacy Official of a large academic medical center, and also has extensive background in both the professional and technical components of CPT/HCPCS and ICD-9-CM coding. She teaches CPT coding and is an approved instructor of the Professional Medical Coding Curriculum, awarded by the AAPC. She has spoken frequently on health care compliance and health information management issues at regional and national professional conferences. Ms. Harrington holds a Bachelor of Science degree in Health Care Administration from Empire State College and a Master of Science degree in Health Systems Administration from the Rochester Institute of Technology. She is a member of the AAPC and a former member of its National Advisory Board, a member of the American Health Information Management Association (AHIMA) and the Health Care Compliance Association (HCCA), and is an associate of the American College of Healthcare Executives (ACHE).

Karen M. Prescott Adkins, CPC, CPC-I, CCS-P

Ms. Adkins has more than 18 years of experience in the health care profession. She has an extensive background in professional component coding and billing. Her prior experience includes establishing and maintaining a coding and billing service, directing physician practice start ups, functioning as director of physician credentialing, negotiating insurance contracts, and functioning as a health care consultant. Her areas of expertise include coding and reimbursement, documentation education, compliance, practice management, and revenue cycle management. Ms. Adkins is a member of the American Academy of Professional Coders (AAPC), and the American Health Information Management Association (AHIMA).

Contents

Coding Companion for OB/GYN

© 2012 OptumInsight, Inc.

Getting Started with Coding Companion

Coding Companion for OB/GYN is designed to be a guide to the specialty procedures classified in the CPT book. It is structured to help coders understand procedures and translate physician narrative into correct CPT codes by combining many clinical resources into one, easy-to-use source book.

The book also allows coders to validate the intended code selection by providing an easy-to-understand explanation of the procedure and associated conditions or indications for performing the various procedures. As a result, data quality and reimbursement will be improved by providing code-specific clinical information and helpful tips regarding the coding of procedures.

For ease of use, *Coding Companion* lists the CPT codes in ascending numeric order. Included in the code set are all surgery, radiology, laboratory, medicine, and evaluation and management (E/M) codes pertinent to the specialty. Each CPT code is followed by its official CPT code description.

Providers

The AMA advises coders that while a particular service or procedure may be assigned to a specific section, the service or procedure itself is not limited to use only by that specialty group (see paragraphs 2 and 3 under "Instructions for Use of the CPT Codebook" on page x of the CPT Book). Additionally, the procedures and services listed throughout the book are for use by any qualified physician or other qualified health care professional or entity (e.g., hospitals, laboratories, or home health agencies).

The use of the phrase "physician or other qualified health care professional" (OQHCP) was adopted to identify a health care provider other than a physician. This type of provider is further described in CPT as an individual "qualified by education, training, licensure/regulation (when applicable), and facility privileging (when applicable)" State licensure guidelines determine the scope of practice and a qualified health care professional must practice within these guidelines, even if more restrictive than the CPT guidelines. The qualified health care professional may report services independently or under incident-to guidelines. The professionals within this definition are separate from "clinical staff" and are able to practice independently. CPT defines clinical staff as "a person who works under the supervision of a physician or other qualified health care professional and who is allowed, by law, regulation, and facility policy to perform or assist in the performance of a specified professional service, but who does not individually report that professional service." Keep in mind that there may be other policies or guidance that can affect who may report a specific service.

Resequencing of CPT Codes

The American Medical Association (AMA) employed a resequenced numbering methodology beginning with *CPT 2010*. According to the AMA, there are instances where a new code is needed within an existing grouping of codes, but an unused code number is not available to keep the range sequential. In the instance where the existing codes were not changed or had only minimal changes, the AMA assigned a code out of numeric sequence with the other related codes being grouped together. The resequenced codes and their descriptions have been placed with their related codes, out of numeric sequence.

CPT codes within the Optum *Coding Companion* series display in their resequenced order. Resequenced codes are enclosed in brackets for easy identification.

Surgery Codes

A full page is dedicated to each surgical procedure or to a series of similar procedures. Following the specific CPT code and its narrative, is a combination of features. A sample is shown on iii. The black boxes with numbers in them correspond to the information on the following page of the sample.

Supplies

Some payers may allow physicians to separately report drugs and other supplies when reporting the place of service as office or other nonfacility setting. Drugs and supplies are to be reported by the facility only when performed in a facility setting.

Appendix

Some CPT codes are presented in a less comprehensive format in the appendix.

Category II and III Codes and Descriptions

Category II codes, which are published January 1 and July 1 of each year, are supplemental tracking codes used for performance measurement only. They describe components usually included in an evaluation and management service or test results that are part of a laboratory test. Use of these codes is voluntary. However, they are not to be used in lieu of Category I codes. Category II codes will not be published in this book. Refer to the CPT book for code description.

In this section, each Category III code appropriate to the specialty is provided, with the official CPT code descriptions. The codes are presented in numeric order, and each code is followed by an easy-to-understand description of the Category III procedure.

These codes are temporary tracking codes to identify new and emerging technologies. This allows health care professionals to indicate emerging technologies, services, and procedures for clinical efficacy, utilization, and outcomes.

Radiology Codes and Descriptions

In this section, each CPT radiology code appropriate to the specialty is provided, with the official CPT code description. The codes are presented in numeric order, and each code is followed by an easy-to-understand lay description of the radiological procedure.

Remember that radiology codes have a technical and a professional component. When physicians do not own their own radiology equipment and send their patients to outside testing facilities, they should append modifier 26 to the radiology procedural code to indicate they performed only the professional component.

Pathology and Laboratory Codes and Descriptions

In this section, each CPT pathology and laboratory code appropriate to the specialty is provided, with the official CPT code description. The codes are presented in numeric order, and each code is followed by an easy-to-understand lay description of the pathology or laboratory procedure.

Medicine Codes and Descriptions

Some medicine codes are expanded into full-page formats, similar to the surgical codes. Only the codes that are directly related to the specialty will be included in this format; general codes that apply across many specialties might be in the appendix in the back of the book. In the appendix section, additional CPT medicine codes appropriate to the specialty are provided, with the official CPT code description. The codes are presented in numeric order, and each code is followed by an easy-to-understand lay description of the medicine service or procedure.

ICD-9-CM Coding System

This section provides a list of codes commonly reported by obstetrics and gynecology.

ICD-9-CM to ICD-10-CM Transition

The codes within ICD-9-CM fall woefully short of today's medical reporting needs. ICD-9-CM was created more than 25 years ago as a modern and expandable system that was then only partially filled. Thousands of codes have been added to ICD-9-CM over the years to classify new procedures and diseases, and today the remaining space in ICD-9-CM procedure and diagnosis coding systems cannot accommodate new technologies or new understanding of diseases.

In response to ICD-9-CM's shortcomings, new coding systems were developed and soon will be implemented in the United States. The World Health Organization (WHO) created and adopted ICD-10 in 1994 and it has been used in much of the world ever since. This system is the basis for the new U.S. diagnosis coding system, International Classification of Diseases, 10th Revision, Clinical Modification (ICD-10-CM).

On January 16, 2009, the Department of Health and Human Services published a final rule in the *Federal Register*, 45 CFR part 162, "HIPAA Administrative Simplification: Modifications to Medical Data Code Set Standards to Adopt ICD-10-CM and ICD-10-PCS" (downloadable at http://edocket.access.gpo.gov/2009/pdf/ E9-743.pdf). This final rule adopts modifications to standard medical data code sets for coding diagnoses and inpatient hospital procedures by adopting ICD-10-CM for diagnosis coding, including the Official ICD-10-CM Guidelines for Coding and Reporting, and ICD-10-PCS for inpatient hospital procedure coding. It is important to note that the implementation of ICD-10-CM and PCS has been delayed. The final rule, released August 24, 2012, confirmed that the new implementation date is October 1, 2014. The most current 2012 draft update release is available for public viewing, and additional updates are expected before implementation. At this time, ICD-10-CM codes are not valid for any purpose or use other than for reporting mortality data for death certificates. This does not mean it is not time to begin preparing, however. Now is the time to prepare, as the 2014 date is approaching rapidly, and there will be no grace period for using the new codes.

Everyone in facilities will be affected: coders, human resources staff, accountants, information systems staff, physicians—just to name a few. The proposed codes provide tremendous opportunities for disease and procedure tracking but also create enormous challenges. Computer hardware and software, medical documentation, and the revenue cycle are just three elements of medical reimbursement that will be shaken when implementation occurs.

Understanding the changes the World Health Organization made in moving from ICD-9-CM to ICD-10-CM is a good basis for learning about the clinical modifications to ICD-10-CM. The first clue to the revisions is in the full title: International Statistical Classification of Diseases and Related Health Problems.

Overall, the 10th revision goes into greater clinical detail than does ICD-9-CM and addresses information about previously classified diseases, as well as those diseases discovered since the last revision. Conditions are grouped with general epidemiological purposes and the evaluation of health care in mind. New features have been added, and conditions have been reorganized, although the format and conventions of the classification remain unchanged for the most part.

CCI Edit Updates

The *Coding Companion* series includes the most up-to-date ICD-9-CM, CPT, and HCPCS codes available at print time. The codes in the Correct Coding Initiative (CCI) section are from version 18.3, the most current version available at press time. Optum maintains a website to accompany the *Coding Companions* series and posts updated CCI edits on this website so that current information is available before the next edition. The website address is www.optumcoding.com.

Evaluation and Management

This resource provides documentation guidelines and tables showing evaluation and management (E/M) codes for different levels of care. The components that should be considered when selecting an E/M code are also indicated.

Index

A comprehensive index is provided for easy access to the codes. The index entries have several axes. A code can be looked up by its procedural name or by the diagnoses commonly associated with it. Codes are also indexed anatomically. For example:

69501   Transmastoid antrotomy (simple mastoidectomy)

could be found in the index under the following main terms:

Antrotomy
Transmastoid, 69501

Excision
Mastoid
Simple, 69501

56501-56515 [1]

56501 Destruction of lesion(s), vulva; simple (eg, laser surgery, electrosurgery, cryosurgery, chemosurgery)

56515 extensive (eg, laser surgery, electrosurgery, cryosurgery, chemosurgery)

[2]

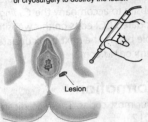

The physician may use laser, fulguration, or cryosurgery to destroy the lesion

Lesion

Report 56501 for simple or single lesions or 56515 for multiple or complicated lesions

Explanation [3]

The vulva includes the labia majora, labia minora, mons pubis, bulb of the vestibule, vestibule of the vagina, greater and lesser vestibular glands, and vaginal orifice. The physician destroys one or more lesions of the vulva. After examining the lower genital tract and perianal area with a colposcope, the physician destroys any lesions of the vulva by any method including laser surgery, electrosurgery, chemosurgery, or cryosurgery.Use 56501 to report single, simple lesion destruction, or 56515 to report multiple or complicated destruction of extensive vulvar lesions.

Coding Tips [4]

For removal or destruction by electric current (fulguration) of Skene's glands, see 53270. For destruction of vaginal lesions, see 57061–57065. For lysis of labial adhesions, see 56441.

ICD-9-CM Procedural [5]

71.3   Other local excision or destruction of vulva and perineum

Anesthesia [6]

00940

ICD-9-CM Diagnostic [7]

054.11 Herpetic vulvovaginitis
054.12 Herpetic ulceration of vulva
078.11 Condyloma acuminatum
078.19 Other specified viral warts
184.4   Malignant neoplasm of vulva, unspecified site
198.82 Secondary malignant neoplasm of genital organs
221.2   Benign neoplasm of vulva
228.01 Hemangioma of skin and subcutaneous tissue
233.30 Carcinoma in situ, unspecified female genital organ
233.31 Carcinoma in situ, vagina
233.32 Carcinoma in situ, vulva
233.39 Carcinoma in situ, other female genital organ
236.3   Neoplasm of uncertain behavior of other and unspecified female genital organs
239.5   Neoplasm of unspecified nature of other genitourinary organs
456.6   Vulval varices
616.81 Mucositis (ulcerative) of cervix, vagina, and vulva — (Use additional code to identify organism: 041.00-041.09, 041.10-041.19) (Use additional E code to identify adverse effects of therapy: E879.2, E930.7, E933.1)
616.89 Other inflammatory disease of cervix, vagina and vulva — (Use additional code to identify organism: 041.00-041.09, 041.10-041.19)
624.01 Vulvar intraepithelial neoplasia I [VIN I]
624.02 Vulvar intraepithelial neoplasia II [VIN II]
624.09 Other dystrophy of vulva
624.6   Polyp of labia and vulva
624.8   Other specified noninflammatory disorder of vulva and perineum
625.8   Other specified symptom associated with female genital organs
698.1   Pruritus of genital organs
701.0   Circumscribed scleroderma
701.5   Other abnormal granulation tissue
709.9   Unspecified disorder of skin and subcutaneous tissue
752.49 Other congenital anomaly of cervix, vagina, and external female genitalia

Terms To Know [8]

carcinoma in situ. Malignancy that arises from the cells of the vessel, gland, or organ of origin that remains confined to that site or has not invaded neighboring tissue.

condyloma. Infectious tumor-like growth caused by the human papilloma virus, with a branching connective tissue core and epithelial covering that occurs on the skin and mucous membranes of the perianal region and external genitalia.

cryosurgery. Application of intense cold, usually produced using liquid nitrogen, to locally freeze diseased or unwanted tissue and induce tissue necrosis without causing harm to adjacent tissue.

electrocautery. Division or cutting of tissue using high-frequency electrical current to produce heat, which destroys cells.

laser surgery. Use of concentrated, sharply defined light beams to cut, cauterize, coagulate, seal, or vaporize tissue.

varices. Enlarged, dilated, or twisted, turning veins.

CCI Version 18.3 [9]

00940, 0213T, 0216T, 0228T, 0230T, 12001-12007, 12011-12057, 13100-13153, 36000, 36400-36410, 36420-36430, 36440, 36600, 36640, 37202, 43752, 51701-51703, 56820, 57100, 57180, 57410, 57500, 57800, 58100, 62310-62319, 64400-64435, 64445-64450, 64479, 64483, 64490, 64493, 64505-64530, 69990, 93000-93010, 93040-93042, 93318, 94002, 94200, 94250, 94680-94690, 94770, 95812-95816, 95819, 95822, 95829, 95955, 96360, 96365, 96372, 96374-96376, 99148-99149, 99150, J0670, J2001

Also not with 56501: 55815❖, 56441❖

Also not with 56515: 53270, 56441, 56501, 56605

Note: These CCI edits are used for Medicare. Other payers may reimburse on codes listed above.

Medicare Edits [10]

	Fac RVU	Non-Fac RVU	FUD	Status
56501	3.42	3.9	10	A
56515	5.93	6.68	10	A

	MUE		Modifiers		
56501	1	51	N/A	N/A	N/A
56515	1	51	N/A	N/A	N/A

* with documentation

Medicare References: 100-3,140.5

1. CPT Codes and Descriptions

This edition of *Coding Companion* is updated with CPT codes for year 2013.

2. Illustrations

The illustrations that accompany the *Coding Companion* series provide coders a better understanding of the medical procedures referenced by the codes and data. The graphics offer coders a visual link between the technical language of the operative report and the cryptic descriptions accompanying the codes.

3. Explanation

Every CPT code or series of similar codes is presented with its official CPT code description. However, sometimes these descriptions do not provide the coder with sufficient information to make a proper code selection. In *Coding Companion*, a step-by-step clinical description of the procedure is provided, in simple terms. Technical language that might be used by the physician is included and defined. *Coding Companion* describes the most common method of performing each procedure.

4. Coding and Reimbursement Tips

Coding and reimbursement tips provide information on how the code should be used, provides related CPT codes, and offers help concerning common billing errors, modifier usage, and anesthesia. This information comes from consultants and technical editors at Optum and from the coding guidelines provided in the CPT book.

5. ICD-9-CM Procedural Codes

Volume 3 of ICD-9-CM lists procedural codes hospitals use in reporting charges to the government. In this field, the CPT code is cross-referenced to its corresponding ICD-9-CM Volume 3 code or codes.

6. Anesthesia Codes

The appropriate CPT anesthesia code(s) for the procedure being referenced is listed in this field. There are procedures, however, for which specific codes cannot be indicated, or anesthesia is already included in the surgery code. In these instances, the following abbreviated indicator appears in this field:

Not Applicable (N/A): Some procedures are performed without any type of anesthesia or are performed with a local anesthetic that, by CPT guideline definition of the global surgical package, is included with the surgery.

7. ICD-9-CM Diagnostic Codes

ICD-9-CM diagnostic codes listed are common diagnoses or reasons the procedure may be necessary. This list in most cases is inclusive to the specialty. In some cases, not every possible code is listed and the ICD-9-CM book should be referenced for other valid codes.

8. Terms to Know

Some codes are accompanied by general information pertinent to the procedure, labeled "Terms to Know." This information is not critical to code selection, but is a useful supplement to coders hoping to expand their knowledge of the specialty.

9. Correct Coding Initiative (CCI)

This section includes a list of codes from the official Centers for Medicare and Medicaid Services' National Correct Coding Policy Manual for Part B Medicare Contractors that are considered to be an integral part of the comprehensive code or mutually exclusive of it and should not be reported separately. Mutually exclusive codes are identified with an icon (⚡).

To conserve space, the codes are listed in ranges whenever possible. The two codes listed and any codes that fall into the numeric sequence between the two codes listed, are considered part of the National CCI unbundle edit.

The *Coding Companion* includes the most up-to-date ICD-9-CM, CPT, and HCPCS codes. The codes in the CCI are from version 18.3 (10-1 through 12-31-12), the most current version available at press time. Optum maintains a website to accompany the *Coding Companions*. Optum posts updated CCI edits on this website so that current information is available before the next book update. The website address is www.optumcoding.com.

10. Medicare Information

Medicare edits are provided for most codes. These Medicare edits were current in November 2012.

Relative Value Units

In a resource based relative value scale (RBRVS), services are ranked based on the relative costs of the resources required to provide those services as opposed to the average fee for the service, or average prevailing Medicare charge. The Medicare RBRVS defines three distinct components affecting the value of each service or procedure:

- Physician work component, reflecting the physician's time and skill
- Practice expense (PE) component, reflecting the physician's rent, staff, supplies, equipment, and other overhead
- Malpractice insurance component, reflecting the relative risk or liability associated with the service

There are two RVUs listed for each CPT code. The first RVU is for nonfacilities (Non-fac Total), which includes services provided in physician offices, patients' homes, or other nonhospital settings. The second RVU is for facilities (Fac Total), which represents services provided in hospitals, ambulatory surgical centers, or skilled nursing facilities.

Medicare Follow-Up Days (FUD)

Information on the Medicare global period is provided here. The global period is the time following a surgery during which routine care by the physician is considered postoperative and included in the surgical fee. Office visits or other routine care related to the original surgery cannot be separately reported if they occur during the global period.

Status

The Medicare status indicates if the service is separately payable by Medicare. The Medicare RBRVS includes:

A   Active code—separate payment may be made

B   Bundled code—payment is bundled into other service

C   Carrier priced—individual carrier will price the code

I   Not valid—Medicare uses another code for this service

N   Non-covered—service is not covered by Medicare

R   Restricted—special coverage instructions apply

T   Injections—separately payable if no other services on same date

X   Statutory exclusion—no RVUs or payment

Medically Unlikely Edits

This column provides the maximum number of units allowed by Medicare. However, it is also important to note that not every code has a Medically Unlikely Edit (MUE) available. Medicare has assigned some MUE values that are not available. If there is not any information in the MUE column for a particular code, this doesn't mean that there is no MUE. It may simply mean that CMS has not released information on that MUE. Watch the remittance advice for possible details on MUE denials related to those codes. If there is not a published MUE, a dash will display in the field.

Modifiers

Medicare identifies some modifiers that are required or appropriate to report with the CPT code. When the modifiers are not appropriate, it will be indicated with N/A. Four modifiers are included.

50   Bilateral Procedures
This modifier is used to identify when the same procedure is performed bilaterally. Medicare requires one line with modifier 50 and the reimbursement is 50 percent of the allowable. Other payers may require two lines and will reduce the second procedure.

51   Multiple Procedure
Medicare and other payers reduce the reimbursement of second and subsequent procedures performed at the same session to 50 percent of the allowable. For endoscopic procedures, the reimbursement is reduced by the value of the endoscopic base code.

62*   Co-surgeons
Medicare identifies procedures that may be performed by co-surgeons. The reimbursement is split between both providers. Both surgeons must report the same code when using this modifier.

80*   Assistant Surgeon
An assistant surgeon is allowed if modifier 80 is listed. Reimbursement is usually 20 percent of the allowable. For Medicare it is 16 percent to account for the patient's co-pay amount.

   * with documentation

Modifiers 62 and 80 may require supporting documentation to justify the assist.

Medicare Official Regulatory Information

Medicare official regulatory information provides official regulatory guidelines. Also known as the CMS Online Manual System, the Internet-only Manuals (IOM) contain official CMS information pertaining to program issuances, instructions, policies, and procedures based on statutes, regulations, guidelines, models, and directives. Optum has provided the reference for the surgery codes. The full text of guidelines can be found online at http://www.cms.hhs.gov/manuals.

10060-10061

10060 Incision and drainage of abscess (eg, carbuncle, suppurative hidradenitis, cutaneous or subcutaneous abscess, cyst, furuncle, or paronychia); simple or single

10061 complicated or multiple

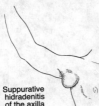

Suppurative hidradenitis is a disease process stemming from clogged specialized sweat glands of the axilla and groin

Suppurative hidradenitis of the axilla

Explanation

The physician makes a small incision through the skin overlying an abscess for incision and drainage (e.g., carbuncle, cyst, furuncle, paronychia, hidradenitis). The abscess or cyst is opened with a surgical instrument, allowing the contents to drain. The lesion may be curetted and irrigated. The physician leaves the surgical wound open to allow for continued drainage or the physician may place a Penrose latex drain or gauze strip packing to allow continued drainage. Report 10060 for incision and drainage of a simple or single abscess. Report 10061 for complex or multiple cysts. Complex or multiple cysts may require surgical closure at a later date.

Coding Tips

These codes are not for reporting incision and drainage of a pilonidal cyst, perineal abscess, or postoperative wound infection. For incision and drainage of a pilonidal cyst, see 10080–10081. For incision and drainage of a wound abscess or infection postoperatively, see 10180. For incision and drainage of an abscess on the perineum or vulva, see 56405. For incision and drainage of a vaginal abscess, see 57010. Surgical trays, A4550, are not separately reimbursed by Medicare; however, other third-party payers may cover them. Check with the specific payer to determine coverage.

ICD-9-CM Procedural

86.04 Other incision with drainage of skin and subcutaneous tissue

Anesthesia

00300, 00400

ICD-9-CM Diagnostic

680.2 Carbuncle and furuncle of trunk

680.5 Carbuncle and furuncle of buttock

682.2 Cellulitis and abscess of trunk — (Use additional code to identify organism, such as 041.1, etc.)

682.5 Cellulitis and abscess of buttock — (Use additional code to identify organism, such as 041.1, etc.)

682.8 Cellulitis and abscess of other specified site — (Use additional code to identify organism, such as 041.1, etc.)

686.00 Unspecified pyoderma — (Use additional code to identify any infectious organism: 041.0-041.8)

686.09 Other pyoderma — (Use additional code to identify any infectious organism: 041.0-041.8)

686.1 Pyogenic granuloma of skin and subcutaneous tissue — (Use additional code to identify any infectious organism: 041.0-041.8)

686.8 Other specified local infections of skin and subcutaneous tissue — (Use additional code to identify any infectious organism: 041.0-041.8)

705.83 Hidradenitis

705.89 Other specified disorder of sweat glands

706.2 Sebaceous cyst

782.2 Localized superficial swelling, mass, or lump

911.3 Trunk blister, infected

958.3 Posttraumatic wound infection not elsewhere classified

998.51 Infected postoperative seroma — (Use additional code to identify organism)

998.59 Other postoperative infection — (Use additional code to identify infection)

Terms To Know

abscess. Circumscribed collection of pus resulting from bacteria, frequently associated with swelling and other signs of inflammation.

carbuncle. Necrotic infection of the skin and subcutaneous tissues, occurring mainly in the neck and back, that produces pus and forms drainage cavities.

furuncle. Inflamed, painful cyst or nodule on the skin caused by bacteria, often staphylococcus, entering along the hair follicle.

hidradenitis. Infection or inflammation of a sweat gland and is usually treated by incision and drainage.

incision and drainage. Cutting open body tissue for the removal of tissue fluids or infected discharge from a wound or cavity.

CCI Version 18.3

0213T, 0216T, 0228T, 0230T, 11055-11057, 11719-11730, 11765, 12001-12007, 12011-12057, 13100-13153, 20005❖, 20500, 29580-29582, 36000, 36400-36410, 36420-36430, 36440, 36600, 36640, 37202, 43752, 51701-51703, 62310-62319, 64400-64435, 64445-64450, 64479, 64483, 64490, 64493, 64505-64530, 69990, 93000-93010, 93040-93042, 93318, 94002, 94200, 94250, 94680-94690, 94770, 95812-95816, 95819, 95822, 95829, 95955, 96360, 96365, 96372, 96374-96376, 97597-97598, 97602-97606, 99148-99149, 99150, G0127, J0670, J2001

Also not with 10060: 11401-11406❖, 11421-11426❖, 11441-11471❖, 11600-11606❖, 11620-11646❖, 11740, 30000❖

Also not with 10061: 10060, 11406❖, 11424-11440❖, 11444-11451❖, 11463-11471❖, 11604-11606❖, 11623-11626❖, 11643-11646❖, 11740-11750, 11760

Note: These CCI edits are used for Medicare. Other payers may reimburse on codes listed above.

Medicare Edits

	Fac RVU	Non-Fac RVU	FUD	Status
10060	2.77	3.32	10	A
10061	5.09	5.81	10	A

	MUE		Modifiers		
10060	1	51	N/A	N/A	N/A
10061	1	51	N/A	N/A	N/A

* with documentation

Medicare References: None

Skin

10080-10081

10080 Incision and drainage of pilonidal cyst; simple

10081 complicated

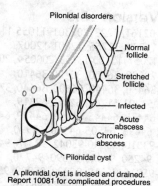

Pilonidal disorders

- Normal follicle
- Stretched follicle
- Infected
- Acute abscess
- Chronic abscess
- Pilonidal cyst

A pilonidal cyst is incised and drained. Report 10081 for complicated procedures

Explanation

Pilonidal cysts are entrapped epithelial tissue located in the sacrococcygeal region above the buttocks. These cysts may produce fluid or exudate into the cystic lining and are usually associated with ingrown hair. An incision is made to allow drainage of cystic fluid or exudate. Curettage is performed to remove the cystic epithelial lining. The wound heals secondarily relying on local wound care. Report 10081 if the procedure is more complicated and requires excision of tissue, primary closure, and/or Z-plasty.

Coding Tips

For excision of a pilonidal cyst, see 11770–11772. For incision and drainage of an abscess, simple or single, other than a pilonidal cyst, see 10060. For incision and drainage of an abscess, complicated or multiple, other than a pilonidal cyst, see 10061. Surgical trays, A4550, are not separately reimbursed by Medicare; however, other third-party payers may cover them. Check with the specific payer to determine coverage.

ICD-9-CM Procedural

86.03 Incision of pilonidal sinus or cyst

Anesthesia

00300

ICD-9-CM Diagnostic

685.0 Pilonidal cyst with abscess

685.1 Pilonidal cyst without mention of abscess

Terms To Know

abscess. Circumscribed collection of pus resulting from bacteria, frequently associated with swelling and other signs of inflammation.

absorbable sutures. Strands prepared from collagen or a synthetic polymer and capable of being absorbed by tissue over time.

closure. Repairing an incision or wound by suture or other means.

curettage. Removal of tissue by scraping.

epithelial tissue. Cells arranged in sheets that cover internal and external body surfaces that can absorb, protect, and/or secrete. Epithelial tissue includes the protective covering for external surfaces (skin), absorptive linings for internal surfaces such as the intestine, and secreting structures such as salivary or sweat glands.

exudate. Fluid or other material, such as debris from cells, that has escaped blood vessel circulation and is deposited in or on tissues and usually occurs due to inflammation.

incision and drainage. Cutting open body tissue for the removal of tissue fluids or infected discharge from a wound or cavity.

nonabsorbable sutures. Strands of natural or synthetic material that resist absorption into living tissue and are removed once healing is under way. Nonabsorbable sutures are commonly used to close skin wounds and repair tendons or collagenous tissue.

pilonidal cyst. Sac or sinus cavity of trapped epithelial tissues in the sacrococcygeal region, usually associated with ingrown hair.

CCI Version 18.3

0213T, 0216T, 0228T, 0230T, 12001-12007, 12011-12057, 13100-13153, 20500, 36000, 36400-36410, 36420-36430, 36440, 36600, 36640, 37202, 43752, 51701-51703, 62310-62319, 64400-64435, 64445-64450, 64479, 64483, 64490, 64493, 64505-64530, 69990, 93000-93010, 93040-93042, 93318, 94002, 94200, 94250, 94680-94690, 94770, 95812-95816, 95819, 95822, 95829, 95955, 96360, 96365, 96372, 96374-96376, 99148-99149, 99150, J0670, J2001

Also not with 10081: 10080

Note: These CCI edits are used for Medicare. Other payers may reimburse on codes listed above.

Medicare Edits

	Fac RVU	Non-Fac RVU	FUD	Status
10080	2.97	5.12	10	A
10081	5.02	7.87	10	A

	MUE		Modifiers		
10080	1	51	N/A	N/A	N/A
10081	1	51	N/A	N/A	N/A

* with documentation

Medicare References: None

Skin

10120-10121

10120 Incision and removal of foreign body, subcutaneous tissues; simple

10121   complicated

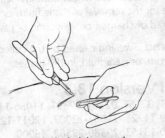

A foreign body is removed through an incision into subcutaneous tissues. Report code 10121 for complicated removal

Explanation

The physician removes a foreign body embedded in subcutaneous tissue. The physician makes a simple incision in the skin overlying the foreign body. The foreign body is retrieved using hemostats or forceps. The skin may be sutured or allowed to heal secondarily. Report 10121 if the procedure is more complicated, requiring dissection of underlying tissues.

Coding Tips

These codes may be used when foreign body removal is confined to the skin and/or subcutaneous tissues. For foreign body removal from the vagina, see 57415. Surgical trays, A4550, are not separately reimbursed by Medicare; however, other third-party payers may cover them. Check with the specific payer to determine coverage.

ICD-9-CM Procedural

86.05 Incision with removal of foreign body or device from skin and subcutaneous tissue

Anesthesia

00300, 00400

ICD-9-CM Diagnostic

709.4 Foreign body granuloma of skin and subcutaneous tissue — (Use additional code to identify foreign body (V90.01-V90.9))

729.6 Residual foreign body in soft tissue — (Use additional code to identify foreign body (V90.01-V90.9))

911.6 Trunk, superficial foreign body (splinter), without major open wound and without mention of infection

911.7 Trunk, superficial foreign body (splinter), without major open wound, infected

912.6 Shoulder and upper arm, superficial foreign body (splinter), without major open wound and without mention of infection

912.7 Shoulder and upper arm, superficial foreign body (splinter), without major open wound, infected

916.6 Hip, thigh, leg, and ankle, superficial foreign body (splinter), without major open wound and without mention of infection

916.7 Hip, thigh, leg, and ankle, superficial foreign body (splinter), without major open wound, infected

919.6 Other, multiple, and unspecified sites, superficial foreign body (splinter), without major open wound and without mention of infection

919.7 Other, multiple, and unspecified sites, superficial foreign body (splinter), without major open wound, infected

998.11 Hemorrhage complicating a procedure

998.4 Foreign body accidentally left during procedure, not elsewhere classified

Terms To Know

dissection. Separating by cutting tissue or body structures apart.

forceps. Tool used for grasping or compressing tissue.

foreign body. Any object or substance found in an organ and tissue that does not belong under normal circumstances.

hemostat. Tool for clamping vessels and arresting hemorrhaging.

incision. Act of cutting into tissue or an organ.

subcutaneous tissue. Sheet or wide band of adipose (fat) and areolar connective tissue in two layers attached to the dermis.

superficial dissection. Cutting through the skin into the subcutaneous fat, but not approaching the fascia.

CCI Version 18.3

0213T, 0216T, 0228T, 0230T, 12001-12007, 12011-12057, 13100-13153, 36000, 36400-36410, 36420-36430, 36440, 36600, 36640, 37202, 43752, 51701-51703, 62310-62319, 64400-64435, 64445-64450, 64479, 64483, 64490, 64493, 64505-64530, 69990, 93000-93010, 93040-93042, 93318, 94002, 94200, 94250, 94680-94690, 94770, 95812-95816, 95819, 95822, 95829, 95955, 96360, 96365, 96372, 96374-96376, 99148-99149, 99150, J0670, J2001

Also not with 10120: 11055-11057, 11719-11721, G0127

Also not with 10121: 10120, 11720-11721

Note: These CCI edits are used for Medicare. Other payers may reimburse on codes listed above.

Medicare Edits

	Fac RVU	Non-Fac RVU	FUD	Status
10120	2.72	4.1	10	A
10121	5.44	7.95	10	A

	MUE		Modifiers		
10120	-	51	N/A	N/A	N/A
10121	-	51	N/A	N/A	N/A

* with documentation

Medicare References: None

Coding Companion for Ob/Gyn

© 2012 OptumInsight, Inc.

Skin

10140

10140 Incision and drainage of hematoma, seroma or fluid collection

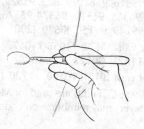

A hematoma, seroma, or fluid collection is incised and drained. A hematoma is a blood pocket and a seroma is a collection of serum, in this instance, within skin tissues

Explanation

The physician makes an incision in the skin to decompress and drain a hematoma, seroma, or other collection of fluid. A hemostat bluntly penetrates the fluid pockets, allowing the fluid to evacuate. A latex drain or gauze packing may be placed into the incision site. This will allow the escape of any fluids that may continue to enter the pocket. A pressure dressing may be placed over the region. Any drain or packing is removed within 48 hours. The incision can be closed primarily or may be left to granulate without closure.

Coding Tips

For puncture aspiration of a hematoma, see 10160. Removal of a drain is not reported separately. For imaging guidance, see 76942, 77012, and 77021. If tissue is transported to an outside laboratory, report 99000 for handling and/or conveyance. Any local anesthesia is not reported separately. Surgical trays, A4550, are not separately reimbursed by Medicare; however, other third-party payers may cover them. Check with the specific payer to determine coverage.

ICD-9-CM Procedural

86.04 Other incision with drainage of skin and subcutaneous tissue

Anesthesia

10140 00300, 00400, 00940

ICD-9-CM Diagnostic

674.30 Other complication of obstetrical surgical wounds, unspecified as to episode of care
674.32 Other complication of obstetrical surgical wounds, with delivery, with mention of postpartum complication
674.34 Other complications of obstetrical surgical wounds, postpartum condition or complication
709.8 Other specified disorder of skin
729.91 Post-traumatic seroma
729.92 Nontraumatic hematoma of soft tissue
767.11 Birth trauma, epicranial subaponeurotic hemorrhage (massive) — (Use additional code(s) to further specify condition)
767.19 Birth trauma, other injuries to scalp — (Use additional code(s) to further specify condition)
767.8 Other specified birth trauma — (Use additional code(s) to further specify condition)
906.3 Late effect of contusion
922.1 Contusion of chest wall
922.2 Contusion of abdominal wall
922.31 Contusion of back
922.32 Contusion of buttock
922.4 Contusion of genital organs
924.00 Contusion of thigh
924.01 Contusion of hip
924.4 Contusion of multiple sites of lower limb
924.5 Contusion of unspecified part of lower limb
924.8 Contusion of multiple sites, not elsewhere classified
959.11 Other injury of chest wall
959.12 Other injury of abdomen
959.14 Other injury of external genitals
959.19 Other injury of other sites of trunk
959.6 Injury, other and unspecified, hip and thigh
959.8 Injury, other and unspecified, other specified sites, including multiple
959.9 Injury, other and unspecified, unspecified site
998.11 Hemorrhage complicating a procedure
998.12 Hematoma complicating a procedure
998.13 Seroma complicating a procedure
998.51 Infected postoperative seroma — (Use additional code to identify organism)

Terms To Know

contusion. Superficial injury (bruising) produced by impact without a break in the skin.

hematoma. Tumor-like collection of blood in some part of the body caused by a break in a blood vessel wall, usually as a result of trauma.

incision and drainage. Cutting open body tissue for the removal of tissue fluids or infected discharge from a wound or cavity.

seroma. Swelling caused by the collection of serum, or clear fluid, in the tissues.

CCI Version 18.3

0213T, 0216T, 0228T, 0230T, 11055-11057, 11719-11721, 12001-12007, 12011-12057, 13100-13153, 29580-29582, 36000, 36400-36410, 36420-36430, 36440, 36600, 36640, 37202, 43752, 51701-51703, 62310-62319, 64400-64435, 64445-64450, 64479, 64483, 64490, 64493, 64505-64530, 69990, 93000-93010, 93040-93042, 93318, 94002, 94200, 94250, 94680-94690, 94770, 95812-95816, 95819, 95822, 95829, 95955, 96360, 96365, 96372, 96374-96376, 99148-99149, 99150, G0127, J0670, J2001

Note: These CCI edits are used for Medicare. Other payers may reimburse on codes listed above.

Medicare Edits

	Fac RVU	Non-Fac RVU	FUD	Status
10140	3.45	4.68	10	A

	MUE		Modifiers		
10140	-	51	N/A	N/A	N/A

* with documentation

Medicare References: 100-4,13,80.1; 100-4,13,80.2

Skin

Coding Companion for Ob/Gyn

10160

10160 Puncture aspiration of abscess, hematoma, bulla, or cyst

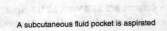
A subcutaneous fluid pocket is aspirated

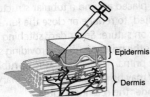
Epidermis
Dermis

Schematic of layers of the skin

Explanation

The physician performs a puncture aspiration of an abscess, hematoma, bulla, or cyst. The palpable collection of fluid is located subcutaneously. The physician cleanses the overlying skin and introduces a large bore needle on a syringe into the fluid space. The fluid is aspirated into the syringe, decompressing the fluid space. A pressure dressing may be placed over the site.

Coding Tips

For incision and drainage of a cutaneous or subcutaneous abscess, carbuncle, suppurative hidradenitis, cyst, furuncle, or paronychia, see 10060–10061. For incision and drainage of a hematoma, see 10140. For incision and drainage of a vaginal hematoma, see 57022–57023. For imaging guidance, see 76942, 77012, and 77021. Surgical trays, A4550, are not separately reimbursed by Medicare; however, other third-party payers may cover them. Check with the specific payer to determine coverage.

ICD-9-CM Procedural

75.91 Evacuation of obstetrical incisional hematoma of perineum

75.92 Evacuation of other hematoma of vulva or vagina

86.01 Aspiration of skin and subcutaneous tissue

Anesthesia

10160 00300, 00400

ICD-9-CM Diagnostic

674.30 Other complication of obstetrical surgical wounds, unspecified as to episode of care

674.32 Other complication of obstetrical surgical wounds, with delivery, with mention of postpartum complication

674.34 Other complications of obstetrical surgical wounds, postpartum condition or complication

682.2 Cellulitis and abscess of trunk — (Use additional code to identify organism, such as 041.1, etc.)

682.5 Cellulitis and abscess of buttock — (Use additional code to identify organism, such as 041.1, etc.)

682.6 Cellulitis and abscess of leg, except foot — (Use additional code to identify organism, such as 041.1, etc.)

705.89 Other specified disorder of sweat glands

706.2 Sebaceous cyst

767.11 Birth trauma, epicranial subaponeurotic hemorrhage (massive) — (Use additional code(s) to further specify condition)

767.19 Birth trauma, other injuries to scalp — (Use additional code(s) to further specify condition)

767.8 Other specified birth trauma — (Use additional code(s) to further specify condition)

906.3 Late effect of contusion

922.1 Contusion of chest wall

922.2 Contusion of abdominal wall

922.31 Contusion of back

922.32 Contusion of buttock

922.4 Contusion of genital organs

923.09 Contusion of multiple sites of shoulder and upper arm

923.8 Contusion of multiple sites of upper limb

924.00 Contusion of thigh

924.01 Contusion of hip

959.11 Other injury of chest wall

959.12 Other injury of abdomen

959.14 Other injury of external genitals

959.19 Other injury of other sites of trunk

959.6 Injury, other and unspecified, hip and thigh

998.12 Hematoma complicating a procedure

Terms To Know

abscess. Circumscribed collection of pus resulting from bacteria, frequently associated with swelling and other signs of inflammation.

bulla. Large, elevated, membranous sac or blister on the skin containing serous or seropurulent fluid, usually treated by incision and drainage or puncture aspiration.

cyst. Elevated encapsulated mass containing fluid, semisolid, or solid material with a membranous lining.

hematoma. Tumor-like collection of blood in some part of the body caused by a break in a blood vessel wall, usually as a result of trauma.

CCI Version 18.3

0213T, 0216T, 0228T, 0230T, 10061❖, 10140❖, 11055-11057, 11719-11721, 12001-12007, 12011-12057, 13100-13153, 29580-29582, 36000, 36400-36410, 36420-36430, 36440, 36600, 36640, 37202, 43752, 51701-51703, 62310-62319, 64400-64435, 64445-64450, 64479, 64483, 64490, 64493, 64505-64530, 69990, 93000-93010, 93040-93042, 93318, 94002, 94200, 94250, 94680-94690, 94770, 95812-95816, 95819, 95822, 95829, 95955, 96360, 96365, 96372, 96374-96376, 99148-99149, 99150, G0127, J0670, J2001

Note: These CCI edits are used for Medicare. Other payers may reimburse on codes listed above.

Medicare Edits

	Fac RVU	Non-Fac RVU	FUD	Status
10160	2.8	3.76	10	A

	MUE	Modifiers			
10160	-	51	N/A	N/A	N/A

* with documentation

Medicare References: 100-4,13,80.1; 100-4,13,80.2

10180

10180 Incision and drainage, complex, postoperative wound infection

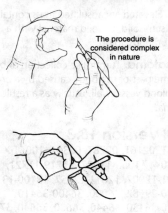

An operation site that has become infected is incised and the wound is drained

The procedure is considered complex in nature

Explanation

This procedure treats an infected postoperative wound. A more complex than usual incision and drainage procedure is necessary to remove the fluid and allow the surgical wound to heal. The physician first removes the surgical sutures or staples and/or makes additional incisions into the skin. The wound is drained of infected fluid. Any necrotic tissue is removed from the surgical site and the wound is irrigated. The wound may be sutured closed or packed open with gauze to allow additional drainage. If closed, the surgical site may have suction or latex drains placed into the wound. If packed open, the wound may be sutured again during a later procedure.

Coding Tips

For simple secondary closure of a surgical wound, see 12020–12021. For extensive or complicated secondary closure of a surgical wound or dehiscence, see 13160. Surgical trays, A4550, are not separately reimbursed by Medicare; however, other third-party payers may cover them. Check with the specific payer to determine coverage.

ICD-9-CM Procedural

86.04 Other incision with drainage of skin and subcutaneous tissue

Anesthesia

10180 00300, 00400

ICD-9-CM Diagnostic

040.42 Wound botulism

674.30 Other complication of obstetrical surgical wounds, unspecified as to episode of care

674.32 Other complication of obstetrical surgical wounds, with delivery, with mention of postpartum complication

674.34 Other complications of obstetrical surgical wounds, postpartum condition or complication

780.62 Postprocedural fever

998.51 Infected postoperative seroma — (Use additional code to identify organism)

998.59 Other postoperative infection — (Use additional code to identify infection)

Terms To Know

classification of surgical wounds.
Surgical wounds fall into four categories that determine treatment methods and outcomes: **1)** Clean wound: No inflammation or contamination; treatment performed with no break in sterile technique; no alimentary, respiratory, or genitourinary tracts involved in the surgery; infection rate = up to five percent. **2)** Clean-contaminated wound: No inflammation; treatment performed with minor break in surgical technique; no unusual contamination resulting when alimentary, respiratory, genitourinary, or oropharyngeal cavity is entered; infection rate = up to 11 percent. **3)** Contaminated wound: Less than four hours old with acute, nonpurulent inflammation; treatment performed with major break in surgical technique; gross contamination resulting from the gastrointestinal tract; infection rate = up to 20 percent. **4)** Dirty and infected wound: More than four hours old with existing infection, inflammation, abscess, and nonsterile conditions due to perforated viscus, fecal contamination, necrotic tissue, or foreign body; infection rate = up to 40 percent.

infection. Presence of microorganisms in body tissues that may result in cellular damage.

necrosis. Death of cells or tissue within a living organ or structure.

seroma. Swelling caused by the collection of serum, or clear fluid, in the tissues.

suture. Numerous stitching techniques employed in wound closure: 1) Buried suture: Continuous or interrupted suture placed under the skin for a layered closure. 2) Continuous suture: Running stitch with tension evenly distributed across a single strand to provide a leakproof closure line. 3) Interrupted suture: Series of single stitches with tension isolated at each stitch, in which all stitches are not affected if one becomes loose, and the isolated sutures cannot act as a wick to transport an infection. 4) Purse-string suture: Continuous suture placed around a tubular structure and tightened, to reduce or close the lumen. 5) Retention suture: Secondary stitching that bridges the primary suture, providing support for the primary repair; a plastic or rubber bolster may be placed over the primary repair and under the retention sutures.

wound. Injury to living tissue often involving a cut or break in the skin.

CCI Version 18.3

0213T, 0216T, 0228T, 0230T, 11720-11721, 12001-12007, 12011-12057, 13100-13153, 20500, 36000, 36400-36410, 36420-36430, 36440, 36600, 36640, 37202, 43752, 51701-51703, 62310-62319, 64400-64435, 64445-64450, 64479, 64483, 64490, 64493, 64505-64530, 69990, 93000-93010, 93040-93042, 93318, 94002, 94200, 94250, 94680-94690, 94770, 95812-95816, 95819, 95822, 95829, 95955, 96360, 96365, 96372, 96374-96376, 99148-99149, 99150, J0670, J2001

Note: These CCI edits are used for Medicare. Other payers may reimburse on codes listed above.

Medicare Edits

	Fac RVU	Non-Fac RVU	FUD	Status
10180	5.25	7.15	10	A

	MUE		Modifiers		
10180	3	51	N/A	N/A	N/A

* with documentation

Medicare References: None

Skin

11004-11006

11004 Debridement of skin, subcutaneous tissue, muscle and fascia for necrotizing soft tissue infection; external genitalia and perineum

11005 abdominal wall, with or without fascial closure

11006 external genitalia, perineum and abdominal wall, with or without fascial closure

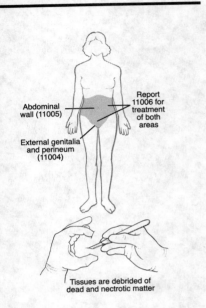

Abdominal wall (11005)

Report 11006 for treatment of both areas

External genitalia and perineum (11004)

Tissues are debrided of dead and nectrotic matter

Explanation

Debridement is carried out for a severe type of tissue infection that causes gangrenous changes, systemic disease, and tissue death. These types of infections are caused by virulent strains of bacteria, such as "flesh-eating" streptococcus, and affect the skin, subcutaneous fat, muscle tissue, and muscle fascia. Surgery is performed immediately upon diagnosis to open and drain the infected area or excise the dead or necrotic tissue. Report 11004 for surgical debridement of necrotic soft tissue in the external genitalia and perineum; 11005 for the abdominal wall, with or without surgical closure of the abdominal fascia; and 11006 for both areas, with or without surgical closure of the abdominal fascia.

Coding Tips

This type of debridement is done on high-risk patients who have a life-threatening infection such as Fournier's gangrene. Necrosis is often caused by infection from a combination of dangerously virulent micro-organisms. Fistulas, herniations, and organ destruction may occur, requiring an extensive level of repair involved with the debridement. Tissue flaps or skin grafting are reported separately when used

for repair or closure. For removal of prosthetic material or mesh from the abdominal wall, see 11008. Report skin grafts or flaps separately when performed for closure at the same session as 11004–11006. When reporting debridement of a single wound, the deepest level of tissue removed determines the correct code. The debridement of multiple wounds at the same tissue level may be added together to determine the appropriate code. Different tissue depths should not be added together for code selection. According to the AMA, the debridement of skin (epidermis/dermis) is reported with the codes describing active wound care management (97597 or 97598). Surgical trays, A4550, are not separately reimbursed by Medicare; however, other third-party payers may cover them. Check with the specific payer to determine coverage.

ICD-9-CM Procedural

54.3 Excision or destruction of lesion or tissue of abdominal wall or umbilicus

83.44 Other fasciectomy

83.45 Other myectomy

86.22 Excisional debridement of wound, infection, or burn

Anesthesia

11004 00400
11005 00400, 00700, 00800
11006 00400

ICD-9-CM Diagnostic

035 Erysipelas

040.0 Gas gangrene

040.3 Necrobacillosis

040.42 Wound botulism

041.11 Methicillin susceptible Staphylococcus aureus — (Note: This code is to be used as an additional code to identify the bacterial agent in diseases classified elsewhere and bacterial infections of unspecified nature or site)

041.12 Methicillin resistant Staphylococcus aureus

616.11 Vaginitis and vulvovaginitis in diseases classified elsewhere — (Use additional code to identify organism: 041.00-041.09, 041.10-041.19) (Code first underlying disease: 127.4)

616.4 Other abscess of vulva — (Use additional code to identify organism: 041.00-041.09, 041.10-041.19)

616.50 Unspecified ulceration of vulva — (Use additional code to identify organism: 041.00-041.09, 041.10-041.19)

616.51 Ulceration of vulva in disease classified elsewhere — (Use additional code to identify organism: 041.00-041.09, 041.10-041.19) (Code first underlying disease: 016.7, 136.1)

728.86 Necrotizing fasciitis — (Use additional code to identify infectious organism, 041.00-041.89, 785.4, if applicable)

785.4 Gangrene — (Code first any associated underlying condition)

Terms To Know

fascia. Fibrous sheet or band of tissue that envelops organs, muscles, and groupings of muscles.

necrotic. Pathological condition of death occurring in a group of cells or tissues within a living part or organism.

CCI Version 18.3

0183T, 0213T, 0216T, 0228T, 0230T, 10060-10061, 11000, 11010-11012, 11042-11044, 11100, 12001-12007, 12011-12057, 13100-13153, 15777, 20552-20553, 36000, 36400-36410, 36420-36430, 36440, 36600, 36640, 37202, 43752, 51701-51703, 62310-62319, 64400-64435, 64445-64450, 64479, 64483, 64490, 64493, 64505-64530, 69990, 93000-93010, 93040-93042, 93318, 94002, 94200, 94250, 94680-94690, 94770, 95812-95816, 95819, 95822, 95829, 95955, 96360, 96365, 96372, 96374-96376, 97597-97598, 99148-99149, 99150, G0168

Also not with 11005: 11004

Also not with 11006: 11004-11005

Note: These CCI edits are used for Medicare. Other payers may reimburse on codes listed above.

Medicare Edits

	Fac RVU	Non-Fac RVU	FUD	Status
11004	17.09	17.09	0	A
11005	23.02	23.02	0	A
11006	20.82	20.82	0	A

	MUE		Modifiers		
11004	1	51	N/A	N/A	N/A
11005	1	N/A	N/A	N/A	80*
11006	1	51	N/A	N/A	N/A

* with documentation

Medicare References: None

11008

11008 Removal of prosthetic material or mesh, abdominal wall for infection (eg, for chronic or recurrent mesh infection or necrotizing soft tissue infection) (List separately in addition to code for primary procedure)

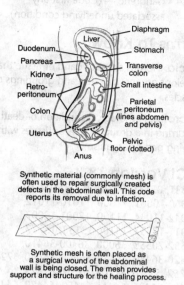

Synthetic material (commonly mesh) is often used to repair surgically created defects in the abdominal wall. This code reports its removal due to infection.

Synthetic mesh is often placed as a surgical wound of the abdominal wall is being closed. The mesh provides support and structure for the healing process.

Explanation

The physician removes prosthetic material or mesh previously placed in the abdominal wall. This may be done due to the presence of a chronic infection, a necrotizing soft tissue infection, or a recurrent mesh infection. Surgery is performed immediately after diagnosis and usually under general anesthesia. The skin is incised and the tissue dissected exposing the prosthetic material. Debridement of the tissue adjacent to or incorporated in the mesh may be performed with instruments or irrigation. Unincorporated or infected areas of the mesh are excised and removed with any remaining areas of infection or necrotic tissue. Incorporated mesh that is not infected may be left in the wound. The area is irrigated and the wound is sutured.

Coding Tips

As an "add-on" code, 11008 is not subject to multiple procedure rules. No reimbursement reduction or modifier 51 is applied. "Add-on" codes describe additional intra-service work associated with the primary procedure. They are performed by the same physician on the same date of service as the primary service/procedure, and must never be reported as a stand-alone code. Report 11008 in combination with 11004–11006 since the necrotizing soft tissue infection must also be debrided at the same time as the previously placed prosthetic material is removed.

ICD-9-CM Procedural

54.0   Incision of abdominal wall

Anesthesia

11008 N/A

ICD-9-CM Diagnostic

The ICD-9-CM diagnostic code(s) would be the same as the actual procedure performed because these are in-addition-to codes.

Terms To Know

chronic. Persistent, continuing, or recurring.

debride. To remove all foreign objects and devitalized or infected tissue from a burn or wound to prevent infection and promote healing.

deep fascia. Sheet of dense, fibrous tissue holding muscle groups together below the hypodermis layer or subcutaneous fat layer that lines the extremities and trunk.

infection. Presence of microorganisms in body tissues that may result in cellular damage.

mesh. Synthetic fabric used as a prosthetic patch in hernia repair.

necrotic. Pathological condition of death occurring in a group of cells or tissues within a living part or organism.

prosthetic. Device that replaces all or part of an internal body organ or body part, or that replaces part of the function of a permanently inoperable or malfunctioning internal body organ or body part.

CCI Version 18.3

No CCI Edits apply to this code.

Medicare Edits

	Fac RVU	Non-Fac RVU	FUD	Status
11008	8.08	8.08	N/A	A

	MUE			Modifiers	
11008	1	N/A	N/A	N/A	80*

* with documentation

Medicare References: None

Skin

11420-11426

11420 Excision, benign lesion including margins, except skin tag (unless listed elsewhere), scalp, neck, hands, feet, genitalia; excised diameter 0.5 cm or less
11421 excised diameter 0.6 to 1.0 cm
11422 excised diameter 1.1 to 2.0 cm
11423 excised diameter 2.1 to 3.0 cm
11424 excised diameter 3.1 to 4.0 cm
11426 excised diameter over 4.0 cm

Code removal according to the following:
11420 for excised diameter .5 cm or less
11421 for excised diameter .6 to 1 cm
11422 for excised diameter 1.1 to 2 cm
11423 for excised diameter 2.1 to 3 cm
11424 for excised diameter 3.1 to 4 cm
11426 for excised diameter greater than 4 cm

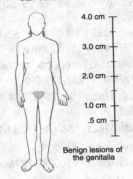

Benign lesions of the genitalia

Explanation

The physician excises a benign (noncancerous) lesion, including the margins, except a skin tag, from the genitalia. After administering a local anesthetic, the physician makes a full-thickness incision through the dermis with a scalpel, usually in an elliptical shape around and under the lesion, and removes it. The physician may suture the wound simply. Complex or layered closure is reported separately, if required. Report 11420 for an excised diameter 0.5 cm or less; 11421 for 0.6 cm to 1 cm; 11422 for 1.1 cm to 2 cm; 11423 for 2.1 cm to 3 cm; 11424 for 3.1 cm to 4 cm; and 11426 if the excised diameter is greater than 4 cm.

Coding Tips

For excision of a malignant lesion, see 11620–11626. If significant additional time and effort is documented, append modifier 22 and submit a cover letter and operative report. Surgical trays, A4550, are not separately reimbursed by Medicare; however, other third-party payers may cover them. Check with the specific payer to determine coverage.

ICD-9-CM Procedural

71.3 Other local excision or destruction of vulva and perineum
86.3 Other local excision or destruction of lesion or tissue of skin and subcutaneous tissue

Anesthesia
00300, 00400, 00940

ICD-9-CM Diagnostic

214.1 Lipoma of other skin and subcutaneous tissue
216.7 Benign neoplasm of skin of lower limb, including hip
216.8 Benign neoplasm of other specified sites of skin
221.2 Benign neoplasm of vulva
221.8 Benign neoplasm of other specified sites of female genital organs
228.01 Hemangioma of skin and subcutaneous tissue
236.3 Neoplasm of uncertain behavior of other and unspecified female genital organs
238.2 Neoplasm of uncertain behavior of skin
448.1 Nevus, non-neoplastic
624.4 Old laceration or scarring of vulva
686.1 Pyogenic granuloma of skin and subcutaneous tissue — (Use additional code to identify any infectious organism: 041.0-041.8)
701.1 Acquired keratoderma
701.4 Keloid scar
701.5 Other abnormal granulation tissue
701.8 Other specified hypertrophic and atrophic condition of skin
702.0 Actinic keratosis
702.11 Inflamed seborrheic keratosis
702.19 Other seborrheic keratosis
702.8 Other specified dermatoses
706.2 Sebaceous cyst
709.1 Vascular disorder of skin
709.2 Scar condition and fibrosis of skin
709.4 Foreign body granuloma of skin and subcutaneous tissue — (Use additional code to identify foreign body (V90.01-V90.9))
757.32 Congenital vascular hamartomas
757.33 Congenital pigmentary anomaly of skin
782.2 Localized superficial swelling, mass, or lump

Terms To Know

lipoma. Benign tumor containing fat cells and the most common of soft tissue lesions, which are usually painless and asymptomatic, with the exception of an angiolipoma.

nevus (plural nevi). Colored (pigmented) skin lesion including dilated blood vessels (telangiectasis) radiating out from a point (vascular spiders), hemangiomas, and moles.

CCI Version 18.3

00400, 0213T, 0216T, 0228T, 0230T, 11100, 11900-11901, 12001-12007, 17250, 36000, 36400-36410, 36420-36430, 36440, 36600, 36640, 37202, 43752, 51701-51703, 62310-62319, 64400-64435, 64445-64450, 64479, 64483, 64490, 64493, 64505-64530, 69990, 93000-93010, 93040-93042, 93318, 94002, 94200, 94250, 94680-94690, 94770, 95812-95816, 95819, 95822, 95829, 95955, 96360, 96365, 96372, 96374-96376, 96405-96406, 99148-99149, 99150, G0168, J0670, J2001

Also not with 11420: 10060-10061❖, 11719, 12011-12057, 13100-13153
Also not with 11421: 10061❖, 11719, 12011-12018
Also not with 11422: 10061❖, 12011-12018
Also not with 11423: 10061❖, 12011-12018
Also not with 11424: 12011-12018
Also not with 11426: 12011-12018

Note: These CCI edits are used for Medicare. Other payers may reimburse on codes listed above.

Medicare Edits

	Fac RVU	Non-Fac RVU	FUD	Status
11420	2.39	3.55	10	A
11421	3.25	4.58	10	A
11422	3.96	5.1	10	A
11423	4.61	5.89	10	A
11424	5.25	6.78	10	A
11426	8.0	9.66	10	A

	MUE		Modifiers		
11420	-	51	N/A	N/A	N/A
11421	-	51	N/A	N/A	N/A
11422	-	51	N/A	N/A	N/A
11423	-	51	N/A	N/A	N/A
11424	-	51	N/A	N/A	N/A
11426	-	51	N/A	N/A	N/A

* with documentation

Medicare References: None

11620-11626

11620	Excision, malignant lesion including margins, scalp, neck, hands, feet, genitalia; excised diameter 0.5 cm or less
11621	excised diameter 0.6 to 1.0 cm
11622	excised diameter 1.1 to 2.0 cm
11623	excised diameter 2.1 to 3.0 cm
11624	excised diameter 3.1 to 4.0 cm
11626	excised diameter over 4.0 cm

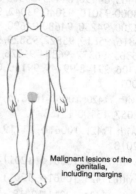

Code removal according to the following:
11620 for excised diameter .5 cm or less
11621 for excised diameter .6 to 1 cm
11622 for excised diameter 1.1 to 2 cm
11623 for excised diameter 2.1 to 3 cm
11624 for excised diameter 3.1 to 4 cm
11626 for excised diameter greater than 4 cm

Malignant lesions of the genitalia, including margins

Explanation

The physician removes a malignant lesion, including the margins, from the genitalia. After administering a local anesthetic, the physician makes a full-thickness incision through the skin, usually in an elliptical shape around and under the lesion. The lesion and a rim of normal tissue are removed. The skin incision is sutured simply. Complex or layered closure is reported separately, if required. Immediate reconstruction with local flaps may be necessary and is also reported separately. Report 11620 for an excised diameter 0.5 cm or less; 11621 for 0.6 cm to 1 cm; 11622 for 1.1 cm to 2 cm; 11623 for 2.1 cm to 3 cm; 11624 for 3.1 cm to 4 cm; and 11626 if the excised diameter is greater than 4 cm.

Coding Tips

For excision of a benign lesion, see 11420–11426. For lesion excision requiring intermediate repair, see 12041–12047; complex repair, see 13131–13133. For any flaps/adjacent tissue transfers, see 14040–14041. For destruction of a malignant lesion, any method, see 17270–17276. Surgical trays, A4550, are not separately reimbursed by Medicare; however, other third-party payers may cover them. Check with the specific payer to determine coverage.

ICD-9-CM Procedural

71.3	Other local excision or destruction of vulva and perineum
86.3	Other local excision or destruction of lesion or tissue of skin and subcutaneous tissue

Anesthesia

00300, 00400, 00940

ICD-9-CM Diagnostic

172.8	Malignant melanoma of other specified sites of skin
173.50	Unspecified malignant neoplasm of skin of trunk, except scrotum
173.51	Basal cell carcinoma of skin of trunk, except scrotum
173.52	Squamous cell carcinoma of skin of trunk, except scrotum
173.59	Other specified malignant neoplasm of skin of trunk, except scrotum
184.0	Malignant neoplasm of vagina
184.1	Malignant neoplasm of labia majora
184.2	Malignant neoplasm of labia minora
184.3	Malignant neoplasm of clitoris
184.4	Malignant neoplasm of vulva, unspecified site
184.8	Malignant neoplasm of other specified sites of female genital organs
198.2	Secondary malignant neoplasm of skin
198.82	Secondary malignant neoplasm of genital organs
209.36	Merkel cell carcinoma of other sites
209.75	Secondary Merkel cell carcinoma
232.7	Carcinoma in situ of skin of lower limb, including hip
232.8	Carcinoma in situ of other specified sites of skin
233.30	Carcinoma in situ, unspecified female genital organ
233.31	Carcinoma in situ, vagina
233.32	Carcinoma in situ, vulva
233.39	Carcinoma in situ, other female genital organ
236.3	Neoplasm of uncertain behavior of other and unspecified female genital organs

Terms To Know

carcinoma in situ. Malignancy that arises from the cells of the vessel, gland, or organ of origin that remains confined to that site or has not invaded neighboring tissue.

excision. Surgical removal of an organ or tissue.

malignant. Any condition tending to progress toward death, specifically an invasive tumor with a loss of cellular differentiation that has the ability to spread or metastasize to other areas in the body.

CCI Version 18.3

00400, 0213T, 0216T, 0228T, 0230T, 11100, 11900-11901, 12001-12007, 12011-12018, 17250, 36000, 36400-36410, 36420-36430, 36440, 36600, 36640, 37202, 43752, 51701-51703, 62310-62319, 64400-64435, 64445-64450, 64479, 64483, 64490, 64493, 64505-64530, 69990, 93000-93010, 93040-93042, 93318, 94002, 94200, 94250, 94680-94690, 94770, 95812-95816, 95819, 95822, 95829, 95955, 96360, 96365, 96372, 96374-96376, 99148-99149, 99150, G0168, J0670, J2001

Also not with 11620: 10061❖, 17262-17266❖, 17271-17276❖, 17281-17286❖

Also not with 11621: 10061❖, 17266❖, 17273-17276❖, 17282-17286❖

Also not with 11622: 10061❖, 17274-17276❖, 17283-17286❖

Also not with 11623: 17276❖, 17284-17286❖

Also not with 11624: 17286❖

Also not with 11626: 15002❖, 17286❖

Note: These CCI edits are used for Medicare. Other payers may reimburse on codes listed above.

Medicare Edits

	Fac RVU	Non-Fac RVU	FUD	Status
11620	3.53	5.64	10	A
11621	4.42	6.72	10	A
11622	5.07	7.52	10	A
11623	6.25	8.8	10	A
11624	7.08	9.91	10	A
11626	8.7	11.97	10	A

	MUE		Modifiers		
11620	-	51	N/A	N/A	N/A
11621	-	51	N/A	N/A	N/A
11622	-	51	N/A	N/A	N/A
11623	-	51	N/A	N/A	N/A
11624	-	51	N/A	N/A	N/A
11626	-	51	N/A	N/A	N/A

* with documentation

Medicare References: None

Skin

11770-11772

11770 Excision of pilonidal cyst or sinus; simple
11771 extensive
11772 complicated

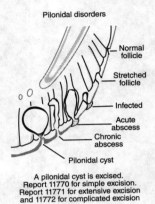

Pilonidal disorders

- Normal follicle
- Stretched follicle
- Infected
- Acute abscess
- Chronic abscess
- Pilonidal cyst

A pilonidal cyst is excised.
Report 11770 for simple excision.
Report 11771 for extensive excision
and 11772 for complicated excision

Explanation

A pilonidal cyst or sinus is entrapped epithelial tissue located in the sacrococcygeal region above the buttocks. These lesions are usually associated with ingrown hair. A sinus cavity is present and may have a fluid-producing cystic lining. With a small or simple sinus in 11770, the physician uses a scalpel to completely excise the involved tissue. The wound is sutured in a single layer. In 11771, the extensive sinus is superficial to the underlying fascia but has subcutaneous extensions. The physician uses a scalpel to completely excise the lesion. The wound may be sutured in several layers. In 11772, the sinus is more complicated and has many subcutaneous extensions. The physician uses a scalpel to completely excise the involved tissue. Local soft tissue flaps (i.e., Z-plasty) may be required for closure of a large defect or the wound may be left open to heal by granulation.

Coding Tips

Closure of the defect is included in this code and should not be reported separately. For incision and drainage of a pilonidal cyst, see 10080–10081. When medically necessary, report moderate (conscious) sedation provided by the performing physician with 99143–99145. When moderate (conscious) sedation is provided by another physician, report 99148–99150. Surgical trays, A4550, are not separately reimbursed by Medicare; however, other third-party payers may cover

them. Check with the specific payer to determine coverage.

ICD-9-CM Procedural

86.21   Excision of pilonidal cyst or sinus

Anesthesia

00300

ICD-9-CM Diagnostic

685.0   Pilonidal cyst with abscess
685.1   Pilonidal cyst without mention of abscess

Terms To Know

abscess. Circumscribed collection of pus resulting from bacteria, frequently associated with swelling and other signs of inflammation.

absorbable sutures. Strands prepared from collagen or a synthetic polymer and capable of being absorbed by tissue over time.

epithelial tissue. Cells arranged in sheets that cover internal and external body surfaces that can absorb, protect, and/or secrete and includes the protective covering for external surfaces (skin), absorptive linings for internal surfaces such as the intestine, and secreting structures such as salivary or sweat glands.

excision. Surgical removal of an organ or tissue.

granulation. Formation of small, bead-like masses of cytoplasm or granules on the surface of healing wounds of an organ, membrane, or tissue.

nonabsorbable sutures. Strands of natural or synthetic material that resist absorption into living tissue and are removed once healing is under way. Nonabsorbable sutures are commonly used to close skin wounds and repair tendons or collagenous tissue.

pilonidal cyst. Sac or sinus cavity of trapped epithelial tissues in the sacrococcygeal region, usually associated with ingrown hair.

sinus. Open space, cavity, or channel within the body or abnormal cavity, fistula, or channel created by a localized infection to allow the escape of pus.

CCI Version 18.3

0213T, 0216T, 0228T, 0230T, 10080-10081, 11900-11901, 12001-12007, 12011-12057, 13100-13153, 17250, 36000, 36400-36410, 36420-36430, 36440, 36600, 36640, 37202, 43752, 51701-51703, 62310-62319, 64400-64435, 64445-64450, 64479, 64483, 64490, 64493, 64505-64530, 69990, 93000-93010, 93040-93042, 93318, 94002, 94200, 94250, 94680-94690, 94770, 95812-95816, 95819, 95822, 95829, 95955, 96360, 96365, 96372, 96374-96376,

96405-96406, 99148-99149, 99150, J0670, J2001
Also not with 11770: 20500
Also not with 11771: 11770, 20500
Also not with 11772: 11770-11771
Note: These CCI edits are used for Medicare. Other payers may reimburse on codes listed above.

Medicare Edits

	Fac RVU	Non-Fac RVU	FUD	Status
11770	5.34	7.97	10	A
11771	12.58	16.5	90	A
11772	16.67	20.01	90	A

	MUE		Modifiers		
11770	1	51	N/A	N/A	N/A
11771	1	51	N/A	N/A	N/A
11772	1	51	N/A	N/A	N/A

* with documentation

Medicare References: None

Coding Companion for Ob/Gyn

11976

11976 Removal, implantable contraceptive capsules

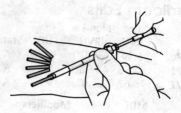

Capsules inserted through trocar under skin of upper arm

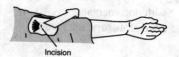

Capsules are surgically removed

Incision

Explanation

The physician makes a small incision in the skin on the inside of the upper arm of a female patient and removes contraceptive capsules previously implanted subdermally. The incision is closed.

Coding Tips

Because this procedure is usually not done out of medical necessity, the patient may be responsible for charges. Verify with the insurance carrier for coverage. Local anesthesia is included in this service. For removal of contraceptive capsules with subsequent reinsertion, report 11976 in conjunction with 11981. The cost of the contraceptive is not included and should be reported separately using the appropriate HCPCS Level II code. Surgical trays, A4550, are not separately reimbursed by Medicare; however, other third-party payers may cover them. Check with the specific payer to determine coverage. Supplies used when providing this service may be reported with 99070 or the appropriate HCPCS Level II code. Check with the specific payer to determine coverage.

ICD-9-CM Procedural

86.05 Incision with removal of foreign body or device from skin and subcutaneous tissue

Anesthesia

11976 00400

ICD-9-CM Diagnostic

V25.43 Surveillance of previously prescribed implantable subdermal contraceptive

Terms To Know

insertion. Placement or implantation into a body part.

levonorgestrel. Drug inhibiting ovulation and preventing sperm from penetrating cervical mucus. It is delivered subcutaneously in polysiloxone capsules. The capsules can be effective for up to five years, and provide a cumulative pregnancy rate of less than 2 percent. The capsules are not biodegradable, and therefore must be removed. Removal is more difficult than insertion of levonorgestrel capsules because fibrosis develops around the capsules. Normal hormonal activity and a return to fertility begins immediately upon removal.

subdermal. Below the skin surface.

trocar. Cannula or a sharp pointed instrument used to puncture and aspirate fluid from cavities.

CCI Version 18.3

0213T, 0216T, 0228T, 0230T, 12001-12007, 12011-12057, 13100-13153, 36000, 36400-36410, 36420-36430, 36440, 36600, 36640, 37202, 43752, 51701-51703, 62310-62319, 64400-64435, 64445-64450, 64479, 64483, 64490, 64493, 64505-64530, 93000-93010, 93040-93042, 93318, 94002, 94200, 94250, 94680-94690, 94770, 95812-95816, 95819, 95822, 95829, 95955, 96360, 96365, 96372, 96374-96376, 99148-99149, 99150, J2001

Note: These CCI edits are used for Medicare. Other payers may reimburse on codes listed above.

Medicare Edits

	Fac RVU	Non-Fac RVU	FUD	Status
11976	2.84	4.28	0	R

	MUE			Modifiers	
11976	1	51	N/A	N/A	80*

* with documentation

Medicare References: None

Implant

11980

11980 Subcutaneous hormone pellet implantation (implantation of estradiol and/or testosterone pellets beneath the skin)

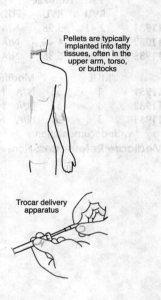

Pellets are typically implanted into fatty tissues, often in the upper arm, torso, or buttocks

Trocar delivery apparatus

Explanation

Biodegradable time-release medication pellets are implanted subcutaneously for the slow delivery of hormones. The physician makes a small incision in the skin with a scalpel. A trocar and cannula are inserted into the incised area. Hormone pellets are inserted through the cannula and the cannula is withdrawn. Pressure is applied to the incised area until any bleeding is stopped, and the incision is closed with Steri-strips. The time-release medication is typically used for women who require hormone replacement therapy during menopause. One method is to implant pellets of testosterone and/or estradiol (taken in conjunction with progesterone) into the fatty tissue of the buttocks. New pellets may be inserted whenever symptoms recur, usually in six to nine months.

Coding Tips

When 11980 is performed with another separately identifiable procedure, the highest dollar value code is listed as the primary procedure and subsequent procedures are appended with modifier 51. Report supplies and materials separately using 99070 or the appropriate HCPCS Level II code for the cost of the capsule. Local anesthesia is included in this service. Surgical trays, A4550, are not separately reimbursed by Medicare; however, other third-party payers may cover them. Check with the specific payer to determine coverage. For insertion of implantable contraceptive capsules, see 11981.

ICD-9-CM Procedural

99.23   Injection of steroid

Anesthesia
11980   00400

ICD-9-CM Diagnostic

253.4   Other anterior pituitary disorders

253.7   Iatrogenic pituitary disorders — (Use additional E code to identify cause)

256.2   Postablative ovarian failure — (Use additional code for states associated with artificial menopause: 627.4)

256.31   Premature menopause — (Use additional code for states associated with natural menopause: 627.2)

256.39   Other ovarian failure — (Use additional code for states associated with natural menopause: 627.2)

256.8   Other ovarian dysfunction

256.9   Unspecified ovarian dysfunction

259.0   Delay in sexual development and puberty, not elsewhere classified

259.1   Precocious sexual development and puberty, not elsewhere classified

346.40   Menstrual migraine, without mention of intractable migraine without mention of status migrainosus

346.41   Menstrual migraine, with intractable migraine, so stated, without mention of status migrainosus

346.42   Menstrual migraine, without mention of intractable migraine with status migrainosus

346.43   Menstrual migraine, with intractable migraine, so stated, with status migrainosus

597.80   Unspecified urethritis

627.0   Premenopausal menorrhagia

627.1   Postmenopausal bleeding

627.2   Symptomatic menopausal or female climacteric states

627.3   Postmenopausal atrophic vaginitis

627.4   Symptomatic states associated with artificial menopause

627.8   Other specified menopausal and postmenopausal disorder

627.9   Unspecified menopausal and postmenopausal disorder

733.00   Unspecified osteoporosis — (Use additional code to identify major osseous defect, if applicable: 731.3) (Use additional code to identify personal history of pathologic (healed) fracture: V13.51)

733.01   Senile osteoporosis — (Use additional code to identify major osseous defect, if applicable: 731.3) (Use additional code to identify personal history of pathologic (healed) fracture: V13.51)

Terms To Know

estradiol. Principal and most potent mammalian estrogen produced by the ovaries, which prepares the uterus for implantation after fertilization and is responsible for female reproductive organ maturation.

hormone. Chemical substance produced by the body that has a regulatory effect on the function of its specific target organ(s).

CCI Version 18.3

0213T, 0216T, 0228T, 0230T, 11900, 12001-12007, 12011-12057, 13100-13153, 36000, 36400-36410, 36420-36430, 36440, 36600, 36640, 37202, 43752, 51701-51703, 62310-62319, 64400-64435, 64445-64450, 64479, 64483, 64490, 64493, 64505-64530, 93000-93010, 93040-93042, 93318, 94002, 94200, 94250, 94680-94690, 94770, 95812-95816, 95819, 95822, 95829, 95955, 96360, 96365, 96372, 96374-96376, 99148-99149, 99150, J0670, J2001

Note: These CCI edits are used for Medicare. Other payers may reimburse on codes listed above.

Medicare Edits

	Fac RVU	Non-Fac RVU	FUD	Status
11980	2.38	3.05	0	A

	MUE		Modifiers		
11980	1	51	N/A	N/A	N/A

* with documentation

Medicare References: None

© 2012 OptumInsight, Inc.

Implant

11981-11983

11981 Insertion, non-biodegradable drug delivery implant

11982 Removal, non-biodegradable drug delivery implant

11983 Removal with reinsertion, non-biodegradable drug delivery implant

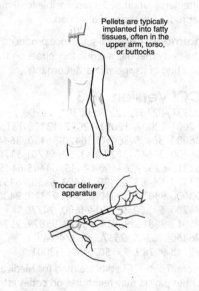

Pellets are typically implanted into fatty tissues, often in the upper arm, torso, or buttocks

Trocar delivery apparatus

Explanation

A non-biodegradable drug delivery implant is inserted to deliver a therapeutic dose of the drug continuously at a predetermined rate of release. One such system works via a semipermeable membrane at one end of the subcutaneous cylinder that permits the entrance of fluid; the drug is delivered from a port at the other end of the cylinder at a controlled rate appropriate to the specific therapeutic agent. The physician injects local anesthesia and makes a small incision in the skin with a scalpel to insert the miniature drug-containing titanium, surgical grade stainless steel, or polymeric cylinder. Various types of medications for different indications may be administered via a non-biodegradable drug delivery implant system that may come in other forms. In 11982, the physician removes a previously implanted, miniature drug-containing titanium cylinder through a small incision. In 11983, the physician removes a previously implanted, miniature drug-containing titanium cylinder through a small incision and inserts a replacement cylinder. The cylinders are held in place with sutures tied by a knot or secured by a single running stitch. The wounds are sutured closed.

Coding Tips

The cost of the drug is not included in these codes and should be reported separately using the appropriate HCPCS Level II code. Surgical trays, A4550, are not separately reimbursed by Medicare; however, other third-party payers may cover them. Check with the specific payer to determine coverage. Supplies used when providing this service may be reported with 99070 or the appropriate HCPCS Level II code. Check with the specific payer to determine coverage. Contraceptive capsules are not usually provided out of medical necessity; the patient may be responsible for charges. Verify with the insurance carrier for coverage. Anesthesia is included in these services. For removal of implantable contraceptive capsules, see 11976. For removal and subsequent insertion of implantable contraceptive capsules, report 11976 (for the removal) in conjunction with 11981 (for the insertion of contraceptive capsules).

ICD-9-CM Procedural

86.05 Incision with removal of foreign body or device from skin and subcutaneous tissue

99.23 Injection of steroid

Anesthesia

00400

ICD-9-CM Diagnostic

V25.5 Insertion of implantable subdermal contraceptive

Terms To Know

implant. Material or device inserted or placed within the body for therapeutic, reconstructive, or diagnostic purposes.

insertion. Placement or implantation into a body part.

levonorgestrel. Drug inhibiting ovulation and preventing sperm from penetrating cervical mucus. It is delivered subcutaneously in polysiloxone capsules. The capsules can be effective for up to five years, and provide a cumulative pregnancy rate of less than 2 percent. The capsules are not biodegradable, and therefore must be removed. Removal is more difficult than insertion of levonorgestrel capsules because fibrosis develops around the capsules. Normal hormonal activity and a return to fertility begins immediately upon removal.

CCI Version 18.3

0213T, 0216T, 36000, 36410, 37202, 62318-62319, 64415-64417, 64450, 64490, 64493, 96360, 96365, 96372, 96374-96376, J0670, J2001

Also not with 11981: 11982❖

Also not with 11982: 11976❖

Also not with 11983: 11976, 11981-11982

Note: These CCI edits are used for Medicare. Other payers may reimburse on codes listed above.

Medicare Edits

	Fac RVU	Non-Fac RVU	FUD	Status
11981	2.41	3.98	N/A	A
11982	2.87	4.47	N/A	A
11983	5.04	6.35	N/A	A

	MUE		Modifiers		
11981	1	51	N/A	N/A	80*
11982	1	51	N/A	N/A	80*
11983	1	51	N/A	N/A	80*

* with documentation

Medicare References: None

12001-12007

■ 12001 Simple repair of superficial wounds of scalp, neck, axillae, external genitalia, trunk and/or extremities (including hands and feet); 2.5 cm or less
12002 2.6 cm to 7.5 cm
12004 7.6 cm to 12.5 cm
12005 12.6 cm to 20.0 cm
12006 20.1 cm to 30.0 cm
12007 over 30.0 cm

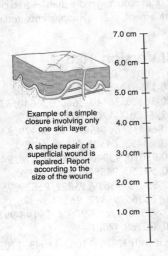

Example of a simple closure involving only one skin layer

A simple repair of a superficial wound is repaired. Report according to the size of the wound

Explanation

The physician sutures superficial lacerations of the external genitalia. A local anesthetic is injected around the laceration and the wound is cleansed, explored, and often irrigated with a saline solution. The physician performs a simple, one-layer repair of the epidermis, dermis, or subcutaneous tissues with sutures. With multiple wounds of the same complexity and in the same anatomical area, the length of all wounds sutured is summed and reported as one total length. Report 12001 for a total length of 2.5 cm or less; 12002 for 2.6 cm to 7.5 cm; 12004 for 7.6 cm to 12.5 cm; 12005 for 12.6 cm to 20 cm; 12006 for 20.1 cm to 30 cm; and 12007 if the total length is greater than 30 cm.

Coding Tips

Wounds treated with tissue glue or staples qualify as a simple repair even if they are not closed with sutures. Suture removal is included in this procedure. Single-layer closure of a wound requiring extensive cleaning or removal of contaminated foreign matter or damaged tissue is classified as an intermediate repair. Surgical trays, A4550, may be separately reimbursed by third-party payers. Check with the specific payer to determine

coverage. When medically necessary, report moderate (conscious) sedation provided by the performing physician with 99143–99145. When moderate (conscious) sedation is provided by another physician, report 99148–99150.

ICD-9-CM Procedural

71.71 Suture of laceration of vulva or perineum
71.79 Other repair of vulva and perineum
85.81 Suture of laceration of breast
86.59 Closure of skin and subcutaneous tissue of other sites

Anesthesia

00300, 00400, 00940

ICD-9-CM Diagnostic

629.20 Female genital mutilation status, unspecified
878.4 Open wound of vulva, without mention of complication
878.6 Open wound of vagina, without mention of complication
878.8 Open wound of other and unspecified parts of genital organs, without mention of complication
879.0 Open wound of breast, without mention of complication
879.2 Open wound of abdominal wall, anterior, without mention of complication
879.4 Open wound of abdominal wall, lateral, without mention of complication
879.6 Open wound of other and unspecified parts of trunk, without mention of complication
880.02 Open wound of axillary region, without mention of complication
890.0 Open wound of hip and thigh, without mention of complication
894.0 Multiple and unspecified open wound of lower limb, without mention of complication

Terms To Know

laceration. Tearing injury; a torn, ragged-edged wound.

repair. Surgical closure of a wound. The wound may be a result of injury/trauma or it may be a surgically created defect. Repairs are divided into three categories: simple, intermediate, and complex.

superficial. On the skin surface or near the surface of any involved structure or field of interest.

CCI Version 18.3

0213T, 0216T, 0228T, 0230T, 11100, 11900-11901, 36000, 36400-36410, 36420-36430, 36440, 36600, 36640, 37202, 43752, 51701-51703, 62310-62319, 64400-64435, 64445-64450, 64479, 64483, 64490, 64493, 64505-64530, 69990, 93000-93010, 93040-93042, 93318, 94002, 94200, 94250, 94680-94690, 94770, 95812-95816, 95819, 95822, 95829, 95955, 96360, 96365, 96372, 96374-96376, 97597-97598, 97602-97606, 99148-99149, 99150, G0168, J0670, J2001

Also not with 12001: 11042, 11055-11056, 11719, 11740-11750, 12011❖

Also not with 12002: 11042, 11740, 12001, 12013-12014❖

Also not with 12004: 11042, 12001-12002, 12015❖

Also not with 12005: 11042-11043, 12001-12004, 12016❖

Also not with 12006: 11042-11043, 12001-12005, 12017❖

Also not with 12007: 12001-12006, 12018❖

Note: These CCI edits are used for Medicare. Other payers may reimburse on codes listed above.

Medicare Edits

	Fac RVU	Non-Fac RVU	FUD	Status
12001	1.46	2.75	0	A
12002	1.9	3.28	0	A
12004	2.34	3.87	0	A
12005	3.12	5.0	0	A
12006	3.81	6.03	0	A
12007	4.65	7.0	0	A

	MUE		Modifiers		
12001	1	51	N/A	N/A	N/A
12002	1	51	N/A	N/A	N/A
12004	1	51	N/A	N/A	N/A
12005	1	51	N/A	N/A	N/A
12006	1	51	N/A	N/A	N/A
12007	1	51	N/A	62*	N/A

* with documentation

Medicare References: None

Coding Companion for Ob/Gyn

© 2012 OptumInsight, Inc.

12020-12021

12020 Treatment of superficial wound dehiscence; simple closure
12021 with packing

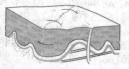

Example of a simple closure involving only one skin layer

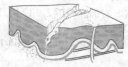

Example of wound with packing

Dehiscence is the failure of a wound to heal. In some instances, the wound will be a sutured surgical site. Others may be unstitched trauma sites. The margins of the wound tend to gape open. Report 12020 for treatment of the wound with simple closure. Report 12021 when packing is placed in the wound to promote drainage of infection

Explanation

There has been a breakdown of the healing skin either before or after suture removal. The skin margins have opened. The physician cleanses the wound with irrigation and antimicrobial solutions. The skin margins may be trimmed to initiate bleeding surfaces. Report 12020 if the wound is sutured in a single layer. Report 12021 if the wound is left open and packed with gauze strips due to the presence of infection. This allows infection to drain from the wound and the skin closure will be delayed until the infection is resolved.

Coding Tips

For extensive or complicated secondary wound closure, see 13160. Medicare and some other payers may require G0168 be reported for wound closure by tissue adhesives only. Surgical trays, A4550, are not separately reimbursed by Medicare; however, other third-party payers may cover them. Check with the specific payer to determine coverage.

ICD-9-CM Procedural

85.81 Suture of laceration of breast
86.59 Closure of skin and subcutaneous tissue of other sites
96.59 Other irrigation of wound

Anesthesia

00300, 00400, 00940

ICD-9-CM Diagnostic

674.10 Disruption of cesarean wound, unspecified as to episode of care
674.12 Disruption of cesarean wound, with delivery, with mention of postpartum complication
674.14 Disruption of cesarean wound, postpartum condition or complication
674.20 Disruption of perineal wound, unspecified as to episode of care in pregnancy
674.22 Disruption of perineal wound, with delivery, with mention of postpartum complication
674.24 Disruption of perineal wound, postpartum condition or complication
780.62 Postprocedural fever
998.30 Disruption of wound, unspecified
998.32 Disruption of external operation (surgical) wound
998.33 Disruption of traumatic injury wound repair
998.59 Other postoperative infection — (Use additional code to identify infection)
998.83 Non-healing surgical wound

Terms To Know

dehiscence. Complication of healing in which the surgical wound ruptures or bursts open, superficially or through multiple layers.

infection. Presence of microorganisms in body tissues that may result in cellular damage.

irrigation. To wash out or cleanse a body cavity, wound, or tissue with water or other fluid.

perineal. Pertaining to the pelvic floor area between the thighs; the diamond-shaped area bordered by the pubic symphysis in front, the ischial tuberosities on the sides, and the coccyx in back.

subcutaneous. Below the skin.

superficial. On the skin surface or near the surface of any involved structure or field of interest.

wound repair. Surgical closure of a wound is divided into three categories: simple, intermediate, and complex. *Simple repair:* Surgical closure of a superficial wound, requiring single layer suturing of the skin epidermis, dermis, or subcutaneous tissue. *Intermediate repair:* Surgical closure of a wound requiring closure of one or more of the deeper subcutaneous tissue and non-muscle fascia layers in addition to suturing the skin; contaminated wounds with single layer closure that need extensive cleaning or foreign body removal. *Complex repair:* Repair of wounds requiring more than layered closure (debridement, scar revision, stents, retention sutures).

CCI Version 18.3

0213T, 0216T, 0228T, 0230T, 11100, 11900-11901, 36000, 36400-36410, 36420-36430, 36440, 36600, 36640, 37202, 43752, 51701-51703, 62310-62319, 64400-64435, 64445-64450, 64479, 64483, 64490, 64493, 64505-64530, 69990, 93000-93010, 93040-93042, 93318, 94002, 94200, 94250, 94680-94690, 94770, 95812-95816, 95819, 95822, 95829, 95955, 96360, 96365, 96372, 96374-96376, 97597-97598, 97602-97606, 99148-99149, 99150, G0168, J2001

Also not with 12020: 11042-11043, 12021, J0670

Also not with 12021: 11042

Note: These CCI edits are used for Medicare. Other payers may reimburse on codes listed above.

Medicare Edits

	Fac RVU	Non-Fac RVU	FUD	Status
12020	5.49	8.05	10	A
12021	4.13	4.86	10	A

	MUE		Modifiers		
12020	3	51	N/A	N/A	N/A
12021	3	51	N/A	N/A	N/A

* with documentation

Medicare References: None

12031-12037

2031 Repair, intermediate, wounds of scalp, axillae, trunk and/or extremities (excluding hands and feet); 2.5 cm or less
2032 2.6 cm to 7.5 cm
2034 7.6 cm to 12.5 cm
2035 12.6 cm to 20.0 cm
2036 20.1 cm to 30.0 cm
2037 over 30.0 cm

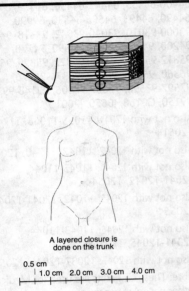

A layered closure is done on the trunk

0.5 cm
| 1.0 cm 2.0 cm 3.0 cm 4.0 cm

Explanation

The physician performs an intermediate repair of a laceration of the scalp, axillae, trunk, and/or extremities (except hands and feet) using layered closure. A local anesthetic is injected around the laceration, and the wound is cleansed, explored, and often irrigated with a saline solution. Due to deeper or more complex lacerations, deep subcutaneous or layered suturing techniques are required. The physician closes tissue layers under the skin with dissolvable sutures before suturing the skin. Extensive cleaning or removal of foreign matter from a heavily contaminated wound that is closed with a single layer may also be reported as an intermediate repair. With multiple wounds of the same complexity and in the same anatomical area, the length of all wounds sutured is summed and reported as one total length. Report 12031 for a total length of 2.5 cm or less; 12032 for 2.6 cm to 7.5 cm; 12034 for 7.6 cm to 12.5 cm; 12035 for 12.6 cm to 20 cm; 12036 for 20.1 cm to 30 cm; and 12037 if the total length is greater than 30 cm.

Coding Tips

Intermediate repair includes the repair of wounds that require layered closure of one or more of the deeper layers of subcutaneous tissue and superficial fascia, in addition to skin closure. Single-layer closure of a wound requiring extensive cleaning or removal of contaminated foreign matter or damaged tissue is classified as an intermediate repair. For simple repairs, see 12001–12007; complex repairs, see 13100–13160. Surgical trays, A4550, are not separately reimbursed by Medicare; however, other third-party payers may cover them. Check with the specific payer to determine coverage.

ICD-9-CM Procedural

85.81 Suture of laceration of breast
86.59 Closure of skin and subcutaneous tissue of other sites

Anesthesia

00300, 00400

ICD-9-CM Diagnostic

172.5 Malignant melanoma of skin of trunk, except scrotum
172.7 Malignant melanoma of skin of lower limb, including hip
172.8 Malignant melanoma of other specified sites of skin
173.50 Unspecified malignant neoplasm of skin of trunk, except scrotum
173.51 Basal cell carcinoma of skin of trunk, except scrotum
173.52 Squamous cell carcinoma of skin of trunk, except scrotum
173.59 Other specified malignant neoplasm of skin of trunk, except scrotum
209.35 Merkel cell carcinoma of the trunk
209.36 Merkel cell carcinoma of other sites
209.75 Secondary Merkel cell carcinoma
214.1 Lipoma of other skin and subcutaneous tissue
216.5 Benign neoplasm of skin of trunk, except scrotum
216.7 Benign neoplasm of skin of lower limb, including hip
232.5 Carcinoma in situ of skin of trunk, except scrotum
448.1 Nevus, non-neoplastic
701.5 Other abnormal granulation tissue
709.1 Vascular disorder of skin
709.2 Scar condition and fibrosis of skin
757.32 Congenital vascular hamartomas
876.0 Open wound of back, without mention of complication
877.0 Open wound of buttock, without mention of complication
879.0 Open wound of breast, without mention of complication
879.2 Open wound of abdominal wall, anterior, without mention of complication
890.0 Open wound of hip and thigh, without mention of complication

CCI Version 18.3

0213T, 0216T, 0228T, 0230T, 11100, 11900-11901, 36000, 36400-36410, 36420-36430, 36440, 36600, 36640, 37202, 43752, 51701-51703, 62310-62319, 64400-64435, 64445-64450, 64479, 64483, 64490, 64493, 64505-64530, 69990, 93000-93010, 93040-93042, 93318, 94002, 94200, 94250, 94680-94690, 94770, 95812-95816, 95819, 95822, 95829, 95955, 96360, 96365, 96372, 96374-96376, 97597-97598, 97602-97606, 99148-99149, 99150, G0168, J0670, J2001

Also not with 12031: 11042, 11055-11056, 12041❖, 12051❖

Also not with 12032: 11042-11043, 12031, 12042❖, 12052-12053❖

Also not with 12034: 11042-11043, 12031-12032, 12044❖, 12054❖

Also not with 12035: 11042-11044, 12031-12034, 12045❖, 12055❖

Also not with 12036: 11043, 12031-12035, 12046❖, 12056❖

Also not with 12037: 11043-11044, 12031-12036, 12057❖

Note: These CCI edits are used for Medicare. Other payers may reimburse on codes listed above.

Medicare Edits

	Fac RVU	Non-Fac RVU	FUD	Status
12031	4.5	6.91	10	A
12032	5.77	8.95	10	A
12034	6.06	9.08	10	A
12035	7.05	11.11	10	A
12036	8.26	12.34	10	A
12037	9.64	13.85	10	A

	MUE		Modifiers		
12031	1	51	N/A	N/A	N/A
12032	1	51	N/A	N/A	N/A
12034	1	51	N/A	N/A	N/A
12035	1	51	N/A	N/A	N/A
12036	1	51	N/A	N/A	N/A
12037	1	51	N/A	62*	80*

* with documentation

Medicare References: None

Coding Companion for Ob/Gyn

12041-12047

12041 Repair, intermediate, wounds of neck, hands, feet and/or external genitalia; 2.5 cm or less

12042 2.6 cm to 7.5 cm
12044 7.6 cm to 12.5 cm
12045 12.6 cm to 20.0 cm
12046 20.1 cm to 30.0 cm
12047 over 30.0 cm

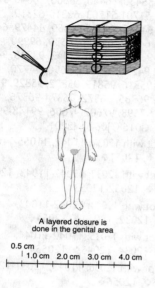

A layered closure is
done in the genital area

0.5 cm
1.0 cm 2.0 cm 3.0 cm 4.0 cm

Explanation

The physician performs an intermediate repair of a laceration of the external genitalia using layered closure. A local anesthetic is injected around the laceration, and the wound is cleansed, explored, and often irrigated with a saline solution. Due to deeper or more complex lacerations, deep subcutaneous or layered suturing techniques are required. The physician closes tissue layers under the skin with dissolvable sutures before suturing the skin. Extensive cleaning or removal of foreign matter from a heavily contaminated wound that is closed with a single layer may also be reported as an intermediate repair. With multiple wounds of the same complexity and in the same anatomical area, the length of all wounds sutured is summed and reported as one total length. Report 12041 for a total length of 2.5 cm or less; 12042 for 2.6 cm to 7.5 cm; 12044 for 7.6 cm to 12.5 cm; 12045 for 12.6 cm to 20 cm; 12046 for 20.1 cm to 30 cm; and 12047 if the total length is greater than 30 cm.

Coding Tips

Single-layer closure of a wound requiring extensive cleaning or removal of contaminated foreign matter or damaged tissue is classified as an intermediate repair. Surgical trays, A4550, are not separately reimbursed by Medicare; however, other third-party payers may cover them. Check with the specific payer to determine coverage.

ICD-9-CM Procedural

71.71 Suture of laceration of vulva or perineum
86.59 Closure of skin and subcutaneous tissue of other sites

Anesthesia

00300, 00400, 00940

ICD-9-CM Diagnostic

172.8 Malignant melanoma of other specified sites of skin
184.1 Malignant neoplasm of labia majora
184.2 Malignant neoplasm of labia minora
184.4 Malignant neoplasm of vulva, unspecified site
209.36 Merkel cell carcinoma of other sites
209.75 Secondary Merkel cell carcinoma
214.1 Lipoma of other skin and subcutaneous tissue
221.2 Benign neoplasm of vulva
228.01 Hemangioma of skin and subcutaneous tissue
232.8 Carcinoma in situ of other specified sites of skin
233.30 Carcinoma in situ, unspecified female genital organ
233.31 Carcinoma in situ, vagina
233.32 Carcinoma in situ, vulva
233.39 Carcinoma in situ, other female genital organ
629.20 Female genital mutilation status, unspecified
629.21 Female genital mutilation, Type I status
629.22 Female genital mutilation, Type II status
686.1 Pyogenic granuloma of skin and subcutaneous tissue — (Use additional code to identify any infectious organism: 041.0-041.8)
701.1 Acquired keratoderma
701.4 Keloid scar
878.4 Open wound of vulva, without mention of complication
878.5 Open wound of vulva, complicated

Terms To Know

genitalia. External organs related to reproduction.

repair. Surgical closure of a wound. The wound may be a result of injury/trauma or may be a surgically created defect. Repairs are divided into three categories: simple, intermediate, and complex.

CCI Version 18.3

0213T, 0216T, 0228T, 0230T, 11100, 11900-11901, 36000, 36400-36410, 36420-36430, 36440, 36600, 36640, 37202, 43752, 51701-51703, 62310-62319, 64400-64435, 64445-64450, 64479, 64483, 64490, 64493, 64505-64530, 69990, 93000-93010, 93040-93042, 93318, 94002, 94200, 94250, 94680-94690, 94770, 95812-95816, 95819, 95822, 95829, 95955, 96360, 96365, 96372, 96374-96376, 97597-97598, 97602-97606, 99148-99149, 99150, G0168, J0670, J2001

Also not with 12041: 11055-11056, 11740, 12051✦

Also not with 12042: 11042, 11740, 12041

Also not with 12044: 11043-11044, 12041-12042, 12054✦

Also not with 12045: 11042, 12041-12044, 12055✦

Also not with 12046: 11043-11044, 12041-12045, 12056✦

Also not with 12047: 12037-12046, 12057✦

Note: These CCI edits are used for Medicare. Other payers may reimburse on codes listed above.

Medicare Edits

	Fac RVU	Non-Fac RVU	FUD	Status
12041	4.61	7.05	10	A
12042	5.9	8.49	10	A
12044	6.3	10.36	10	A
12045	7.77	11.51	10	A
12046	8.88	13.16	10	A
12047	9.98	15.14	10	A

	MUE		Modifiers		
12041	1	51	N/A	N/A	N/A
12042	1	51	N/A	N/A	N/A
12044	1	51	N/A	N/A	N/A
12045	1	51	N/A	N/A	N/A
12046	1	51	N/A	N/A	80*
12047	1	51	N/A	62*	80

* with documentation

Medicare References: None

Coding Companion for Ob/Gyn

13100-13102

13100 Repair, complex, trunk; 1.1 cm to 2.5 cm
13101 2.6 cm to 7.5 cm
13102 each additional 5 cm or less (List separately in addition to code for primary procedure)

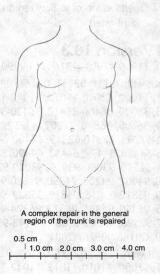

A complex repair in the general region of the trunk is repaired

0.5 cm

1.0 cm 2.0 cm 3.0 cm 4.0 cm

Explanation

The physician repairs complex wounds of the trunk. The physician performs complex, layered suturing of torn, crushed, or deeply lacerated tissue. The physician debrides the wound by removing foreign material or damaged tissue. Irrigation of the wound is performed and antimicrobial solutions are used to decontaminate and cleanse the wound. The physician may trim skin margins with a scalpel or scissors to allow for proper closure. The wound is closed in layers. The physician may perform scar revision, which creates a complex defect requiring repair. Stents or retention sutures may also be used in complex repair of a wound. Reconstructive procedures, such as utilization of local flaps, may be required and are reported separately. Report 13100 for wounds 1.1 cm to 2.5 cm; 13101 for 2.6 cm to 7.5 cm; and 13102 for each additional 5 cm or less.

Coding Tips

As an "add-on" code, 13102 is not subject to multiple procedure rules. No reimbursement reduction or modifier 51 is applied. "Add-on" codes describe additional intra-service work associated with the primary procedure. They are performed by the same physician on the same date of service as the primary service/procedure, and must never be reported as a stand-alone code. When multiple wounds are repaired, the lengths of all wounds in the same classification are added together and reported with one code. Complex repair includes the repair of wounds requiring more than layered closure, such as extensive undermining, stents, or retention sutures. Complex repair may also include creation of the defect in preparation for repairs, or the debridement of complicated lacerations and avulsions. Surgical trays, A4550, are not separately reimbursed by Medicare; however, other third-party payers may cover them. Check with the specific payer to determine coverage.

ICD-9-CM Procedural

85.81 Suture of laceration of breast
86.59 Closure of skin and subcutaneous tissue of other sites

Anesthesia

13100 00300, 00400
13101 00300, 00400
13102 N/A

ICD-9-CM Diagnostic

172.5 Malignant melanoma of skin of trunk, except scrotum
173.50 Unspecified malignant neoplasm of skin of trunk, except scrotum
173.51 Basal cell carcinoma of skin of trunk, except scrotum
173.52 Squamous cell carcinoma of skin of trunk, except scrotum
173.59 Other specified malignant neoplasm of skin of trunk, except scrotum
198.2 Secondary malignant neoplasm of skin
209.35 Merkel cell carcinoma of the trunk
209.75 Secondary Merkel cell carcinoma
214.1 Lipoma of other skin and subcutaneous tissue
216.5 Benign neoplasm of skin of trunk, except scrotum
228.01 Hemangioma of skin and subcutaneous tissue
232.5 Carcinoma in situ of skin of trunk, except scrotum
238.2 Neoplasm of uncertain behavior of skin
448.1 Nevus, non-neoplastic
686.1 Pyogenic granuloma of skin and subcutaneous tissue — (Use additional code to identify any infectious organism: 041.0-041.8)
875.1 Open wound of chest (wall), complicated
877.0 Open wound of buttock, without mention of complication
877.1 Open wound of buttock, complicated
879.1 Open wound of breast, complicated
879.3 Open wound of abdominal wall, anterior, complicated
879.5 Open wound of abdominal wall, lateral, complicated
879.7 Open wound of other and unspecified parts of trunk, complicated

Terms To Know

nevus. Benign, pigmented skin lesion that includes congenital lesions of the skin such as birthmarks, telangiectasias (permanent dilations of small blood vessels), vascular spider veins, hemangiomas, and moles.

CCI Version 18.3

11100, 11900-11901, 13160❖, 69990

Also not with 13100: 0213T, 0216T, 0228T, 0230T, 11000, 11010-11012, 11042-11044, 13102, 36000, 36400-36410, 36420-36430, 36440, 36600, 36640, 37202, 43752, 51701-51703, 62310-62319, 64400-64435, 64445-64450, 64479, 64483, 64490, 64493, 64505-64530, 93000-93010, 93040-93042, 93318, 94002, 94200, 94250, 94680-94690, 94770, 95812-95816, 95819, 95822, 95829, 95955, 96360, 96365, 96372, 96374-96376, 97597-97598, 97602-97606, 99148-99149, 99150, G0168, J0670, J2001

Also not with 13101: 0213T, 0216T, 0228T, 0230T, 11000, 11010-11012, 11042-11044, 13100, 36000, 36400-36410, 36420-36430, 36440, 36600, 36640, 37202, 43752, 51701-51703, 62310-62319, 64400-64435, 64445-64450, 64479, 64483, 64490, 64493, 64505-64530, 93000-93010, 93040-93042, 93318, 94002, 94200, 94250, 94680-94690, 94770, 95812-95816, 95819, 95822, 95829, 95955, 96360, 96365, 96372, 96374-96376, 97597-97598, 97602-97606, 99148-99149, 99150, G0168, J0670, J2001

Note: These CCI edits are used for Medicare. Other payers may reimburse on codes listed above.

Medicare Edits

	Fac RVU	Non-Fac RVU	FUD	Status
13100	6.91	9.2	10	A
13101	8.39	11.67	10	A
13102	2.22	3.2	N/A	A

	MUE		Modifiers		
13100	1	51	N/A	N/A	N/A
13101	1	51	N/A	N/A	N/A
13102	-	N/A	N/A	N/A	N/A

* with documentation

Medicare References: None

© 2012 OptumInsight, Inc.

Repair

13131-13133

13131 Repair, complex, forehead, cheeks, chin, mouth, neck, axillae, genitalia, hands and/or feet; 1.1 cm to 2.5 cm
13132 2.6 cm to 7.5 cm
13133 each additional 5 cm or less (List separately in addition to code for primary procedure)

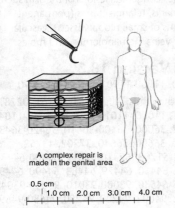

A complex repair is made in the genital area

```
0.5 cm
|   1.0 cm   2.0 cm   3.0 cm   4.0 cm
|-----|-----|-----|-----|
```

Explanation

The physician repairs complex wounds of the genitalia. The physician performs complex, layered suturing of torn, crushed, or deeply lacerated tissue. The physician debrides the wound by removing foreign material or damaged tissue. Irrigation of the wound is performed and antimicrobial solutions are used to decontaminate and cleanse the wound. The physician may trim skin margins with a scalpel or scissors to allow for proper closure. The wound is closed in layers. The physician may perform scar revision, which creates a complex defect requiring repair. Stents or retention sutures may also be used in complex repair of a wound. Reconstructive procedures, such as utilization of local flaps, may be required and are reported separately. Report 13131 for wounds 1.1 cm to 2.5 cm; 13132 for 2.6 cm to 7.5 cm; and 13133 for each additional 5 cm or less.

Coding Tips

As an "add-on" code, 13133 is not subject to multiple procedure rules. No reimbursement reduction or modifier 51 is applied. "Add-on" codes describe additional intra-service work associated with the primary procedure. They are performed by the same physician on the same date of service as the primary service/procedure, and must never be reported as a stand-alone code. When multiple wounds are repaired, the lengths of all wounds in the same classification are added together and reported with one code. Complex repair includes the repair of wounds requiring more than layered closure, such as extensive undermining, stents, or retention sutures. Complex repair may also include creation of the defect in preparation for repairs, or the debridement of complicated lacerations and avulsions. Surgical trays, A4550, are not separately reimbursed by Medicare; however, other third-party payers may cover them. Check with the specific payer to determine coverage.

ICD-9-CM Procedural

71.71 Suture of laceration of vulva or perineum
75.62 Repair of current obstetric laceration of rectum and sphincter ani
75.69 Repair of other current obstetric laceration
86.59 Closure of skin and subcutaneous tissue of other sites
86.89 Other repair and reconstruction of skin and subcutaneous tissue

Anesthesia

13131 00300, 00400, 00940
13132 00300, 00400, 00940
13133 N/A

ICD-9-CM Diagnostic

184.4 Malignant neoplasm of vulva, unspecified site
198.82 Secondary malignant neoplasm of genital organs
209.36 Merkel cell carcinoma of other sites
221.2 Benign neoplasm of vulva
233.30 Carcinoma in situ, unspecified female genital organ
233.31 Carcinoma in situ, vagina
233.32 Carcinoma in situ, vulva
233.39 Carcinoma in situ, other female genital organ
236.3 Neoplasm of uncertain behavior of other and unspecified female genital organs
629.20 Female genital mutilation status, unspecified
629.21 Female genital mutilation, Type I status
629.22 Female genital mutilation, Type II status
629.23 Female genital mutilation, Type III status
629.29 Other female genital mutilation status
629.89 Other specified disorders of female genital organs
878.4 Open wound of vulva, without mention of complication
878.5 Open wound of vulva, complicated
878.9 Open wound of other and unspecified parts of genital organs, complicated
880.12 Open wound of axillary region, complicated

CCI Version 18.3

11100, 11900-11901, 13160❖, 69990

Also not with 13131: 0213T, 0216T, 0228T, 0230T, 11000, 11010-11012, 11042-11044, 13133, 36000, 36400-36410, 36420-36430, 36440, 36600, 36640, 37202, 43752, 51701-51703, 62310-62319, 64400-64435, 64445-64450, 64479, 64483, 64490, 64493, 64505-64530, 93000-93010, 93040-93042, 93318, 94002, 94200, 94250, 94680-94690, 94770, 95812-95816, 95819, 95822, 95829, 95955, 96360, 96365, 96372, 96374-96376, 97597-97598, 97602-97606, 99148-99149, 99150, G0168, J0670, J2001

Also not with 13132: 0213T, 0216T, 0228T, 0230T, 11000, 11010-11012, 11042-11044, 11056, 13131, 36000, 36400-36410, 36420-36430, 36440, 36600, 36640, 37202, 43752, 51701-51703, 62310-62319, 64400-64435, 64445-64450, 64479, 64483, 64490, 64493, 64505-64530, 93000-93010, 93040-93042, 93318, 94002, 94200, 94250, 94680-94690, 94770, 95812-95816, 95819, 95822, 95829, 95955, 96360, 96365, 96372, 96374-96376, 97597-97598, 97602-97606, 99148-99149, 99150, G0168, J0670, J2001

Note: These CCI edits are used for Medicare. Other payers may reimburse on codes listed above.

Medicare Edits

	Fac RVU	Non-Fac RVU	FUD	Status
13131	8.13	10.54	10	A
13132	13.87	17.05	10	A
13133	3.91	4.93	N/A	A

	MUE		Modifiers		
13131	1	51	N/A	N/A	N/A
13132	1	51	N/A	N/A	N/A
13133	-	N/A	N/A	N/A	N/A

* with documentation
Medicare References: None

Repair

13160

13160 Secondary closure of surgical wound or dehiscence, extensive or complicated

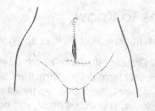

An extensive or complicated surgical wound is closed secondarily or an extensive or complicated dehiscence is treated and closed

Explanation

The physician secondarily repairs a surgical skin closure after an infectious breakdown of the healing skin. After resolution of the infection, the wound is now ready for closure. The physician uses a scalpel to excise granulation and scar tissue. Skin margins are trimmed to bleeding edges. The wound is sutured in several layers.

Coding Tips

For simple closure of secondary wound dehiscence, see 12020; with packing, see 12021. If incision and drainage of a hematoma, seroma, or fluid collection is performed, see 10140. Surgical trays, A4550, are not separately reimbursed by Medicare; however, other third-party payers may cover them. Check with the specific payer to determine coverage.

ICD-9-CM Procedural

N/A

Anesthesia

13160 00300, 00400, 00940

ICD-9-CM Diagnostic

674.10 Disruption of cesarean wound, unspecified as to episode of care

674.12 Disruption of cesarean wound, with delivery, with mention of postpartum complication

674.14 Disruption of cesarean wound, postpartum condition or complication

674.20 Disruption of perineal wound, unspecified as to episode of care in pregnancy

674.22 Disruption of perineal wound, with delivery, with mention of postpartum complication

674.24 Disruption of perineal wound, postpartum condition or complication

958.3 Posttraumatic wound infection not elsewhere classified

998.30 Disruption of wound, unspecified

998.31 Disruption of internal operation (surgical) wound

998.32 Disruption of external operation (surgical) wound

998.83 Non-healing surgical wound

V58.41 Planned postoperative wound closure — (This code should be used in conjunction with other aftercare codes to fully identify the reason for the aftercare encounter)

Terms To Know

classification of surgical wounds. Surgical wounds fall into four categories that determine treatment methods and outcomes: **1)** Clean wound: No inflammation or contamination; treatment performed with no break in sterile technique; no alimentary, respiratory, or genitourinary tracts involved in the surgery; infection rate = up to five percent. **2)** Clean-contaminated wound: No inflammation; treatment performed with minor break in surgical technique; no unusual contamination resulting when alimentary, respiratory, genitourinary, or oropharyngeal cavity is entered; infection rate = up to 11 percent. **3)** Contaminated wound: Less than four hours old with acute, nonpurulent inflammation; treatment performed with major break in surgical technique; gross contamination resulting from the gastrointestinal tract; infection rate = up to 20 percent. **4)** Dirty and infected wound: More than four hours old with existing infection, inflammation, abscess, and nonsterile conditions due to perforated viscus, fecal contamination, necrotic tissue, or foreign body; infection rate = up to 40 percent.

dehiscence. Complication of healing in which the surgical wound ruptures or bursts open, superficially or through multiple layers.

perineal. Pertaining to the pelvic floor area between the thighs; the diamond-shaped area bordered by the pubic symphysis in front, the ischial tuberosities on the sides, and the coccyx in back.

CCI Version 18.3

0213T, 0216T, 0228T, 0230T, 10180, 11000, 11010-11012, 11042-11044, 11100, 11900-11901, 12001-12007, 12011-12057, 36000, 36400-36410, 36420-36430, 36440, 36600, 36640, 37202, 43752, 51701-51703, 62310-62319, 64400-64435, 64445-64450, 64479, 64483, 64490, 64493, 64505-64530, 69990, 93000-93010, 93040-93042, 93318, 94002, 94200, 94250, 94680-94690, 94770, 95812-95816, 95819, 95822, 95829, 95955, 96360, 96365, 96372, 96374-96376, 97597-97598, 97602-97606, 99148-99149, 99150, G0168

Note: These CCI edits are used for Medicare. Other payers may reimburse on codes listed above.

Medicare Edits

	Fac RVU	Non-Fac RVU	FUD	Status
13160	23.82	23.82	90	A

	MUE		Modifiers		
13160	3	51	N/A	N/A	N/A

* with documentation

Medicare References: None

14040-14041

14040 Adjacent tissue transfer or rearrangement, forehead, cheeks, chin, mouth, neck, axillae, genitalia, hands and/or feet; defect 10 sq cm or less

14041 defect 10.1 sq cm to 30.0 sq cm

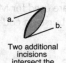

Example of common Z-plasty

Defect is removed with oval-shaped incision

a.

b.

Two additional incisions intersect the removal area

a.

b.

Skin of each incision is reflected back

a.

b.

The flaps are then transposed

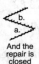

b.

a.

And the repair is closed

Report code 14040 when the defect is 10.0 sq cm or less and 14041 when the defect is 10.1 to 30.0 sq cm

Explanation

The physician transfers or rearranges adjacent tissue to repair traumatic or surgical wounds on the genitalia. This includes, but is not limited to, such rearrangement procedures as Z-plasty, W-plasty, ZY-plasty, or tissue transfers such as rotational flaps or advancement flaps. Report 14040 for defects that are 10 sq cm or less and 14041 for defects that are 10.1 sq cm to 30 sq cm.

Coding Tips

When adjacent tissue transfer or rearrangement is performed in conjunction with excision of a lesion, the lesion excision is not reported separately. When these codes are used to report repair of traumatic wounds, the procedure must have been previously planned and developed by the physician to constitute the repair. These codes do not apply when direct closure or rearrangement of the traumatized tissue itself incidentally results in these configurations. Any skin grafting required to close the secondary defect is reported separately. For intralesional injection to limit scarring, see 11900. Surgical trays, A4550, are not separately reimbursed by Medicare; however, other third-party payers may cover them. Check with the specific payer to determine coverage.

ICD-9-CM Procedural

86.3 Other local excision or destruction of lesion or tissue of skin and subcutaneous tissue

86.70 Pedicle or flap graft, not otherwise specified

86.71 Cutting and preparation of pedicle grafts or flaps

86.72 Advancement of pedicle graft

86.74 Attachment of pedicle or flap graft to other sites

86.84 Relaxation of scar or web contracture of skin

86.89 Other repair and reconstruction of skin and subcutaneous tissue

Anesthesia

00300, 00400, 00940

ICD-9-CM Diagnostic

184.0 Malignant neoplasm of vagina

184.1 Malignant neoplasm of labia majora

184.2 Malignant neoplasm of labia minora

184.3 Malignant neoplasm of clitoris

184.4 Malignant neoplasm of vulva, unspecified site

184.8 Malignant neoplasm of other specified sites of female genital organs

184.9 Malignant neoplasm of female genital organ, site unspecified

209.36 Merkel cell carcinoma of other sites

209.75 Secondary Merkel cell carcinoma

214.1 Lipoma of other skin and subcutaneous tissue

215.6 Other benign neoplasm of connective and other soft tissue of pelvis

228.01 Hemangioma of skin and subcutaneous tissue

629.20 Female genital mutilation status, unspecified

629.21 Female genital mutilation, Type I status

629.22 Female genital mutilation, Type II status

629.23 Female genital mutilation, Type III status

629.29 Other female genital mutilation status

629.89 Other specified disorders of female genital organs

878.4 Open wound of vulva, without mention of complication

878.5 Open wound of vulva, complicated

878.6 Open wound of vagina, without mention of complication

878.7 Open wound of vagina, complicated

878.8 Open wound of other and unspecified parts of genital organs, without mention of complication

880.12 Open wound of axillary region, complicated

959.14 Other injury of external genitals

998.32 Disruption of external operation (surgical) wound

998.83 Non-healing surgical wound

Terms To Know

defect. Imperfection, flaw, or absence.

tissue. Group of similar cells with a similar function that form definite structures and organs. Tissue types include epithelial tissue, muscle tissue, connective tissue, and nervous tissue.

CCI Version 18.3

0213T, 0216T, 0228T, 0230T, 11000, 11042, 11100, 11400-11471, 11600-11606, 11620-11646, 12001-12007, 12011-12057, 13100-13153, 25259, 26340, 29086, 36000, 36400-36410, 36420-36430, 36440, 36600, 36640, 37202, 43752, 51701-51703, 62310-62319, 64400-64435, 64445-64450, 64479, 64483, 64490, 64493, 64505-64530, 69990, 93000-93010, 93040-93042, 93318, 94002, 94200, 94250, 94680-94690, 94770, 95812-95816, 95819, 95822, 95829, 95955, 96360, 96365, 96372, 96374-96376, 97597-97598, 97602-97606, 99148-99149, 99150, G0168, J0670, J2001

Also not with 14040: 11055-11056, 15852, 20526-20553

Also not with 14041: 14040, 20526, 20551-20553

Note: These CCI edits are used for Medicare. Other payers may reimburse on codes listed above.

Medicare Edits

	Fac RVU	Non-Fac RVU	FUD	Status
14040	19.02	22.65	90	A
14041	23.34	27.97	90	A

	MUE		Modifiers		
14040	-	51	N/A	N/A	N/A
14041	-	51	N/A	N/A	N/A

* with documentation

Medicare References: None

Repair

17270-17276

7270 Destruction, malignant lesion (eg, laser surgery, electrosurgery, cryosurgery, chemosurgery, surgical curettement), scalp, neck, hands, feet, genitalia; lesion diameter 0.5 cm or less

7271 lesion diameter 0.6 to 1.0 cm
7272 lesion diameter 1.1 to 2.0 cm
7273 lesion diameter 2.1 to 3.0 cm
7274 lesion diameter 3.1 to 4.0 cm
7276 lesion diameter over 4.0 cm

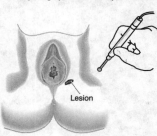

The physician may use laser, fulguration, or cryosurgery, etc. to destroy the lesion

Lesion

Report according to the area of destruction

Explanation

he physician destroys a malignant lesion of he genitalia. Destruction may be accomplished by using a laser or electrocautery to burn the lesion, cryotherapy o freeze the lesion, chemicals to destroy the esion, or surgical curettement to remove the esion. Report 17270 for a lesion diameter 0.5 m or less; 17271 for 0.6 cm to 1 cm; 17272 or 1.1 cm to 2 cm; 17273 for 2.1 cm to 3 m; 17274 for 3.1 cm to 4 cm; and 17276 if he lesion diameter is greater than 4 cm.

Coding Tips

hese codes are appropriate for reporting this rocedure when performed with any echnique or combination of techniques (e.g., ser, hot cautery). Local anesthesia is included these services. For destruction of benign esions other than skin tags or cutaneous ascular lesions, see 17110–17111. For xcision of a malignant lesion, see 1620–11626.

CD-9-CM Procedural

1.3 Other local excision or destruction of vulva and perineum

86.3 Other local excision or destruction of lesion or tissue of skin and subcutaneous tissue

Anesthesia
00300, 00400, 00940

ICD-9-CM Diagnostic

184.0 Malignant neoplasm of vagina
184.1 Malignant neoplasm of labia majora
184.2 Malignant neoplasm of labia minora
184.3 Malignant neoplasm of clitoris
184.4 Malignant neoplasm of vulva, unspecified site
184.8 Malignant neoplasm of other specified sites of female genital organs
209.36 Merkel cell carcinoma of other sites
233.30 Carcinoma in situ, unspecified female genital organ
233.31 Carcinoma in situ, vagina
233.32 Carcinoma in situ, vulva
233.39 Carcinoma in situ, other female genital organ
236.3 Neoplasm of uncertain behavior of other and unspecified female genital organs

Terms To Know

chemosurgery. Application of chemical agents to destroy tissue, originally referring to the in situ chemical fixation of premalignant or malignant lesions to facilitate surgical excision.

cryosurgery. Application of intense cold, usually produced using liquid nitrogen, to locally freeze diseased or unwanted tissue and induce tissue necrosis without causing harm to adjacent tissue.

destruction. Ablation or eradication of a structure or tissue.

electrocautery. Division or cutting of tissue using high-frequency electrical current to produce heat, which destroys cells.

electrosurgery. Use of electric currents to generate heat in performing surgery.

malignant. Any condition tending to progress toward death, specifically an invasive tumor with a loss of cellular differentiation that has the ability to spread or metastasize to other areas in the body.

neoplasm. New abnormal growth, tumor.

CCI Version 18.3

0213T, 0216T, 0228T, 0230T, 11100, 11900-11901, 12001-12007, 12011-12057, 13100-13153, 36000, 36400-36410, 36420-36430, 36440, 36600, 36640, 37202,

43752, 51701-51703, 62310-62319, 64400-64435, 64445-64450, 64479, 64483, 64490, 64493, 64505-64530, 69990, 93000-93010, 93040-93042, 93318, 94002, 94200, 94250, 94680-94690, 94770, 95812-95816, 95819, 95822, 95829, 95955, 96360, 96365, 96372, 96374-96376, 99148-99149, 99150, J0670, J2001

Also not with 17270: 11600-11606❖, 11620-11646❖

Also not with 17271: 11601-11606❖, 11621-11646❖

Also not with 17272: 11601-11606❖, 11621-11626❖, 11641-11646❖

Also not with 17273: 11602-11606❖, 11622-11626❖, 11641-11646❖

Also not with 17274: 11606❖, 11623-11626❖, 11642-11646❖

Also not with 17276: 11606❖, 11624-11626❖, 11643-11646❖

Note: These CCI edits are used for Medicare. Other payers may reimburse on codes listed above.

Medicare Edits

	Fac RVU	Non-Fac RVU	FUD	Status
17270	2.96	4.42	10	A
17271	3.3	4.82	10	A
17272	3.8	5.49	10	A
17273	4.29	6.12	10	A
17274	5.24	7.22	10	A
17276	6.3	8.39	10	A

	MUE		Modifiers		
17270	-	51	N/A	N/A	N/A
17271	-	51	N/A	N/A	N/A
17272	-	51	N/A	N/A	N/A
17273	-	51	N/A	N/A	N/A
17274	-	51	N/A	N/A	N/A
17276	3	51	N/A	N/A	N/A

* with documentation

Medicare References: 100-3,140.5

19000-19001

19000 Puncture aspiration of cyst of breast;

19001 each additional cyst (List separately in addition to code for primary procedure)

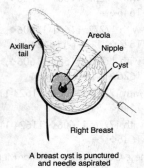

Axillary tail
Areola
Nipple
Cyst
Right Breast

A breast cyst is punctured and needle aspirated

Explanation

The physician punctures with a syringe needle the skin of the breast overlying a cyst. The needle is inserted into the cyst and fluid is evacuated into the syringe, thus reducing the size of the cyst. The physician withdraws the needle and applies pressure to the puncture wound to stop the bleeding. Report 19001 for aspiration of each additional cyst of the breast.

Coding Tips

As an "add-on" code, 19001 is not subject to multiple procedure rules. No reimbursement reduction or modifier 51 is applied. "Add-on" codes describe additional intraservice work associated with the primary procedure. They are performed by the same physician on the same date of service as the primary service/procedure, and must never be reported as a stand-alone code. When imaging guidance is used, report 76942, 77021, or 77031–77032. For a percutaneous needle core breast biopsy without imaging guidance, see 19100. To report an open, incisional breast biopsy, see 19101. For a percutaneous needle core biopsy with imaging guidance, report 19102. For percutaneous breast biopsy using automated vacuum assisted or rotating biopsy device with imaging guidance, see 19103. Surgical trays, A4550, are not separately reimbursed by Medicare; however, other third-party payers may cover them. Check with the specific payer to determine coverage.

ICD-9-CM Procedural

85.91 Aspiration of breast

Anesthesia

19000 00400

19001 N/A

ICD-9-CM Diagnostic

610.0 Solitary cyst of breast

610.1 Diffuse cystic mastopathy

610.8 Other specified benign mammary dysplasias

611.5 Galactocele

611.72 Lump or mass in breast

611.89 Other specified disorders of breast

793.80 Unspecified abnormal mammogram

793.89 Other (abnormal) findings on radiological examination of breast

Terms To Know

cyst. Elevated encapsulated mass containing fluid, semisolid, or solid material with a membranous lining.

dysplasia. Abnormality or alteration in the size, shape, and organization of cells from their normal pattern of development.

galactocele. Tumor or cyst-like enlargement of the milk-containing gland in the breast.

mastopathy. Disease or disorder of the breast or lactiferous (mammary) glands.

puncture aspiration. Use of a knife or needle to pierce a fluid-filled cavity and then withdraw the fluid using a syringe or suction device.

CCI Version 18.3

J2001

Also not with 19000: 00400, 0213T, 0216T, 0228T, 0230T, 12001-12007, 12011-12057, 13100-13153, 36000, 36400-36410, 36420-36430, 36440, 36600, 36640, 37202, 43752, 51701-51703, 62310-62319, 64400-64435, 64445-64450, 64479, 64483, 64490, 64493, 64505-64530, 69990, 93000-93010, 93040-93042, 93318, 94002, 94200, 94250, 94680-94690, 94770, 95812-95816, 95819, 95822, 95829, 95955, 96360, 96365, 96372, 96374-96376, 99148-99149, 99150, J0670

Note: These CCI edits are used for Medicare. Other payers may reimburse on codes listed above.

Medicare Edits

	Fac RVU	Non-Fac RVU	FUD	Status
19000	1.28	3.23	0	A
19001	0.63	0.77	N/A	A

	MUE		Modifiers		
19000	2	51	N/A	N/A	N/A
19001	5	N/A	N/A	N/A	N/A

* with documentation

Medicare References: 100-4,13,80.1

19020

19020 Mastotomy with exploration or drainage of abscess, deep

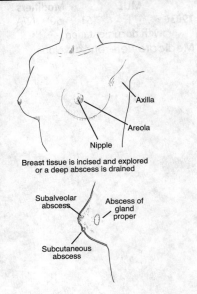

Breast tissue is incised and explored or a deep abscess is drained

Subalveolar abscess

Abscess of gland proper

Subcutaneous abscess

Explanation

The physician makes an incision in the skin of the breast over the site of an abscess or suspicious tissue for exploration or drainage. The infected cavity is accessed and specimens for culture are taken before the cavity is irrigated with warm saline solution. Bleeding vessels may be tied or cauterized. If no abscess or suspicious tissue is found, the wound is closed with sutures. In the case of an abscess, the wound is usually loosely packed with gauze to promote free drainage rather than being closed with sutures.

Coding Tips

For aspiration of a breast cyst, see 19000. For open, incisional breast biopsy, see 19101. For percutaneous needle core breast biopsy with imaging guidance, see 19102; using automated vacuum assisted or rotating biopsy device, see 19103. Excision of a breast lesion(s) may be reported with 19120.

ICD-9-CM Procedural

85.0   Mastotomy

Anesthesia

19020   00400

ICD-9-CM Diagnostic

611.0   Inflammatory disease of breast

675.10   Abscess of breast associated with childbirth, unspecified as to episode of care

675.11   Abscess of breast associated with childbirth, delivered, with or without mention of antepartum condition

675.12   Abscess of breast associated with childbirth, delivered, with mention of postpartum complication

675.13   Abscess of breast, antepartum

675.14   Abscess of breast, postpartum condition or complication

996.69   Infection and inflammatory reaction due to other internal prosthetic device, implant, and graft — (Use additional code to identify specified infections)

998.51   Infected postoperative seroma — (Use additional code to identify organism)

998.59   Other postoperative infection — (Use additional code to identify infection)

Terms To Know

abscess. Circumscribed collection of pus resulting from bacteria, frequently associated with swelling and other signs of inflammation.

cauterize. Heat or chemicals used to burn or cut.

cyst. Elevated encapsulated mass containing fluid, semisolid, or solid material with a membranous lining.

dysplasia. Abnormality or alteration in the size, shape, and organization of cells from their normal pattern of development.

exploration. Examination for diagnostic purposes.

mastitis. Inflammation of the breast. Acute mastitis is caused by a bacterial infection; chronic mastitis is caused by hormonal changes.

mastodynia. Pain, discomfort, or tenderness in the breast, often due to hormonal changes.

mastopathy. Disease or disorder of the breast or lactiferous (mammary) glands.

CCI Version 18.3

00400, 0213T, 0216T, 0228T, 0230T, 12001-12007, 12011-12057, 13100-13153, 20500, 36000, 36400-36410, 36420-36430, 36440, 36600, 36640, 37202, 43752, 51701-51703, 62310-62319, 64400-64435, 64445-64450, 64479, 64483, 64490, 64493, 64505-64530, 69990, 93000-93010, 93040-93042, 93318, 94002, 94200, 94250, 94680-94690, 94770, 95812-95816, 95819, 95822, 95829, 95955, 96360, 96365, 96372, 96374-96376, 99148-99149, 99150, J0670, J2001

Note: These CCI edits are used for Medicare. Other payers may reimburse on codes listed above.

Medicare Edits

	Fac RVU	Non-Fac RVU	FUD	Status
19020	8.85	13.66	90	A

	MUE		Modifiers		
19020	2	51	50	N/A	N/A

* with documentation

Medicare References: None

Coding Companion for Ob/Gyn

Breast

19030

19030 Injection procedure only for mammary ductogram or galactogram

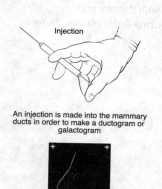
Injection

An injection is made into the mammary ducts in order to make a ductogram or galactogram

Explanation

The physician performs an injection procedure for mammary ductogram or galactogram. A cannula or needle is inserted into the duct of the breast. Contrast media is introduced into the breast duct for the purpose of radiographic study. A dissecting microscope may be used to aid in placing the cannula. The needle or cannula is removed once the study has been completed.

Coding Tips

Radiological supervision and interpretation is reported with codes 77053 and 77054.

ICD-9-CM Procedural

87.35   Contrast radiogram of mammary ducts

Anesthesia

19030   00400

ICD-9-CM Diagnostic

217   Benign neoplasm of breast
610.0   Solitary cyst of breast
610.1   Diffuse cystic mastopathy
610.4   Mammary duct ectasia
610.8   Other specified benign mammary dysplasias
611.0   Inflammatory disease of breast
611.1   Hypertrophy of breast
611.5   Galactocele
611.6   Galactorrhea not associated with childbirth
611.71   Mastodynia
611.72   Lump or mass in breast
611.79   Other sign and symptom in breast
611.89   Other specified disorders of breast

Terms To Know

cannula. Tube inserted into a blood vessel, duct, or body cavity to facilitate passage.

cystic mastopathy. Mammary dysplasia involving inflammation and the formation of fluid-filled nodular cysts in the breast tissue.

dysplasia. Abnormality or alteration in the size, shape, and organization of cells from their normal pattern of development.

galactocele. Tumor or cyst-like enlargement of the milk-containing gland in the breast.

galactogram. Following injection of a radiopaque dye into the ducts of the breast, radiographic pictures are taken of the milk-producing mammary ducts.

hypertrophy of breast. Overgrowth of normal breast tissue.

mammary duct ectasia. Condition characterized by dilated ducts of the mammary gland.

mastitis. Inflammation of the breast. Acute mastitis is caused by a bacterial infection; chronic mastitis is caused by hormonal changes.

mastodynia. Pain, discomfort, or tenderness in the breast, often due to hormonal changes.

mastopathy. Disease or disorder of the breast or lactiferous (mammary) glands.

CCI Version 18.3

00400, 0213T, 0216T, 0228T, 0230T, 12001-12007, 12011-12057, 13100-13153, 36000, 36400-36410, 36420-36430, 36440, 36600, 36640, 37202, 43752, 51701-51703, 62310-62319, 64400-64435, 64445-64450, 64479, 64483, 64490, 64493, 64505-64530, 69990, 76000-76001, 77001-77002, 93000-93010, 93040-93042, 93318, 94002, 94200, 94250, 94680-94690, 94770, 95812-95816, 95819, 95822, 95829, 95955, 96360, 96365, 96372, 96374-96376, 99148-99149, 99150

Note: These CCI edits are used for Medicare. Other payers may reimburse on codes listed above.

Medicare Edits

	Fac RVU	Non-Fac RVU	FUD	Status
19030	2.25	4.72	0	A

	MUE		Modifiers		
19030	1	51	50	N/A	N/A

* with documentation

Medicare References: None

19100

19100 Biopsy of breast; percutaneous, needle core, not using imaging guidance (separate procedure)

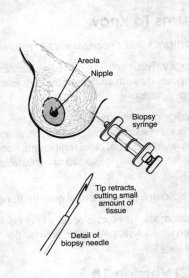

Areola
Nipple
Biopsy syringe

Tip retracts, cutting small amount of tissue

Detail of biopsy needle

Explanation

The physician inserts a large gauge needle through the skin of the breast and into the suspect breast tissue. The needle is removed along with a core of breast tissue. Pressure is applied to the puncture site to stop any bleeding.

Coding Tips

This separate procedure by definition is usually a component of a more complex service and is not identified separately. When performed alone or with other unrelated procedures or services it may be reported. If performed alone, list the code; if performed with other procedures/services, list the code and append modifier 59. This is a unilateral procedure. If performed bilaterally, some payers require that the service be reported twice with modifier 50 appended to the second code while others require identification of the service only once with modifier 50 appended. Check with individual payers. Modifier 50 identifies a procedure performed identically on the opposite side of the body (mirror image). For aspiration of a breast cyst, see 19000. For open, incisional breast biopsy, see 19101. For a percutaneous needle core breast biopsy with imaging guidance, see 19102; using an automated vacuum assisted device or a rotating biopsy device, see 19103. For excision of a breast lesion(s), see 19120.

ICD-9-CM Procedural

85.11   Closed (percutaneous) (needle) biopsy of breast
85.12   Open biopsy of breast

Anesthesia
19100   00400

ICD-9-CM Diagnostic

174.0   Malignant neoplasm of nipple and areola of female breast — (Use additional code to identify estrogen receptor status: V86.0-V86.1)
174.1   Malignant neoplasm of central portion of female breast — (Use additional code to identify estrogen receptor status: V86.0-V86.1)
174.2   Malignant neoplasm of upper-inner quadrant of female breast — (Use additional code to identify estrogen receptor status: V86.0-V86.1)
174.3   Malignant neoplasm of lower-inner quadrant of female breast — (Use additional code to identify estrogen receptor status: V86.0-V86.1)
174.4   Malignant neoplasm of upper-outer quadrant of female breast — (Use additional code to identify estrogen receptor status: V86.0-V86.1)
174.5   Malignant neoplasm of lower-outer quadrant of female breast — (Use additional code to identify estrogen receptor status: V86.0-V86.1)
174.6   Malignant neoplasm of axillary tail of female breast — (Use additional code to identify estrogen receptor status: V86.0-V86.1)
174.8   Malignant neoplasm of other specified sites of female breast — (Use additional code to identify estrogen receptor status: V86.0-V86.1)
198.81 Secondary malignant neoplasm of breast
217   Benign neoplasm of breast
233.0   Carcinoma in situ of breast
238.3   Neoplasm of uncertain behavior of breast
239.3   Neoplasm of unspecified nature of breast
610.0   Solitary cyst of breast
610.1   Diffuse cystic mastopathy
610.2   Fibroadenosis of breast
610.3   Fibrosclerosis of breast
610.8   Other specified benign mammary dysplasias
611.0   Inflammatory disease of breast

611.72 Lump or mass in breast
611.89 Other specified disorders of breast
793.80 Unspecified abnormal mammogram
793.81 Mammographic microcalcification
793.89 Other (abnormal) findings on radiological examination of breast
V10.3   Personal history of malignant neoplasm of breast
V16.3   Family history of malignant neoplasm of breast

Terms To Know

benign mammary dysplasias. Noncancerous fibrous or cystic growths in the breast.

core biopsy. Large-bore biopsy needle is inserted into a mass and a core of tissue is removed for diagnostic study.

cyst. Elevated encapsulated mass containing fluid, semisolid, or solid material with a membranous lining.

mastopathy. Disease or disorder of the breast or lactiferous (mammary) glands.

CCI Version 18.3

00400, 0213T, 0216T, 0228T, 0230T, 10021-10022, 12001-12007, 12011-12057, 13100-13153, 19290, 19295, 36000, 36400-36410, 36420-36430, 36440, 36600, 36640, 37202, 43752, 51701-51703, 62310-62319, 64400-64435, 64445-64450, 64479, 64483, 64490, 64493, 64505-64530, 69990, 76942, 77012, 77021, 77031-77032, 93000-93010, 93040-93042, 93318, 94002, 94200, 94250, 94680-94690, 94770, 95812-95816, 95819, 95822, 95829, 95955, 96360, 96365, 96372, 96374-96376, 99148-99149, 99150, J0670, J2001

Note: These CCI edits are used for Medicare. Other payers may reimburse on codes listed above.

Medicare Edits

	Fac RVU	Non-Fac RVU	FUD	Status
19100	2.03	4.35	0	A

	MUE		Modifiers		
19100	-	51	50	N/A	N/A

* with documentation

Medicare References: 100-4,12,40.7; 100-4,13,80.1

19101

19101 Biopsy of breast; open, incisional

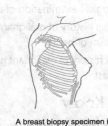
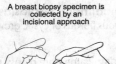

A breast biopsy specimen is collected by an incisional approach

Explanation

The physician removes tissue for biopsy. The physician makes an incision in the skin of the breast near the site of the suspect mass. The mass is identified and a sample of the lesion is removed. This specimen is often examined immediately. If the lesion is benign, the incision is repaired with layered closure. If malignant, the incision may be closed pending a separate, more extensive surgical session, or a more extensive surgery may occur immediately, in which case this code would not be reported.

Coding Tips

This is a unilateral procedure. If performed bilaterally, some payers require that the service be reported twice with modifier 50 appended to the second code while others require identification of the service only once with modifier 50 appended. Check with individual payers. Modifier 50 identifies a procedure performed identically on the opposite side of the body (mirror image). For aspiration of a breast cyst, see 19000. For breast biopsy, incisional, open, see 19101; needle core, percutaneous, with imaging guidance, see 19102; using an automated vacuum assisted device or a rotating biopsy device, see 19103. For excision of a breast lesion(s), see 19120.

ICD-9-CM Procedural

85.11 Closed (percutaneous) (needle) biopsy of breast

85.12 Open biopsy of breast

87.37 Other mammography

Anesthesia

19101 00400

ICD-9-CM Diagnostic

174.0 Malignant neoplasm of nipple and areola of female breast — (Use additional code to identify estrogen receptor status: V86.0-V86.1)

174.1 Malignant neoplasm of central portion of female breast — (Use additional code to identify estrogen receptor status: V86.0-V86.1)

174.2 Malignant neoplasm of upper-inner quadrant of female breast — (Use additional code to identify estrogen receptor status: V86.0-V86.1)

174.3 Malignant neoplasm of lower-inner quadrant of female breast — (Use additional code to identify estrogen receptor status: V86.0-V86.1)

174.4 Malignant neoplasm of upper-outer quadrant of female breast — (Use additional code to identify estrogen receptor status: V86.0-V86.1)

174.5 Malignant neoplasm of lower-outer quadrant of female breast — (Use additional code to identify estrogen receptor status: V86.0-V86.1)

174.6 Malignant neoplasm of axillary tail of female breast — (Use additional code to identify estrogen receptor status: V86.0-V86.1)

174.8 Malignant neoplasm of other specified sites of female breast — (Use additional code to identify estrogen receptor status: V86.0-V86.1)

198.81 Secondary malignant neoplasm of breast

217 Benign neoplasm of breast

233.0 Carcinoma in situ of breast

238.3 Neoplasm of uncertain behavior of breast

239.3 Neoplasm of unspecified nature of breast

610.0 Solitary cyst of breast

610.1 Diffuse cystic mastopathy

610.2 Fibroadenosis of breast

610.3 Fibrosclerosis of breast

610.8 Other specified benign mammary dysplasias

611.0 Inflammatory disease of breast

611.72 Lump or mass in breast

611.89 Other specified disorders of breast

793.80 Unspecified abnormal mammogram

793.81 Mammographic microcalcification

793.89 Other (abnormal) findings on radiological examination of breast

V10.3 Personal history of malignant neoplasm of breast

V16.3 Family history of malignant neoplasm of breast

Terms To Know

benign. Mild or nonmalignant in nature.

biopsy. Tissue or fluid removed for diagnostic purposes through analysis of the cells in the biopsy material.

malignant. Any condition tending to progress toward death, specifically an invasive tumor with a loss of cellular differentiation that has the ability to spread or metastasize to other areas in the body.

neoplasm. New abnormal growth, tumor.

specimen. Tissue cells or sample of fluid taken for analysis, pathologic examination, and diagnosis.

CCI Version 18.3

00400, 0213T, 0216T, 0228T, 0230T, 10021-10022, 12001-12007, 12011-12057, 13100-13153, 19100, 19290, 19295, 36000, 36400-36410, 36420-36430, 36440, 36600, 36640, 37202, 43752, 51701-51703, 62310-62319, 64400-64435, 64445-64450, 64479, 64483, 64490, 64493, 64505-64530, 69990, 76942, 77012, 77021, 77031-77032, 88172, 93000-93010, 93040-93042, 93318, 94002, 94200, 94250, 94680-94690, 94770, 95812-95816, 95819, 95822, 95829, 95955, 96360, 96365, 96372, 96374-96376, 99148-99149, 99150, J0670, J2001

Note: These CCI edits are used for Medicare. Other payers may reimburse on codes listed above.

Medicare Edits

	Fac RVU	Non-Fac RVU	FUD	Status
19101	6.44	9.92	10	A

	MUE		Modifiers		
19101	3	51	50	N/A	N/A

* with documentation

Medicare References: None

Breast

19102-19103

19102 Biopsy of breast; percutaneous, needle core, using imaging guidance

19103 percutaneous, automated vacuum assisted or rotating biopsy device, using imaging guidance

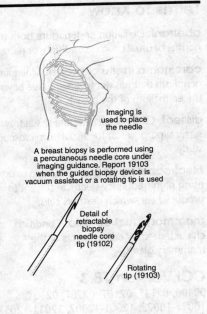

Imaging is used to place the needle

A breast biopsy is performed using a percutaneous needle core under imaging guidance. Report 19103 when the guided biopsy device is vacuum assisted or a rotating tip is used

Detail of retractable biopsy needle core tip (19102)

Rotating tip (19103)

Explanation

The physician performs a breast biopsy with image guidance using a percutaneous needle core in 19102, and an automated vacuum assisted or rotating biopsy device, in 19103. In 19102, under image guidance, the physician inserts a large gauge (e.g., 14 gauge), hollow core biopsy needle through the skin of the breast and into the suspicious breast tissue. The physician takes five or more cores of tissue to obtain a sufficient amount of tissue for diagnosis. In 19103, under image guidance, an automated vacuum assisted or rotating biopsy device is inserted through the skin into the suspicious breast tissue and a core of suspect tissue is removed for biopsy. The needle or automated vacuum assisted or rotating biopsy device is withdrawn. Pressure and bandages are applied to the puncture site.

Coding Tips

These are unilateral procedures. If performed bilaterally, some payers require that the service be reported twice with modifier 50 appended to the second code while others require identification of the service only once with modifier 50 appended. Check with individual payers. Modifier 50 identifies a procedure performed identically on the opposite side of the body (mirror image). For placement of a percutaneous localization clip, see 19295. For imaging guidance performed with these procedures, see 76942, 77012, 77021, or 77031–77032. For aspiration of a breast cyst, see 19000. For breast biopsy, incisional, open, see 19101; needle core, percutaneous, with imaging guidance, see 19102; using an automated vacuum assisted device or a rotating biopsy device, see 19103. For excision of a breast lesion(s), see 19120.

ICD-9-CM Procedural

85.11 Closed (percutaneous) (needle) biopsy of breast

87.37 Other mammography

Anesthesia

00400

ICD-9-CM Diagnostic

174.0 Malignant neoplasm of nipple and areola of female breast — (Use additional code to identify estrogen receptor status: V86.0-V86.1)

174.1 Malignant neoplasm of central portion of female breast — (Use additional code to identify estrogen receptor status: V86.0-V86.1)

174.2 Malignant neoplasm of upper-inner quadrant of female breast — (Use additional code to identify estrogen receptor status: V86.0-V86.1)

174.3 Malignant neoplasm of lower-inner quadrant of female breast — (Use additional code to identify estrogen receptor status: V86.0-V86.1)

174.4 Malignant neoplasm of upper-outer quadrant of female breast — (Use additional code to identify estrogen receptor status: V86.0-V86.1)

174.5 Malignant neoplasm of lower-outer quadrant of female breast — (Use additional code to identify estrogen receptor status: V86.0-V86.1)

174.6 Malignant neoplasm of axillary tail of female breast — (Use additional code to identify estrogen receptor status: V86.0-V86.1)

174.8 Malignant neoplasm of other specified sites of female breast — (Use additional code to identify estrogen receptor status: V86.0-V86.1)

198.81 Secondary malignant neoplasm of breast

217 Benign neoplasm of breast

233.0 Carcinoma in situ of breast

238.3 Neoplasm of uncertain behavior of breast

239.3 Neoplasm of unspecified nature of breast

610.0 Solitary cyst of breast

610.1 Diffuse cystic mastopathy

610.2 Fibroadenosis of breast

610.3 Fibrosclerosis of breast

610.8 Other specified benign mammary dysplasias

611.0 Inflammatory disease of breast

611.72 Lump or mass in breast

611.89 Other specified disorders of breast

793.80 Unspecified abnormal mammogram

793.81 Mammographic microcalcification

793.89 Other (abnormal) findings on radiological examination of breast

V10.3 Personal history of malignant neoplasm of breast

V16.3 Family history of malignant neoplasm of breast

Terms To Know

core biopsy. Large-bore biopsy needle is inserted into a mass and a core of tissue is removed for diagnostic study.

malignant. Any condition tending to progress toward death, specifically an invasive tumor with a loss of cellular differentiation that has the ability to spread or metastasize to other areas in the body.

CCI Version 18.3

00400, 0213T, 0216T, 0228T, 0230T, 10021-10022, 12001-12007, 12011-12057, 13100-13153, 19100-19101❖, 36000, 36400-36410, 36420-36430, 36440, 36600, 36640, 37202, 43752, 51701-51703, 62310-62319, 64400-64435, 64445-64450, 64479, 64483, 64490, 64493, 64505-64530, 69990, 88172, 93000-93010, 93040-93042, 93318, 94002, 94200, 94250, 94680-94690, 94770, 95812-95816, 95819, 95822, 95829, 95955, 96360, 96365, 96372, 96374-96376, 99148-99149, 99150, J0670, J2001

Also not with 19102: 19103❖

Note: These CCI edits are used for Medicare. Other payers may reimburse on codes listed above.

Medicare Edits

	Fac RVU	Non-Fac RVU	FUD	Status
19102	2.98	6.23	0	A
19103	5.57	16.11	0	A

	MUE		Modifiers		
19102	-	51	50	N/A	N/A
19103	-	51	50	N/A	N/A

* with documentation

Medicare References: 100-3,220.13; 100-4,13,80.1; 100-4,13,80.2

Breast

19120

19120 Excision of cyst, fibroadenoma, or other benign or malignant tumor, aberrant breast tissue, duct lesion, nipple or areolar lesion (except 19300), open, male or female, 1 or more lesions

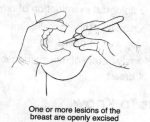

One or more lesions of the breast are openly excised

Explanation

The physician excises breast tissue for biopsy. The physician makes an incision in the skin of the breast overlying the site of the mass. Skin and tissue are dissected from the site of the defective tissue. The lesion is removed without attention to obtaining clean margins. Bleeding vessels are controlled with electrocautery or ligated with sutures. A drain may be inserted into the wound. The incision is sutured in layered closure and a light pressure dressing is applied.

Coding Tips

This is a unilateral procedure. If performed bilaterally, some payers require that the service be reported twice with modifier 50 appended to the second code while others require identification of the service only once with modifier 50 appended. Check with individual payers. Modifier 50 identifies a procedure performed identically on the opposite side of the body (mirror image). For aspiration of a breast cyst, see 19000. For breast biopsy, incisional, open, see 19101; needle core, percutaneous needle, see 19100; with imaging, see 19102; using an automated vacuum assisted device or a rotating biopsy device, see 19103. For excision of a breast lesion(s), see 19120.

ICD-9-CM Procedural

85.20	Excision or destruction of breast tissue, not otherwise specified
85.21	Local excision of lesion of breast
85.24	Excision of ectopic breast tissue
85.25	Excision of nipple

Anesthesia

19120 00400

ICD-9-CM Diagnostic

174.0	Malignant neoplasm of nipple and areola of female breast — (Use additional code to identify estrogen receptor status: V86.0-V86.1)
174.1	Malignant neoplasm of central portion of female breast — (Use additional code to identify estrogen receptor status: V86.0-V86.1)
174.2	Malignant neoplasm of upper-inner quadrant of female breast — (Use additional code to identify estrogen receptor status: V86.0-V86.1)
174.3	Malignant neoplasm of lower-inner quadrant of female breast — (Use additional code to identify estrogen receptor status: V86.0-V86.1)
174.4	Malignant neoplasm of upper-outer quadrant of female breast — (Use additional code to identify estrogen receptor status: V86.0-V86.1)
174.5	Malignant neoplasm of lower-outer quadrant of female breast — (Use additional code to identify estrogen receptor status: V86.0-V86.1)
174.6	Malignant neoplasm of axillary tail of female breast — (Use additional code to identify estrogen receptor status: V86.0-V86.1)
174.8	Malignant neoplasm of other specified sites of female breast — (Use additional code to identify estrogen receptor status: V86.0-V86.1)
198.81	Secondary malignant neoplasm of breast
217	Benign neoplasm of breast
233.0	Carcinoma in situ of breast
238.3	Neoplasm of uncertain behavior of breast
239.3	Neoplasm of unspecified nature of breast
610.0	Solitary cyst of breast
610.1	Diffuse cystic mastopathy
610.2	Fibroadenosis of breast
610.3	Fibrosclerosis of breast
610.4	Mammary duct ectasia
610.8	Other specified benign mammary dysplasias
611.0	Inflammatory disease of breast
611.72	Lump or mass in breast
611.79	Other sign and symptom in breast
611.89	Other specified disorders of breast

Terms To Know

aberrant. Deviation or departure from the normal or usual course, condition, or pattern.

carcinoma in situ of breast. Malignant neoplasm that has not invaded tissue beyond the epithelium of the breast.

dissect. Cut apart or separate tissue for surgical purposes or for visual or microscopic study.

electrocautery. Division or cutting of tissue using high-frequency electrical current to produce heat, which destroys cells.

mammary duct ectasia. Condition characterized by dilated ducts of the mammary gland.

CCI Version 18.3

00400, 0213T, 0216T, 0228T, 0230T, 10021-10022, 12001-12007, 12011-12057, 13100-13153, 19100, 19102-19103, 19110-19112, 19290, 19295, 36000, 36400-36410, 36420-36430, 36440, 36600, 36640, 37202, 43752, 51701-51703, 62310-62319, 64400-64435, 64445-64450, 64479, 64483, 64490, 64493, 64505-64530, 69990, 76942, 77031-77032, 93000-93010, 93040-93042, 93318, 94002, 94200, 94250, 94680-94690, 94770, 95812-95816, 95819, 95822, 95829, 95955, 96360, 96365, 96372, 96374-96376, 99148-99149, 99150, J0670, J2001

Note: These CCI edits are used for Medicare. Other payers may reimburse on codes listed above.

Medicare Edits

	Fac RVU	Non-Fac RVU	FUD	Status
19120	11.94	14.21	90	A

	MUE		Modifiers		
19120	1	51	50	N/A	N/A

* with documentation

Medicare References: None

Breast

19125–19126

19125 Excision of breast lesion identified by preoperative placement of radiological marker, open; single lesion

19126 each additional lesion separately identified by a preoperative radiological marker (List separately in addition to code for primary procedure)

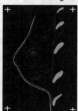

A breast lesion has been identified by placement of radiological marker

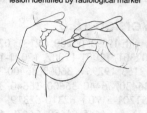

A single lesion is excised. Report code 19126 for removal of each additional lesion identified by radiological marker

Explanation

The physician uses radiologic markers to identify breast tissue to be excised for biopsy. The physician makes an incision in the skin of the breast over the site of the lesion marked for excision by preoperative placement of a radiological marker. The lesion and marker are excised, without attention to obtaining clean margins. Bleeding vessels are controlled with electrocautery or ligated with sutures. A drain may be inserted into the wound. The incision is sutured in layered closure and a light dressing is applied. Report 19126 for each additional lesion identified by a preoperative marker and removed during the same surgical session.

Coding Tips

As an "add-on" code, 19126 is not subject to multiple procedure rules. No reimbursement reduction or modifier 51 is applied. "Add-on" codes describe additional intra-service work associated with the primary procedure. They are performed by the same physician on the same date of service as the primary service or procedure, and must never be reported as a stand-alone code. For preoperative placement of a breast needle localization wire, see 19290–19291. For excision of a breast lesion(s), see 19120.

ICD-9-CM Procedural

85.21 Local excision of lesion of breast

Anesthesia

19125 00400
19126 N/A

ICD-9-CM Diagnostic

174.0 Malignant neoplasm of nipple and areola of female breast — (Use additional code to identify estrogen receptor status: V86.0-V86.1)

174.1 Malignant neoplasm of central portion of female breast — (Use additional code to identify estrogen receptor status: V86.0-V86.1)

174.2 Malignant neoplasm of upper-inner quadrant of female breast — (Use additional code to identify estrogen receptor status: V86.0-V86.1)

174.3 Malignant neoplasm of lower-inner quadrant of female breast — (Use additional code to identify estrogen receptor status: V86.0-V86.1)

174.4 Malignant neoplasm of upper-outer quadrant of female breast — (Use additional code to identify estrogen receptor status: V86.0-V86.1)

174.5 Malignant neoplasm of lower-outer quadrant of female breast — (Use additional code to identify estrogen receptor status: V86.0-V86.1)

174.6 Malignant neoplasm of axillary tail of female breast — (Use additional code to identify estrogen receptor status: V86.0-V86.1)

174.8 Malignant neoplasm of other specified sites of female breast — (Use additional code to identify estrogen receptor status: V86.0-V86.1)

198.81 Secondary malignant neoplasm of breast

217 Benign neoplasm of breast

233.0 Carcinoma in situ of breast

238.3 Neoplasm of uncertain behavior of breast

239.3 Neoplasm of unspecified nature of breast

610.0 Solitary cyst of breast

610.1 Diffuse cystic mastopathy

610.3 Fibrosclerosis of breast

611.0 Inflammatory disease of breast

611.72 Lump or mass in breast

611.79 Other sign and symptom in breast

611.89 Other specified disorders of breast

793.81 Mammographic microcalcification

793.89 Other (abnormal) findings on radiological examination of breast

Terms To Know

cystic mastopathy. Mammary dysplasia involving inflammation and the formation of fluid-filled nodular cysts in the breast tissue.

dysplasia. Abnormality or alteration in the size, shape, and organization of cells from their normal pattern of development.

excision. Surgical removal of an organ or tissue.

ligate. To tie off a blood vessel or duct with a suture or a soft, thin wire (ligature wire).

neoplasm. New abnormal growth, tumor.

CCI Version 18.3

19295

Also not with 19125: 00400, 0213T, 0216T, 0228T, 0230T, 10021-10022, 12001-12007, 12011-12057, 13100-13153, 19100-19103, 19110-19120, 36000, 36400-36410, 36420-36430, 36440, 36600, 36640, 37202, 43752, 51701-51703, 62310-62319, 64400-64435, 64445-64450, 64479, 64483, 64490, 64493, 64505-64530, 69990, 93000-93010, 93040-93042, 93318, 94002, 94200, 94250, 94680-94690, 94770, 95812-95816, 95819, 95822, 95829, 95955, 96360, 96365, 96372, 96374-96376, 99148-99149, 99150, J0670, J2001

Also not with 19126: 19102-19103

Note: These CCI edits are used for Medicare. Other payers may reimburse on codes listed above.

Medicare Edits

	Fac RVU	Non-Fac RVU	FUD	Status
19125	13.26	15.76	90	A
19126	4.7	4.7	N/A	A

	MUE	Modifiers			
19125	1	51	50	62*	N/A
19126	3	N/A	N/A	62*	N/A

* with documentation

Medicare References: None

Breast

19290-19291

19290 Preoperative placement of needle localization wire, breast;

19291 each additional lesion (List separately in addition to code for primary procedure)

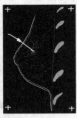

A needle localization wire is placed under flouroscopic guidance into breast tissue. Dye may be released through the needle, or the needle alone may be used to mark the lesion

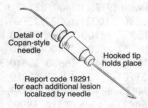

Detail of Copan-style needle

Hooked tip holds place

Report code 19291 for each additional lesion localized by needle

Explanation

Placement of a needle localization wire into a breast lesion is performed to assist in operative identification of the suspect tissue. The physician punctures the skin overlying a breast mass and inserts a needle threaded with a guide wire. Using radiological guidance to facilitate placement, the physician inserts the wire into the mass. Sometimes dye is also injected into the suspect tissue. The wire will help identify a nonpalpable mass that is to be removed from the patient during a separate operative session. Report 19291 for each additional lesion localization wire placed.

Coding Tips

As an "add-on" code, 19291 is not subject to multiple procedure rules. No reimbursement reduction or modifier 51 is applied. "Add-on" codes describe additional intra-service work associated with the primary procedure. They are performed by the same physician on the same date of service as the primary service or procedure, and must never be reported as a stand-alone code. Radiological supervision and interpretation is reported with 76942 or 77031–77032, when performed. Surgical trays, A4550, are not separately reimbursed by Medicare; however, other third-party payers may cover them. Check with the specific payer to determine coverage.

ICD-9-CM Procedural

85.99 Other operations on the breast

Anesthesia

19290 00400
19291 N/A

ICD-9-CM Diagnostic

174.0 Malignant neoplasm of nipple and areola of female breast — (Use additional code to identify estrogen receptor status: V86.0-V86.1)

174.1 Malignant neoplasm of central portion of female breast — (Use additional code to identify estrogen receptor status: V86.0-V86.1)

174.2 Malignant neoplasm of upper-inner quadrant of female breast — (Use additional code to identify estrogen receptor status: V86.0-V86.1)

174.3 Malignant neoplasm of lower-inner quadrant of female breast — (Use additional code to identify estrogen receptor status: V86.0-V86.1)

174.4 Malignant neoplasm of upper-outer quadrant of female breast — (Use additional code to identify estrogen receptor status: V86.0-V86.1)

174.5 Malignant neoplasm of lower-outer quadrant of female breast — (Use additional code to identify estrogen receptor status: V86.0-V86.1)

174.6 Malignant neoplasm of axillary tail of female breast — (Use additional code to identify estrogen receptor status: V86.0-V86.1)

174.8 Malignant neoplasm of other specified sites of female breast — (Use additional code to identify estrogen receptor status: V86.0-V86.1)

198.81 Secondary malignant neoplasm of breast

217 Benign neoplasm of breast

233.0 Carcinoma in situ of breast

238.3 Neoplasm of uncertain behavior of breast

239.3 Neoplasm of unspecified nature of breast

610.0 Solitary cyst of breast

610.1 Diffuse cystic mastopathy

611.0 Inflammatory disease of breast

611.72 Lump or mass in breast

611.79 Other sign and symptom in breast

611.89 Other specified disorders of breast

V10.3 Personal history of malignant neoplasm of breast

V16.3 Family history of malignant neoplasm of breast

V84.01 Genetic susceptibility to malignant neoplasm of breast — (Use additional code, if applicable, for any associated family history of the disease: V16-V19. Code first, if applicable, any current malignant neoplasms: 140.0-195.8, 200.0-208.9, 230.0-234.9. Use additional code, if applicable, for any personal history of malignant neoplasm: V10.0-V10.9)

Terms To Know

carcinoma in situ of breast. Malignant neoplasm that has not invaded tissue beyond the epithelium of the breast.

cyst. Elevated encapsulated mass containing fluid, semisolid, or solid material with a membranous lining.

neoplasm. New abnormal growth, tumor.

CCI Version 18.3

Also not with 19290: 00400, 0213T, 0216T, 0228T, 0230T, 12001-12007, 12011-12057, 13100-13153, 19295❖, 36000, 36400-36410, 36420-36430, 36440, 36600, 36640, 37202, 43752, 51701-51703, 62310-62319, 64400-64435, 64445-64450, 64479, 64483, 64490, 64493, 64505-64530, 69990, 93000-93010, 93040-93042, 93318, 94002, 94200, 94250, 94680-94690, 94770, 95812-95816, 95819, 95822, 95829, 95955, 96360, 96365, 96372, 96374-96376, 99148-99149, 99150, J0670, J2001

Note: These CCI edits are used for Medicare. Other payers may reimburse on codes listed above.

Medicare Edits

	Fac RVU	Non-Fac RVU	FUD	Status
19290	1.87	4.69	0	A
19291	0.92	1.99	N/A	A

	MUE		Modifiers		
19290	3	51	50	N/A	N/A
19291	-	N/A	N/A	N/A	N/A

* with documentation

Medicare References: 100-4,12,40.7; 100-4,13,80.1; 100-4,13,80.2

Breast

19295

19295 Image guided placement, metallic localization clip, percutaneous, during breast biopsy/aspiration (List separately in addition to code for primary procedure)

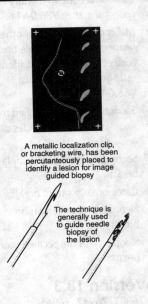

A metallic localization clip, or bracketing wire, has been percutaneously placed to identify a lesion for image guided biopsy

The technique is generally used to guide needle biopsy of the lesion

Explanation

The physician places a metallic clip prior to a breast biopsy or aspiration. Using image guidance, the physician places a metallic clip adjacent to a breast lesion to mark the site for a separately reportable breast biopsy or aspiration.

Coding Tips

Code 19295 is reported with the appropriate code for the breast biopsy or aspiration performed. This code reports only the clip placement under image guidance for the purpose of localizing the biopsy or aspiration site. As an "add-on" code, 19295 is not subject to multiple procedure rules. No reimbursement reduction or modifier 51 is applied. "Add-on" codes describe additional intra-service work associated with the primary procedure. They are performed by the same physician on the same date of service as the primary service or procedure, and must never be reported as a stand-alone code. Report this code with 10022, 19102, or 19103.

ICD-9-CM Procedural

87.37   Other mammography

88.73   Diagnostic ultrasound of other sites of thorax

Anesthesia

19295   N/A

ICD-9-CM Diagnostic

This is an add-on code. Refer to the corresponding primary procedure code for ICD-9-CM diagnosis code links.

Terms To Know

biopsy. Tissue or fluid removed for diagnostic purposes through analysis of the cells in the biopsy material.

localization. Limitation to one area.

percutaneous. Through the skin.

ultrasound. Imaging using ultra-high sound frequency bounced off body structures.

CCI Version 18.3

No CCI Edits apply to this code.

Medicare Edits

	Fac RVU	Non-Fac RVU	FUD	Status
19295	2.68	2.68	N/A	A

	MUE		Modifiers		
19295	-	N/A	N/A	N/A	80*

* with documentation

Medicare References: 100-3,220.13; 100-4,13,80.1; 100-4,13,80.2

Coding Companion for Ob/Gyn

Breast

19296-19297

19296 Placement of radiotherapy afterloading expandable catheter (single or multichannel) into the breast for interstitial radioelement application following partial mastectomy, includes imaging guidance; on date separate from partial mastectomy

19297 concurrent with partial mastectomy (List separately in addition to code for primary procedure)

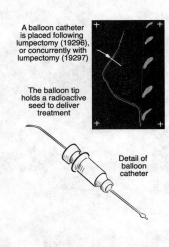

A balloon catheter is placed following lumpectomy (19296), or concurrently with lumpectomy (19297)

The balloon tip holds a radioactive seed to deliver treatment

Detail of balloon catheter

Explanation

A remote single or multichannel afterloading expandable catheter for interstitial radiotherapy treatment is placed in the breast following partial mastectomy. A catheter is placed at a later date, separate from the lumpectomy surgery in 19296, and concurrently with the lumpectomy in 19297. This is a single catheter with an expandable balloon tip that holds the radioactive seed or treatment source, which is loaded and removed for each session. The catheter can be single or multichannel, depending on the treatment delivery requirements. During the lumpectomy surgery, an uninflated balloon catheter is inserted into the recently created tumor cavity and positioned under imaging with a portion of the catheter remaining outside of the body. If a separate procedure is done after surgery, a small incision is first made and the uninflated balloon catheter is guided into position under imaging. After correct placement is determined, the balloon is inflated with saline to fit snugly into the lumpectomy cavity, and the breast is bandaged. The catheter remains until radiotherapy treatment sessions are complete.

Coding Tips

As an "add-on" code, 19297 is not subject to multiple procedure rules. No reimbursement reduction or modifier 51 is applied. "Add-on" codes describe additional intra-service work associated with the primary procedure. They are performed by the same physician on the same date of service as the primary service or procedure, and must never be reported as a stand-alone code. Report 19297 in conjunction with 19301 or 19302 for partial mastectomy. These codes report only the radiotherapy balloon catheter placement and subsequent catheter removal for interstitial brachytherapy. Preparation of the isodose plan is reported separately, see 77326–77328. For remote afterloading of the actual radiotherapy source through the catheter, see 77785–77787.

ICD-9-CM Procedural

85.0 Mastotomy

92.27 Implantation or insertion of radioactive elements

Anesthesia

19296 00400
19297 N/A

ICD-9-CM Diagnostic

174.0 Malignant neoplasm of nipple and areola of female breast — (Use additional code to identify estrogen receptor status: V86.0-V86.1)

174.1 Malignant neoplasm of central portion of female breast — (Use additional code to identify estrogen receptor status: V86.0-V86.1)

174.2 Malignant neoplasm of upper-inner quadrant of female breast — (Use additional code to identify estrogen receptor status: V86.0-V86.1)

174.3 Malignant neoplasm of lower-inner quadrant of female breast — (Use additional code to identify estrogen receptor status: V86.0-V86.1)

174.4 Malignant neoplasm of upper-outer quadrant of female breast — (Use additional code to identify estrogen receptor status: V86.0-V86.1)

174.5 Malignant neoplasm of lower-outer quadrant of female breast — (Use additional code to identify estrogen receptor status: V86.0-V86.1)

174.6 Malignant neoplasm of axillary tail of female breast — (Use additional code to identify estrogen receptor status: V86.0-V86.1)

174.8 Malignant neoplasm of other specified sites of female breast — (Use additional code to identify estrogen receptor status: V86.0-V86.1)

175.0 Malignant neoplasm of nipple and areola of male breast — (Use additional code to identify estrogen receptor status: V86.0-V86.1)

175.9 Malignant neoplasm of other and unspecified sites of male breast — (Use additional code to identify estrogen receptor status: V86.0-V86.1)

196.3 Secondary and unspecified malignant neoplasm of lymph nodes of axilla and upper limb

198.81 Secondary malignant neoplasm of breast

233.0 Carcinoma in situ of breast

238.3 Neoplasm of uncertain behavior of breast

239.3 Neoplasm of unspecified nature of breast

CCI Version 18.3

76000-76001, 76942, 76965

Also not with 19296: 0213T, 0216T, 0228T, 0230T, 12001-12007, 12011-12057, 13100-13153, 19297❖, 36000, 36400-36410, 36420-36430, 36440, 36600, 36640, 37202, 43752, 51701-51703, 62310-62319, 64400-64435, 64445-64450, 64479, 64483, 64490, 64493, 64505-64530, 69990, 77001-77002, 77012, 77021, 77031-77032, 93000-93010, 93040-93042, 93318, 94002, 94200, 94250, 94680-94690, 94770, 95812-95816, 95819, 95822, 95829, 95955, 96360, 96365, 96372, 96374-96376, 99148-99149, 99150, J0670, J2001

Also not with 19297: 77001

Note: These CCI edits are used for Medicare. Other payers may reimburse on codes listed above.

Medicare Edits

	Fac RVU	Non-Fac RVU	FUD	Status
19296	6.12	120.63	0	A
19297	2.75	2.75	N/A	A

	MUE		Modifiers		
19296	1	51	50	N/A	80*
19297	2	N/A	N/A	N/A	80*

* with documentation

Medicare References: 100-4,12,40.7; 100-4,13,80.2

Breast

19298

19298 Placement of radiotherapy afterloading brachytherapy catheters (multiple tube and button type) into the breast for interstitial radioelement application following (at the time of or subsequent to) partial mastectomy, includes imaging guidance

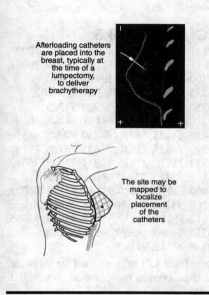

Afterloading catheters are placed into the breast, typically at the time of a lumpectomy, to deliver brachytherapy

The site may be mapped to localize placement of the catheters

Explanation

Using imaging guidance, at the time of a partial mastectomy, or subsequent to a partial mastectomy having been performed, remote afterloading catheters are placed into the breast for interstitial radiotherapy application. The lumpectomy site is identified. A template with pre-drilled holes that function as coordinates for catheter placement around the surgical area may be applied for imaging. Brachytherapy needles are first inserted into the chosen coordinates. The brachytherapy catheters are fed into position through the needles, which are removed. A catheter button is positioned to hold each catheter in place and imaging confirms their position. These remain in place until the actual loading of the radioactive material for treatment. This code reports only the placement of the catheters.

Coding Tips

Moderate sedation performed with 19298 is considered to be an integral part of the procedure and is not reported separately. However, anesthesia services (00100–01999) may be billed separately when performed by a physician (or other qualified provider) other than the physician performing the procedure. This code reports only the placement and subsequent removal of multiple tube and

button type catheters for interstitial brachytherapy. Preparation of the isodose plan is reported separately with 77326–77328. For remote afterloading of the actual radiotherapy source through the catheter, see 77785–77787.

ICD-9-CM Procedural

85.0	Mastotomy
92.27	Implantation or insertion of radioactive elements

Anesthesia

19298 00400

ICD-9-CM Diagnostic

174.0	Malignant neoplasm of nipple and areola of female breast — (Use additional code to identify estrogen receptor status: V86.0-V86.1)
174.1	Malignant neoplasm of central portion of female breast — (Use additional code to identify estrogen receptor status: V86.0-V86.1)
174.2	Malignant neoplasm of upper-inner quadrant of female breast — (Use additional code to identify estrogen receptor status: V86.0-V86.1)
174.3	Malignant neoplasm of lower-inner quadrant of female breast — (Use additional code to identify estrogen receptor status: V86.0-V86.1)
174.4	Malignant neoplasm of upper-outer quadrant of female breast — (Use additional code to identify estrogen receptor status: V86.0-V86.1)
174.5	Malignant neoplasm of lower-outer quadrant of female breast — (Use additional code to identify estrogen receptor status: V86.0-V86.1)
174.6	Malignant neoplasm of axillary tail of female breast — (Use additional code to identify estrogen receptor status: V86.0-V86.1)
174.8	Malignant neoplasm of other specified sites of female breast — (Use additional code to identify estrogen receptor status: V86.0-V86.1)
175.0	Malignant neoplasm of nipple and areola of male breast — (Use additional code to identify estrogen receptor status: V86.0-V86.1)
175.9	Malignant neoplasm of other and unspecified sites of male breast — (Use additional code to identify estrogen receptor status: V86.0-V86.1)
196.3	Secondary and unspecified malignant neoplasm of lymph nodes of axilla and upper limb
198.81	Secondary malignant neoplasm of breast
238.3	Neoplasm of uncertain behavior of breast
239.3	Neoplasm of unspecified nature of breast

Terms To Know

brachytherapy. Form of radiation therapy in which radioactive pellets or seeds are implanted directly into the tissue being treated to deliver their dose of radiation in a more directed fashion and over a longer period of time. Brachytherapy provides radiation to the prescribed body area while minimizing exposure to normal tissue. The most common indications are for treatment of cancers of the prostate.

interstitial radiation. Radioactive source placed into the tissue being treated.

CCI Version 18.3

0213T, 0216T, 0228T, 0230T, 12001-12007, 12011-12057, 13100-13153, 19296-19297❖, 36000, 36400-36410, 36420-36430, 36440, 36600, 36640, 37202, 43752, 51701-51703, 62310-62319, 64400-64435, 64445-64450, 64479, 64483, 64490, 64493, 64505-64530, 69990, 76000-76001, 76942, 76965, 77001-77002, 77012, 77021, 77031-77032, 93000-93010, 93040-93042, 93318, 94002, 94200, 94250, 94680-94690, 94770, 95812-95816, 95819, 95822, 95829, 95955, 96360, 96365, 96372, 96374-96376, 99143-99149, 99150, J0670, J2001

Note: These CCI edits are used for Medicare. Other payers may reimburse on codes listed above.

Medicare Edits

	Fac RVU	Non-Fac RVU	FUD	Status
19298	9.38	34.04	0	A

	MUE		Modifiers		
19298	1	51	50	N/A	80*

* with documentation

Medicare References: 100-4,12,40.7; 100-4,13,80.1; 100-4,13,80.2

Breast

35840

35840 Exploration for postoperative hemorrhage, thrombosis or infection; abdomen

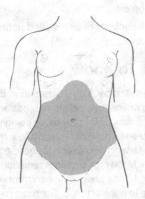

A previous surgery involving the abdominal area has been performed. A surgical exploration is performed in the abdominal cavity for the purpose of finding and identifying postoperative hemorrhage, thrombosis (clotting), or infection

Explanation

The physician reopens the original incision site and inspects the operative area for active bleeding, hematoma, thrombus, and exudate. The physician removes or debrides any observed hematoma, thrombus, and infected tissues. The physician looks for and corrects any active bleeding sites using electrocautery or ligation of bleeding vessels. The physician may leave an infected wound open, but generally closes the incision, leaving drains in place.

Coding Tips

This code is used to report exploration for postoperative hemorrhage, thrombosis, or infection of veins and arteries of the abdomen only.

ICD-9-CM Procedural

38.00 Incision of vessel, unspecified site
38.06 Incision of abdominal arteries
39.41 Control of hemorrhage following vascular surgery
39.98 Control of hemorrhage, not otherwise specified
54.19 Other laparotomy

Anesthesia

35840 00770

ICD-9-CM Diagnostic

338.18 Other acute postoperative pain — (Use additional code to identify pain associated with psychological factors: 307.89)
444.81 Embolism and thrombosis of iliac artery
444.89 Embolism and thrombosis of other specified artery
445.89 Atheroembolism of other site
557.0 Acute vascular insufficiency of intestine
593.81 Vascular disorders of kidney
997.2 Peripheral vascular complications — (Use additional code to identify complications)
997.49 Other digestive system complications
997.5 Urinary complications — (Use additional code to identify complications)
997.71 Vascular complications of mesenteric artery — (Use additional code to identify complications)
997.72 Vascular complications of renal artery — (Use additional code to identify complications)
997.79 Vascular complications of other vessels — (Use additional code to identify complications)
998.11 Hemorrhage complicating a procedure
998.12 Hematoma complicating a procedure
998.13 Seroma complicating a procedure
998.31 Disruption of internal operation (surgical) wound
998.32 Disruption of external operation (surgical) wound
998.51 Infected postoperative seroma — (Use additional code to identify organism)
998.59 Other postoperative infection — (Use additional code to identify infection)

Terms To Know

debride. To remove all foreign objects and devitalized or infected tissue from a burn or wound to prevent infection and promote healing.

electrocautery. Division or cutting of tissue using high-frequency electrical current to produce heat, which destroys cells.

embolism. Obstruction of a blood vessel resulting from a clot or foreign substance.

exudate. Fluid or other material, such as debris from cells, that has escaped blood vessel circulation and is deposited in or on tissues and usually occurs due to inflammation.

hematoma. Tumor-like collection of blood in some part of the body caused by a break in a blood vessel wall, usually as a result of trauma.

ligation. Tying off a blood vessel or duct with a suture or a soft, thin wire.

seroma. Swelling caused by the collection of serum, or clear fluid, in the tissues.

thrombosis. Condition arising from the presence or formation of blood clots within a blood vessel that may cause vascular obstruction and insufficient oxygenation.

CCI Version 18.3

0213T, 0216T, 0228T, 0230T, 12001-12007, 12011-12057, 13100-13153, 36000, 36002, 36400-36410, 36420-36430, 36440, 36595-36596❖, 36600, 36640, 37202, 43752, 49000-49002, 51701-51703, 62310-62319, 64400-64435, 64445-64450, 64479, 64483, 64490, 64493, 64505-64530, 69990, 75625, 75630, 75635, 75726, 75731, 75733, 75810, 75825, 75831, 75833, 75840, 75842, 75885, 75887, 75889, 75891, 93000-93010, 93040-93042, 93318, 94002, 94200, 94250, 94680-94690, 94770, 95812-95816, 95819, 95822, 95829, 95955, 96360, 96365, 96372, 96374-96376, 99148-99149, 99150

Note: These CCI edits are used for Medicare. Other payers may reimburse on codes listed above.

Medicare Edits

	Fac RVU	Non-Fac RVU	FUD	Status
35840	34.54	34.54	90	A

	MUE		Modifiers		
35840	2	51	N/A	62*	80

* with documentation

Medicare References: None

36415-36416

36415 Collection of venous blood by venipuncture

36416 Collection of capillary blood specimen (eg, finger, heel, ear stick)

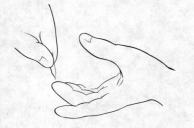

Capillary blood is collected. The specimen is typically collected by finger stick

Explanation

A needle is inserted into the skin over a vein to puncture the blood vessel and withdraw blood for venous collection in 36415. In 36416, a prick is made into the finger, heel, or ear and capillary blood that pools at the puncture site is collected in a pipette. In either case, the blood is used for diagnostic study and no catheter is placed.

Coding Tips

These procedures do not include laboratory analysis. If a specimen is transported to an outside laboratory, report 99000. Modifier 63 should not be reported in conjunction with 36415.

ICD-9-CM Procedural

38.99 Other puncture of vein

Anesthesia

N/A

ICD-9-CM Diagnostic

The application of this code is too broad to adequately present ICD-9-CM diagnostic code links here. Refer to your ICD-9-CM book.

Terms To Know

capillary. Tiny, minute blood vessel that connects the arterioles (smallest arteries) and the venules (smallest veins) and acts as a semipermeable membrane between the blood and the tissue fluid.

diagnostic. Examination or procedure to which the patient is subjected, or which is performed on materials derived from a hospital outpatient, to obtain information to aid in the assessment of a medical condition or the identification of a disease. Among these examinations and tests are diagnostic laboratory services such as hematology and chemistry, diagnostic x-rays, isotope studies, EKGs, pulmonary function studies, thyroid function tests, psychological tests, and other tests given to determine the nature and severity of an ailment or injury.

specimen. Tissue cells or sample of fluid taken for analysis, pathologic examination, and diagnosis.

venipuncture. Piercing a vein through the skin by a needle and syringe or sharp-ended cannula or catheter to draw blood, start an intravenous infusion, instill medication, or inject another substance such as radiopaque dye.

venous. Relating to the veins.

CCI Version 18.3

No CCI Edits apply to this code.

Medicare Edits

	Fac RVU	Non-Fac RVU	FUD	Status
36415	0.0	0.0	N/A	X
36416	0.0	0.0	N/A	B

	MUE		Modifiers		
36415	-	N/A	N/A	N/A	N/A
36416	-	N/A	N/A	N/A	N/A

* with documentation

Medicare References: None

36460

36460 Transfusion, intrauterine, fetal

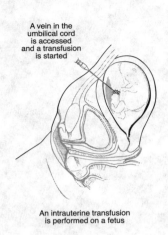

A vein in the umbilical cord is accessed and a transfusion is started

An intrauterine transfusion is performed on a fetus

Arteries and Veins

Explanation

The physician performs a blood transfusion to a fetus. The physician uses separately reportable ultrasound guidance to locate the umbilical vein. A needle is directed through the abdominal wall into the amniotic cavity. The umbilical vein is pierced and fetal blood is exchanged with transfused blood. The needle is withdrawn and the fetus is observed under separately reportable ultrasound.

Coding Tips

Radiological supervision and interpretation is reported with code 76941. Modifier 63 should not be reported in conjunction with 36460.

ICD-9-CM Procedural

75.2   Intrauterine transfusion

Anesthesia

36460   00840

ICD-9-CM Diagnostic

656.13   Rhesus isoimmunization affecting management of mother, antepartum condition

656.23   Isoimmunization from other and unspecified blood-group incompatibility, affecting management of mother, antepartum

Terms To Know

blood transfusion. Introduction of blood or blood products from another source into a vein or an artery.

fetus. Unborn offspring past the embryonic stage that has developed major structures. It is the period defined from nine weeks after fertilization until birth.

ultrasound. Imaging using ultra-high sound frequency bounced off body structures.

CCI Version 18.3

69990

Note: These CCI edits are used for Medicare. Other payers may reimburse on codes listed above.

Medicare Edits

	Fac RVU	Non-Fac RVU	FUD	Status
36460	10.57	10.57	N/A	A

	MUE		Modifiers		
36460	-	51	N/A	N/A	80

* with documentation

Medicare References: 100-1,3,20.5.2; 100-3,110.5; 100-3,110.7; 100-3,110.8; 100-4,3,40.2.2

37210

37210 Uterine fibroid embolization (UFE, embolization of the uterine arteries to treat uterine fibroids, leiomyomata), percutaneous approach inclusive of vascular access, vessel selection, embolization, and all radiological supervision and interpretation, intraprocedural roadmapping, and imaging guidance necessary to complete the procedure

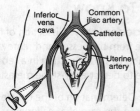

The catheter is inserted in the femoral artery at the groin, and advanced to branches of the uterine artery

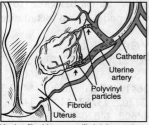

Uterine fibroid tumors will shrink over time after granules injected into arterial branches stop the blood flow to the fibroids

Explanation

In an endovascular procedure using angiographic guidance, the physician occludes branches of the uterine arteries to block the blood supply to uterine fibroid tumors. Through an incision in the left femoral artery, the physician advances a catheter containing granules of polyvinyl alcohol (PVA) to the branches of the contralateral (right) uterine artery adjacent to the fibroid tumors. PVA granules are released into these branches and they effectively block blood flow to the fibroid tumors. The catheter is retracted and the femoral incision treated with compression or sutured. This procedure is repeated from the right femoral artery advancing the catheter to the contralateral (left) uterine artery.

Coding Tips

All catheterizations and intraprocedural imaging required to confirm the presence of previously known fibroids and to roadmap vascular anatomy in order to enable appropriate therapy are included in this service and should not be reported separately. Do not report 36200, 36245–36248, 37204, 75894, or 75898 with this code. For all other

non-central nervous system embolization procedures, see 37204. Moderate (conscious) sedation performed with 37210 is considered to be an integral part of the procedure and is not reported separately. However, anesthesia services (00100–01999) may be reported separately when performed by an anesthesiologist (or other qualified provider) other than the physician performing the procedure.

ICD-9-CM Procedural

68.24   Uterine artery embolization [UAE] with coils

68.25   Uterine artery embolization [UAE] without coils

Anesthesia

37210   00880, 01924

ICD-9-CM Diagnostic

218.0   Submucous leiomyoma of uterus

218.1   Intramural leiomyoma of uterus

218.2   Subserous leiomyoma of uterus

218.9   Leiomyoma of uterus, unspecified

Terms To Know

embolization. Placement of a clotting agent, such as a coil, plastic particles, gel, foam, etc., into an area of hemorrhage to stop the bleeding or to block blood flow to a problem area, such as an aneurysm or a tumor.

fibrous tissue. Connective tissues.

leiomyoma. Benign tumor consisting of smooth muscle in the uterus.

supervision and interpretation. Radiology services that usually contain an invasive component and are reported by the radiologist for supervision of the procedure and the personnel involved with performing the examination, reading the film, and preparing the written report.

uterine fibroid tumor. Benign tumor consisting of smooth muscle in the uterus classified according to the site of the growth: intramural or interstitial tumors are found in the wall of the uterus; subserous fibromas are found beneath the serous membrane lining the uterus; and submucosal fibromas are found beneath the inner lining of the uterus. Although often asymptomatic, these fibroid tumors can cause reproductive problems, pain and pressure, and abnormal menstruation.

CCI Version 18.3

00840, 00860, 01916, 01924, 0213T, 0216T, 0228T, 0230T, 12001-12007, 12011-12057, 13100-13153, 35226, 35256, 35286, 36000, 36140, 36200, 36245-36247, 36400-36410,

36420-36430, 36440, 36600, 36640, 37202, 37204, 43752, 51701-51703, 62310-62319, 64400-64435, 64445-64450, 64479, 64483, 64490, 64493, 64505-64530, 69990, 75726, 75736, 75894, 75896, 75898, 76000-76001, 76942, 76998, 77001-77002, 77012, 77021, 93000-93010, 93040-93042, 93318, 94002, 94200, 94250, 94680-94690, 94770, 95812-95816, 95819, 95822, 95829, 95955, 96360, 96365, 96372, 96374-96376, 99143-99149, 99150, J0670, J1644, J2001

Note: These CCI edits are used for Medicare. Other payers may reimburse on codes listed above.

Medicare Edits

	Fac RVU	Non-Fac RVU	FUD	Status
37210	15.74	107.62	0	A

	MUE		Modifiers		
37210	1	51	N/A	N/A	N/A

* with documentation

Medicare References: None

38562

38562 Limited lymphadenectomy for staging (separate procedure); pelvic and para-aortic

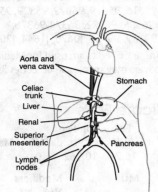

Aorta and vena cava
Stomach
Celiac trunk
Liver
Renal
Superior mesenteric
Pancreas
Lymph nodes

The aorta and other structures of the posterior abdominal cavity are lined with lymph nodes. The code 38562 reports the limited removal of aortic or pelvic nodes in a surgical procedure to determine the stage of a malignancy

Explanation

The physician makes a midline abdominal incision just below the navel. The surrounding tissue, nerves, and blood vessels are dissected away, and the pelvic and/or para-aortic lymph nodes are visualized. The nodes are removed. The wound is closed with sutures or staples.

Coding Tips

This separate procedure by definition is usually a component of a more complex service and is not identified separately. When performed alone or with other unrelated procedures or services it may be reported. If performed alone, list the code; if performed with other procedures or services, list the code and append modifier 59. For extensive retroperitoneal transabdominal lymphadenectomy, see 38780.

ICD-9-CM Procedural

40.3   Regional lymph node excision
40.9   Other operations on lymphatic structures

Anesthesia

38562   00840, 00860

ICD-9-CM Diagnostic

151.5   Malignant neoplasm of lesser curvature of stomach, unspecified
151.8   Malignant neoplasm of other specified sites of stomach
152.0   Malignant neoplasm of duodenum
153.7   Malignant neoplasm of splenic flexure
154.0   Malignant neoplasm of rectosigmoid junction
154.1   Malignant neoplasm of rectum
156.1   Malignant neoplasm of extrahepatic bile ducts
158.0   Malignant neoplasm of retroperitoneum
180.0   Malignant neoplasm of endocervix
180.1   Malignant neoplasm of exocervix
180.8   Malignant neoplasm of other specified sites of cervix
180.9   Malignant neoplasm of cervix uteri, unspecified site
181   Malignant neoplasm of placenta
182.0   Malignant neoplasm of corpus uteri, except isthmus
182.1   Malignant neoplasm of isthmus
182.8   Malignant neoplasm of other specified sites of body of uterus
183.0   Malignant neoplasm of ovary — (Use additional code to identify any functional activity)
183.2   Malignant neoplasm of fallopian tube
183.3   Malignant neoplasm of broad ligament of uterus
183.4   Malignant neoplasm of parametrium of uterus
183.5   Malignant neoplasm of round ligament of uterus
183.8   Malignant neoplasm of other specified sites of uterine adnexa
188.0   Malignant neoplasm of trigone of urinary bladder
188.1   Malignant neoplasm of dome of urinary bladder
188.2   Malignant neoplasm of lateral wall of urinary bladder
188.3   Malignant neoplasm of anterior wall of urinary bladder
188.4   Malignant neoplasm of posterior wall of urinary bladder
188.5   Malignant neoplasm of bladder neck
188.6   Malignant neoplasm of ureteric orifice
189.0   Malignant neoplasm of kidney, except pelvis
189.1   Malignant neoplasm of renal pelvis
189.2   Malignant neoplasm of ureter
189.3   Malignant neoplasm of urethra
189.4   Malignant neoplasm of paraurethral glands
195.3   Malignant neoplasm of pelvis
196.2   Secondary and unspecified malignant neoplasm of intra-abdominal lymph nodes
196.6   Secondary and unspecified malignant neoplasm of intrapelvic lymph nodes
197.5   Secondary malignant neoplasm of large intestine and rectum
197.6   Secondary malignant neoplasm of retroperitoneum and peritoneum
197.8   Secondary malignant neoplasm of other digestive organs and spleen
230.4   Carcinoma in situ of rectum

Terms To Know

lymphadenectomy. Dissection of lymph nodes free from the vessels and removal for examination by frozen section in a separate procedure to detect early-stage metastases.

staging. Determination of the course of a disease, as in the case of a malignancy, to determine whether the malignancy is confined to the primary tumor, has spread to one or more lymph nodes, or has metastasized.

CCI Version 18.3

0213T, 0216T, 0228T, 0230T, 12001-12007, 12011-12057, 13100-13153, 36000, 36400-36410, 36420-36430, 36440, 36600, 36640, 37202, 43752, 44005, 44180, 44602-44605, 44820-44850, 44950, 44970, 49000-49010, 49255, 49320, 49570, 51701-51703, 62310-62319, 64400-64435, 64445-64450, 64479, 64483, 64490, 64493, 64505-64530, 69990, 93000-93010, 93040-93042, 93318, 94002, 94200, 94250, 94680-94690, 94770, 95812-95816, 95819, 95822, 95829, 95955, 96360, 96365, 96372, 96374-96376, 99148-99149, 99150

Note: These CCI edits are used for Medicare. Other payers may reimburse on codes listed above.

Medicare Edits

	Fac RVU	Non-Fac RVU	FUD	Status
38562	20.55	20.55	90	A

	MUE		Modifiers		
38562	1	51	N/A	62*	80

* with documentation

Medicare References: None

Lymph Nodes

38747

38747 Abdominal lymphadenectomy, regional, including celiac, gastric, portal, peripancreatic, with or without para-aortic and vena caval nodes (List separately in addition to code for primary procedure)

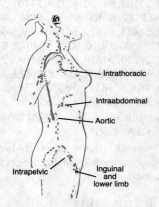

Code 38747 reports regional resection of abdominal lymph nodes. This includes nodes from around the celiac trunk and pancreas, the gastric and portal arterial and venous groupings, with or without nodes from around the aorta or vena cava. Report 38747 in addition to the code for the primary procedure

Explanation

The physician makes a midline abdominal incision. The abdominal contents are exposed, allowing the physician to locate the lymph nodes. Each lymph node grouping, with or without para-aortic and vena caval nodes, is dissected away from the surrounding tissue, nerves, and blood vessels, and removed. The incision is closed with sutures or staples.

Coding Tips

As an "add-on" code, 38747 is not subject to multiple procedure rules. No reimbursement reduction or modifier 51 is applied. "Add-on" codes describe additional intra-service work associated with the primary procedure. They are performed by the same physician on the same date of service as the primary service or procedure, and must never be reported as a stand-alone code. For extensive retroperitoneal transabdominal lymphadenectomy, see 38780.

ICD-9-CM Procedural

40.29   Simple excision of other lymphatic structure

40.3   Regional lymph node excision

40.50   Radical excision of lymph nodes, not otherwise specified

40.52   Radical excision of periaortic lymph nodes

40.59   Radical excision of other lymph nodes

Anesthesia

38747   N/A

ICD-9-CM Diagnostic

This is an add-on code. Refer to the corresponding primary procedure code for ICD-9-CM diagnosis code links.

Terms To Know

abdominal lymphadenectomy. Surgical removal of the abdominal lymph nodes grouping, with or without para-aortic and vena cava nodes.

dissect. Cut apart or separate tissue for surgical purposes or for visual or microscopic study.

excision. Surgical removal of an organ or tissue.

lymphadenectomy. Dissection of lymph nodes free from the vessels and removal for examination by frozen section in a separate procedure to detect early-stage metastases.

CCI Version 18.3

38500, 38570, 44950, 44970, 49000-49002

Note: These CCI edits are used for Medicare. Other payers may reimburse on codes listed above.

Medicare Edits

	Fac RVU	Non-Fac RVU	FUD	Status		
38747	7.79	7.79	N/A	A		
	MUE		Modifiers			
38747	1	N/A	N/A	62*	80

* with documentation

Medicare References: None

Lymph Nodes

38760-38765

38760 Inguinofemoral lymphadenectomy, superficial, including Cloquets node (separate procedure)

38765 Inguinofemoral lymphadenectomy, superficial, in continuity with pelvic lymphadenectomy, including external iliac, hypogastric, and obturator nodes (separate procedure)

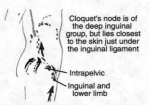

Cloquet's node is of the deep inguinal group, but lies closest to the skin just under the inguinal ligament

Intrapelvic

Inguinal and lower limb

Superficial nodes of the inguinal region are removed along with certain pelvic nodes. Report 38765 when nodes lying deep in the pelvic abdomen (internal iliac) are removed

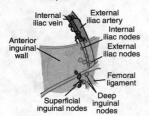

Internal iliac vein

External iliac artery

Anterior inguinal wall

Internal iliac nodes

External iliac nodes

Femoral ligament

Superficial inguinal nodes

Deep inguinal nodes

Explanation

The physician makes an incision across the groin area. The surrounding tissue, nerves, and blood vessels are dissected away, and the inguinal and femoral lymph nodes are visualized. The nodes are removed by group. The wound is closed with sutures or staples. Report 38765 if performing pelvic lymphadenectomy concurrently.

Coding Tips

These separate procedures by definition are usually a component of a more complex service and are not identified separately. When performed alone or with other unrelated procedures/services they may be reported. These are unilateral procedures. If performed bilaterally, some payers require that the service be reported twice with modifier 50 appended to the second code while others require identification of the service only once with modifier 50 appended. Check with individual payers. Modifier 50 identifies a procedure performed identically on the opposite side of the body (mirror image).

ICD-9-CM Procedural

40.24   Excision of inguinal lymph node

40.3   Regional lymph node excision

Anesthesia

38760   00400, 00840, 00860
38765   00840, 00860

ICD-9-CM Diagnostic

154.0   Malignant neoplasm of rectosigmoid junction

154.1   Malignant neoplasm of rectum

180.0   Malignant neoplasm of endocervix

180.1   Malignant neoplasm of exocervix

180.8   Malignant neoplasm of other specified sites of cervix

180.9   Malignant neoplasm of cervix uteri, unspecified site

181   Malignant neoplasm of placenta

182.0   Malignant neoplasm of corpus uteri, except isthmus

182.1   Malignant neoplasm of isthmus

182.8   Malignant neoplasm of other specified sites of body of uterus

183.0   Malignant neoplasm of ovary — (Use additional code to identify any functional activity)

183.2   Malignant neoplasm of fallopian tube

183.3   Malignant neoplasm of broad ligament of uterus

183.4   Malignant neoplasm of parametrium of uterus

183.5   Malignant neoplasm of round ligament of uterus

183.8   Malignant neoplasm of other specified sites of uterine adnexa

183.9   Malignant neoplasm of uterine adnexa, unspecified site

184.0   Malignant neoplasm of vagina

184.1   Malignant neoplasm of labia majora

184.2   Malignant neoplasm of labia minora

184.3   Malignant neoplasm of clitoris

184.4   Malignant neoplasm of vulva, unspecified site

184.8   Malignant neoplasm of other specified sites of female genital organs

184.9   Malignant neoplasm of female genital organ, site unspecified

209.36   Merkel cell carcinoma of other sites

230.4   Carcinoma in situ of rectum

Terms To Know

dissect. Cut apart or separate tissue for surgical purposes or for visual or microscopic study.

incision. Act of cutting into tissue or an organ.

lymphadenectomy. Dissection of lymph nodes free from the vessels and removal for examination by frozen section in a separate procedure to detect early-stage metastases.

CCI Version 18.3

0213T, 0216T, 0228T, 0230T, 12001-12007, 12011-12057, 13100-13153, 36000, 36400-36410, 36420-36430, 36440, 36600, 36640, 37202, 38500, 43752, 51701-51703, 62310-62319, 64400-64435, 64445-64450, 64479, 64483, 64490, 64493, 64505-64530, 69990, 93000-93010, 93040-93042, 93318, 94002, 94200, 94250, 94680-94690, 94770, 95812-95816, 95819, 95822, 95829, 95955, 96360, 96365, 96372, 96374-96376, 99148-99149, 99150

Also not with 38765: 38562, 38571, 38760, 38770, J0670, J2001

Note: These CCI edits are used for Medicare. Other payers may reimburse on codes listed above.

Medicare Edits

	Fac RVU	Non-Fac RVU	FUD	Status
38760	24.65	24.65	90	A
38765	37.66	37.66	90	A

	MUE		Modifiers		
38760	1	51	50	62*	80
38765	1	51	50	62*	80

* with documentation

Medicare References: None

Lymph Nodes

38770

38770 Pelvic lymphadenectomy, including external iliac, hypogastric, and obturator nodes (separate procedure)

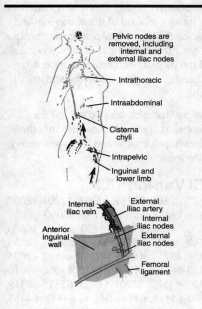

Pelvic nodes are removed, including internal and external iliac nodes

- Intrathoracic
- Intraabdominal
- Cisterna chyli
- Intrapelvic
- Inguinal and lower limb

Internal iliac vein
External iliac artery
Internal iliac nodes
Anterior inguinal wall
External iliac nodes
Femoral ligament

Explanation

The physician makes a low abdominal vertical incision. The surrounding tissue, nerves, and blood vessels are dissected away, and the pelvic lymph nodes are visualized. The nodes are removed by group. The wound is closed with sutures or staples.

Coding Tips

This separate procedure by definition is usually a component of a more complex service and is not identified separately. When performed alone or with other unrelated procedures/services it may be reported. If performed alone, list the code; if performed with other procedures/services, list the code and append modifier 59. This is a unilateral procedure. If performed bilaterally, some payers require that the service be reported twice with modifier 50 appended to the second code while others require identification of the service only once with modifier 50 appended. Check with individual payers. Modifier 50 identifies a procedure performed identically on the opposite side of the body (mirror image). For limited pelvic and para-aortic lymphadenectomy staging procedure, see 38562.

ICD-9-CM Procedural

- 40.3 Regional lymph node excision
- 40.53 Radical excision of iliac lymph nodes

Anesthesia

38770 00840, 00860

ICD-9-CM Diagnostic

- 180.0 Malignant neoplasm of endocervix
- 180.1 Malignant neoplasm of exocervix
- 180.8 Malignant neoplasm of other specified sites of cervix
- 182.0 Malignant neoplasm of corpus uteri, except isthmus
- 182.1 Malignant neoplasm of isthmus
- 183.0 Malignant neoplasm of ovary — (Use additional code to identify any functional activity)
- 183.2 Malignant neoplasm of fallopian tube
- 183.3 Malignant neoplasm of broad ligament of uterus
- 183.4 Malignant neoplasm of parametrium of uterus
- 183.5 Malignant neoplasm of round ligament of uterus
- 183.8 Malignant neoplasm of other specified sites of uterine adnexa
- 184.0 Malignant neoplasm of vagina
- 184.1 Malignant neoplasm of labia majora
- 184.2 Malignant neoplasm of labia minora
- 184.3 Malignant neoplasm of clitoris
- 184.4 Malignant neoplasm of vulva, unspecified site
- 184.8 Malignant neoplasm of other specified sites of female genital organs
- 196.6 Secondary and unspecified malignant neoplasm of intrapelvic lymph nodes

Terms To Know

staging in carcinoma of the uterus.

Carcinoma of the corpus uteri is classified by stage:

Stage 1A: Endometrial tumor.

Stage 1B: Invasion to less than half of the myometrium.

Stage 2A: Endocervical involvement.

Stage 2B: Cervical stromal invasion.

Stage 3A: Positive peritoneal cytology and/or serosal and/or adnexal invasion.

Stage 3B: Vaginal metastasis.

Stage 3C: Pelvic and/or paraaortic lymph node metastases.

Stage 4A: Invasion of bladder and/or rectal mucosa.

Stage 4B: Invasion of distant organs.

Note: This staging does not apply to melanoma or secondary malignances.

staging of carcinoma of the vagina.

Carcinoma of the vagina is classified by stage:

Stage 0: Carcinoma in situ (intraepithelial).

Stage 1: Carcinoma limited to subvaginal wall.

Stage 2: Carcinoma involving subvaginal wall but not pelvic wall.

Stage 3: Carcinoma involving subvaginal and pelvic wall.

Stage 4: Carcinoma extending into anal or rectal mucosa, or beyond pelvis.

Stage 4A: Carcinoma spread to adjacent organs.

Stage 4B: Carcinoma spread to distant organs.

Note: This staging does not apply to melanoma or secondary malignancies.

CCI Version 18.3

0213T, 0216T, 0228T, 0230T, 12001-12007, 12011-12057, 13100-13153, 36000, 36400-36410, 36420-36430, 36440, 36600, 36640, 37202, 38500, 38562-38564, 38571, 38760, 43752, 44005, 44180, 44602-44605, 44820-44850, 44950, 44970, 49000-49010, 49320, 49570, 51701-51703, 62310-62319, 64400-64435, 64445-64450, 64479, 64483, 64490, 64493, 64505-64530, 69990, 93000-93010, 93040-93042, 93318, 94002, 94200, 94250, 94680-94690, 94770, 95812-95816, 95819, 95822, 95829, 95955, 96360, 96365, 96372, 96374-96376, 99148-99149, 99150

Note: These CCI edits are used for Medicare. Other payers may reimburse on codes listed above.

Medicare Edits

	Fac RVU	Non-Fac RVU	FUD	Status
38770	23.59	23.59	90	A

	MUE			Modifiers	
38770	1	51	50	62*	80

* with documentation

Medicare References: None

38780

38780 Retroperitoneal transabdominal lymphadenectomy, extensive, including pelvic, aortic, and renal nodes (separate procedure)

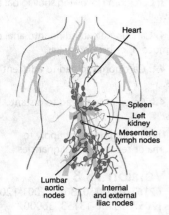

Extensive removal of lymph nodes of the retroperitoneal area is performed by a transabdominal approach

Explanation

The physician makes a large midline abdominal incision. The surrounding tissue, nerves, and blood vessels are dissected away, and the lymph nodes are visualized. The nodes are then removed by group. Some surrounding tissues may also be removed. The wound is closed with sutures or staples.

Coding Tips

This separate procedure by definition is usually a component of a more complex service and is not identified separately. When performed alone or with other unrelated procedures or services it may be reported. If performed alone, list the code; if performed with other procedures or services, list the code and append modifier 59. For pelvic lymphadenectomy, see 38770. For a limited pelvic and para-aortic lymphadenectomy staging procedure, see 38562. For excision and repair of lymphedematous skin and subcutaneous tissue, see 15004–15005 or 15570–15650.

ICD-9-CM Procedural

40.3 Regional lymph node excision
40.54 Radical groin dissection

Anesthesia

38780 00860

ICD-9-CM Diagnostic

180.0 Malignant neoplasm of endocervix
180.1 Malignant neoplasm of exocervix
180.8 Malignant neoplasm of other specified sites of cervix
180.9 Malignant neoplasm of cervix uteri, unspecified site
182.0 Malignant neoplasm of corpus uteri, except isthmus
182.1 Malignant neoplasm of isthmus
182.8 Malignant neoplasm of other specified sites of body of uterus
183.0 Malignant neoplasm of ovary — (Use additional code to identify any functional activity)
183.2 Malignant neoplasm of fallopian tube
183.3 Malignant neoplasm of broad ligament of uterus
183.4 Malignant neoplasm of parametrium of uterus
183.5 Malignant neoplasm of round ligament of uterus
183.8 Malignant neoplasm of other specified sites of uterine adnexa
183.9 Malignant neoplasm of uterine adnexa, unspecified site
188.0 Malignant neoplasm of trigone of urinary bladder
188.1 Malignant neoplasm of dome of urinary bladder
188.2 Malignant neoplasm of lateral wall of urinary bladder
188.3 Malignant neoplasm of anterior wall of urinary bladder
188.4 Malignant neoplasm of posterior wall of urinary bladder
188.5 Malignant neoplasm of bladder neck
188.6 Malignant neoplasm of ureteric orifice
189.1 Malignant neoplasm of renal pelvis
189.2 Malignant neoplasm of ureter
189.3 Malignant neoplasm of urethra
189.4 Malignant neoplasm of paraurethral glands
196.2 Secondary and unspecified malignant neoplasm of intra-abdominal lymph nodes

Terms To Know

abdominal lymphadenectomy. Surgical removal of the abdominal lymph nodes grouping, with or without para-aortic and vena cava nodes.

corpus uteri. Main body of the uterus, which is located above the isthmus and below the openings of the fallopian tubes.

malignant neoplasm. Any cancerous tumor or lesion exhibiting uncontrolled tissue growth that can progressively invade other parts of the body with its disease-generating cells.

peritoneum. Strong, continuous membrane that forms the lining of the abdominal and pelvic cavity. The parietal peritoneum, or outer layer, is attached to the abdominopelvic walls and the visceral peritoneum, or inner layer, surrounds the organs inside the abdominal cavity.

retroperitoneal. Located behind the peritoneum, the membrane that lines the abdominopelvic walls and forms a covering for the internal organs.

CCI Version 18.3

0213T, 0216T, 0228T, 0230T, 12001-12007, 12011-12057, 13100-13153, 36000, 36400-36410, 36420-36430, 36440, 36600, 36640, 37202, 38500, 38562-38572, 38765, 38770, 43752, 44005, 44180, 44602-44605, 44820-44850, 44950, 44970, 49000-49010, 49320, 49570, 51701-51703, 62310-62319, 64400-64435, 64445-64450, 64479, 64483, 64490, 64493, 64505-64530, 69990, 93000-93010, 93040-93042, 93318, 94002, 94200, 94250, 94680-94690, 94770, 95812-95816, 95819, 95822, 95829, 95955, 96360, 96365, 96372, 96374-96376, 99148-99149, 99150

Note: These CCI edits are used for Medicare. Other payers may reimburse on codes listed above.

Medicare Edits

	Fac RVU	Non-Fac RVU	FUD	Status
38780	30.27	30.27	90	A

	MUE		Modifiers		
38780	1	51	N/A	62*	80

* with documentation

Medicare References: None

Coding Companion for Ob/Gyn

Lymph Nodes

44180

44180 Laparoscopy, surgical, enterolysis (freeing of intestinal adhesion) (separate procedure)

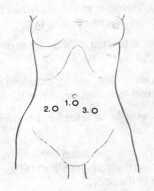

1. Laparoscope is inserted near the umbilicus
2. and 3. Ports for trocars and surgical instruments

Explanation

The physician performs laparoscopic enterolysis to free intestinal adhesions. With the patient under anesthesia, the physician places a trocar at the umbilicus into the abdominal or retroperitoneal space and insufflates the abdominal cavity. The physician places a laparoscope through the umbilical incision and additional trocars are placed into the abdomen. Intestinal adhesions are identified and instruments are passed through to dissect and remove the adhesions. The trocars are removed and the incisions are closed with sutures.

Coding Tips

This separate procedure by definition is usually a component of a more complex service and is not identified separately. When performed alone or with other unrelated procedures/services it may be reported. If performed alone, list the code; if performed with other procedures/services, list the code and append modifier 59. Surgical laparoscopy always includes diagnostic laparoscopy. For diagnostic laparoscopy only, see 49320. To report laparoscopic salpingolysis, ovariolysis, see 58660.

ICD-9-CM Procedural

54.51 Laparoscopic lysis of peritoneal adhesions

Anesthesia

44180 00790, 00840

ICD-9-CM Diagnostic

338.18 Other acute postoperative pain — (Use additional code to identify pain associated with psychological factors: 307.89)

338.28 Other chronic postoperative pain — (Use additional code to identify pain associated with psychological factors: 307.89)

560.81 Intestinal or peritoneal adhesions with obstruction (postoperative) (postinfection)

568.0 Peritoneal adhesions (postoperative) (postinfection)

614.6 Pelvic peritoneal adhesions, female (postoperative) (postinfection) — (Use additional code to identify organism: 041.00-041.09, 041.10-041.19) (Use additional code to identify any associated infertility: 628.2)

617.5 Endometriosis of intestine

751.4 Congenital anomalies of intestinal fixation

789.00 Abdominal pain, unspecified site

789.01 Abdominal pain, right upper quadrant

789.02 Abdominal pain, left upper quadrant

789.03 Abdominal pain, right lower quadrant

789.04 Abdominal pain, left lower quadrant

789.05 Abdominal pain, periumbilic

789.06 Abdominal pain, epigastric

789.07 Abdominal pain, generalized

789.09 Abdominal pain, other specified site

789.30 Abdominal or pelvic swelling, mass or lump, unspecified site

789.31 Abdominal or pelvic swelling, mass, or lump, right upper quadrant

789.32 Abdominal or pelvic swelling, mass, or lump, left upper quadrant

789.33 Abdominal or pelvic swelling, mass, or lump, right lower quadrant

789.34 Abdominal or pelvic swelling, mass, or lump, left lower quadrant

789.35 Abdominal or pelvic swelling, mass or lump, periumbilic

789.36 Abdominal or pelvic swelling, mass, or lump, epigastric

789.37 Abdominal or pelvic swelling, mass, or lump, generalized

789.39 Abdominal or pelvic swelling, mass, or lump, other specified site

908.1 Late effect of internal injury to intra-abdominal organs

908.2 Late effect of internal injury to other internal organs

908.6 Late effect of certain complications of trauma

909.3 Late effect of complications of surgical and medical care

V64.41 Laparoscopic surgical procedure converted to open procedure

Terms To Know

dissect. Cut apart or separate tissue for surgical purposes or for visual or microscopic study.

endometriosis. Aberrant uterine mucosal tissue appearing in areas of the pelvic cavity outside of its normal location, lining the uterus and inflaming surrounding tissues, and can result in infertility and spontaneous abortion.

insufflation. Blowing air or gas into a body cavity.

laparoscopy. Direct visualization of the peritoneal cavity, outer fallopian tubes, uterus, and ovaries utilizing a laparoscope, a thin, flexible fiberoptic tube.

trocar. Cannula or a sharp pointed instrument used to puncture and aspirate fluid from cavities.

CCI Version 18.3

0213T, 0216T, 0228T, 0230T, 12001-12007, 12011-12057, 13100-13153, 36000, 36400-36410, 36420-36430, 36440, 36600, 36640, 37202, 43752, 44701, 49320, 51701-51703, 62310-62319, 64400-64435, 64445-64450, 64479, 64483, 64490, 64493, 64505-64530, 69990, 76000-76001, 77001-77002, 93000-93010, 93040-93042, 93318, 94002, 94200, 94250, 94680-94690, 94770, 95812-95816, 95819, 95822, 95829, 95955, 96360, 96365, 96372, 96374-96376, 99148-99149, 99150

Note: These CCI edits are used for Medicare. Other payers may reimburse on codes listed above.

Medicare Edits

	Fac RVU	Non-Fac RVU	FUD	Status
44180	26.89	26.89	90	A

	MUE			Modifiers	
44180	1	51	N/A	62*	80

* with documentation

Medicare References: None

Intestines

45560

45560 Repair of rectocele (separate procedure)

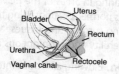

The posterior wall of the vagina is opened directly over the rectocele. The walls of both structures are repaired. A rectocele is a herniated protrusion of part of the rectum into the vagina

Rectum descends and protrudes through posterior wall of vagina

Explanation

The physician repairs a rectocele, a herniation of the rectum against the vaginal wall. The physician makes an incision in the mucosa of the posterior vaginal wall over the rectocele. The rectocele is dissected free of surrounding structures and the levator muscles are identified. The rectum is plicated to surrounding fascia with multiple sutures and the levator muscles are reapproximated. The vaginal mucosa is excised and the incision is closed.

Coding Tips

This separate procedure by definition is usually a component of a more complex service and is not identified separately. When performed alone or with other unrelated procedures or services it may be reported. If performed alone, list the code; if performed with other procedures or services, list the code and append modifier 59. For posterior colporrhaphy with repair of a rectocele, with or without perineorrhaphy, see 57250. For combined anteroposterior colporrhaphy, see 57260; with enterocele repair, see 57265.

ICD-9-CM Procedural

70.52   Repair of rectocele

Anesthesia

45560   00902

ICD-9-CM Diagnostic

569.1   Rectal prolapse

569.44 Dysplasia of anus

569.49 Other specified disorder of rectum and anus — (Use additional code for any associated fecal incontinence (787.60-787.63))

618.00 Unspecified prolapse of vaginal walls without mention of uterine prolapse — (Use additional code to identify urinary incontinence: 625.6, 788.31, 788.33-788.39)

618.04 Rectocele without mention of uterine prolapse — (Use additional code to identify urinary incontinence: 625.6, 788.31, 788.33-788.39) (Use additional code for any associated fecal incontinence: 787.60-787.63)

618.2   Uterovaginal prolapse, incomplete — (Use additional code to identify urinary incontinence: 625.6, 788.31, 788.33-788.39)

618.3   Uterovaginal prolapse, complete — (Use additional code to identify urinary incontinence: 625.6, 788.31, 788.33-788.39)

618.4   Uterovaginal prolapse, unspecified — (Use additional code to identify urinary incontinence: 625.6, 788.31, 788.33-788.39)

618.5   Prolapse of vaginal vault after hysterectomy — (Use additional code to identify urinary incontinence: 625.6, 788.31, 788.33-788.39)

618.82 Incompetence or weakening of rectovaginal tissue — (Use additional code to identify urinary incontinence: 625.6, 788.31, 788.33-788.39)

618.89 Other specified genital prolapse — (Use additional code to identify urinary incontinence: 625.6, 788.31, 788.33-788.39)

Terms To Know

closure. Repairing an incision or wound by suture or other means.

dissection. Separating by cutting tissue or body structures apart.

excision. Surgical removal of an organ or tissue.

fascia. Fibrous sheet or band of tissue that envelops organs, muscles, and groupings of muscles.

incision. Act of cutting into tissue or an organ.

mucous membranes. Thin sheets of tissue that secrete mucous and absorb water, salt, and other solutes. Mucous membranes cover or line cavities or canals of the body that open to the outside, such as linings of the mouth, respiratory and genitourinary passages, and the digestive tube.

plication. Surgical technique involving folding, tucking, or pleating to reduce the size of a hollow structure or organ.

posterior. Located in the back part or caudal end of the body.

prolapse. Falling, sliding, or sinking of an organ from its normal location in the body.

rectocele. Rectal tissue herniation into the vaginal wall.

urethra. Small tube lined with mucous membrane that leads from the bladder to the exterior of the body.

uterovaginal prolapse. Uterus displaces downward and is exposed in the external genitalia.

CCI Version 18.3

0213T, 0216T, 0226T, 0228T, 0230T, 0288T, 12001-12007, 12011-12057, 13100-13153, 15777, 36000, 36400-36410, 36420-36430, 36440, 36600, 36640, 37202, 43752, 44602-44605, 44701, 45900-45990, 46040, 46080, 46220, 46600, 46940-46942, 49000-49002, 49320, 51701-51703, 62310-62319, 64400-64435, 64445-64450, 64479, 64483, 64490, 64493, 64505-64530, 69990, 93000-93010, 93040-93042, 93318, 94002, 94200, 94250, 94680-94690, 94770, 95812-95816, 95819, 95822, 95829, 95955, 96360, 96365, 96372, 96374-96376, 99148-99149, 99150

Note: These CCI edits are used for Medicare. Other payers may reimburse on codes listed above.

Medicare Edits

	Fac RVU	Non-Fac RVU	FUD	Status
45560	20.56	20.56	90	A

	MUE		Modifiers	
45560	1	51	N/A	62*	80

* with documentation

Medicare References: None

Coding Companion for Ob/Gyn

Anus

46083

46083 Incision of thrombosed hemorrhoid, external

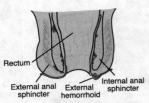

Rectum

External anal sphincter   External hemorrhoid   Internal anal sphincter

External hemorrhoids are varicosities of the inferior rectal veins and are covered by skin. Code 46083 reports the direct incision of an external hemorrhoid. This is usually performed to remove a thrombus

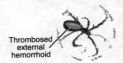

Thrombosed external hemorrhoid

Explanation

The physician performs incision of a thrombosed external hemorrhoid. The physician identifies the thrombosed external hemorrhoid. An incision is made in the skin over the hemorrhoid and the thrombus is removed. The incision is left open for continued drainage.

Coding Tips

Selection of codes for hemorrhoid treatment depends on the site of the hemorrhoid (internal or external) and the nature of the surgical procedure (injection, destruction, incision, ligation, or excision). For external hemorrhoidectomy, 2 or more columns/groups, see 46250. For excision of external anal papilla or tag, single, see 46220; multiple, see 46230. For excision of an external thrombosed hemorrhoid, see 46320. For an internal hemorrhoidectomy by rubber band(s) ligation, see 46221. For injection of a hemorrhoidal sclerosing agent, see 46500. Surgical trays, A4550, are not separately reimbursed by Medicare; however, other third-party payers may cover them. Check with the specific payer to determine coverage.

ICD-9-CM Procedural

49.47   Evacuation of thrombosed hemorrhoids

Anesthesia

46083   00902

ICD-9-CM Diagnostic

455.4   External thrombosed hemorrhoids

Terms To Know

hemorrhoid. Dilated, varicose vein in the anal region caused by continually increased venous pressure. Reversed blood flow and clotted blood within a vein that extends beyond the anus.

incision. Act of cutting into tissue or an organ.

sphincter. Ring-like band of muscle that surrounds a bodily opening, constricting and relaxing as required for normal physiological functioning.

thrombosed hemorrhoid. Dilated, varicose vein in the anal region that has clotted blood within it.

thrombus. Stationary blood clot inside a blood vessel.

CCI Version 18.3

00902, 0213T, 0216T, 0226T, 0228T, 0230T, 0288T, 12001-12007, 12011-12057, 13100-13153, 36000, 36400-36410, 36420-36430, 36440, 36600, 36640, 37202, 43752, 45900-45990, 46040, 46080, 46220, 46600, 46940-46942, 51701-51703, 62310-62319, 64400-64435, 64445-64450, 64479, 64483, 64490, 64493, 64505-64530, 69990, 93000-93010, 93040-93042, 93318, 94002, 94200, 94250, 94680-94690, 94770, 95812-95816, 95819, 95822, 95829, 95955, 96360, 96365, 96372, 96374-96376, 99148-99149, 99150, J0670, J2001

Note: These CCI edits are used for Medicare. Other payers may reimburse on codes listed above.

Medicare Edits

	Fac RVU	Non-Fac RVU	FUD	Status
46083	3.13	5.19	10	A

	MUE		Modifiers		
46083	2	51	N/A	N/A	N/A

* with documentation

Medicare References: None

46221

46221 Hemorrhoidectomy, internal, by rubber band ligation(s)

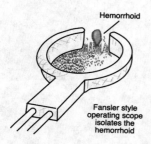

Hemorrhoid

Fansler style operating scope isolates the hemorrhoid

The hemorrhoid is ligated

The hemorrhoid is identified and isolated. A banding device is used to place a rubber band around the base of the hemorrhoid. The hemorrhoid is left to slough off as the elastic strangulates blood flow

Explanation

The physician performs hemorrhoidectomy by tying off (ligating) an internal hemorrhoid. The physician identifies the internal hemorrhoid. The hemorrhoid is ligated at its base with a rubber band. The hemorrhoid tissue is allowed to slough over time.

Coding Tips

Selection of codes for hemorrhoid treatment depends on the site of the hemorrhoid (internal or external) and the nature of the surgical procedure (injection, destruction, incision, ligation, or excision). For incision of an external thrombosed hemorrhoid, see 46083; excision, see 46320. For excision of external anal papilla or tag, single, see 46220; multiple, see 46230. For external hemorrhoidectomy, 2 or more columns/groups, see 46250. For injection of a hemorrhoidal sclerosing agent, see 46500.

ICD-9-CM Procedural

49.45   Ligation of hemorrhoids

Anesthesia

46221   00902

ICD-9-CM Diagnostic

455.0   Internal hemorrhoids without mention of complication
455.1   Internal thrombosed hemorrhoids
455.2   Internal hemorrhoids with other complication

569.1   Rectal prolapse
569.41 Ulcer of anus and rectum
569.44 Dysplasia of anus

Terms To Know

hemorrhoid. Dilated, varicose vein in the anal region caused by continually increased venous pressure. Reversed blood flow and clotted blood within a vein that extends beyond the anus.

ligate. To tie off a blood vessel or duct with a suture or a soft, thin wire (ligature wire).

prolapse. Falling, sliding, or sinking of an organ from its normal location in the body.

thrombosed hemorrhoid. Dilated, varicose vein in the anal region that has clotted blood within it.

CCI Version 18.3

00902, 0213T, 0216T, 0226T-0228T, 0230T, 0249T, 0288T, 12001-12007, 12011-12057, 13100-13153, 36000, 36400-36410, 36420-36430, 36440, 36600, 36640, 37202, 43752, 45300, 45303, 45317, 45330, 45334, 45340, 45900-45990, 46040, 46220, 46500, 46600, 46604-46606, 46614, 46930❖, 46940-46942, 51701-51703, 62310-62319, 64400-64435, 64445-64450, 64479, 64483, 64490, 64493, 64505-64530, 69990, 93000-93010, 93040-93042, 93318, 94002, 94200, 94250, 94680-94690, 94770, 95812-95816, 95819, 95822, 95829, 95955, 96360, 96365, 96372, 96374-96376, 99148-99149, 99150, J0670, J2001

Note: These CCI edits are used for Medicare. Other payers may reimburse on codes listed above.

Medicare Edits

	Fac RVU	Non-Fac RVU	FUD	Status
46221	5.57	7.78	10	A

	MUE		Modifiers		
46221	1	51	N/A	N/A	N/A

* with documentation

Medicare References: None

Anus

Coding Companion for Ob/Gyn

(46220)

46220 Excision of single external papilla or tag, anus

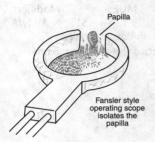

Papilla

Fansler style operating scope isolates the papilla

A papillectomy is performed

Report 46220 excision of a single papilla or skin tag. Report 46230 for excision of multiple papilla or skin tags

Explanation

The physician performs excision of a single external anal papilla or skin tag. The physician identifies the anal skin tag or papilla, which is usually associated with the external edge of a fissure or fistula. An incision is made around the skin tag or papilla and the lesion is dissected from the underlying sphincter muscle and removed. The incision is closed with sutures or may be left partially open to drain.

Coding Tips

This code is a resequenced code and will not display in numeric order. For excision of multiple external anal papillae or tags, see 46230. For external hemorrhoidectomy, 2 or more columns/groups, see 46250. For an internal hemorrhoidectomy by rubber band(s) ligation, see 46221. For incision of an external thrombosed hemorrhoid, see 46083. For injection of a hemorrhoidal sclerosing agent, see 46500. Surgical trays, A4550, are not separately reimbursed by Medicare; however, other third-party payers may cover them. Check with the specific payer to determine coverage.

ICD-9-CM Procedural

49.03 Excision of perianal skin tags

49.39 Other local excision or destruction of lesion or tissue of anus

Anesthesia

46220 00400

ICD-9-CM Diagnostic

455.3 External hemorrhoids without mention of complication

455.5 External hemorrhoids with other complication

455.9 Residual hemorrhoidal skin tags

565.0 Anal fissure

565.1 Anal fistula

569.0 Anal and rectal polyp

569.41 Ulcer of anus and rectum

569.44 Dysplasia of anus

569.49 Other specified disorder of rectum and anus — (Use additional code for any associated fecal incontinence (787.60-787.63))

787.99 Other symptoms involving digestive system

Terms To Know

anal fissure. Slit, crack, or tear of the anal mucosa that can cause pain, bleeding, and infection.

anal papilla. Skin tag protruding up from the area between the skin and the inside lining of the anus. Anal papillae frequently occur with anal fissures and are often detected during a digital examination of the anus or with a scope.

benign. Mild or nonmalignant in nature.

dissect. Cut apart or separate tissue for surgical purposes or for visual or microscopic study.

excision. Surgical removal of an organ or tissue.

fistula. Abnormal tube-like passage between two body cavities or organs or from an organ to the outside surface.

neoplasm. New abnormal growth, tumor.

skin tag. Small skin-colored or brown appendage appearing on the neck and upper chest resembling a little epithelial polyp.

CCI Version 18.3

00902, 0213T, 0216T, 0226T, 0228T, 0230T, 0288T, 12001-12007, 12011-12057, 13100-13153, 36000, 36400-36410, 36420-36430, 36440, 36600, 36640, 37202, 43752, 45300, 46040, 46600, 46940-46942, 51701-51703, 62310-62319, 64400-64435, 64445-64450, 64479, 64483, 64490, 64493, 64505-64530, 69990, 93000-93010, 93040-93042, 93318, 94002, 94200, 94250, 94680-94690, 94770, 95812-95816, 95819, 95822, 95829, 95955, 96360, 96365, 96372, 96374-96376, 99148-99149, 99150, J0670, J2001

Note: These CCI edits are used for Medicare. Other payers may reimburse on codes listed above.

Medicare Edits

	Fac RVU	Non-Fac RVU	FUD	Status
46220	3.47	5.97	10	A

	MUE		Modifiers		
46220	2	51	N/A	N/A	N/A

* with documentation

Medicare References: None

Anus

46230

46230 Excision of multiple external papillae or tags, anus

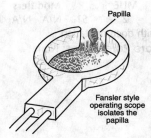

Papilla

Fansler style operating scope isolates the papilla

A papillectomy is performed

Report 46220 excision of a single papilla or skin tag. Report 46230 for excision of multiple papilla or skin tags

Explanation

The physician performs an excision of multiple external anal papillae or tags. Papillae are often associated with the external edge of an anal fissure or fistula. Once the physician has identified the external tags or papillae, incisions are made around the lesions. The lesions are dissected from the underlying sphincter muscle and removed. The incisions are closed with sutures or may be left partially open to drain.

Coding Tips

For excision of a single external anal papilla or tag, see 46220. For external hemorrhoidectomy, 2 or more columns/groups, see 46250. For incision of an external thrombosed hemorrhoid, see 46083; excision, see 46320. For internal hemorrhoidectomy by rubber band(s) ligation, see 46221. For injection of a hemorrhoidal sclerosing agent, see 46500.

ICD-9-CM Procedural

49.03   Excision of perianal skin tags
49.39   Other local excision or destruction of lesion or tissue of anus

Anesthesia

46230   00400, 00902

ICD-9-CM Diagnostic

455.3   External hemorrhoids without mention of complication

455.5   External hemorrhoids with other complication
455.9   Residual hemorrhoidal skin tags
565.0   Anal fissure
565.1   Anal fistula
569.0   Anal and rectal polyp
569.41   Ulcer of anus and rectum
569.44   Dysplasia of anus
569.49   Other specified disorder of rectum and anus — (Use additional code for any associated fecal incontinence (787.60-787.63))
787.99   Other symptoms involving digestive system

Terms To Know

anal fissure. Slit, crack, or tear of the anal mucosa that can cause pain, bleeding, and infection.

anal papilla. Skin tag protruding up from the area between the skin and the inside lining of the anus. Anal papillae frequently occur with anal fissures and are often detected during a digital examination of the anus or with a scope.

dissect. Cut apart or separate tissue for surgical purposes or for visual or microscopic study.

excision. Surgical removal of an organ or tissue.

fistula. Abnormal tube-like passage between two body cavities or organs or from an organ to the outside surface.

hemorrhoid. Dilated, varicose vein in the anal region caused by continually increased venous pressure. Reversed blood flow and clotted blood within a vein that extends beyond the anus.

suture. Stitching technique employed in wound closure.

CCI Version 18.3

00902, 0213T, 0216T, 0226T, 0228T, 0230T, 0249T, 0288T, 12001-12007, 12011-12057, 13100-13153, 36000, 36400-36410, 36420-36430, 36440, 36600, 36640, 37202, 43752, 45900-45990, 46040, 46080, 46220-46221, 46600, 46940-46942, 51701-51703, 62310-62319, 64400-64435, 64445-64450, 64479, 64483, 64490, 64493, 64505-64530, 69990, 93000-93010, 93040-93042, 93318, 94002, 94200, 94250, 94680-94690, 94770, 95812-95816, 95819, 95822, 95829, 95955, 96360, 96365, 96372, 96374-96376, 99148-99149, 99150, J0670, J2001

Note: These CCI edits are used for Medicare. Other payers may reimburse on codes listed above.

Medicare Edits

	Fac RVU	Non-Fac RVU	FUD	Status
46230	5.05	7.93	10	A

	MUE		Modifiers		
46230	1	51	N/A	N/A	N/A

* with documentation

Medicare References: None

(46320)

46320 Excision of thrombosed hemorrhoid, external

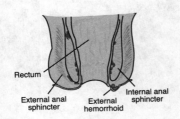

Rectum

External anal sphincter

External hemorrhoid

Internal anal sphincter

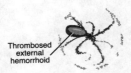

Thrombosed external hemorrhoid

External hemorrhoids are varicosities of the inferior rectal veins and are covered by skin. Code 46320 reports incision of an external hemorrhoid with removal of the thrombosis or complete excision

Explanation

The physician performs an excision of an external hemorrhoid that has become clotted with blood (thrombosed). Following appropriate anesthesia, the physician exposes the thrombosed external hemorrhoid. The hemorrhoid is completely excised with a scalpel. The site of the excision may be closed or left open to allow continued drainage.

Coding Tips

This code is a resequenced code and will not display in numeric order. Selection of codes depends on the site of the hemorrhoid (internal or external) and the nature of the surgical procedure (injection, destruction, incision, ligation, excision, excision with other procedures). For excision of external anal papilla or tag, single, see 46220; multiple, see 46230. For an internal hemorrhoidectomy by rubber band(s) ligation, see 46221. For external hemorrhoidectomy, 2 or more columns/groups, see 46250. To report an internal and external hemorrhoidectomy, single column or group, see 46255.

ICD-9-CM Procedural

49.46 Excision of hemorrhoids

49.47 Evacuation of thrombosed hemorrhoids

Anesthesia

46320 00902

ICD-9-CM Diagnostic

455.4 External thrombosed hemorrhoids

Terms To Know

excision. Surgical removal of an organ or tissue.

external thrombosed hemorrhoid. Reversed blood flow and clotted blood within a vein that extends beyond the anus.

hemorrhage. Internal or external bleeding with loss of significant amounts of blood.

incision and drainage. Cutting open body tissue for the removal of tissue fluids or infected discharge from a wound or cavity.

sphincter. Ring-like band of muscle that surrounds a bodily opening, constricting and relaxing as required for normal physiological functioning.

thrombus. Stationary blood clot inside a blood vessel.

CCI Version 18.3

00902, 0213T, 0216T, 0226T, 0228T, 0230T, 0288T, 12001-12007, 12011-12057, 13100-13153, 36000, 36400-36410, 36420-36430, 36440, 36600, 36640, 37202, 43752, 45900-45990, 46040, 46083, 46220, 46600, 46940-46942, 51701-51703, 62310-62319, 64400-64435, 64445-64450, 64479, 64483, 64490, 64493, 64505-64530, 69990, 93000-93010, 93040-93042, 93318, 94002, 94200, 94250, 94680-94690, 94770, 95812-95816, 95819, 95822, 95829, 95955, 96360, 96365, 96372, 96374-96376, 99148-99149, 99150, J0670, J2001

Note: These CCI edits are used for Medicare. Other payers may reimburse on codes listed above.

Medicare Edits

	Fac RVU	Non-Fac RVU	FUD	Status
46320	3.24	5.32	10	A

	MUE		Modifiers		
46320	2	51	N/A	N/A	N/A

* with documentation

Medicare References: None

46250

46250 Hemorrhoidectomy, external, 2 or more columns/groups

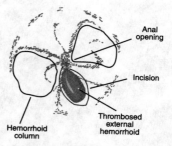

Anal opening

Incision

Thrombosed external hemorrhoid

Hemorrhoid column

An external hemorrhoid is completely excised (46250)

The hemorrhoid is identified and isolated. An incision is made around the lesion and it is dissected free from underlying tissues

Explanation

The physician performs an excision of external hemorrhoids. The physician identifies the external hemorrhoids. Incisions are made around the hemorrhoids and the lesions are dissected from the underlying sphincter muscle and removed. The incisions are closed with sutures.

Coding Tips

Selection of codes for hemorrhoid treatment depends on the site of the hemorrhoid (internal or external) and the nature of the surgical procedure (injection, destruction, incision, ligation, or excision). For hemorrhoidectomy, external, single column/group, see 46999. For incision of an external thrombosed hemorrhoid, see 46083; excision, see 46320. For excision of external anal papilla or tag, single, see 46220; multiple, see 46230. To report an internal hemorrhoidectomy by rubber band(s) ligation, see 46221. For injection of a hemorrhoidal sclerosing agent, see 46500.

ICD-9-CM Procedural

49.46   Excision of hemorrhoids

Anesthesia

46250   00902

ICD-9-CM Diagnostic

455.3   External hemorrhoids without mention of complication

455.4   External thrombosed hemorrhoids

455.5   External hemorrhoids with other complication

455.7   Unspecified thrombosed hemorrhoids

455.9   Residual hemorrhoidal skin tags

569.44   Dysplasia of anus

Terms To Know

dissection. Separating by cutting tissue or body structures apart.

excision. Surgical removal of an organ or tissue.

external thrombosed hemorrhoid. Reversed blood flow and clotted blood within a vein that extends beyond the anus.

incision. Act of cutting into tissue or an organ.

sphincter. Ring-like band of muscle that surrounds a bodily opening, constricting and relaxing as required for normal physiological functioning.

thrombus. Stationary blood clot inside a blood vessel.

CCI Version 18.3

00902, 0213T, 0216T, 0226T, 0228T, 0230T, 0249T, 0288T, 12001-12007, 12011-12057, 13100-13153, 36000, 36400-36410, 36420-36430, 36440, 36600, 36640, 37202, 43752, 45900-45990, 46040, 46080, 46220-46221, 46600, 46940-46942, 51701-51703, 62310-62319, 64400-64435, 64445-64450, 64479, 64483, 64490, 64493, 64505-64530, 69990, 93000-93010, 93040-93042, 93318, 94002, 94200, 94250, 94680-94690, 94770, 95812-95816, 95819, 95822, 95829, 95955, 96360, 96365, 96372, 96374-96376, 99148-99149, 99150, J0670, J2001

Note: These CCI edits are used for Medicare. Other payers may reimburse on codes listed above.

Medicare Edits

	Fac RVU	Non-Fac RVU	FUD	Status
46250	9.12	13.31	90	A

	MUE		Modifiers		
46250	1	51	N/A	N/A	N/A

* with documentation

Medicare References: None

Anus

Coding Companion for Ob/Gyn

46500

46500 Injection of sclerosing solution, hemorrhoids

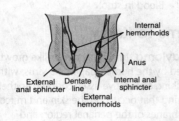

Internal hemorrhoids
Anus
External anal sphincter
Dentate line
Internal anal sphincter
External hemorrhoids

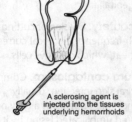

A sclerosing agent is injected into the tissues underlying hemorrhoids

Explanation

The physician performs sclerotherapy of internal hemorrhoids. The physician explores the anal canal and identifies the hemorrhoid columns. Sclerosing solution is injected into the submucosa of the rectal wall under the hemorrhoid columns.

Coding Tips

For external hemorrhoidectomy, 2 or more columns/groups, see 46250. For excision of external anal papilla or tag, single, see 46220; multiple, see 46230. For excision of an external thrombosed hemorrhoid, see 46320. For an internal hemorrhoidectomy by rubber band(s) ligation, see 46221. Surgical trays, A4550, are not separately reimbursed by Medicare; however, other third-party payers may cover them. Check with the specific payer to determine coverage.

ICD-9-CM Procedural

49.42   Injection of hemorrhoids

Anesthesia

46500 00902

ICD-9-CM Diagnostic

455.0   Internal hemorrhoids without mention of complication

455.1   Internal thrombosed hemorrhoids

455.2   Internal hemorrhoids with other complication

455.3   External hemorrhoids without mention of complication

455.4   External thrombosed hemorrhoids

455.5   External hemorrhoids with other complication

455.7   Unspecified thrombosed hemorrhoids

569.3   Hemorrhage of rectum and anus

569.42   Anal or rectal pain

578.1   Blood in stool

Terms To Know

hemorrhoid. Dilated, varicose vein in the anal region caused by continually increased venous pressure. Reversed blood flow and clotted blood within a vein that extends beyond the anus.

injection. Forcing a liquid substance into a body part such as a joint or muscle.

sclerose. To become hard or firm and indurated from increased formation of connective tissue or disease.

sclerotherapy. Injection of a chemical agent that will irritate, inflame, and cause fibrosis in a vein, eventually obliterating hemorrhoids or varicose veins.

thrombosed hemorrhoid. Dilated, varicose vein in the anal region that has clotted blood within it.

CCI Version 18.3

00902, 0213T, 0216T, 0226T, 0228T, 0230T, 0288T, 12001-12007, 12011-12057, 13100-13153, 36000, 36400-36410, 36420-36430, 36440, 36600, 36640, 37202, 43752, 45305, 45331, 45900-45990, 46040, 46080, 46220, 46600, 46930, 46940-46942, 51701-51703, 62310-62319, 64400-64435, 64445-64450, 64479, 64483, 64490, 64493, 64505-64530, 69990, 93000-93010, 93040-93042, 93318, 94002, 94200, 94250, 94680-94690, 94770, 95812-95816, 95819, 95822, 95829, 95955, 96360, 96365, 96372, 96374-96376, 99148-99149, 99150, J0670, J2001

Note: These CCI edits are used for Medicare. Other payers may reimburse on codes listed above.

Medicare Edits

	Fac RVU	Non-Fac RVU	FUD	Status
46500	3.77	6.81	10	A

	MUE		Modifiers		
46500	1	51	N/A	N/A	N/A

* with documentation

Medicare References: None

Anus

46900-46916

46900 Destruction of lesion(s), anus (eg, condyloma, papilloma, molluscum contagiosum, herpetic vesicle), simple; chemical
46910   electrodesiccation
46916   cryosurgery

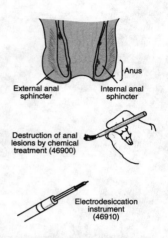

External anal sphincter

Internal anal sphincter

Anus

Destruction of anal lesions by chemical treatment (46900)

Electrodesiccation instrument (46910)

Minor lesions of the anal canal are destroyed using any of a variety of methods. Report code 46900 for simple chemical destruction. Code 46910 reports electrodesiccation. Report 46916 for cryosurgery (freezing)

Explanation

The physician performs destruction of anal lesions with chemicals in 46900. The physician exposes the perianal skin and identifies the lesions. The lesions are painted with destructive chemicals. In 46910, the physician performs destruction of anal lesions with electrodesiccation. The physician exposes the perianal skin and identifies the lesions. The lesions are destroyed with cautery. In 46916, the physician performs destruction of anal lesions with cryosurgery. The physician exposes the perianal skin and identifies the lesions. The lesions are frozen and destroyed, usually with liquid nitrogen.

Coding Tips

Select the code based on the method of destruction (chemical, electrodesiccation, cryosurgery, laser, surgical excision) and the extent of the procedure (simple, extensive). For simple destruction of anal lesions by laser, see 46917; surgical excision, see 46922; extensive, by any method, see 46924. Destruction of internal hemorrhoids by thermal energy is reported with 46930.

ICD-9-CM Procedural

49.39   Other local excision or destruction of lesion or tissue of anus

Anesthesia
00400

ICD-9-CM Diagnostic

054.10 Unspecified genital herpes
078.0   Molluscum contagiosum
078.10 Viral warts, unspecified
078.11 Condyloma acuminatum
078.19 Other specified viral warts
154.1   Malignant neoplasm of rectum
154.2   Malignant neoplasm of anal canal
154.3   Malignant neoplasm of anus, unspecified site
209.17 Malignant carcinoid tumor of the rectum — (Code first any associated multiple endocrine neoplasia syndrome: 258.01-258.03)(Use additional code to identify associated endocrine syndrome, as: carcinoid syndrome: 259.2)
209.29 Malignant carcinoid tumor of other sites — (Code first any associated multiple endocrine neoplasia syndrome: 258.01-258.03)(Use additional code to identify associated endocrine syndrome, as: carcinoid syndrome: 259.2)
209.57 Benign carcinoid tumor of the rectum — (Code first any associated multiple endocrine neoplasia syndrome: 258.01-258.03)(Use additional code to identify associated endocrine syndrome, as: carcinoid syndrome: 259.2)
209.69 Benign carcinoid tumor of other sites — (Code first any associated multiple endocrine neoplasia syndrome: 258.01-258.03)(Use additional code to identify associated endocrine syndrome, as: carcinoid syndrome: 259.2)
211.4   Benign neoplasm of rectum and anal canal
214.9   Lipoma of unspecified site
216.5   Benign neoplasm of skin of trunk, except scrotum
216.9   Benign neoplasm of skin, site unspecified
228.01 Hemangioma of skin and subcutaneous tissue
235.5   Neoplasm of uncertain behavior of other and unspecified digestive organs
238.2   Neoplasm of uncertain behavior of skin
239.0   Neoplasm of unspecified nature of digestive system
455.2   Internal hemorrhoids with other complication
569.3   Hemorrhage of rectum and anus
569.41 Ulcer of anus and rectum
569.42 Anal or rectal pain
569.44 Dysplasia of anus
578.1   Blood in stool

Terms To Know

condyloma. Infectious tumor-like growth caused by the human papilloma virus, with a branching connective tissue core and epithelial covering that occurs on the skin and mucous membranes of the perianal region and external genitalia.

electrocautery. Division or cutting of tissue using high-frequency electrical current to produce heat, which destroys cells.

molluscum contagiosum. Common, benign, viral skin infection, usually self-limiting, that appears as a gray or flesh-colored umbilicated lesion by itself or in groups, and later becomes white with an expulsable core containing the replication bodies. It is often transmitted sexually in adults, by autoinoculation, or close contact in children.

CCI Version 18.3

00902, 0213T, 0216T, 0226T, 0228T, 0230T, 0288T, 12001-12007, 12011-12057, 13100-13153, 36000, 36400-36410, 36420-36430, 36440, 36600, 36640, 37202, 43752, 45900-45990, 46040, 46080, 46220, 46600, 46940-46942, 51701-51703, 62310-62319, 64400-64435, 64445-64450, 64479, 64483, 64490, 64493, 64505-64530, 69990, 93000-93010, 93040-93042, 93318, 94002, 94200, 94250, 94680-94690, 94770, 95812-95816, 95819, 95822, 95829, 95955, 96360, 96365, 96372, 96374-96376, 99148-99149, 99150, J0670, J2001

Note: These CCI edits are used for Medicare. Other payers may reimburse on codes listed above.

Medicare Edits

	Fac RVU	Non-Fac RVU	FUD	Status
46900	4.05	6.99	10	A
46910	3.95	7.39	10	A
46916	4.27	6.84	10	A

	MUE		Modifiers		
46900	1	51	N/A	N/A	N/A
46910	1	51	N/A	N/A	N/A
46916	1	51	N/A	N/A	N/A

* with documentation

Medicare References: 100-3,140.5

46917-46922

46917 Destruction of lesion(s), anus (eg, condyloma, papilloma, molluscum contagiosum, herpetic vesicle), simple; laser surgery

46922   surgical excision

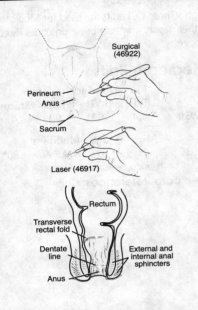

Surgical (46922)

Perineum
Anus

Sacrum

Laser (46917)

Rectum

Transverse rectal fold

Dentate line

External and internal anal sphincters

Anus

Explanation

The physician performs destruction of anal lesions with laser therapy in 46917. The physician exposes the perianal skin and identifies the lesions. The lesions are destroyed by laser ablation or laser excision. In 46922, the physician performs destruction of anal lesions by excision. The physician exposes the perianal skin and identifies the lesions. The lesions are surgically excised. The incisions are closed.

Coding Tips

Select the code based on the method of destruction (chemical, electrodesiccation, cryosurgery, laser, or surgical excision). For simple destruction, by chemical, see 46900; electrodesiccation, see 46910; cryosurgery, see 46916.

ICD-9-CM Procedural

49.39   Other local excision or destruction of lesion or tissue of anus

Anesthesia

46917 00400
46922 00902

ICD-9-CM Diagnostic

054.10 Unspecified genital herpes
078.0   Molluscum contagiosum

078.10 Viral warts, unspecified
078.11 Condyloma acuminatum
078.19 Other specified viral warts
154.1   Malignant neoplasm of rectum
154.2   Malignant neoplasm of anal canal
154.3   Malignant neoplasm of anus, unspecified site
209.17 Malignant carcinoid tumor of the rectum — (Code first any associated multiple endocrine neoplasia syndrome: 258.01-258.03)(Use additional code to identify associated endocrine syndrome, as: carcinoid syndrome: 259.2)
209.29 Malignant carcinoid tumor of other sites — (Code first any associated multiple endocrine neoplasia syndrome: 258.01-258.03)(Use additional code to identify associated endocrine syndrome, as: carcinoid syndrome: 259.2)
209.57 Benign carcinoid tumor of the rectum — (Code first any associated multiple endocrine neoplasia syndrome: 258.01-258.03)(Use additional code to identify associated endocrine syndrome, as: carcinoid syndrome: 259.2)
209.69 Benign carcinoid tumor of other sites — (Code first any associated multiple endocrine neoplasia syndrome: 258.01-258.03)(Use additional code to identify associated endocrine syndrome, as: carcinoid syndrome: 259.2)
211.4   Benign neoplasm of rectum and anal canal
214.9   Lipoma of unspecified site
216.5   Benign neoplasm of skin of trunk, except scrotum
216.9   Benign neoplasm of skin, site unspecified
228.01 Hemangioma of skin and subcutaneous tissue
235.5   Neoplasm of uncertain behavior of other and unspecified digestive organs
238.2   Neoplasm of uncertain behavior of skin
239.0   Neoplasm of unspecified nature of digestive system
455.2   Internal hemorrhoids with other complication
569.3   Hemorrhage of rectum and anus
569.41 Ulcer of anus and rectum
569.42 Anal or rectal pain
569.44 Dysplasia of anus

578.1   Blood in stool

Terms To Know

condyloma. Infectious tumor-like growth caused by the human papilloma virus, with a branching connective tissue core and epithelial covering that occurs on the skin and mucous membranes of the perianal region and external genitalia.

laser surgery. Use of concentrated, sharply defined light beams to cut, cauterize, coagulate, seal, or vaporize tissue.

molluscum contagiosum. Common, benign, viral skin infection, usually self-limiting, that appears as a gray or flesh-colored umbilicated lesion by itself or in groups, and later becomes white with an expulsable core containing the replication bodies. It is often transmitted sexually in adults, by autoinoculation, or close contact in children.

papilloma. Benign skin neoplasm with small branchings from the epithelial surface.

CCI Version 18.3

00902, 0213T, 0216T, 0226T, 0228T, 0230T, 0288T, 12001-12007, 12011-12057, 13100-13153, 36000, 36400-36410, 36420-36430, 36440, 36600, 36640, 37202, 43752, 45900-45990, 46040, 46080, 46220, 46600, 46940-46942, 51701-51703, 62310-62319, 64400-64435, 64445-64450, 64479, 64483, 64490, 64493, 64505-64530, 69990, 93000-93010, 93040-93042, 93318, 94002, 94200, 94250, 94680-94690, 94770, 95812-95816, 95819, 95822, 95829, 95955, 96360, 96365, 96372, 96374-96376, 99148-99149, 99150, J0670, J2001

Note: These CCI edits are used for Medicare. Other payers may reimburse on codes listed above.

Medicare Edits

	Fac RVU	Non-Fac RVU	FUD	Status
46917	3.92	13.65	10	A
46922	3.95	7.73	10	A

	MUE		Modifiers		
46917	1	51	N/A	N/A	N/A
46922	1	51	N/A	N/A	N/A

* with documentation

Medicare References: 100-3,140.5

Coding Companion for Ob/Gyn

© 2012 OptumInsight, Inc.

Anus

46930

46930 Destruction of internal hemorrhoid(s) by thermal energy (eg, infrared coagulation, cautery, radiofrequency)

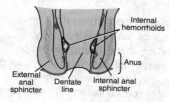

Internal hemorrhoids

External anal sphincter — Dentate line — Internal anal sphincter — Anus

Internal hemorrhoids are destroyed using thermal energy.

Explanation

The physician destroys internal hemorrhoids using various forms of thermal energy. The physician explores the anal canal and identifies the hemorrhoid columns. The hemorrhoids may be destroyed by clamping and cauterization, by employing high-frequency radio waves (radiofrequency), or by infrared or laser coagulation, which causes the hemorrhoidal tissue to harden, deteriorate, and form scar tissue as the area heals. The hemorrhoidal remnants may be removed.

Coding Tips

When medically necessary, report moderate sedation provided by the performing physician with 99143–99145. When provided by another physician, report 99148–99150. For internal hemorrhoidectomy by rubber band(s) ligation, see 46221. For excision of multiple external anal papillae or tags, see 46230. For external hemorrhoidectomy, two or more columns/groups, see 46250; single column/group, see 46999. For an injection of a hemorrhoidal sclerosing agent, see 46500. For an internal hemorrhoidectomy by ligation, other than rubber band, single hemorrhoid column/group, see 46945; two or more hemorrhoid columns/groups, see 46946. For hemorrhoidopexy by stapling, see 46947.

ICD-9-CM Procedural

49.43   Cauterization of hemorrhoids
49.49   Other procedures on hemorrhoids

Anesthesia
46930   00902

ICD-9-CM Diagnostic

209.57   Benign carcinoid tumor of the rectum — (Code first any associated multiple endocrine neoplasia syndrome: 258.01-258.03)(Use additional code to identify associated endocrine syndrome, as: carcinoid syndrome: 259.2)

211.4   Benign neoplasm of rectum and anal canal

455.0   Internal hemorrhoids without mention of complication

455.1   Internal thrombosed hemorrhoids

455.2   Internal hemorrhoids with other complication

564.6   Anal spasm

565.0   Anal fissure

565.1   Anal fistula

566   Abscess of anal and rectal regions

569.3   Hemorrhage of rectum and anus

569.41   Ulcer of anus and rectum

569.42   Anal or rectal pain

569.44   Dysplasia of anus

578.1   Blood in stool

751.5   Other congenital anomalies of intestine

Terms To Know

cauterization. Tissue destruction by means of a hot instrument, an electric current, or a caustic chemical.

clamp. Tool used to grip, compress, join, or fasten body parts.

coagulation. Clot formation.

destruction. Ablation or eradication of a structure or tissue.

hemorrhoid. Dilated, varicose vein in the anal region caused by continually increased venous pressure. Reversed blood flow and clotted blood within a vein that extends beyond the anus.

laser. Concentrated light used to cut or seal tissue.

thrombosed hemorrhoid. Dilated, varicose vein in the anal region that has clotted blood within it.

CCI Version 18.3

00902, 0213T, 0216T, 0226T, 0249T❖, 0288T, 12001-12007, 12011-12057, 13100-13153, 36000, 36400-36410, 36420-36430, 36440, 36600, 36640, 37202, 43752, 45380, 45900-45990, 46040, 46080, 46220, 46600, 46940-46942, 51701-51703, 62310-62319, 64400-64435, 64445-64450, 64479, 64483, 64490, 64493, 64505-64530, 69990, 93000-93010, 93040-93042, 93318, 94002, 94200, 94250, 94680-94690, 94770, 95812-95816, 95819, 95822, 95829, 95955, 96360, 96365, 96372, 96374-96376, 99148-99149, 99150

Note: These CCI edits are used for Medicare. Other payers may reimburse on codes listed above.

Medicare Edits

	Fac RVU	Non-Fac RVU	FUD	Status
46930	4.4	6.1	90	A

	MUE		Modifiers	
46930	1	51	N/A N/A	80*

* with documentation

Medicare References: None

Anus

49000

49000 Exploratory laparotomy, exploratory celiotomy with or without biopsy(s) (separate procedure)

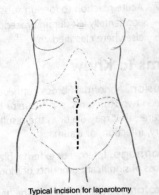

Typical incision for laparotomy

An access incision is made into the abdominal cavity for exploratory purposes. Biopsy samples may be collected during the surgical session. A celiotomy (from the Greek word for belly) implies an incision to access the stomach area. A laparotomy (from the Greek word for loin) implies an incision to access the abdominal area

Explanation

To explore the intra-abdominal organs and structures, the physician makes a large incision extending from just above the pubic hairline to the rib cage. The abdominal cavity is opened for a systematic examination of all organs. The physician may take tissue samples of any or all intra-abdominal organs for diagnosis. The incision is closed with sutures.

Coding Tips

This separate procedure by definition is usually a component of a more complex service and is not identified separately. When performed alone or with other unrelated procedures or services it may be reported. If performed alone, list the code; if performed with other procedures or services, list the code and append modifier 59. When 49000 is performed with another separately identifiable procedure, the highest dollar value code is listed as the primary procedure and subsequent procedures are appended with modifier 51. For diagnostic laparoscopy, see 49320.

ICD-9-CM Procedural

54.11 Exploratory laparotomy

54.23 Biopsy of peritoneum

Anesthesia

49000 00840

ICD-9-CM Diagnostic

The application of this code is too broad to adequately present ICD-9-CM diagnostic code links here. Refer to your ICD-9-CM book.

Terms To Know

celiotomy. Incision into the abdominal cavity.

incision. Act of cutting into tissue or an organ.

intra. Within.

CCI Version 18.3

0213T, 0216T, 0228T, 0230T, 10021-10022, 12001-12007, 12011-12057, 13100-13153, 20102, 36000, 36400-36410, 36420-36430, 36440, 36600, 36640, 37202, 43752, 44015, 44180, 44950, 44970, 49255, 51701-51703, 62310-62319, 64400-64435, 64445-64450, 64479, 64483, 64490, 64493, 64505-64530, 69990, 93000-93010, 93040-93042, 93318, 94002, 94200, 94250, 94680-94690, 94770, 95812-95816, 95819, 95822, 95829, 95955, 96360, 96365, 96372, 96374-96376, 99148-99149, 99150

Note: These CCI edits are used for Medicare. Other payers may reimburse on codes listed above.

Medicare Edits

	Fac RVU	Non-Fac RVU	FUD	Status
49000	22.51	22.51	90	A

	MUE		Modifiers		
49000	1	51	N/A	62*	80

* with documentation

Medicare References: None

Coding Companion for Ob/Gyn

49002

49002 Reopening of recent laparotomy

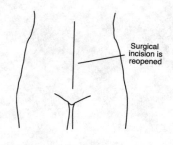

Surgical incision is reopened

Explanation

The physician reopens the incision of a recent laparotomy before the incision has fully healed to control bleeding, remove packing, or drain a postoperative infection.

Coding Tips

This procedure is usually performed within one week of the primary laparotomy. The accompanying diagnosis code(s) needs to support the reason for reopening the laparotomy. When 49002 is performed with another separately identifiable procedure, the highest dollar value code is listed as the primary procedure and subsequent procedures are appended with modifier 51.

ICD-9-CM Procedural

54.12   Reopening of recent laparotomy site

Anesthesia

49002   00840

ICD-9-CM Diagnostic

338.18   Other acute postoperative pain — (Use additional code to identify pain associated with psychological factors: 307.89)

553.21   Incisional hernia without mention of obstruction or gangrene

557.0   Acute vascular insufficiency of intestine

560.81   Intestinal or peritoneal adhesions with obstruction (postoperative) (postinfection)

567.21   Peritonitis (acute) generalized

567.22   Peritoneal abscess

567.23   Spontaneous bacterial peritonitis

567.29   Other suppurative peritonitis

567.89   Other specified peritonitis

568.81   Hemoperitoneum (nontraumatic)

568.9   Unspecified disorder of peritoneum

614.6   Pelvic peritoneal adhesions, female (postoperative) (postinfection) — (Use additional code to identify organism: 041.00-041.09, 041.10-041.19) (Use additional code to identify any associated infertility: 628.2)

628.2   Female infertility of tubal origin — (Use additional code for any associated peritubal adhesions: 614.6)

674.34   Other complications of obstetrical surgical wounds, postpartum condition or complication

780.62   Postprocedural fever

789.01   Abdominal pain, right upper quadrant

789.02   Abdominal pain, left upper quadrant

789.03   Abdominal pain, right lower quadrant

789.04   Abdominal pain, left lower quadrant

789.05   Abdominal pain, periumbilic

789.06   Abdominal pain, epigastric

789.07   Abdominal pain, generalized

789.31   Abdominal or pelvic swelling, mass, or lump, right upper quadrant

789.32   Abdominal or pelvic swelling, mass, or lump, left upper quadrant

789.33   Abdominal or pelvic swelling, mass, or lump, right lower quadrant

789.34   Abdominal or pelvic swelling, mass, or lump, left lower quadrant

789.35   Abdominal or pelvic swelling, mass or lump, periumbilic

789.36   Abdominal or pelvic swelling, mass, or lump, epigastric

789.37   Abdominal or pelvic swelling, mass, or lump, generalized

997.5   Urinary complications — (Use additional code to identify complications)

998.11   Hemorrhage complicating a procedure

998.12   Hematoma complicating a procedure

998.13   Seroma complicating a procedure

998.31   Disruption of internal operation (surgical) wound

998.32   Disruption of external operation (surgical) wound

998.4   Foreign body accidentally left during procedure, not elsewhere classified

998.51   Infected postoperative seroma — (Use additional code to identify organism)

998.59   Other postoperative infection — (Use additional code to identify infection)

998.7   Acute reaction to foreign substance accidentally left during procedure, not elsewhere classified

Terms To Know

adhesion. Abnormal fibrous connection between two structures, soft tissue or bony structures, that may occur as the result of surgery, infection, or trauma.

hemorrhage. Internal or external bleeding with loss of significant amounts of blood.

laparotomy. Incision through the flank or abdomen for therapeutic or diagnostic purposes.

seroma. Swelling caused by the collection of serum, or clear fluid, in the tissues.

CCI Version 18.3

0213T, 0216T, 0228T, 0230T, 12001-12007, 12011-12057, 13100-13153, 20102, 36000, 36400-36410, 36420-36430, 36440, 36600, 36640, 37202, 43752, 44005, 44180, 44820-44850, 44950, 44970, 49000, 49010, 49021, 49255, 49570, 51701-51703, 62310-62319, 64400-64435, 64445-64450, 64479, 64483, 64490, 64493, 64505-64530, 69990, 93000-93010, 93040-93042, 93318, 94002, 94200, 94250, 94680-94690, 94770, 95812-95816, 95819, 95822, 95829, 95955, 96360, 96365, 96372, 96374-96376, 99148-99149, 99150

Note: These CCI edits are used for Medicare. Other payers may reimburse on codes listed above.

Medicare Edits

	Fac RVU	Non-Fac RVU	FUD	Status
49002	30.43	30.43	90	A

	MUE			Modifiers	
49002	1	51	N/A	62*	80

* with documentation

Medicare References: None

49020-49021

49020 Drainage of peritoneal abscess or localized peritonitis, exclusive of appendiceal abscess; open

49021 percutaneous

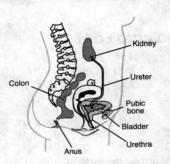

Peritonitis is an infectious irritation of the peritoneum, the lining of internal organs and abdominal walls. A localized irritation may form or an abscess may develop. These codes report treatment measures for this type of condition when appendicitis is ruled out

Report 49020 for an open approach to the infection. Drains may be placed, usually by an additional incision or stab wound through the abdominal wall

Report 49021 when the drainage is accomplished percutaneously

Explanation

In 49020, the physician makes an open abdominal or flank incision (laparotomy) to gain access to the peritoneal cavity. The peritoneum is explored and the abscess or isolated area of peritoneal inflammation is identified. The abscess is incised and drained, and inflamed peritoneal tissue may be excised. The abscess and surrounding peritoneal cavity may be irrigated. A drain may be placed whereby a separate abdominal incision is made and the drain is drawn through it and sutured in place. The physician may completely reapproximate the abdominal incision or leave a portion of the incision open to allow for further drainage. In 49021, to avoid exposure of the abdominal cavity, the physician makes a small skin incision in the abdomen or flank. Percutaneous needle aspiration and closed catheter drainage using computer tomographic (CT) or ultrasound guidance is performed. A needle, guidewire, or pigtail catheter is placed within the abscess. Specimens taken during these procedures are typically sent to microbiology for identification and to determine antibiotic suitability. If a drain is placed, it is removed at a later date. These procedures do not apply to abscess of the appendix.

Coding Tips

Moderate sedation performed with 49021 is considered to be an integral part of the

procedure and is not reported separately. However, anesthesia services may be billed separately when performed by a physician (or other qualified provider) other than the physician performing the procedure. For radiological supervision and interpretation for percutaneous drainage of an abscess with catheter placement, see 75989. If an indwelling catheter is not placed, append modifier 52 to the radiology code.

ICD-9-CM Procedural

54.19   Other laparotomy

54.91   Percutaneous abdominal drainage

Anesthesia

49020   00840

49021   00800

ICD-9-CM Diagnostic

562.13   Diverticulitis of colon with hemorrhage — (Use additional code to identify any associated peritonitis: 567.0-567.9)

567.0   Peritonitis in infectious diseases classified elsewhere — (Code first underlying disease)

567.1   Pneumococcal peritonitis

567.22   Peritoneal abscess

567.23   Spontaneous bacterial peritonitis

567.29   Other suppurative peritonitis

567.38   Other retroperitoneal abscess

567.81   Choleperitonitis

567.89   Other specified peritonitis

567.9   Unspecified peritonitis

568.81   Hemoperitoneum (nontraumatic)

568.82   Peritoneal effusion (chronic)

568.89   Other specified disorder of peritoneum

569.5   Abscess of intestine

569.83   Perforation of intestine

614.5   Acute or unspecified pelvic peritonitis, female — (Use additional code to identify organism: 041.00-041.09, 041.10-041.19)

614.7   Other chronic pelvic peritonitis, female — (Use additional code to identify organism: 041.00-041.09, 041.10-041.19)

670.00   Major puerperal infection, unspecified, unspecified as to episode of care or not applicable

863.95   Appendix injury with open wound into cavity

879.2   Open wound of abdominal wall, anterior, without mention of complication

998.51   Infected postoperative seroma — (Use additional code to identify organism)

998.59   Other postoperative infection — (Use additional code to identify infection)

Terms To Know

abscess. Circumscribed collection of pus resulting from bacteria, frequently associated with swelling and other signs of inflammation.

peritonitis. Inflammation and infection within the peritoneal cavity, the space between the membrane lining the abdominopelvic walls and covering the internal organs.

CCI Version 18.3

0213T, 0216T, 0228T, 0230T, 12001-12007, 12011-12057, 13100-13153, 36000, 36400-36410, 36420-36430, 36440, 36600, 36640, 37202, 43752, 44602-44605, 49320, 49402, 51701-51703, 62310-62319, 64400-64435, 64445-64450, 64479, 64483, 64490, 64493, 64505-64530, 69990, 76000-76001, 77001-77002, 93000-93010, 93040-93042, 93318, 94002, 94200, 94250, 94680-94690, 94770, 95812-95816, 95819, 95822, 95829, 95955, 96360, 96365, 96372, 96374-96376, 99150

Also not with 49020: 20102, 44005, 44180, 44820-44850, 44950, 44970, 49000-49010, 49203-49204, 49255, 49424, 49570, 99148-99149

Also not with 49021: 49000, 49010-49020❖, 49040, 49082-49084, 49180, 49400, 49423-49424, 76942, 99143-99149, J0670, J2001

Note: These CCI edits are used for Medicare. Other payers may reimburse on codes listed above.

Medicare Edits

	Fac RVU	Non-Fac RVU	FUD	Status
49020	46.39	46.39	90	A
49021	4.94	26.47	0	A

	MUE		Modifiers		
49020	2	51	N/A	N/A	80
49021	3	51	N/A	N/A	N/A

* with documentation

Medicare References: None

Coding Companion for Ob/Gyn

© 2012 OptumInsight, Inc.

49082-49083

49082 Abdominal paracentesis (diagnostic or therapeutic); without imaging guidance

49083 with imaging guidance

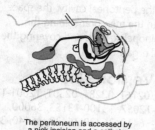

The peritoneum is accessed by a nick incision and a catheter is introduced into the cavity

Explanation

The physician inserts a needle or catheter into the abdominal cavity and withdraws and drains fluid for diagnostic or therapeutic purposes. The needle or catheter is removed at the completion of the procedure. Report 49082 if imaging guidance is not used and 49083 if imaging guidance is used.

Coding Tips

Code 49083 includes imaging guidance. Do not report 76942, 77002, 77012, or 77021 with 49083. For peritoneal lavage, see 49084.

ICD-9-CM Procedural

00.31 Computer assisted surgery with CT/CTA

00.32 Computer assisted surgery with MR/MRA

00.33 Computer assisted surgery with fluoroscopy

00.34 Imageless computer assisted surgery

00.35 Computer assisted surgery with multiple datasets

00.39 Other computer assisted surgery

54.25 Peritoneal lavage

54.91 Percutaneous abdominal drainage

Anesthesia

00700, 00800

ICD-9-CM Diagnostic

095.2 Syphilitic peritonitis

457.8 Other noninfectious disorders of lymphatic channels

567.0 Peritonitis in infectious diseases classified elsewhere — (Code first underlying disease)

567.1 Pneumococcal peritonitis

567.21 Peritonitis (acute) generalized

567.22 Peritoneal abscess

567.23 Spontaneous bacterial peritonitis

567.29 Other suppurative peritonitis

567.81 Choleperitonitis

567.89 Other specified peritonitis

567.9 Unspecified peritonitis

568.82 Peritoneal effusion (chronic)

789.51 Malignant ascites

789.59 Other ascites

998.4 Foreign body accidentally left during procedure, not elsewhere classified

998.7 Acute reaction to foreign substance accidentally left during procedure, not elsewhere classified

Terms To Know

diagnostic. Examination or procedure to which the patient is subjected, or which is performed on materials derived from a hospital outpatient, to obtain information to aid in the assessment of a medical condition or the identification of a disease. Among these examinations and tests are diagnostic laboratory services such as hematology and chemistry, diagnostic x-rays, isotope studies, EKGs, pulmonary function studies, thyroid function tests, psychological tests, and other tests given to determine the nature and severity of an ailment or injury.

imaging. Radiologic means of producing pictures for clinical study of the internal structures and functions of the body, such as x-ray, ultrasound, magnetic resonance, or positron emission tomography.

paracentesis. Surgical puncture of a body cavity with a specialized needle or hollow tubing to aspirate fluid for diagnostic or therapeutic reasons.

therapeutic. Act meant to alleviate a medical or mental condition.

CCI Version 18.3

0213T, 0216T, 0228T, 0230T, 12001-12007, 12011-12057, 13100-13153, 20102, 36000, 36400-36410, 36420-36430, 36440, 36600, 36640, 37202, 43752, 51701-51703, 62310-62319, 64400-64435, 64445-64450, 64479, 64483, 64490, 64493, 64505-64530, 69990, 76000-76001, 76942, 76998, 77001-77002, 77012, 77021, 93000-93010, 93040-93042, 93318, 94002, 94200, 94250, 94680-94690, 94770, 95812-95816, 95819, 95822, 95829, 95955, 96360, 96365, 96372, 96374-96376, 99148-99149, 99150

Note: These CCI edits are used for Medicare. Other payers may reimburse on codes listed above.

Medicare Edits

	Fac RVU	Non-Fac RVU	FUD	Status
49082	2.05	4.82	0	A
49083	3.16	9.09	0	A

	MUE		Modifiers		
49082	1	51	N/A	N/A	N/A
49083	1	51	N/A	N/A	N/A

* with documentation

Medicare References: None

49084

49084 Peritoneal lavage, including imaging guidance, when performed

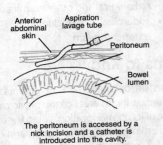

Anterior abdominal skin
Aspiration lavage tube
Peritoneum
Bowel lumen

The peritoneum is accessed by a nick incision and a catheter is introduced into the cavity.

Explanation

Peritoneal lavage is usually performed to determine the presence and/or extent of internal bleeding within the peritoneum. The physician makes a small incision to insert a catheter into the abdominal cavity. Fluids are infused into the cavity and subsequently aspirated for diagnostic testing. The catheter is removed at the completion of the procedure and the incision is closed.

Coding Tips

Imaging is included in this procedure and should not be reported separately.

ICD-9-CM Procedural

00.31	Computer assisted surgery with CT/CTA
00.32	Computer assisted surgery with MR/MRA
00.33	Computer assisted surgery with fluoroscopy
00.34	Imageless computer assisted surgery
00.35	Computer assisted surgery with multiple datasets
00.39	Other computer assisted surgery
54.25	Peritoneal lavage
54.91	Percutaneous abdominal drainage

Anesthesia

49084 00700, 00800

ICD-9-CM Diagnostic

095.2	Syphilitic peritonitis
457.8	Other noninfectious disorders of lymphatic channels
567.0	Peritonitis in infectious diseases classified elsewhere — (Code first underlying disease)
567.1	Pneumococcal peritonitis
567.21	Peritonitis (acute) generalized
567.22	Peritoneal abscess
567.23	Spontaneous bacterial peritonitis
567.29	Other suppurative peritonitis
567.81	Choleperitonitis
567.89	Other specified peritonitis
567.9	Unspecified peritonitis
568.82	Peritoneal effusion (chronic)
789.51	Malignant ascites
789.59	Other ascites
998.4	Foreign body accidentally left during procedure, not elsewhere classified
998.7	Acute reaction to foreign substance accidentally left during procedure, not elsewhere classified

Terms To Know

lavage. Washing.

peritoneal. Space between the lining of the abdominal wall, or parietal peritoneum, and the surface layer of the abdominal organs, or visceral peritoneum. It contains a thin, watery fluid that keeps the peritoneal surfaces moist.

CCI Version 18.3

0213T, 0216T, 0228T, 0230T, 12001-12007, 12011-12057, 13100-13153, 20102, 36000, 36400-36410, 36420-36430, 36440, 36600, 36640, 37202, 43752, 51701-51703, 62310-62319, 64400-64435, 64445-64450, 64479, 64483, 64490, 64493, 64505-64530, 69990, 76000-76001, 76942, 76998, 77001-77002, 77012, 77021, 93000-93010, 93040-93042, 93318, 94002, 94200, 94250, 94680-94690, 94770, 95812-95816, 95819, 95822, 95829, 95955, 96360, 96365, 96372, 96374-96376, 99148-99149, 99150

Note: These CCI edits are used for Medicare. Other payers may reimburse on codes listed above.

Medicare Edits

	Fac RVU	Non-Fac RVU	FUD	Status
49084	2.89	2.89	0	A

	MUE		Modifiers		
49084	1	51	N/A	N/A	N/A

* with documentation

Medicare References: None

Coding Companion for Ob/Gyn

49180

49180 Biopsy, abdominal or retroperitoneal mass, percutaneous needle

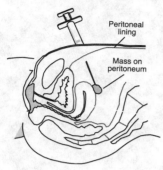

Biopsy needle guided to mass with aid of radiology (fluoroscope, CT, ultrasound)

Peritoneal lining

Mass on peritoneum

Explanation

Using radiological supervision, the physician locates the mass within or immediately outside the peritoneal lining of the abdominal cavity. A biopsy needle is then passed into the mass, a tissue sample is removed, and the needle is withdrawn. This may be repeated several times. No incision is necessary.

Coding Tips

If multiple areas are biopsied, report 49180 for each site taken and append modifier 51 to additional codes. Report radiology services separately; for radiological supervision and interpretation, see 77002, 77012, 77021 and 76942. The code is dependent on the type of radiological guidance used. For cytopathology of smears for specimens obtained by percutaneous needle biopsy, see 88160–88162. Local anesthesia is included in the service. However, general anesthesia may be administered depending on the age or condition of the patient.

ICD-9-CM Procedural

54.24 Closed (percutaneous) (needle) biopsy of intra-abdominal mass

Anesthesia

49180 00800, 00820

ICD-9-CM Diagnostic

158.0 Malignant neoplasm of retroperitoneum

158.8 Malignant neoplasm of specified parts of peritoneum

158.9 Malignant neoplasm of peritoneum, unspecified

159.8 Malignant neoplasm of other sites of digestive system and intra-abdominal organs

183.0 Malignant neoplasm of ovary — (Use additional code to identify any functional activity)

183.8 Malignant neoplasm of other specified sites of uterine adnexa

195.2 Malignant neoplasm of abdomen

196.2 Secondary and unspecified malignant neoplasm of intra-abdominal lymph nodes

196.6 Secondary and unspecified malignant neoplasm of intrapelvic lymph nodes

197.6 Secondary malignant neoplasm of retroperitoneum and peritoneum

209.74 Secondary neuroendocrine tumor of peritoneum

211.8 Benign neoplasm of retroperitoneum and peritoneum

220 Benign neoplasm of ovary — (Use additional code to identify any functional activity: 256.0-256.1)

228.04 Hemangioma of intra-abdominal structures

235.4 Neoplasm of uncertain behavior of retroperitoneum and peritoneum

236.2 Neoplasm of uncertain behavior of ovary — (Use additional code to identify any functional activity)

236.3 Neoplasm of uncertain behavior of other and unspecified female genital organs

256.0 Hyperestrogenism

256.1 Other ovarian hyperfunction

614.6 Pelvic peritoneal adhesions, female (postoperative) (postinfection) — (Use additional code to identify organism: 041.00-041.09, 041.10-041.19) (Use additional code to identify any associated infertility: 628.2)

617.0 Endometriosis of uterus

617.3 Endometriosis of pelvic peritoneum

617.9 Endometriosis, site unspecified

628.2 Female infertility of tubal origin — (Use additional code for any associated peritubal adhesions: 614.6)

789.31 Abdominal or pelvic swelling, mass, or lump, right upper quadrant

789.32 Abdominal or pelvic swelling, mass, or lump, left upper quadrant

789.33 Abdominal or pelvic swelling, mass, or lump, right lower quadrant

789.34 Abdominal or pelvic swelling, mass, or lump, left lower quadrant

789.35 Abdominal or pelvic swelling, mass or lump, periumbilic

789.36 Abdominal or pelvic swelling, mass, or lump, epigastric

793.6 Nonspecific (abnormal) findings on radiological and other examination of abdominal area, including retroperitoneum

Terms To Know

endometriosis. Aberrant uterine mucosal tissue appearing in areas of the pelvic cavity outside of its normal location, lining the uterus and inflaming surrounding tissues, and can result in infertility and spontaneous abortion.

peritoneum. Strong, continuous membrane that forms the lining of the abdominal and pelvic cavity. The parietal peritoneum, or outer layer, is attached to the abdominopelvic walls and the visceral peritoneum, or inner layer, surrounds the organs inside the abdominal cavity.

retroperitoneal. Located behind the peritoneum, the membrane that lines the abdominopelvic walls and forms a covering for the internal organs.

CCI Version 18.3

0213T, 0216T, 0228T, 0230T, 10021-10022, 12001-12007, 12011-12057, 13100-13153, 36000, 36400-36410, 36420-36430, 36440, 36600, 36640, 37202, 43752, 44950, 44970, 51701-51703, 62310-62319, 64400-64435, 64445-64450, 64479, 64483, 64490, 64493, 64505-64530, 69990, 93000-93010, 93040-93042, 93318, 94002, 94200, 94250, 94680-94690, 94770, 95812-95816, 95819, 95822, 95829, 95955, 96360, 96365, 96372, 96374-96376, 99148-99149, 99150, J0670, J1642, J2001

Note: These CCI edits are used for Medicare. Other payers may reimburse on codes listed above.

Medicare Edits

	Fac RVU	Non-Fac RVU	FUD	Status
49180	2.54	4.75	0	A

	MUE		Modifiers		
49180	3	51	N/A	N/A	N/A

* with documentation

Medicare References: None

49203-49205

49203 Excision or destruction, open, intra-abdominal tumors, cysts or endometriomas, 1 or more peritoneal, mesenteric, or retroperitoneal primary or secondary tumors; largest tumor 5 cm diameter or less

49204 largest tumor 5.1-10.0 cm diameter

49205 largest tumor greater than 10.0 cm diameter

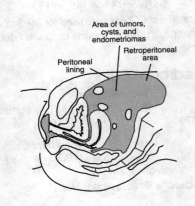

Area of tumors, cysts, and endometriomas

Retroperitoneal area

Peritoneal lining

Explanation

The physician removes or destroys intraabdominal tumors, cysts, or endometriomas (displaced endometrial tissue) or primary or secondary mesenteric, peritoneal, or retroperitoneal tumors. The physician makes a large incision extending from just above the pubic hairline to the rib cage. The growths are removed using a laser, electric cautery, or a scalpel. The incision is closed with sutures. Report 49203 when the diameter of the largest tumor is 5 cm or smaller, 49204 when the diameter is 5.1 to 10 cm, and 49205 when the diameter is larger than 10 cm.

Coding Tips

For laparoscopic fulguration (destruction) or excision of lesions of the ovary, pelvic viscera, or peritoneal surface, see 58662. For resection of recurrent ovarian, tubal, primary peritoneal, or uterine malignancy, see 58957–58958. Do not report these codes with 38770, 38780, 49000, 49010, 49215, 50010, 50205, 50225, 50236, 50250, 50290, or 58900–58960.

ICD-9-CM Procedural

54.3 Excision or destruction of lesion or tissue of abdominal wall or umbilicus

54.4 Excision or destruction of peritoneal tissue

68.23 Endometrial ablation

Anesthesia
00790, 00840

ICD-9-CM Diagnostic

154.0 Malignant neoplasm of rectosigmoid junction

158.0 Malignant neoplasm of retroperitoneum

158.8 Malignant neoplasm of specified parts of peritoneum

171.5 Malignant neoplasm of connective and other soft tissue of abdomen

171.6 Malignant neoplasm of connective and other soft tissue of pelvis

183.0 Malignant neoplasm of ovary — (Use additional code to identify any functional activity)

183.3 Malignant neoplasm of broad ligament of uterus

183.4 Malignant neoplasm of parametrium of uterus

183.5 Malignant neoplasm of round ligament of uterus

183.9 Malignant neoplasm of uterine adnexa, unspecified site

195.2 Malignant neoplasm of abdomen

195.3 Malignant neoplasm of pelvis

197.6 Secondary malignant neoplasm of retroperitoneum and peritoneum

214.3 Lipoma of intra-abdominal organs

228.04 Hemangioma of intra-abdominal structures

235.4 Neoplasm of uncertain behavior of retroperitoneum and peritoneum

614.6 Pelvic peritoneal adhesions, female (postoperative) (postinfection) — (Use additional code to identify organism: 041.00-041.09, 041.10-041.19) (Use additional code to identify any associated infertility: 628.2)

617.0 Endometriosis of uterus

617.1 Endometriosis of ovary

617.2 Endometriosis of fallopian tube

617.3 Endometriosis of pelvic peritoneum

617.5 Endometriosis of intestine

617.8 Endometriosis of other specified sites

789.31 Abdominal or pelvic swelling, mass, or lump, right upper quadrant

789.32 Abdominal or pelvic swelling, mass, or lump, left upper quadrant

789.33 Abdominal or pelvic swelling, mass, or lump, right lower quadrant

789.34 Abdominal or pelvic swelling, mass, or lump, left lower quadrant

789.35 Abdominal or pelvic swelling, mass or lump, periumbilic

CCI Version 18.3
0213T, 0216T, 0228T, 0230T, 12001-12007, 12011-12057, 13100-13153, 36000, 36400-36410, 36420-36430, 36440, 36600, 36640, 37202, 38500, 38770, 38780, 43752, 43832, 44005, 44602-44605, 44820-44850, 44950, 44970, 49040, 49255, 49320, 49322-49323, 49560-49566, 49570-49572, 49580, 49582-49587, 50010, 50205, 50592-50593, 58700-58720, 58805, 58900-58940, 60540-60545, 62310-62319, 64400-64435, 64445-64450, 64479, 64483, 64490, 64493, 64505-64530, 69990, 93000-93010, 93040-93042, 93318, 94002, 94200, 94250, 94680-94690, 94770, 95812-95816, 95819, 95822, 95829, 95955, 96360, 96365, 96372, 96374-96376, 99148-99149, 99150

Also not with 49203: 44180, 47382❖, 49000-49010, 50220, 50280-50290, 58950, 58960

Also not with 49204: 44160-44180, 47370-47371❖, 47380-47382❖, 49000-49010, 49203, 50220-50234, 50250-50290, 50542, 50715, 58200, 58943, 58950-58951, 58956, 58960

Also not with 49205: 44160-44180, 47370-47371❖, 47380-47382❖, 49000-49020, 49203-49204, 50220-50236, 50250-50290, 50542, 50715, 58200, 58943, 58950-58952, 58956-58960

Note: These CCI edits are used for Medicare. Other payers may reimburse on codes listed above.

Medicare Edits

	Fac RVU	Non-Fac RVU	FUD	Status
49203	34.9	34.9	90	A
49204	44.45	44.45	90	A
49205	51.01	51.01	90	A

	MUE			Modifiers	
49203	1	51	N/A	62*	80
49204	1	51	N/A	62*	80
49205	1	51	N/A	62*	80

* with documentation

Medicare References: None

49320

49320 Laparoscopy, abdomen, peritoneum, and omentum, diagnostic, with or without collection of specimen(s) by brushing or washing (separate procedure)

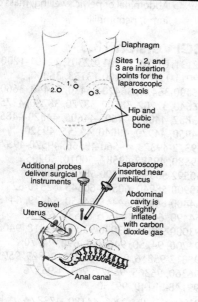

Sites 1, 2, and 3 are insertion points for the laparoscopic tools

Diaphragm

Hip and pubic bone

Additional probes deliver surgical instruments

Laparoscope inserted near umbilicus

Abdominal cavity is slightly inflated with carbon dioxide gas

Bowel Uterus

Anal canal

Explanation

The physician makes a 1.0-centimeter incision in the umbilicus through which the abdomen is inflated and a fiberoptic laparoscope is inserted. Other incisions are also made through which trocars can be passed into the abdominal cavity to deliver instruments, a video camera, and when needed an additional light source. The physician manipulates the tools so that the pelvic organs, peritoneum, abdomen, and omentum can be viewed through the laparoscope and/or video monitor. Biopsy from any or all of the areas observed are obtained by brushing the surface and collecting the cells or by washing (bathing) the area with a saline solution, and suctioning out the cell rich solution. When the procedure is complete, the laparoscope, instruments, and light source are removed and the incisions are closed with sutures. If biopsy of pelvic organs is performed, the physician may also insert an instrument through the vagina to grasp the cervix and pass another instrument through the cervix, into the uterus to manipulate the uterus.

Coding Tips

This separate procedure by definition is usually a component of a more complex service and is not identified separately. When performed alone or with other unrelated procedures or services it may be reported. If performed alone, list the code; if performed with other procedures or services, list the code and append modifier 59. For exploratory laparotomy (open approach), exploratory celiotomy, with or without biopsies, see 49000. For surgical laparoscopy, report a code from the appropriate anatomical section in CPT.

ICD-9-CM Procedural

54.21 Laparoscopy

54.23 Biopsy of peritoneum

54.24 Closed (percutaneous) (needle) biopsy of intra-abdominal mass

65.14 Other laparoscopic diagnostic procedures on ovaries

Anesthesia

49320 00840

ICD-9-CM Diagnostic

The application of this code is too broad to adequately present ICD-9-CM diagnostic code links here. Refer to your ICD-9-CM book.

Terms To Know

biopsy. Tissue or fluid removed for diagnostic purposes through analysis of the cells in the biopsy material.

diagnostic. Examination or procedure to which the patient is subjected, or which is performed on materials derived from a hospital outpatient, to obtain information to aid in the assessment of a medical condition or the identification of a disease. Among these examinations and tests are diagnostic laboratory services such as hematology and chemistry, diagnostic x-rays, isotope studies, EKGs, pulmonary function studies, thyroid function tests, psychological tests, and other tests given to determine the nature and severity of an ailment or injury.

laparoscopy. Direct visualization of the peritoneal cavity, outer fallopian tubes, uterus, and ovaries utilizing a laparoscope, a thin, flexible fiberoptic tube.

omentum. Fold of peritoneal tissue suspended between the stomach and neighboring visceral organs of the abdominal cavity.

peritoneum. Strong, continuous membrane that forms the lining of the abdominal and pelvic cavity. The parietal peritoneum, or outer layer, is attached to the abdominopelvic walls and the visceral peritoneum, or inner layer, surrounds the organs inside the abdominal cavity.

specimen. Tissue cells or sample of fluid taken for analysis, pathologic examination, and diagnosis.

trocar. Cannula or a sharp pointed instrument used to puncture and aspirate fluid from cavities.

CCI Version 18.3

0213T, 0216T, 0228T, 0230T, 12001-12007, 12011-12057, 13100-13153, 36000, 36400-36410, 36420-36430, 36440, 36600, 36640, 37202, 43752, 44005, 47001, 50715, 51701-51703, 57410, 62310-62319, 64400-64435, 64445-64450, 64479, 64483, 64490, 64493, 64505-64530, 69990, 76000-76001, 77001-77002, 93000-93010, 93040-93042, 93318, 94002, 94200, 94250, 94680-94690, 94770, 95812-95816, 95819, 95822, 95829, 95955, 96360, 96365, 96372, 96374-96376, 99148-99149, 99150

Note: These CCI edits are used for Medicare. Other payers may reimburse on codes listed above.

Medicare Edits

	Fac RVU	Non-Fac RVU	FUD	Status
49320	9.59	9.59	10	A

	MUE		Modifiers		
49320	1	51	N/A	N/A	80

* with documentation

Medicare References: None

49321

49321 Laparoscopy, surgical; with biopsy (single or multiple)

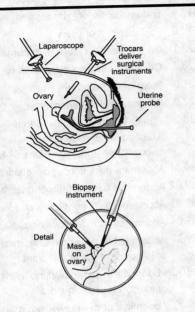

Explanation

The physician makes a 1.0-centimeter incision in the umbilicus through which the abdomen is inflated and a fiberoptic laparoscope is inserted. Other incisions are also made through which trocars can be passed into the abdominal cavity to deliver instruments, a video camera, and when needed an additional light source. The physician manipulates the tools so that the pelvic organs, peritoneum, abdomen and omentum can be viewed through the laparoscope and/or video monitor. Biopsy from any or all of the areas observed are obtained by grasping a sample with a biopsy forceps that is capable of "biting off" small pieces of tissue. When the procedure is complete, the laparoscope, instruments, and light source are removed and the incisions are closed with sutures. If biopsy of pelvic organs is performed, the physician may also insert an instrument through the vagina to grasp the cervix and pass another instrument through the cervix, into the uterus to manipulate the uterus.

Coding Tips

Surgical laparoscopy always includes diagnostic laparoscopy. To report a diagnostic laparoscopy (peritoneoscopy), see 49320. For laparoscopic aspiration (single or multiple), see 49322. For exploratory laparotomy, exploratory celiotomy, with or without biopsies, see 49000.

ICD-9-CM Procedural

54.23	Biopsy of peritoneum
54.24	Closed (percutaneous) (needle) biopsy of intra-abdominal mass
65.14	Other laparoscopic diagnostic procedures on ovaries

Anesthesia

49321 00840

ICD-9-CM Diagnostic

The application of this code is too broad to adequately present ICD-9-CM diagnostic code links here. Refer to your ICD-9-CM book.

Terms To Know

biopsy. Tissue or fluid removed for diagnostic purposes through analysis of the cells in the biopsy material.

forceps. Tool used for grasping or compressing tissue.

laparoscopy. Direct visualization of the peritoneal cavity, outer fallopian tubes, uterus, and ovaries utilizing a laparoscope, a thin, flexible fiberoptic tube.

omentum. Fold of peritoneal tissue suspended between the stomach and neighboring visceral organs of the abdominal cavity.

peritoneum. Strong, continuous membrane that forms the lining of the abdominal and pelvic cavity. The parietal peritoneum, or outer layer, is attached to the abdominopelvic walls and the visceral peritoneum, or inner layer, surrounds the organs inside the abdominal cavity.

trocar. Cannula or a sharp pointed instrument used to puncture and aspirate fluid from cavities.

CCI Version 18.3

0213T, 0216T, 0228T, 0230T, 12001-12007, 12011-12057, 13100-13153, 36000, 36400-36410, 36420-36430, 36440, 36600, 36640, 37202, 43653, 43752, 44005, 44180, 44602-44605, 44950, 44970, 47001, 49320, 50715, 51701-51703, 57410, 62310-62319, 64400-64435, 64445-64450, 64479, 64483, 64490, 64493, 64505-64530, 69990, 76000-76001, 77001-77002, 93000-93010, 93040-93042, 93318, 94002, 94200, 94250, 94680-94690, 94770, 95812-95816, 95819, 95822, 95829, 95955, 96360, 96365, 96372, 96374-96376, 99148-99149, 99150

Note: These CCI edits are used for Medicare. Other payers may reimburse on codes listed above.

Medicare Edits

	Fac RVU	Non-Fac RVU	FUD	Status
49321	10.15	10.15	10	A

	MUE		Modifiers		
49321	1	51	N/A	62	80

* with documentation

Medicare References: None

49322

49322 Laparoscopy, surgical; with aspiration of cavity or cyst (eg, ovarian cyst) (single or multiple)

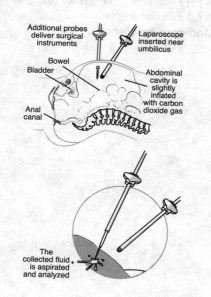

Additional probes deliver surgical instruments

Laparoscope inserted near umbilicus

Bowel
Bladder

Abdominal cavity is slightly inflated with carbon dioxide gas

Anal canal

The collected fluid is aspirated and analyzed

Explanation

The physician makes a 1.0-centimeter incision in the umbilicus through which the abdomen is inflated and a fiberoptic laparoscope is inserted. A second incision is made directly below the umbilicus, just above the pubic hairline, through which a trocar can be passed into the abdominal cavity to deliver instruments. The physician manipulates the tools to view the pelvic organs through the laparoscope. An additional incision may be needed for a second light source. Once the biopsy site is viewed through the laparoscope, a 5.0-centimeter incision is made just above the site. Through this incision, the physician uses an aspirating probe to aspirate a cavity or cyst or to collect fluid for culture. The instruments are removed and the incisions are sutured.

Coding Tips

Surgical laparoscopy always includes diagnostic laparoscopy. For diagnostic laparoscopy only, see 49320. For laparoscopic fulguration or excision of lesions of the ovary, pelvic viscera, or peritoneal surface by any method, see 58662.

ICD-9-CM Procedural

65.11 Aspiration biopsy of ovary
65.91 Aspiration of ovary
66.91 Aspiration of fallopian tube

Anesthesia

49322 00840

ICD-9-CM Diagnostic

179 Malignant neoplasm of uterus, part unspecified
183.0 Malignant neoplasm of ovary — (Use additional code to identify any functional activity)
183.2 Malignant neoplasm of fallopian tube
183.4 Malignant neoplasm of parametrium of uterus
183.9 Malignant neoplasm of uterine adnexa, unspecified site
184.8 Malignant neoplasm of other specified sites of female genital organs
220 Benign neoplasm of ovary — (Use additional code to identify any functional activity: 256.0-256.1)
256.0 Hyperestrogenism
614.0 Acute salpingitis and oophoritis — (Use additional code to identify organism: 041.00-041.09, 041.10-041.19)
614.1 Chronic salpingitis and oophoritis — (Use additional code to identify organism: 041.00-041.09, 041.10-041.19)
614.2 Salpingitis and oophoritis not specified as acute, subacute, or chronic — (Use additional code to identify organism: 041.00-041.09, 041.10-041.19)
614.3 Acute parametritis and pelvic cellulitis — (Use additional code to identify organism: 041.00-041.09, 041.10-041.19)
614.4 Chronic or unspecified parametritis and pelvic cellulitis — (Use additional code to identify organism: 041.00-041.09, 041.10-041.19)
614.6 Pelvic peritoneal adhesions, female (postoperative) (postinfection) — (Use additional code to identify organism: 041.00-041.09, 041.10-041.19) (Use additional code to identify any associated infertility: 628.2)
614.7 Other chronic pelvic peritonitis, female — (Use additional code to identify organism: 041.00-041.09, 041.10-041.19)
614.8 Other specified inflammatory disease of female pelvic organs and tissues — (Use additional code to identify organism: 041.00-041.09, 041.10-041.19)
617.0 Endometriosis of uterus

617.1 Endometriosis of ovary
617.2 Endometriosis of fallopian tube
617.3 Endometriosis of pelvic peritoneum
617.8 Endometriosis of other specified sites
617.9 Endometriosis, site unspecified
620.0 Follicular cyst of ovary
620.1 Corpus luteum cyst or hematoma
620.2 Other and unspecified ovarian cyst
621.0 Polyp of corpus uteri
627.0 Premenopausal menorrhagia
628.2 Female infertility of tubal origin — (Use additional code for any associated peritubal adhesions: 614.6)
789.01 Abdominal pain, right upper quadrant
789.02 Abdominal pain, left upper quadrant
789.03 Abdominal pain, right lower quadrant
789.04 Abdominal pain, left lower quadrant
789.31 Abdominal or pelvic swelling, mass, or lump, right upper quadrant
789.32 Abdominal or pelvic swelling, mass, or lump, left upper quadrant
789.33 Abdominal or pelvic swelling, mass, or lump, right lower quadrant
789.34 Abdominal or pelvic swelling, mass, or lump, left lower quadrant

CCI Version 18.3

0213T, 0216T, 0228T, 0230T, 12001-12007, 12011-12057, 13100-13153, 36000, 36400-36410, 36420-36430, 36440, 36600, 36640, 37202, 43653, 43752, 44005, 44180, 44602-44605, 44950, 44970, 49320, 50715, 51701-51703, 57410, 62310-62319, 64400-64435, 64445-64450, 64479, 64483, 64490, 64493, 64505-64530, 69990, 76000-76001, 77001-77002, 93000-93010, 93040-93042, 93318, 94002, 94200, 94250, 94680-94690, 94770, 95812-95816, 95819, 95822, 95829, 95955, 96360, 96365, 96372, 96374-96376, 99148-99149, 99150

Note: These CCI edits are used for Medicare. Other payers may reimburse on codes listed above.

Medicare Edits

	Fac RVU	Non-Fac RVU	FUD	Status
49322	10.89	10.89	10	A

	MUE		Modifiers		
49322	1	51	N/A	62	80

* with documentation

Medicare References: None

49324-49325

49324 Laparoscopy, surgical; with insertion of tunneled intraperitoneal catheter

49325   with revision of previously placed intraperitoneal cannula or catheter, with removal of intraluminal obstructive material if performed

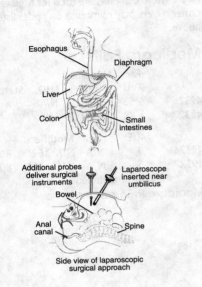

Esophagus

Diaphragm

Liver

Colon

Small intestines

Additional probes deliver surgical instruments

Laparoscope inserted near umbilicus

Bowel

Anal canal

Spine

Side view of laparoscopic surgical approach

Explanation

A permanent intraperitoneal catheter is inserted laparoscopically using a tunneling technique. The physician makes a 1 cm incision in the umbilicus through which the abdomen is inflated and a fiberoptic laparoscope is inserted. Other incisions are also made through which trocars can be passed into the abdominal cavity to deliver additional instruments. The physician manipulates the tools so that the pelvic organs, peritoneum, abdomen, and omentum can be viewed through the laparoscope and/or video monitor. Using various tunneling techniques, the physician inserts the intraperitoneal catheter, positioning the tip inside the peritoneal cavity. A separately reportable subcutaneous extension of the catheter with a remote chest exit site may also be performed. If the physician is revising an intraperitoneal catheter, the catheter is inspected and freed of occlusion or blockage. When either procedure is complete, the laparoscope and other instruments are removed and the incisions are closed with sutures. Report 49324 for the tunneled insertion of an intraperitoneal cannula or catheter and 49325 for its revision.

Coding Tips

Surgical laparoscopy always includes diagnostic laparoscopy. To report a diagnostic laparoscopy (peritoneoscopy), see 49320. Subcutaneous extension of intraperitoneal catheter with remote chest exit site is reported separately, see 49435. For open insertion of permanent tunneled intraperitoneal cannula or catheter, see 49418–49419.

ICD-9-CM Procedural

54.93   Creation of cutaneoperitoneal fistula

54.99   Other operations of abdominal region

Anesthesia

00790, 00840

ICD-9-CM Diagnostic

158.0   Malignant neoplasm of retroperitoneum

158.8   Malignant neoplasm of specified parts of peritoneum

159.9   Malignant neoplasm of ill-defined sites of digestive organs and peritoneum

182.0   Malignant neoplasm of corpus uteri, except isthmus

182.1   Malignant neoplasm of isthmus

182.8   Malignant neoplasm of other specified sites of body of uterus

183.0   Malignant neoplasm of ovary — (Use additional code to identify any functional activity)

183.2   Malignant neoplasm of fallopian tube

183.5   Malignant neoplasm of round ligament of uterus

183.8   Malignant neoplasm of other specified sites of uterine adnexa

184.8   Malignant neoplasm of other specified sites of female genital organs

197.6   Secondary malignant neoplasm of retroperitoneum and peritoneum

198.6   Secondary malignant neoplasm of ovary

789.00 Abdominal pain, unspecified site

789.01 Abdominal pain, right upper quadrant

789.02 Abdominal pain, left upper quadrant

789.03 Abdominal pain, right lower quadrant

789.04 Abdominal pain, left lower quadrant

789.05 Abdominal pain, periumbilic

789.06 Abdominal pain, epigastric

789.07 Abdominal pain, generalized

789.09 Abdominal pain, other specified site

998.59 Other postoperative infection — (Use additional code to identify infection)

Terms To Know

cannula. Tube inserted into a blood vessel, duct, or body cavity to facilitate passage.

catheter. Flexible tube inserted into an area of the body for introducing or withdrawing fluid.

intraperitoneal. Within the cavity or space created by the double-layered sac that lines the abdominopelvic walls and forms a covering for the internal organs.

laparoscopy. Direct visualization of the peritoneal cavity, outer fallopian tubes, uterus, and ovaries utilizing a laparoscope, a thin, flexible fiberoptic tube.

CCI Version 18.3

0213T, 0216T, 0228T, 0230T, 12001-12007, 12011-12057, 13100-13153, 36000, 36400-36410, 36420-36430, 36440, 36600, 36640, 37202, 43653, 43752, 44005, 44180, 44602-44605, 44950, 44970, 49000, 49320, 49400, 49421-49422❖, 50715, 51701-51703, 58660, 62310-62319, 64400-64435, 64445-64450, 64479, 64483, 64490, 64493, 64505-64530, 69990, 76000-76001, 77001-77002, 93000-93010, 93040-93042, 93318, 94002, 94200, 94250, 94680-94690, 94770, 95812-95816, 95819, 95822, 95829, 95955, 96360, 96365, 96372, 96374-96376, 99148-99149, 99150

Also not with 49324: 49436

Also not with 49325: 49324❖

Note: These CCI edits are used for Medicare. Other payers may reimburse on codes listed above.

Medicare Edits

	Fac RVU	Non-Fac RVU	FUD	Status
49324	11.55	11.55	10	A
49325	12.33	12.33	10	A

	MUE		Modifiers		
49324	1	51	N/A	62	80
49325	1	51	N/A	62	80

  * with documentation

Medicare References: None

Coding Companion for Ob/Gyn

© 2012 OptumInsight, Inc.

49326-49327

Abdomen

49326 Laparoscopy, surgical; with omentopexy (omental tacking procedure) (List separately in addition to code for primary procedure)

49327 with placement of interstitial device(s) for radiation therapy guidance (eg, fiducial markers, dosimeter), intra-abdominal, intrapelvic, and/or retroperitoneum, including imaging guidance, if performed, single or multiple (List separately in addition to code for primary procedure)

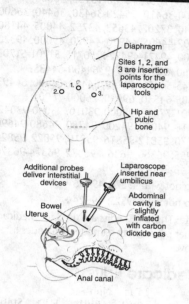

Explanation

Omentum is a strong and highly vascularized serous membrane in the abdomen. The physician makes a 1 cm incision in the umbilicus through which the abdomen is inflated and a fiberoptic laparoscope is inserted. Other incisions are also made through which trocars can be passed into the abdominal cavity to deliver instruments, a video camera, and, when needed, an additional light source. The physician manipulates the tools so the pelvic organs, peritoneum, abdomen, and omentum can be viewed through the laparoscope and/or video monitor. In 49326, the physician isolates the omentum at the stomach and intestine and may cut, suture, or plicate omental tissue to achieve the desired effect. When the procedure is complete, the laparoscope, instruments, and light source are removed and the incisions are closed with sutures. In 49327, the physician, using image guidance if necessary, places one or more interstitial devices such as gold seeds (fiducial markers) for radiation therapy guidance or a dosimeter

to gauge the amount of radiation received into the targeted soft tissue tumor. Allowing for precision in targeting radiation and/or for measuring the radiation doses received, a fiducial marker is visible by ultrasound and fluoroscopy and permits accurate triangulation of the tissue to be treated. A capsule dosimeter relays radiation dose information so that the clinical team can monitor for any deviation between the radiation plan and the actual radiation received. When the procedure is complete, the laparoscope, instruments, and light source are removed and the incisions are closed with sutures.

Coding Tips

As "add-on" codes, 49326 and 49327 are not subject to multiple procedure rules. No reimbursement reduction or modifier 51 is applied. Add-on codes describe additional intra-service work associated with the primary procedure. They are performed by the same physician on the same date of service as the primary service/procedure, and must never be reported as a stand-alone code. Report 49326 in conjunction with 49324 and 49325. Report 49327 in conjunction with laparoscopic abdominal, pelvic, or retroperitoneal procedures performed concurrently. Surgical laparoscopy always includes diagnostic laparoscopy. To report a diagnostic laparoscopy (peritoneoscopy), see 49320. For placement of interstitial devices percutaneously, see 49411; for placement by open method, see 49412.

ICD-9-CM Procedural

54.74 Other repair of omentum

Anesthesia
N/A

ICD-9-CM Diagnostic

The ICD-9-CM diagnostic code(s) would be the same as the actual procedure performed because these are in-addition-to codes.

Terms To Know

interstitial. Within the small spaces or gaps occurring in tissue or organs.

laparoscopy. Direct visualization of the peritoneal cavity, outer fallopian tubes, uterus, and ovaries utilizing a laparoscope, a thin, flexible fiberoptic tube. Laparoscopy can be performed for diagnostic purposes alone or included as part of other surgical procedures accomplished by this approach.

omentum. Fold of peritoneal tissue suspended between the stomach and neighboring visceral organs of the abdominal cavity.

trocar. Cannula or a sharp pointed instrument used to puncture and aspirate fluid from cavities.

CCI Version 18.3

Also not with 49327: 43653, 44005, 44180, 44970, 49320, 50715, 57410, 58660, 76000-76001, 76942, 76998, 77002, 77012, 77021

Note: These CCI edits are used for Medicare. Other payers may reimburse on codes listed above.

Medicare Edits

	Fac RVU	Non-Fac RVU	FUD	Status
49326	5.53	5.53	N/A	A
49327	3.83	3.83	N/A	A

	MUE		Modifiers		
49326	1	N/A	N/A	62*	80
49327	1	N/A	N/A	62*	80

* with documentation

Medicare References: None

Coding Companion for Ob/Gyn

49402

49402 Removal of peritoneal foreign body from peritoneal cavity

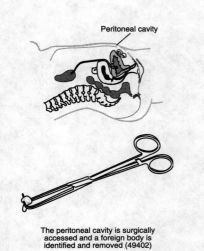
Peritoneal cavity

The peritoneal cavity is surgically accessed and a foreign body is identified and removed (49402)

Explanation
The physician removes a foreign body from the abdominal cavity. The physician makes an abdominal incision and explores the abdominal cavity. The foreign body is identified and removed. The incision is closed.

Coding Tips
For lysis of intestinal adhesions, see 44005.

ICD-9-CM Procedural
54.92 Removal of foreign body from peritoneal cavity

Anesthesia
49402 00790, 00840

ICD-9-CM Diagnostic
789.00 Abdominal pain, unspecified site

868.10 Injury to unspecified intra-abdominal organ, with open wound into cavity

868.13 Peritoneum injury with open wound into cavity

868.19 Injury to other and multiple intra-abdominal organs, with open wound into cavity

996.60 Infection and inflammatory reaction due to unspecified device, implant, and graft — (Use additional code to identify specified infections)

996.62 Infection and inflammatory reaction due to other vascular device, implant,

and graft — (Use additional code to identify specified infections)

996.70 Other complications due to unspecified device, implant, and graft — (Use additional code to identify complication: 338.18-338.19, 338.28-338.29)

998.4 Foreign body accidentally left during procedure, not elsewhere classified

Terms To Know

foreign body. Any object or substance found in an organ and tissue that does not belong under normal circumstances.

peritoneal cavity. Space between the lining of the abdominal wall, or parietal peritoneum, and the surface layer of the abdominal organs, or visceral peritoneum. It contains a thin, watery fluid that keeps the peritoneal surfaces moist.

removal. Process of moving out of or away from, or the fact of being removed.

CCI Version 18.3
0213T, 0216T, 12001-12007, 12011-12057, 13100-13153, 20102, 36000, 36400-36410, 36420-36430, 36440, 36600, 36640, 37202, 43752, 44005, 44180, 44602-44605, 44820-44850, 44950, 44970, 49000-49010, 49255, 49320, 49429, 49560-49566, 49570-49572, 49580, 49582-49587, 51701-51703, 62310-62319, 64400-64435, 64445-64450, 64479, 64483, 64490, 64493, 64505-64530, 69990, 93000-93010, 93040-93042, 93318, 94002, 94200, 94250, 94680-94690, 94770, 95812-95816, 95819, 95822, 95829, 95955, 96360, 96365, 96372, 96374-96376, 99148-99149, 99150

Note: These CCI edits are used for Medicare. Other payers may reimburse on codes listed above.

Medicare Edits

	Fac RVU	Non-Fac RVU	FUD	Status
49402	24.93	24.93	90	A

	MUE		Modifiers		
49402	1	51	N/A	62*	N/A

* with documentation

Medicare References: None

© 2012 OptumInsight, Inc.

49412

49412 Placement of interstitial device(s) for radiation therapy guidance (eg, fiducial markers, dosimeter), open, intra-abdominal, intrapelvic, and/or retroperitoneum, including image guidance, if performed, single or multiple (List separately in addition to code for primary procedure)

Abdomen

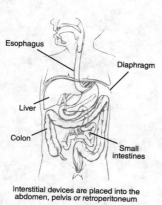

Interstitial devices are placed into the abdomen, pelvis or retroperitoneum

Explanation

The physician places one or more interstitial devices such as gold seeds (fiducial markers) for radiation therapy guidance or a dosimeter to gauge the amount of radiation received into a targeted intra-abdominal, intrapelvic, or retroperitoneal soft tissue tumor. Implanted in conjunction with an open abdominal, pelvic, or retroperitoneal procedure performed concurrently, these act as radiographic landmarks to define the position of the target lesion. Using image guidance if necessary, the physician places a small capsule or seed into the targeted tissue. Allowing for precision in targeting radiation and/or for measuring the radiation doses received, a fiducial marker is visible by ultrasound and fluoroscopy and permits accurate triangulation of the tissue to be treated. A capsule dosimeter relays radiation dose information so that the clinical team can monitor for any deviation between the radiation plan and the actual radiation received. When the procedures are complete, the incisions are closed with sutures.

Coding Tips

As an "add-on" code, 49412 is not subject to multiple procedure rules. No reimbursement reduction or modifier 51 is applied. Add-on

codes describe additional intra-service work associated with the primary procedure. They are performed by the same physician on the same date of service as the primary service/procedure, and must never be reported as a stand-alone code. This code should be reported in conjunction with open abdominal, pelvic, or retroperitoneal procedures performed during the same operative session. When placement of interstitial devices is performed laparoscopically, see 49327; percutaneous placement is reported using 49411. This code includes imaging guidance if performed.

ICD-9-CM Procedural

54.0 Incision of abdominal wall
54.19 Other laparotomy
54.95 Incision of peritoneum
54.99 Other operations of abdominal region
92.29 Other radiotherapeutic procedure

Anesthesia

49412 N/A

ICD-9-CM Diagnostic

The application of this code is too broad to adequately present ICD-9-CM diagnostic code links here. Refer to your ICD-9-CM book.

Terms To Know

dosimetry. Component in the administration of radiation oncology therapy in which a radiation dose is calculated to a specific site, including implant or beam orientation and exposure, isodose strengths, tissue inhomogeneities, and volume.

interstitial. Within the small spaces or gaps occurring in tissue or organs.

intra. Within.

CCI Version 18.3

49327, 76000-76001, 76942, 76998, 77002, 77012, 77021

Note: These CCI edits are used for Medicare. Other payers may reimburse on codes listed above.

Medicare Edits

	Fac RVU	Non-Fac RVU	FUD	Status
49412	2.38	2.38	N/A	A

	MUE		Modifiers	
49412	1	N/A	N/A 62*	80*

* with documentation

Medicare References: None

49435

49435 Insertion of subcutaneous extension to intraperitoneal cannula or catheter with remote chest exit site (List separately in addition to code for primary procedure)

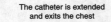

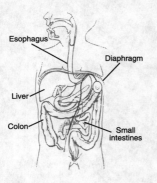

The catheter is extended and exits the chest

Esophagus
Diaphragm
Liver
Colon
Small intestines

List in addition to primary procedure

Explanation

A permanent, subcutaneous intraperitoneal catheter is lengthened with an extension and brought to the surface of the skin during the primary procedure in which a catheter/cannula is established. In the primary procedure, the physician makes a small abdominal incision, opens the peritoneum, and establishes the cannula. In 49435, the physician fits an extension to the cannula and tunnels subcutaneously to accommodate the extension. The physician makes a separate incision in the chest as an exit site for the extension. The extension is brought out through the skin and may be attached to the drug delivery system. The operative incision is closed.

Coding Tips

As an "add-on" code, 49435 is not subject to multiple procedure rules. No reimbursement reduction or modifier 51 is applied. "Add-on" codes describe additional intra-service work associated with the primary procedure. They are performed by the same physician on the same date of service as the primary service/procedure, and must never be reported as a stand-alone code. Report 49435 in conjunction with 49324 or 49421.

ICD-9-CM Procedural

54.99   Other operations of abdominal region

Anesthesia

49435   N/A

ICD-9-CM Diagnostic

The ICD-9-CM diagnostic code(s) would be the same as the actual procedure performed because these are in-addition-to codes.

Terms To Know

cannula. Tube inserted into a blood vessel, duct, or body cavity to facilitate passage.

catheter. Flexible tube inserted into an area of the body for introducing or withdrawing fluid.

insertion. Placement or implantation into a body part.

intraperitoneal. Within the cavity or space created by the double-layered sac that lines the abdominopelvic walls and forms a covering for the internal organs.

subcutaneous. Below the skin.

CCI Version 18.3

No CCI Edits apply to this code.

Medicare Edits

	Fac RVU	Non-Fac RVU	FUD	Status
49435	3.53	3.53	N/A	A

	MUE		Modifiers	
49435	1	N/A	N/A 62*	80

* with documentation

Medicare References: None

Coding Companion for Ob/Gyn

49436

49436 Delayed creation of exit site from embedded subcutaneous segment of intraperitoneal cannula or catheter

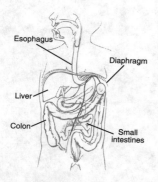

Esophagus
Diaphragm
Liver
Colon
Small intestines

An exit site for the intraperitoneal catheter is created in a subsequent operative session

Explanation

A previously implanted, permanent subcutaneous intraperitoneal catheter is brought to the surface of the skin. The physician makes a small abdominal incision, opens the peritoneum, and locates the end of the existing intraperitoneal cannula. An extension may be fitted to the existing cannula. The physician makes a separate incision as an exit site for the cannula. The cannula is brought out through the skin and may be attached to the drug delivery system. The operative incision is closed.

Coding Tips

To indicate that this is a staged or related procedure performed during the postoperative period by the same physician, append modifier 58. For laparoscopic insertion of intraperitoneal cannula or catheter, see 49324. For revision of previously placed intraperiteonal cannula or catheter with removal of intraluminal obstructive material if performed, see 49325; with omentectomy, see 49326. For insertion of subcutaneous extension at time of laparoscopic placement of intraperitoneal catheter, see 49435.

ICD-9-CM Procedural

54.99   Other operations of abdominal region

Anesthesia

49436   00840

ICD-9-CM Diagnostic

996.74   Other complications due to other vascular device, implant, and graft — (Use additional code to identify complication: 338.18-338.19, 338.28-338.29)

998.59   Other postoperative infection — (Use additional code to identify infection)

Terms To Know

cannula. Tube inserted into a blood vessel, duct, or body cavity to facilitate passage.

catheter. Flexible tube inserted into an area of the body for introducing or withdrawing fluid.

intraperitoneal. Within the cavity or space created by the double-layered sac that lines the abdominopelvic walls and forms a covering for the internal organs.

subcutaneous. Below the skin.

CCI Version 18.3

0213T, 0216T, 12001-12007, 12011-12057, 13100-13153, 36000, 36400-36410, 36420-36430, 36440, 36600, 36640, 37202, 43752, 51701-51703, 62310-62319, 64400-64435, 64445-64450, 64479, 64483, 64490, 64493, 64505-64530, 69990, 93000-93010, 93040-93042, 93318, 94002, 94200, 94250, 94680-94690, 94770, 95812-95816, 95819, 95822, 95829, 95955, 96360, 96365, 96372, 96374-96376, 99148-99149, 99150

Note: These CCI edits are used for Medicare. Other payers may reimburse on codes listed above.

Medicare Edits

	Fac RVU	Non-Fac RVU	FUD	Status
49436	5.44	5.44	10	A

	MUE		Modifiers		
49436	1	51	N/A	62*	80

* with documentation

Medicare References: None

Coding Companion for Ob/Gyn

49904-49905

49904 Omental flap, extra-abdominal (eg, for reconstruction of sternal and chest wall defects)

49905 Omental flap, intra-abdominal (List separately in addition to code for primary procedure)

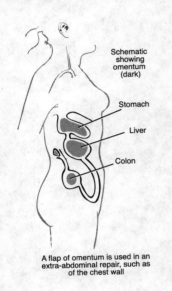

Schematic showing omentum (dark)

Stomach

Liver

Colon

A flap of omentum is used in an extra-abdominal repair, such as of the chest wall

Explanation

The physician mobilizes an omental flap for reconstruction of a defect. The surgical recipient site of the flap is prepared. An upper abdominal transverse or midline incision is made. A laparotomy and manual exploration of the abdominal cavity is done first and the omentum and transverse colon are delivered from the cavity. The omentum is dissected from the transverse colon from left to right and small vessels are ligated. When completely separated from the transverse colon, the omentum is dissected from the stomach with careful clamping, division, and ligation of vessels. The omentum is fully mobilized and pedicled on the right or left gastroepiploic vessel, depending on the purpose. More incisions and tunneling may be necessary to bring the flap into its new location to fill a defect. The flap may be used as a pedicled transposition flap or a free microvascular transfer flap. Report 49904 when the flap is transpositioned to repair an extra-abdominal defect, such as chest wounds after radiation and mastectomy or lower extremity trauma wounds. Report 49905 when the omental flap is repositioned to repair a defect intra-abdominally.

Coding Tips

As an "add-on" code, 49905 is not subject to multiple procedure rules. No reimbursement reduction or modifier 51 is applied. "Add-on" codes describe additional intra-service work associated with the primary procedure. They are performed by the same physician on the same date of service as the primary service/procedure, and must never be reported as a stand-alone code. Harvesting and transfer of the flap are included in 49904. If another surgeon harvests the flap, then both should report 49904 with modifier 62, denoting two surgeons.

ICD-9-CM Procedural

34.79 Other repair of chest wall

53.9 Other hernia repair

54.74 Other repair of omentum

Anesthesia

49904 00790

49905 N/A

ICD-9-CM Diagnostic

171.4 Malignant neoplasm of connective and other soft tissue of thorax

172.5 Malignant melanoma of skin of trunk, except scrotum

174.0 Malignant neoplasm of nipple and areola of female breast — (Use additional code to identify estrogen receptor status: V86.0-V86.1)

174.1 Malignant neoplasm of central portion of female breast — (Use additional code to identify estrogen receptor status: V86.0-V86.1)

174.2 Malignant neoplasm of upper-inner quadrant of female breast — (Use additional code to identify estrogen receptor status: V86.0-V86.1)

174.3 Malignant neoplasm of lower-inner quadrant of female breast — (Use additional code to identify estrogen receptor status: V86.0-V86.1)

174.4 Malignant neoplasm of upper-outer quadrant of female breast — (Use additional code to identify estrogen receptor status: V86.0-V86.1)

174.5 Malignant neoplasm of lower-outer quadrant of female breast — (Use additional code to identify estrogen receptor status: V86.0-V86.1)

174.6 Malignant neoplasm of axillary tail of female breast — (Use additional code to identify estrogen receptor status: V86.0-V86.1)

174.8 Malignant neoplasm of other specified sites of female breast — (Use

additional code to identify estrogen receptor status: V86.0-V86.1)

174.9 Malignant neoplasm of breast (female), unspecified site — (Use additional code to identify estrogen receptor status: V86.0-V86.1)

756.6 Congenital anomaly of diaphragm

875.0 Open wound of chest (wall), without mention of complication

875.1 Open wound of chest (wall), complicated

879.2 Open wound of abdominal wall, anterior, without mention of complication

879.3 Open wound of abdominal wall, anterior, complicated

879.5 Open wound of abdominal wall, lateral, complicated

998.31 Disruption of internal operation (surgical) wound

998.32 Disruption of external operation (surgical) wound

998.83 Non-healing surgical wound

CCI Version 18.3

43752, 44005, 44180, 44602-44605, 44820-44850, 49255, 49320, 49400, 49570, 69990

Also not with 49904: 0213T, 0216T, 0228T, 0230T, 12001-12007, 12011-12057, 13100-13153, 36000, 36400-36410, 36420-36430, 36440, 36600, 36640, 37202, 49000-49010, 49905-49906❖, 51701-51703, 62310-62319, 64400-64435, 64445-64450, 64479, 64483, 64490, 64493, 64505-64530, 93000-93010, 93040-93042, 93318, 94002, 94200, 94250, 94680-94690, 94770, 95812-95816, 95819, 95822, 95829, 95955, 96360, 96365, 96372, 96374-96376, 99148-99149, 99150

Also not with 49905: 49000, 49010, 49906❖

Note: These CCI edits are used for Medicare. Other payers may reimburse on codes listed above.

Medicare Edits

	Fac RVU	Non-Fac RVU	FUD	Status
49904	42.98	42.98	90	A
49905	10.33	10.33	N/A	A

	MUE		Modifiers		
49904	1	51	N/A	62*	N/A
49905	1	N/A	N/A	62	80

* with documentation

Medicare References: None

Coding Companion for Ob/Gyn

50722

50722 Ureterolysis for ovarian vein syndrome

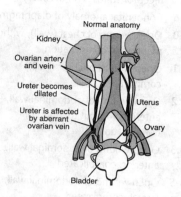

Normal anatomy
Kidney
Ovarian artery and vein
Ureter becomes dilated
Ureter is affected by aberrant ovarian vein
Uterus
Ovary
Bladder

Physician surgically frees ureter from obstruction caused by ovarian vein syndrome

Explanation

The physician surgically frees the ureter from ureteral obstruction caused by aberrant ovarian veins (ovarian vein syndrome). To access the ureter, the physician makes an incision in the skin above the pubic hairline, and cuts the muscles, fat, and fibrous membranes (fascia) overlying the ureter. The physician incises surrounding adhesions to free the ureter from the obstructing ovarian veins. The physician places a drain tube, bringing it out through a separate stab incision in the skin, and performs a layered closure.

Coding Tips

For excision of urethral diverticulum, see 53230. For excision of urethral polyps, see 53260.

ICD-9-CM Procedural

59.02 Other lysis of perirenal or periureteral adhesions

Anesthesia

50722 00860

ICD-9-CM Diagnostic

593.4 Other ureteric obstruction

593.89 Other specified disorder of kidney and ureter

Terms To Know

aberrant. Deviation or departure from the normal or usual course, condition, or pattern.

adhesion. Abnormal fibrous connection between two structures, soft tissue or bony structures, that may occur as the result of surgery, infection, or trauma.

lysis. Destruction, breakdown, dissolution, or decomposition of cells or substances by a specific catalyzing agent.

obstruction. Blockage that prevents normal function of the valve or structure.

ovarian vein syndrome. Retroperitoneal structures involving and often obstructing the ureters following certain types of chemical treatment; there is no identified cause.

ureterolysis. Surgical procedure to release or free the ureter from surrounding obstructive retroperitoneal fibrotic tissue (CPT code 50715), free the ureter from adhesions caused by obstructive ovarian veins (50722), or divide and reconnect to free the ureter from an obstructive aberrant position behind the vena cava (50725).

CCI Version 18.3

00910, 0213T, 0216T, 0228T, 0230T, 12001-12007, 12011-12057, 13100-13153, 36000, 36400-36410, 36420-36430, 36440, 36600, 36640, 37202, 43752, 44602-44605, 44850, 44950, 44970, 49000-49010, 50600-50605, 50715, 50900, 51701-51703, 62310-62319, 64400-64435, 64445-64450, 64479, 64483, 64490, 64493, 64505-64530, 69990, 93000-93010, 93040-93042, 93318, 94002, 94200, 94250, 94680-94690, 94770, 95812-95816, 95819, 95822, 95829, 95955, 96360, 96365, 96372, 96374-96376, 99148-99149, 99150

Note: These CCI edits are used for Medicare. Other payers may reimburse on codes listed above.

Medicare Edits

	Fac RVU	Non-Fac RVU	FUD	Status
50722	31.11	31.11	90	A

	MUE		Modifiers	
50722	1	51	N/A	62*	80

* with documentation

Medicare References: None

51020-51030

51020 Cystotomy or cystostomy; with fulguration and/or insertion of radioactive material

51030 with cryosurgical destruction of intravesical lesion

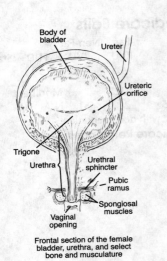

Frontal section of the female bladder, urethra, and select bone and musculature

Explanation

The physician makes an incision (cystotomy) or creates an opening (cystostomy) into the bladder to destroy abnormal tissue. To access the bladder, the physician makes an incision in the skin of the lower abdomen and cuts the corresponding muscles, fat, fibrous membranes (fascia), and bladder wall. Report 51020 if the physician uses electric current (fulguration) or (usually with the aid of a radiation oncologist) inserts radioactive material to destroy a lesion on the bladder. Report 51030 if the physician uses cryosurgery to destroy the lesion. The bladder wall and lower abdomen is sutured closed. If a cystostomy is made, the cystostomy tube is sutured in place and the bladder and abdominal wall is closed.

Coding Tips

For a cystotomy with insertion of a ureteral catheter or stent, see 51045.

ICD-9-CM Procedural

57.18 Other suprapubic cystostomy

57.19 Other cystotomy

92.27 Implantation or insertion of radioactive elements

Anesthesia

00860

ICD-9-CM Diagnostic

188.0 Malignant neoplasm of trigone of urinary bladder

188.1 Malignant neoplasm of dome of urinary bladder

188.2 Malignant neoplasm of lateral wall of urinary bladder

188.3 Malignant neoplasm of anterior wall of urinary bladder

188.4 Malignant neoplasm of posterior wall of urinary bladder

188.5 Malignant neoplasm of bladder neck

188.6 Malignant neoplasm of ureteric orifice

188.7 Malignant neoplasm of urachus

188.8 Malignant neoplasm of other specified sites of bladder

198.1 Secondary malignant neoplasm of other urinary organs

223.3 Benign neoplasm of bladder

233.7 Carcinoma in situ of bladder

236.7 Neoplasm of uncertain behavior of bladder

239.4 Neoplasm of unspecified nature of bladder

596.9 Unspecified disorder of bladder — (Use additional code to identify urinary incontinence: 625.6, 788.30-788.39)

788.99 Other symptoms involving urinary system

Terms To Know

benign. Mild or nonmalignant in nature.

carcinoma in situ. Malignancy that arises from the cells of the vessel, gland, or organ of origin that remains confined to that site or has not invaded neighboring tissue.

cryosurgery. Application of intense cold, usually produced using liquid nitrogen, to locally freeze diseased or unwanted tissue and induce tissue necrosis without causing harm to adjacent tissue.

cystostomy. Formation of an opening through the abdominal wall into the bladder.

cystotomy. Surgical incision into the gallbladder or urinary bladder.

destruction. Ablation or eradication of a structure or tissue.

electrocautery. Division or cutting of tissue using high-frequency electrical current to produce heat, which destroys cells.

fulguration. Destruction of living tissue by using sparks from a high-frequency electric current.

malignant. Any condition tending to progress toward death, specifically an invasive tumor with a loss of cellular differentiation that has the ability to spread or metastasize to other areas in the body.

CCI Version 18.3

00910, 0213T, 0216T, 0228T, 0230T, 12001-12007, 12011-12057, 13100-13153, 36000, 36400-36410, 36420-36430, 36440, 36600, 36640, 37202, 43752, 44602-44605, 44950, 44970, 49000-49002, 49320, 50715, 51045, 51100-51102, 51520-51525, 51701-51703, 62310-62319, 64400-64435, 64445-64450, 64479, 64483, 64490, 64493, 64505-64530, 69990, 93000-93010, 93040-93042, 93318, 94002, 94200, 94250, 94680-94690, 94770, 95812-95816, 95819, 95822, 95829, 95955, 96360, 96365, 96372, 96374-96376, 99148-99149, 99150

Note: These CCI edits are used for Medicare. Other payers may reimburse on codes listed above.

Medicare Edits

	Fac RVU	Non-Fac RVU	FUD	Status
51020	13.92	13.92	90	A
51030	13.75	13.75	90	A

	MUE			Modifiers	
51020	1	51	N/A	62*	80
51030	1	51	N/A	N/A	80*

* with documentation

Medicare References: None

Coding Companion for Ob/Gyn

51045

51045 Cystotomy, with insertion of ureteral catheter or stent (separate procedure)

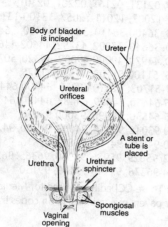

Body of bladder is incised

Ureter

Ureteral orifices

A stent or tube is placed

Urethra

Urethral sphincter

Spongiosal muscles

Vaginal opening

Bladder

Explanation

The physician makes an incision in the bladder to insert a catheter or slender tube (stent) into the ureter. To access the bladder and ureters, the physician makes a midline incision in the skin of the abdomen and cuts the corresponding muscles, fat, and fibrous membranes (fascia). The physician incises the bladder (cystotomy) and inserts a stent or catheter in the ureter. Insertion of a ureteral catheter requires that the physician bring the tube end out through the urethra or bladder incision. The physician inserts a drain tube and performs a layered closure.

Coding Tips

This separate procedure by definition is usually a component of a more complex service and is not identified separately. When performed alone or with other unrelated procedures or services it may be reported. If performed alone, list the code; if performed with other procedures or services, list the code and append modifier 59. For a bladder incision for drainage, fulguration, insertion of radioactive material, and/or cryosurgical destruction of lesions, see 51020–51030.

ICD-9-CM Procedural

57.19   Other cystotomy

Anesthesia

51045   00860

ICD-9-CM Diagnostic

592.1   Calculus of ureter
593.3   Stricture or kinking of ureter
593.4   Other ureteric obstruction
593.5   Hydroureter
593.82   Ureteral fistula
599.60   Urinary obstruction, unspecified — (Use additional code to identify urinary incontinence: 625.6, 788.30-788.39)
599.69   Urinary obstruction, not elsewhere classified — (Use additional code to identify urinary incontinence: 625.6, 788.30-788.39. Code, if applicable, any causal condition first: 600.0-600.9, with fifth-digit 1)
599.70   Hematuria, unspecified
599.71   Gross hematuria
599.72   Microscopic hematuria
867.2   Ureter injury without mention of open wound into cavity
867.3   Ureter injury with open wound into cavity

Terms To Know

calculus. Abnormal, stone-like concretion of calcium, cholesterol, mineral salts, or other substances that forms in any part of the body.

catheter. Flexible tube inserted into an area of the body for introducing or withdrawing fluid.

cystotomy. Surgical incision into the gallbladder or urinary bladder.

fistula. Abnormal tube-like passage between two body cavities or organs or from an organ to the outside surface.

hematuria. Blood in urine, which may present as gross visible blood or as the presence of red blood cells visible only under a microscope.

hydroureter. Abnormal enlargement or distension of the ureter with water or urine caused by an obstruction.

stent. Tube to provide support in a body cavity or lumen.

stricture. Narrowing of an anatomical structure.

CCI Version 18.3

00910, 0213T, 0216T, 0228T, 0230T, 12001-12007, 12011-12057, 13100-13153, 36000, 36400-36410, 36420-36430, 36440, 36600, 36640, 37202, 43752, 44602-44605, 44950, 44970, 49000-49002, 49320, 50715, 51701-51703, 62310-62319, 64400-64435, 64445-64450, 64479, 64483, 64490, 64493,

64505-64530, 69990, 93000-93010, 93040-93042, 93318, 94002, 94200, 94250, 94680-94690, 94770, 95812-95816, 95819, 95822, 95829, 95955, 96360, 96365, 96372, 96374-96376, 99148-99149, 99150

Note: These CCI edits are used for Medicare. Other payers may reimburse on codes listed above.

Medicare Edits

	Fac RVU	Non-Fac RVU	FUD	Status
51045	14.5	14.5	90	A

	MUE		Modifiers		
51045	2	51	N/A	N/A	80

* with documentation

Medicare References: None

51100-51102

51100 Aspiration of bladder; by needle
51101 by trocar or intracatheter
51102 with insertion of suprapubic catheter

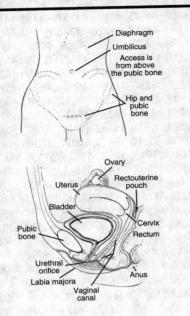

Diaphragm
Umbilicus
Access is from above the pubic bone
Hip and pubic bone

Ovary
Rectouterine pouch
Uterus
Bladder
Cervix
Rectum
Pubic bone
Urethral orifice
Anus
Labia majora
Vaginal canal

Explanation
In 51100, the physician inserts a needle through the skin into the bladder to withdraw urine. In 51101, the physician inserts a trocar or intracatheter through the skin into the bladder. In 51102, a suprapubic catheter is placed into the bladder. This procedure may also be performed after the abdomen has been surgically incised.

Coding Tips
Local anesthesia is included in these services. However, these procedures may be performed under general anesthesia, depending on the age and/or condition of the patient. If a specimen is transported to an outside laboratory, report 99000 for handling or conveyance.

ICD-9-CM Procedural
57.11 Percutaneous aspiration of bladder
57.17 Percutaneous cystostomy
57.18 Other suprapubic cystostomy

Anesthesia
00800

ICD-9-CM Diagnostic
188.0 Malignant neoplasm of trigone of urinary bladder
188.2 Malignant neoplasm of lateral wall of urinary bladder

188.3 Malignant neoplasm of anterior wall of urinary bladder
188.4 Malignant neoplasm of posterior wall of urinary bladder
188.5 Malignant neoplasm of bladder neck
188.6 Malignant neoplasm of ureteric orifice
344.61 Cauda equina syndrome with neurogenic bladder
590.00 Chronic pyelonephritis without lesion of renal medullary necrosis — (Use additional code to identify organism, such as E. coli, 041.41-041.49. Code if applicable, any causal condition first)
590.3 Pyeloureteritis cystica — (Use additional code to identify organism, such as E. coli, 041.41-041.49)
590.81 Pyelitis or pyelonephritis in diseases classified elsewhere — (Use additional code to identify organism, such as E. coli, 041.41-041.49. Code first underlying disease: 016.0)
593.70 Vesicoureteral reflux, unspecified or without reflex nephropathy
595.0 Acute cystitis — (Use additional code to identify organism, such as E. coli: 041.41-041.49)
595.1 Chronic interstitial cystitis — (Use additional code to identify organism, such as E. coli: 041.41-041.49)
595.3 Trigonitis — (Use additional code to identify organism, such as E. coli: 041.41-041.49)
595.4 Cystitis in diseases classified elsewhere — (Use additional code to identify organism, such as E. coli: 041.41-041.49. Code first underlying disease: 006.8, 039.8, 120.0-120.9, 122.3, 122.6)
599.0 Urinary tract infection, site not specified — (Use additional code to identify organism, such as E. coli: 041.41-041.49)
599.70 Hematuria, unspecified
599.71 Gross hematuria
599.72 Microscopic hematuria
625.6 Female stress incontinence
753.6 Congenital atresia and stenosis of urethra and bladder neck
783.5 Polydipsia
788.1 Dysuria
788.21 Incomplete bladder emptying — (Code, if applicable, any causal condition first, such as: 600.0-600.9, with fifth digit 1)

788.29 Other specified retention of urine — (Code, if applicable, any causal condition first, such as: 600.0-600.9, with fifth digit 1)
788.41 Urinary frequency — (Code, if applicable, any causal condition first, such as: 600.0-600.9, with fifth digit 1)
788.42 Polyuria — (Code, if applicable, any causal condition first, such as: 600.0-600.9, with fifth digit 1)
788.43 Nocturia — (Code, if applicable, any causal condition first, such as: 600.0-600.9, with fifth digit 1)
788.63 Urgency of urination — (Code, if applicable, any causal condition first, such as: 600.0-600.9, with fifth digit 1)
867.0 Bladder and urethra injury without mention of open wound into cavity
997.5 Urinary complications — (Use additional code to identify complications)

CCI Version 18.3
00910, 0213T, 0216T, 0228T, 0230T, 12001-12007, 12011-12057, 13100-13153, 36000, 36400-36410, 36420-36430, 36440, 36600, 36640, 37202, 43752, 44970, 62310-62319, 64400-64435, 64445-64450, 64479, 64483, 64490, 64493, 64505-64530, 69990, 93000-93010, 93040-93042, 93318, 94002, 94200, 94250, 94680-94690, 94770, 95812-95816, 95819, 95822, 95829, 95955, 96360, 96365, 96372, 96374-96376, 99148-99149, 99150, J0670, J2001

Also not with 51100: 51701

Also not with 51101: 51100, 51701, 76000-76001, 77001

Also not with 51102: 51100-51101❖, 51701-51702, 52281, 76000-76001, 77001

Note: These CCI edits are used for Medicare. Other payers may reimburse on codes listed above.

Medicare Edits

	Fac RVU	Non-Fac RVU	FUD	Status
51100	1.15	1.81	0	A
51101	1.56	3.76	0	A
51102	4.34	6.81	0	A

	MUE		Modifiers		
51100	1	51	N/A	N/A	N/A
51101	1	51	N/A	N/A	N/A
51102	1	51	N/A	N/A	N/A

* with documentation

Medicare References: None

Bladder

51597

51597 Pelvic exenteration, complete, for vesical, prostatic or urethral malignancy, with removal of bladder and ureteral transplantations, with or without hysterectomy and/or abdominoperineal resection of rectum and colon and colostomy, or any combination thereof

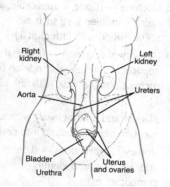

A complete pelvic exenteration is performed. The bladder is removed and the distal ureters are transplanted. A hysterectomy may be performed, as well as resection of the rectum and colon with construction of colostomy

Explanation

The physician removes the bladder, lower ureters, lymph nodes, urethra, prostate (if applicable), colon, and rectum, due to a vesical, prostatic, or urethral malignancy. To access the bladder and ureters, the physician makes a midline incision in the skin of the abdomen and cuts the corresponding muscles, fat, and fibrous membranes (fascia). The physician dissects and ligates the hypogastric and vesical vessels, and severs the bladder, urethra, lower ureters, lymph nodes, and prostate (if applicable) from surrounding structures. The physician removes the bladder and diverts urine flow by transplanting the ureters to the skin or colon. The vagina and uterus (if applicable) and/or rectum and part of the colon may be removed and an artificial abdominal opening in the skin surface created for waste (colostomy). After completing the urinary diversion procedure, the physician inserts drain tubes and performs a layered closure.

Coding Tips

Pelvic exenteration for a gynecological malignancy is reported with 58240.

ICD-9-CM Procedural

40.3   Regional lymph node excision

40.54   Radical groin dissection
46.13   Permanent colostomy
48.50   Abdominoperineal resection of the rectum, not otherwise specified
48.52   Open abdominoperineal resection of the rectum
48.59   Other abdominoperineal resection of the rectum
56.61   Formation of other cutaneous ureterostomy
56.71   Urinary diversion to intestine
57.71   Radical cystectomy
68.8   Pelvic evisceration

Anesthesia

51597   00848

ICD-9-CM Diagnostic

188.0   Malignant neoplasm of trigone of urinary bladder
188.1   Malignant neoplasm of dome of urinary bladder
188.2   Malignant neoplasm of lateral wall of urinary bladder
188.3   Malignant neoplasm of anterior wall of urinary bladder
188.4   Malignant neoplasm of posterior wall of urinary bladder
188.5   Malignant neoplasm of bladder neck
188.6   Malignant neoplasm of ureteric orifice
188.8   Malignant neoplasm of other specified sites of bladder
188.9   Malignant neoplasm of bladder, part unspecified
189.3   Malignant neoplasm of urethra
197.5   Secondary malignant neoplasm of large intestine and rectum
198.1   Secondary malignant neoplasm of other urinary organs
198.6   Secondary malignant neoplasm of ovary
198.82 Secondary malignant neoplasm of genital organs

Terms To Know

exenteration. Surgical removal of the entire contents of a body cavity, such as the pelvis or orbit.

malignant neoplasm. Any cancerous tumor or lesion exhibiting uncontrolled tissue growth that can progressively invade other parts of the body with its disease-generating cells.

secondary. Second in order of occurrence or importance, or appearing during the course of another disease or condition.

CCI Version 18.3

00910, 0213T, 0216T, 0226T, 0228T, 0230T, 0249T, 0288T, 12001-12007, 12011-12057, 13100-13153, 36000, 36400-36410, 36420-36430, 36440, 36600, 36640, 37202, 38562-38564, 38571-38572, 38770, 38780, 43752, 44005, 44140-44151, 44155-44158, 44180, 44188, 44320-44346, 44602-44605, 44620-44625, 44820-44850, 44950-44970, 45110-45135, 45160, 45171-45172, 45190, 45395-45397, 45505, 45540, 46080-46200, 46220-46280, 46285, 46600, 46940-46942, 46947, 49000-49020, 49040, 49082-49084, 49203-49205, 49255, 49320, 49560-49566, 49570, 49580, 49582-49587, 50650, 50715, 50800, 50810-50815, 50820, 50860, 51040-51045, 51520-51525, 51550-51596, 51701-51703, 55821-55845, 55866, 57106, 57410, 57530-57556, 58100, 58120-58200, 58210-58263, 58267-58280, 58290-58294, 58541-58544, 58548, 58558, 58570-58573, 58660, 58662, 58950-58958, 62310-62319, 64400-64435, 64445-64450, 64479, 64483, 64490, 64493, 64505-64530, 69990, 93000-93010, 93040-93042, 93318, 94002, 94200, 94250, 94680-94690, 94770, 95812-95816, 95819, 95822, 95829, 95955, 96360, 96365, 96372, 96374-96376, 99148-99149, 99150, P9612

Note: These CCI edits are used for Medicare. Other payers may reimburse on codes listed above.

Medicare Edits

	Fac RVU	Non-Fac RVU	FUD	Status
51597	67.91	67.91	90	A

	MUE			Modifiers	
51597	1	51	N/A	62*	80

* with documentation

Medicare References: None

Coding Companion for Ob/Gyn

51701-51703

51701 Insertion of non-indwelling bladder catheter (eg, straight catheterization for residual urine)

51702 Insertion of temporary indwelling bladder catheter; simple (eg, Foley)

51703 complicated (eg, altered anatomy, fractured catheter/balloon)

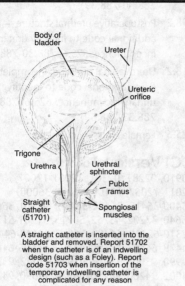

A straight catheter is inserted into the bladder and removed. Report 51702 when the catheter is of an indwelling design (such as a Foley). Report code 51703 when insertion of the temporary indwelling catheter is complicated for any reason

Explanation

The patient is catheterized with a non-indwelling bladder catheter (e.g., for residual urine) in 51701; simple catheterization with a temporary indwelling bladder catheter (Foley) is performed in 51702. The area is properly cleaned and sterilized. A water-soluble lubricant may be injected into the urethra before catheterization begins. The distal part of the catheter is coated with lubricant. The catheter is gently inserted until urine is noted. With an indwelling catheter, insertion continues into the bladder until the retention balloon can be inflated. The catheter is gently pulled until the retention balloon is snuggled against the neck of the bladder. The catheter is secured to the abdomen or thigh and the drainage bag is secured below bladder level. Report 51703 if a change in anatomy or a fractured catheter or balloon complicate the catheterization process.

Coding Tips

Codes 51701 and 51702 should not be reported in addition to any other procedure that includes catheter insertion as a component. Report 51701 and 51702 only when performed independently. Supplies used when providing this procedure may be reported with the appropriate HCPCS Level II

code. Check with the specific payer to determine coverage.

ICD-9-CM Procedural

57.94 Insertion of indwelling urinary catheter

57.95 Replacement of indwelling urinary catheter

57.99 Other operations on bladder

Anesthesia
00910

ICD-9-CM Diagnostic

188.2 Malignant neoplasm of lateral wall of urinary bladder

188.3 Malignant neoplasm of anterior wall of urinary bladder

188.4 Malignant neoplasm of posterior wall of urinary bladder

189.3 Malignant neoplasm of urethra

233.7 Carcinoma in situ of bladder

593.3 Stricture or kinking of ureter

594.0 Calculus in diverticulum of bladder

594.2 Calculus in urethra

595.0 Acute cystitis — (Use additional code to identify organism, such as E. coli: 041.41-041.49)

595.1 Chronic interstitial cystitis — (Use additional code to identify organism, such as E. coli: 041.41-041.49)

595.2 Other chronic cystitis — (Use additional code to identify organism, such as E. coli: 041.41-041.49)

596.4 Atony of bladder — (Use additional code to identify urinary incontinence: 625.6, 788.30-788.39)

596.51 Hypertonicity of bladder — (Use additional code to identify urinary incontinence: 625.6, 788.30-788.39)

598.2 Postoperative urethral stricture — (Use additional code to identify urinary incontinence: 625.6, 788.30-788.39)

599.1 Urethral fistula

599.5 Prolapsed urethral mucosa

599.71 Gross hematuria

599.72 Microscopic hematuria

618.01 Cystocele without mention of uterine prolapse, midline — (Use additional code to identify urinary incontinence: 625.6, 788.31, 788.33-788.39)

618.02 Cystocele without mention of uterine prolapse, lateral — (Use additional code to identify urinary incontinence: 625.6, 788.31, 788.33-788.39)

618.03 Urethrocele without mention of uterine prolapse — (Use additional

code to identify urinary incontinence: 625.6, 788.31, 788.33-788.39)

618.81 Incompetence or weakening of pubocervical tissue — (Use additional code to identify urinary incontinence: 625.6, 788.31, 788.33-788.39)

618.82 Incompetence or weakening of rectovaginal tissue — (Use additional code to identify urinary incontinence: 625.6, 788.31, 788.33-788.39)

618.83 Pelvic muscle wasting — (Use additional code to identify urinary incontinence: 625.6, 788.31, 788.33-788.39)

625.6 Female stress incontinence

788.1 Dysuria

788.21 Incomplete bladder emptying — (Code, if applicable, any causal condition first, such as: 600.0-600.9, with fifth digit 1)

788.41 Urinary frequency — (Code, if applicable, any causal condition first, such as: 600.0-600.9, with fifth digit 1)

788.42 Polyuria — (Code, if applicable, any causal condition first, such as: 600.0-600.9, with fifth digit 1)

788.91 Functional urinary incontinence

CCI Version 18.3

13102, 13122, 13133, 13153, 36400-36406, 36420-36430, 36440, 36600, 69990, 93000-93010, 93040-93042, 93318, 94002, 94200, 94250, 94680-94690, 94770, 95812-95816, 95819, 95822, 95829, 95955, 96360, 96365, 96372, 96374-96376, 99148-99149, 99150, J0670, J2001

Also not with 51701: P9612-P9615❖

Also not with 51702: 51701, P9612

Also not with 51703: 37202, 51700-51702, 53080, 62318-62319, 64415, 64417, 64450, P9612

Note: These CCI edits are used for Medicare. Other payers may reimburse on codes listed above.

Medicare Edits

	Fac RVU	Non-Fac RVU	FUD	Status
51701	0.81	1.68	0	A
51702	0.89	2.17	0	A
51703	2.41	3.93	0	A

	MUE		Modifiers		
51701	2	51	N/A	N/A	N/A
51702	2	51	N/A	N/A	N/A
51703	2	51	N/A	N/A	N/A

* with documentation

Medicare References: None

Coding Companion for Ob/Gyn

© 2012 OptumInsight, Inc.

Bladder

51725-51729

51725 Simple cystometrogram (CMG) (eg, spinal manometer)

51726 Complex cystometrogram (ie, calibrated electronic equipment);

51727 with urethral pressure profile studies (ie, urethral closure pressure profile), any technique

51728 with voiding pressure studies (ie, bladder voiding pressure), any technique

51729 with voiding pressure studies (ie, bladder voiding pressure) and urethral pressure profile studies (ie, urethral closure pressure profile), any technique

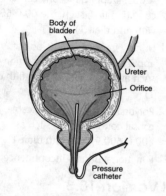

A pressure catheter is introduced into the bladder and connected to a manometer to measure pressure in the lower urinary tract (51725)

Explanation

A cystometrogram (a graphic record of urinary bladder pressure at different volumes) is used to distinguish bladder outlet obstruction from other voiding dysfunctions. For a simple cystometrogram (51725), the physician inserts a pressure catheter into the bladder and connects it to a manometer line filled with fluid to measure pressure and flow in the lower urinary tract. For a complex cystometrogram (51726), the physician typically uses a transurethral catheter to fill the bladder with water or gas while simultaneously obtaining rectal pressure. As the bladder is being filled, intravesical pressure is measured by a microtip transducer or fluid-filled catheter attached to the transducer. Code 51727 reports a complex cystometrogram performed in conjunction with a study for measuring urethral pressure. In one technique, the bladder is filled with fluid and the catheter withdrawn into the urethra while bladder sensations and volume are recorded. Urethral pressure changes are recorded as the patient follows specific instructions (Valsalva maneuver, cough). For voiding pressure studies performed in conjunction with a complex cystometrogram (51728), a transducer is placed into the bladder and the bladder is filled with fluid. The patient is instructed to attempt to void upon the feeling of bladder fullness, and recordings are taken of bladder sensation and volume at specific times. Report 51729 if complex cystometrogram is combined with both voiding pressure studies and urethral pressure profile studies.

Coding Tips

These codes imply that the service is performed by, or under the direct supervision of, a physician or other qualified health care professional. All instruments, equipment, fluids, gases, probes, catheters, technician fees, medications, gloves, trays, tubing, and other sterile supplies are presumed to be provided by the physician. To claim only the professional component of a code, append modifier 26 or for the technical component, append modifier TC. To claim the complete procedure (i.e., both the professional and technical components), submit without a modifier. When multiple procedures are performed during the same operative session, modifier 51 should be reported on all subsequent procedures beyond the primary service.

ICD-9-CM Procedural

89.22 Cystometrogram

89.25 Urethral pressure profile (UPP)

89.29 Other nonoperative genitourinary system measurements

Anesthesia

00910

ICD-9-CM Diagnostic

595.1 Chronic interstitial cystitis — (Use additional code to identify organism, such as E. coli: 041.41-041.49)

595.3 Trigonitis — (Use additional code to identify organism, such as E. coli: 041.41-041.49)

596.0 Bladder neck obstruction — (Use additional code to identify urinary incontinence: 625.6, 788.30-788.39)

596.3 Diverticulum of bladder — (Use additional code to identify urinary incontinence: 625.6, 788.30-788.39)

596.4 Atony of bladder — (Use additional code to identify urinary incontinence: 625.6, 788.30-788.39)

596.51 Hypertonicity of bladder — (Use additional code to identify urinary incontinence: 625.6, 788.30-788.39)

596.52 Low bladder compliance — (Use additional code to identify urinary incontinence: 625.6, 788.30-788.39)

596.53 Paralysis of bladder — (Use additional code to identify urinary incontinence: 625.6, 788.30-788.39)

596.55 Detrusor sphincter dyssynergia — (Use additional code to identify urinary incontinence: 625.6, 788.30-788.39)

598.2 Postoperative urethral stricture — (Use additional code to identify urinary incontinence: 625.6, 788.30-788.39)

618.2 Uterovaginal prolapse, incomplete — (Use additional code to identify urinary incontinence: 625.6, 788.31, 788.33-788.39)

625.6 Female stress incontinence

CCI Version 18.3

00910, 0228T, 0230T, 12001-12007, 12011-12057, 13100-13153, 36000, 36400-36410, 36420-36430, 36440, 36600, 36640, 37202, 43752, 50715, 51701-51703, 62310-62319, 64400-64435, 64445-64450, 64479, 64483, 64490, 64493, 64505-64530, 69990, 93000-93010, 93040-93042, 93318, 94002, 94200, 94250, 94680-94690, 94770, 95812-95816, 95819, 95822, 95829, 95955, 96360, 96365, 96372, 96374-96376, 99148-99149, 99150, P9612

Also not with 51725: 0213T, 0216T

Also not with 51726: 51725

Also not with 51727: 0213T, 0216T, 51725-51726, J0670, J2001

Also not with 51728: 0213T, 0216T, 51725-51727, 90901, J0670, J2001

Also not with 51729: 0213T, 0216T, 51725-51728, 90901, J0670, J2001

Note: These CCI edits are used for Medicare. Other payers may reimburse on codes listed above.

Medicare Edits

	Fac RVU	Non-Fac RVU	FUD	Status
51725	5.87	5.87	0	A
51726	8.61	8.61	0	A
51727	9.28	9.28	0	A
51728	9.24	9.24	0	A
51729	10.08	10.08	0	A

	MUE		Modifiers		
51725	1	51	N/A	N/A	80*
51726	1	51	N/A	N/A	N/A
51727	1	51	N/A	N/A	80*
51728	1	51	N/A	N/A	80*
51729	1	51	N/A	N/A	80*

* with documentation

Medicare References: None

Bladder

51736-51741

51736 Simple uroflowmetry (UFR) (eg, stop-watch flow rate, mechanical uroflowmeter)

51741 Complex uroflowmetry (eg, calibrated electronic equipment)

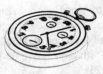

Simple uroflowmetry is performed (51736). Typically, a stopwatch is used to measure the amount of time a patient needs to urinate into a calibrated vessel. The physician assesses the ratio

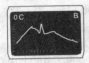

Complex uroflowmetry is performed (51741). Typically, electronic equipment is used to record the volume of urine and elapsed time. The physician assesses the ratio

Explanation

For simple uroflowmetry (51736), the physician assesses the rate of emptying the bladder by stopwatch, recording the volume of urine per time. For complex uroflowmetry, (51741), the physician assesses the rate of emptying of the bladder by electronic equipment, recording the volume of urine per time.

Coding Tips

These codes imply that the service is performed by, or under the direct supervision of, a physician, and that all instruments, equipment, fluids, gases, probes, catheters, technician's fee, medications, gloves, trays, tubing, and other sterile supplies be provided by the physician. Procedures 51736 and 51741 have both a technical and professional component. To claim only the professional component, append modifier 26. To claim only the technical component, append modifier TC. To claim the complete procedure (i.e., both the professional and technical components), submit without a modifier.

ICD-9-CM Procedural

89.24 Uroflowmetry (UFR)

Anesthesia

00910

ICD-9-CM Diagnostic

595.1 Chronic interstitial cystitis — (Use additional code to identify organism, such as E. coli: 041.41-041.49)

595.2 Other chronic cystitis — (Use additional code to identify organism, such as E. coli: 041.41-041.49)

595.81 Cystitis cystica — (Use additional code to identify organism, such as E. coli: 041.41-041.49)

596.0 Bladder neck obstruction — (Use additional code to identify urinary incontinence: 625.6, 788.30-788.39)

596.1 Intestinovesical fistula — (Use additional code to identify urinary incontinence: 625.6, 788.30-788.39)

596.2 Vesical fistula, not elsewhere classified — (Use additional code to identify urinary incontinence: 625.6, 788.30-788.39)

596.3 Diverticulum of bladder — (Use additional code to identify urinary incontinence: 625.6, 788.30-788.39)

596.4 Atony of bladder — (Use additional code to identify urinary incontinence: 625.6, 788.30-788.39)

596.52 Low bladder compliance — (Use additional code to identify urinary incontinence: 625.6, 788.30-788.39)

596.55 Detrusor sphincter dyssynergia — (Use additional code to identify urinary incontinence: 625.6, 788.30-788.39)

598.00 Urethral stricture due to unspecified infection — (Use additional code to identify urinary incontinence: 625.6, 788.30-788.39)

618.03 Urethrocele without mention of uterine prolapse — (Use additional code to identify urinary incontinence: 625.6, 788.31, 788.33-788.39)

618.2 Uterovaginal prolapse, incomplete — (Use additional code to identify urinary incontinence: 625.6, 788.31, 788.33-788.39)

618.5 Prolapse of vaginal vault after hysterectomy — (Use additional code to identify urinary incontinence: 625.6, 788.31, 788.33-788.39)

618.7 Genital prolapse, old laceration of muscles of pelvic floor — (Use additional code to identify urinary incontinence: 625.6, 788.31, 788.33-788.39)

625.6 Female stress incontinence

753.6 Congenital atresia and stenosis of urethra and bladder neck

788.21 Incomplete bladder emptying — (Code, if applicable, any causal condition first, such as: 600.0-600.9, with fifth digit 1)

788.29 Other specified retention of urine — (Code, if applicable, any causal condition first, such as: 600.0-600.9, with fifth digit 1)

788.31 Urge incontinence — (Code, if applicable, any causal condition first: 600.0-600.9, with fifth digit 1; 618.00-618.9; 753.23)

788.33 Mixed incontinence urge and stress (male)(female) — (Code, if applicable, any causal condition first: 600.0-600.9, with fifth digit 1; 618.00-618.9; 753.23)

788.34 Incontinence without sensory awareness — (Code, if applicable, any causal condition first: 600.0-600.9, with fifth digit 1; 618.00-618.9; 753.23)

788.37 Continuous leakage — (Code, if applicable, any causal condition first: 600.0-600.9, with fifth digit 1; 618.00-618.9; 753.23)

788.39 Other urinary incontinence — (Code, if applicable, any causal condition first: 600.0-600.9, with fifth digit 1; 618.00-618.9; 753.23)

CCI Version 18.3

00910, 0213T, 0216T, 0228T, 0230T, 36000, 36400-36410, 36420-36430, 36440, 36600, 36640, 37202, 43752, 50715, 51701-51703, 62310-62319, 64400-64435, 64445-64450, 64479, 64483, 64490, 64493, 64505-64530, 69990, 93000-93010, 93040-93042, 93318, 94002, 94200, 94250, 94680-94690, 94770, 95812-95816, 95819, 95822, 95829, 95955, 96360, 96365, 96372, 96374-96376, 99148-99149, 99150, P9612

Also not with 51741: 51736

Note: These CCI edits are used for Medicare. Other payers may reimburse on codes listed above.

Medicare Edits

	Fac RVU	Non-Fac RVU	FUD	Status
51736	0.64	0.64	N/A	A
51741	0.74	0.74	N/A	A

	MUE			Modifiers	
51736	1	51	N/A	N/A	80*
51741	1	51	N/A	N/A	N/A

* with documentation

Medicare References: None

Coding Companion for Ob/Gyn

© 2012 OptumInsight, Inc.

51840-51841

51840 Anterior vesicourethropexy, or urethropexy (eg, Marshall-Marchetti-Krantz, Burch); simple

51841 complicated (eg, secondary repair)

1. A common approach involves placing sutures from pubic bone to paraurethral tissues

2. The urethrovesical angle is elevated and continence restored

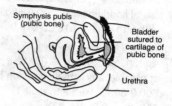

Symphysis pubis (pubic bone)

Bladder sutured to cartilage of pubic bone

Urethra

Bladder

Explanation

The physician performs a vesicourethropexy or urethropexy in the Marshall-Marchetti-Krantz or Burch style. The physician makes a small horizontal incision in the abdomen above the symphysis pubis, which is the midline junction of the pubic bones at the front. The bladder is suspended by placing several sutures through the tissue surrounding the urethra and into the vaginal wall. The sutures are pulled tight so that the tissues are tacked to the symphysis pubis and the urethra is moved forward. The incision is closed by suturing. 51841 is used when the procedure is performed for the second time or if some other factor increases the time or level of complexity.

Coding Tips

When 51840 or 51841 is performed with another separately identifiable procedure, the highest dollar value code is listed as the primary procedure and subsequent procedures are appended with modifier 51. When reporting 51841, the operative and diagnostic documentation should support the complicated procedure. For a urethropexy with a hysterectomy, see 58152 or 58267. Use 57289, 58152, or 58267 if suspension of the urethra is performed with a hysterectomy. For plastic repair and reconstruction of the female urethra only, see 53430.

ICD-9-CM Procedural

59.5 Retropubic urethral suspension

59.79 Other repair of urinary stress incontinence

Anesthesia

00860

ICD-9-CM Diagnostic

599.5 Prolapsed urethral mucosa

618.01 Cystocele without mention of uterine prolapse, midline — (Use additional code to identify urinary incontinence: 625.6, 788.31, 788.33-788.39)

618.02 Cystocele without mention of uterine prolapse, lateral — (Use additional code to identify urinary incontinence: 625.6, 788.31, 788.33-788.39)

618.03 Urethrocele without mention of uterine prolapse — (Use additional code to identify urinary incontinence: 625.6, 788.31, 788.33-788.39)

618.1 Uterine prolapse without mention of vaginal wall prolapse — (Use additional code to identify urinary incontinence: 625.6, 788.31, 788.33-788.39)

618.2 Uterovaginal prolapse, incomplete — (Use additional code to identify urinary incontinence: 625.6, 788.31, 788.33-788.39)

618.3 Uterovaginal prolapse, complete — (Use additional code to identify urinary incontinence: 625.6, 788.31, 788.33-788.39)

618.4 Uterovaginal prolapse, unspecified — (Use additional code to identify urinary incontinence: 625.6, 788.31, 788.33-788.39)

618.5 Prolapse of vaginal vault after hysterectomy — (Use additional code to identify urinary incontinence: 625.6, 788.31, 788.33-788.39)

618.81 Incompetence or weakening of pubocervical tissue — (Use additional code to identify urinary incontinence: 625.6, 788.31, 788.33-788.39)

618.83 Pelvic muscle wasting — (Use additional code to identify urinary incontinence: 625.6, 788.31, 788.33-788.39)

618.84 Cervical stump prolapse — (Use additional code to identify urinary incontinence: 625.6, 788.31, 788.33-788.39)

625.5 Pelvic congestion syndrome

625.6 Female stress incontinence

788.31 Urge incontinence — (Code, if applicable, any causal condition first: 600.0-600.9, with fifth digit 1; 618.00-618.9; 753.23)

788.33 Mixed incontinence urge and stress (male)(female) — (Code, if applicable, any causal condition first: 600.0-600.9, with fifth digit 1; 618.00-618.9; 753.23)

788.34 Incontinence without sensory awareness — (Code, if applicable, any causal condition first: 600.0-600.9, with fifth digit 1; 618.00-618.9; 753.23)

788.35 Post-void dribbling — (Code, if applicable, any causal condition first: 600.0-600.9, with fifth digit 1; 618.00-618.9; 753.23)

788.37 Continuous leakage — (Code, if applicable, any causal condition first: 600.0-600.9, with fifth digit 1; 618.00-618.9; 753.23)

788.38 Overflow incontinence — (Code, if applicable, any causal condition first: 600.0-600.9, with fifth digit 1; 618.00-618.9; 753.23)

CCI Version 18.3

00910, 0213T, 0216T, 0228T, 0230T, 12001-12007, 12011-12057, 13100-13153, 36000, 36400-36410, 36420-36430, 36440, 36600, 36640, 37202, 43752, 44602-44605, 44950, 44970, 49000-49002, 49320, 50715, 51595❖, 51701-51703, 53000-53025, 62310-62319, 64400-64435, 64445-64450, 64479, 64483, 64490, 64493, 64505-64530, 69990, 93000-93010, 93040-93042, 93318, 94002, 94200, 94250, 94680-94690, 94770, 95812-95816, 95819, 95822, 95829, 95955, 96360, 96365, 96372, 96374-96376, 99148-99149, 99150

Also not with 51840: 51040, 52000-52005, 53660-53661

Also not with 51841: 51840, 52000-52001, 57285❖

Note: These CCI edits are used for Medicare. Other payers may reimburse on codes listed above.

Medicare Edits

	Fac RVU	Non-Fac RVU	FUD	Status
51840	19.67	19.67	90	A
51841	23.37	23.37	90	A

	MUE		Modifiers		
51840	1	51	N/A	62*	80
51841	1	51	N/A	62*	80

* with documentation

Medicare References: None

Coding Companion for Ob/Gyn

51845

51845 Abdomino-vaginal vesical neck suspension, with or without endoscopic control (eg, Stamey, Raz, modified Pereyra)

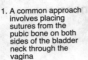

1. A common approach involves placing sutures from the pubic bone on both sides of the bladder neck through the vagina

2. The bladder neck and continence are restored, vagina is suspended

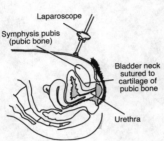

Laparoscope

Symphysis pubis (pubic bone)

Bladder neck sutured to cartilage of pubic bone

Urethra

Explanation

The physician surgically suspends the bladder neck by suturing surrounding tissue to the fibrous membranes (fascia) of the abdomen in a female patient. After inserting a catheter through the urethra to visualize the bladder neck, the physician makes an incision in the vagina, extending it upward toward the base of the bladder. On both sides of the vesical neck, the physician passes a needle through a small incision in the skin above the pubic bone down through the vaginal incision. The physician threads the needle in the vagina and pulls the needle back through the suprapubic incision. Dacron tubing may be threaded onto the sutures to provide extra periurethral support. The physician repeats this process, using an endoscope to ensure proper placement of the suspending sutures. After placing sutures on both sides of the bladder neck, the physician uses moderate upward traction to tighten the bladder neck. The physician inserts a drain tube, bringing it out through a stab incision in the skin, and performs a layered closure.

Coding Tips

Report 51840–51841 if the urethra is suspended from the pubic bone by sutures through the vaginal wall and pubic bone. Use 57289 if a Pereyra type operation is done. For laparoscopic repair of stress incontinence only, see 51990 and 51992.

ICD-9-CM Procedural

59.6 Paraurethral suspension

59.79 Other repair of urinary stress incontinence

Anesthesia

51845 00860

ICD-9-CM Diagnostic

599.5 Prolapsed urethral mucosa

618.01 Cystocele without mention of uterine prolapse, midline — (Use additional code to identify urinary incontinence: 625.6, 788.31, 788.33-788.39)

618.02 Cystocele without mention of uterine prolapse, lateral — (Use additional code to identify urinary incontinence: 625.6, 788.31, 788.33-788.39)

618.03 Urethrocele without mention of uterine prolapse — (Use additional code to identify urinary incontinence: 625.6, 788.31, 788.33-788.39)

618.1 Uterine prolapse without mention of vaginal wall prolapse — (Use additional code to identify urinary incontinence: 625.6, 788.31, 788.33-788.39)

618.2 Uterovaginal prolapse, incomplete — (Use additional code to identify urinary incontinence: 625.6, 788.31, 788.33-788.39)

618.3 Uterovaginal prolapse, complete — (Use additional code to identify urinary incontinence: 625.6, 788.31, 788.33-788.39)

618.4 Uterovaginal prolapse, unspecified — (Use additional code to identify urinary incontinence: 625.6, 788.31, 788.33-788.39)

618.5 Prolapse of vaginal vault after hysterectomy — (Use additional code to identify urinary incontinence: 625.6, 788.31, 788.33-788.39)

618.6 Vaginal enterocele, congenital or acquired — (Use additional code to identify urinary incontinence: 625.6, 788.31, 788.33-788.39)

618.7 Genital prolapse, old laceration of muscles of pelvic floor — (Use additional code to identify urinary incontinence: 625.6, 788.31, 788.33-788.39)

618.81 Incompetence or weakening of pubocervical tissue — (Use additional code to identify urinary incontinence: 625.6, 788.31, 788.33-788.39)

618.83 Pelvic muscle wasting — (Use additional code to identify urinary incontinence: 625.6, 788.31, 788.33-788.39)

625.5 Pelvic congestion syndrome

625.6 Female stress incontinence

788.30 Unspecified urinary incontinence — (Code, if applicable, any causal condition first: 600.0-600.9, with fifth digit 1; 618.00-618.9; 753.23)

788.33 Mixed incontinence urge and stress (male)(female) — (Code, if applicable, any causal condition first: 600.0-600.9, with fifth digit 1; 618.00-618.9; 753.23)

788.34 Incontinence without sensory awareness — (Code, if applicable, any causal condition first: 600.0-600.9, with fifth digit 1; 618.00-618.9; 753.23)

788.35 Post-void dribbling — (Code, if applicable, any causal condition first: 600.0-600.9, with fifth digit 1; 618.00-618.9; 753.23)

788.37 Continuous leakage — (Code, if applicable, any causal condition first: 600.0-600.9, with fifth digit 1; 618.00-618.9; 753.23)

CCI Version 18.3

00910, 0213T, 0216T, 0228T, 0230T, 12001-12007, 12011-12057, 13100-13153, 36000, 36400-36410, 36420-36430, 36440, 36600, 36640, 37202, 43752, 44602-44605, 44820-44850, 44950, 44970, 49000-49010, 49255, 49320, 50715, 51040, 51701-51703, 51840-51841❖, 52000-52005, 52281, 52332, 53660-53661, 57250, 57265, 57289, 62310-62319, 64400-64435, 64445-64450, 64479, 64483, 64490, 64493, 64505-64530, 69990, 93000-93010, 93040-93042, 93318, 94002, 94200, 94250, 94680-94690, 94770, 95812-95816, 95819, 95822, 95829, 95955, 96360, 96365, 96372, 96374-96376, 99148-99149, 99150

Note: These CCI edits are used for Medicare. Other payers may reimburse on codes listed above.

Medicare Edits

	Fac RVU	Non-Fac RVU	FUD	Status
51845	17.5	17.5	90	A

	MUE		Modifiers		
51845	1	51	N/A	62*	80

* with documentation

Medicare References: None

Coding Companion for Ob/Gyn

Bladder

51900

51900 Closure of vesicovaginal fistula, abdominal approach

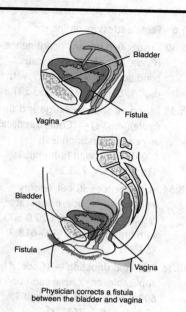

Physician corrects a fistula between the bladder and vagina

Explanation
The physician closes a vesicovaginal fistula, which is an abnormal passage between the bladder and the vagina. This procedure is done through the abdomen. The fistula and surrounding scar tissue of the vaginal wall are usually excised. The physician makes an incision in the skin, muscle, and fascia of the abdomen. The bladder wall is opened and the bladder explored. The fistula is excised along with the surrounding tissue. The resulting defect is closed with sutures in multiple layers. In some cases, a pedicle graft of tissue may be sutured between the bladder and the vagina. A urethral or suprapubic catheter is left in the bladder to prevent distension of the bladder and tension to the sutured areas.

Coding Tips
For a vaginal approach, see 57320 and 57330. For closure of a vesicouterine fistula, see 51920 or 51925.

ICD-9-CM Procedural
57.84   Repair of other fistula of bladder

Anesthesia
51900   00860

ICD-9-CM Diagnostic
619.0   Urinary-genital tract fistula, female

Terms To Know

aberrant. Deviation or departure from the normal or usual course, condition, or pattern.

absorbable sutures. Strands prepared from collagen or a synthetic polymer and capable of being absorbed by tissue over time.

approach. Method or anatomical location used to gain access to a body organ or specific area for procedures. The approach is not coded separately although it may be a specified component of the procedure, such as laparoscopic vs. incisional, or spinal procedures in which the amount of dissection required to expose the spine significantly alters with the site of approach.

excision. Surgical removal of an organ or tissue.

fistula. Abnormal tube-like passage between two body cavities or organs or from an organ to the outside surface.

nonabsorbable sutures. Strands of natural or synthetic material that resist absorption into living tissue and are removed once healing is under way. Nonabsorbable sutures are commonly used to close skin wounds and repair tendons or collagenous tissue.

peritoneum. Strong, continuous membrane that forms the lining of the abdominal and pelvic cavity. The parietal peritoneum, or outer layer, is attached to the abdominopelvic walls and the visceral peritoneum, or inner layer, surrounds the organs inside the abdominal cavity.

vesicovaginal fistula. Abnormal communication between the bladder and the vagina that is the most common genital fistula, often with urinary leakage causing skin irritation of the vulva and thighs, or total incontinence.

CCI Version 18.3
00910, 0213T, 0216T, 0228T, 0230T, 12001-12007, 12011-12057, 13100-13153, 36000, 36400-36410, 36420-36430, 36440, 36600, 36640, 37202, 43752, 44602-44605, 44850, 44950, 44970, 49000-49010, 49255, 49320, 50715, 51701-51703, 51860-51880, 62310-62319, 64400-64435, 64445-64450, 64479, 64483, 64490, 64493, 64505-64530, 69990, 93000-93010, 93040-93042, 93318, 94002, 94200, 94250, 94680-94690, 94770, 95812-95816, 95819, 95822, 95829, 95955, 96360, 96365, 96372, 96374-96376, 99148-99149, 99150

Note: These CCI edits are used for Medicare. Other payers may reimburse on codes listed above.

Medicare Edits

	Fac RVU	Non-Fac RVU	FUD	Status
51900	24.51	24.51	90	A

	MUE		Modifiers		
51900	1	51	N/A	62*	80

* with documentation

Medicare References: None

Bladder

51920-51925

51920 Closure of vesicouterine fistula;
51925   with hysterectomy

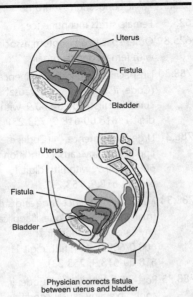

Physician corrects fistula
between uterus and bladder

Explanation

The physician excises an abnormal opening between the uterus and the bladder, then sutures the clean tissues together closing the resulting defect and creating a smooth surface. In 51920, the procedure is done through the bladder with a small abdominal incision or during a laparotomy. In 51925, the physician completes the fistula closure and also removes the uterus through a small horizontal incision just above the pubic hairline. To remove the uterus, the supporting pedicles containing the tubes, ligaments, and arteries are clamped and cut free. The uterus and cervix are removed along with a narrow rim or cuff of vaginal lining. The vaginal defect may be left open for drainage. The abdominal incision is closed by suturing.

Coding Tips

When both a vesicouterine fistula closure and a hysterectomy are performed, only 51925 should be reported. When 51920 or 51925 is performed with another separately identifiable procedure, the highest dollar value code is listed as the primary procedure and subsequent procedures are appended with modifier 51. For closure of a vesicovaginal fistula, abdominal approach, see 51900; by vaginal approach, see 57320 and 57330.

ICD-9-CM Procedural

57.84   Repair of other fistula of bladder
68.59   Other and unspecified vaginal hysterectomy

Anesthesia

51920   00860
51925   00840, 00860

ICD-9-CM Diagnostic

182.8   Malignant neoplasm of other specified sites of body of uterus

183.9   Malignant neoplasm of uterine adnexa, unspecified site

615.9   Unspecified inflammatory disease of uterus — (Use additional code to identify organism: 041.00-041.09, 041.10-041.19)

617.0   Endometriosis of uterus

619.0   Urinary-genital tract fistula, female

621.30   Endometrial hyperplasia, unspecified

621.31   Simple endometrial hyperplasia without atypia

621.32   Complex endometrial hyperplasia without atypia

621.33   Endometrial hyperplasia with atypia

621.34   Benign endometrial hyperplasia

621.35   Endometrial intraepithelial neoplasia [EIN]

Terms To Know

dissection. Separating by cutting tissue or body structures apart.

endometrial cystic hyperplasia. Abnormal cyst-forming overgrowth of the endometrium.

endometriosis. Aberrant uterine mucosal tissue appearing in areas of the pelvic cavity outside of its normal location, lining the uterus and inflaming surrounding tissues, and can result in infertility and spontaneous abortion.

endometrium. Lining of the uterus, which thickens in preparation for fertilization. A fertilized ovum embeds into the thickened endometrium. When no fertilization takes place, the endometrial lining sheds during the process of menstruation.

fistula. Abnormal tube-like passage between two body cavities or organs or from an organ to the outside surface.

malignant neoplasm. Any cancerous tumor or lesion exhibiting uncontrolled tissue growth that can progressively invade other parts of the body with its disease-generating cells.

peritoneum

peritoneum. Strong, continuous membrane that forms the lining of the abdominal and pelvic cavity. The parietal peritoneum, or outer layer, is attached to the abdominopelvic walls and the visceral peritoneum, or inner layer, surrounds the organs inside the abdominal cavity.

CCI Version 18.3

00910, 0213T, 0216T, 0228T, 0230T, 12001-12007, 12011-12057, 13100-13153, 36000, 36400-36410, 36420-36430, 36440, 36600, 36640, 37202, 43752, 44602-44605, 44850, 44950, 44970, 49000-49010, 49255, 49320, 50715, 51701-51703, 51860-51880, 62310-62319, 64400-64435, 64445-64450, 64479, 64483, 64490, 64493, 64505-64530, 69990, 93000-93010, 93040-93042, 93318, 94002, 94200, 94250, 94680-94690, 94770, 95812-95816, 95819, 95822, 95829, 95955, 96360, 96365, 96372, 96374-96376, 99148-99149, 99150

Also not with 51925: 44005, 44180, 51920, 58150-58180, 58260-58263, 58267-58280, 58290-58294

Note: These CCI edits are used for Medicare. Other payers may reimburse on codes listed above.

Medicare Edits

	Fac RVU	Non-Fac RVU	FUD	Status
51920	22.43	22.43	90	A
51925	30.22	30.22	90	A

	MUE			Modifiers	
51920	1		51	N/A	62*	80
51925	1		51	N/A	62*	80

* with documentation

Medicare References: None

Bladder

Coding Companion for Ob/Gyn

51990-51992

51990 Laparoscopy, surgical; urethral suspension for stress incontinence

51992 sling operation for stress incontinence (eg, fascia or synthetic)

Bladder

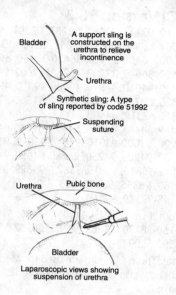

A support sling is constructed on the urethra to relieve incontinence

Bladder

Urethra

Synthetic sling: A type of sling reported by code 51992

Suspending suture

Urethra — Pubic bone

Bladder

Laparoscopic views showing suspension of urethra

Explanation

The physician makes a 1 cm incision just below the umbilicus through which a fiberoptic laparoscope is inserted. A second incision is made on the left or right side of the abdomen and a second instrument is passed into the abdomen. The physician manipulates the tools so that the pelvic organs can be observed through the laparoscope. The bladder is suspended by placing several sutures through the tissue surrounding the urethra and into support structures. The sutures are pulled tight so that the urethra is elevated and moved forward. In 51992, a sling is placed under the junction of the urethra and bladder. A catheter is inserted into the bladder and an incision is made in the anterior wall of the vagina. Tissue is folded and tacked around the urethra. A sling is formed out of synthetic material or from fascia harvested from the sheath of the rectus abdominis muscle. The loop end of the sling is sutured around the junction of the urethra. An incision is made into the lower abdomen and the ends of the sling are grasped with a clamp and pulled into the incision and sutured to the rectus abdominis sheath. The instruments are removed and incisions are closed with sutures.

Coding Tips

Surgical laparoscopy always includes diagnostic laparoscopy. For removal or revision

of sling for stress incontinence, see 57287; open approach for sling procedure, see 57288.

ICD-9-CM Procedural

59.5 Retropubic urethral suspension

Anesthesia

00840, 00860

ICD-9-CM Diagnostic

599.5 Prolapsed urethral mucosa

618.00 Unspecified prolapse of vaginal walls without mention of uterine prolapse — (Use additional code to identify urinary incontinence: 625.6, 788.31, 788.33-788.39)

618.01 Cystocele without mention of uterine prolapse, midline — (Use additional code to identify urinary incontinence: 625.6, 788.31, 788.33-788.39)

618.02 Cystocele without mention of uterine prolapse, lateral — (Use additional code to identify urinary incontinence: 625.6, 788.31, 788.33-788.39)

618.03 Urethrocele without mention of uterine prolapse — (Use additional code to identify urinary incontinence: 625.6, 788.31, 788.33-788.39)

618.1 Uterine prolapse without mention of vaginal wall prolapse — (Use additional code to identify urinary incontinence: 625.6, 788.31, 788.33-788.39)

618.2 Uterovaginal prolapse, incomplete — (Use additional code to identify urinary incontinence: 625.6, 788.31, 788.33-788.39)

618.3 Uterovaginal prolapse, complete — (Use additional code to identify urinary incontinence: 625.6, 788.31, 788.33-788.39)

618.4 Uterovaginal prolapse, unspecified — (Use additional code to identify urinary incontinence: 625.6, 788.31, 788.33-788.39)

618.5 Prolapse of vaginal vault after hysterectomy — (Use additional code to identify urinary incontinence: 625.6, 788.31, 788.33-788.39)

618.6 Vaginal enterocele, congenital or acquired — (Use additional code to identify urinary incontinence: 625.6, 788.31, 788.33-788.39)

618.81 Incompetence or weakening of pubocervical tissue — (Use additional code to identify urinary incontinence: 625.6, 788.31, 788.33-788.39)

618.82 Incompetence or weakening of rectovaginal tissue — (Use additional code to identify urinary incontinence: 625.6, 788.31, 788.33-788.39)

625.5 Pelvic congestion syndrome

625.6 Female stress incontinence

625.8 Other specified symptom associated with female genital organs

788.30 Unspecified urinary incontinence — (Code, if applicable, any causal condition first: 600.0-600.9, with fifth digit 1; 618.00-618.9; 753.23)

788.31 Urge incontinence — (Code, if applicable, any causal condition first: 600.0-600.9, with fifth digit 1; 618.00-618.9; 753.23)

788.33 Mixed incontinence urge and stress (male)(female) — (Code, if applicable, any causal condition first: 600.0-600.9, with fifth digit 1; 618.00-618.9; 753.23)

788.35 Post-void dribbling — (Code, if applicable, any causal condition first: 600.0-600.9, with fifth digit 1; 618.00-618.9; 753.23)

CCI Version 18.3

00910, 0213T, 0216T, 0228T, 0230T, 12001-12007, 12011-12057, 13100-13153, 36000, 36400-36410, 36420-36430, 36440, 36600, 36640, 37202, 43653, 43752, 44005, 44180, 44602-44605, 44950, 44970, 49320, 50715, 51701-51703, 58660, 62310-62319, 64400-64435, 64445-64450, 64479, 64483, 64490, 64493, 64505-64530, 69990, 76000-76001, 77001-77002, 93000-93010, 93040-93042, 93318, 94002, 94200, 94250, 94680-94690, 94770, 95812-95816, 95819, 95822, 95829, 95955, 96360, 96365, 96372, 96374-96376, 99148-99149, 99150

Also not with 51990: 51992❖, 57285

Also not with 51992: 53000-53025

Note: These CCI edits are used for Medicare. Other payers may reimburse on codes listed above.

Medicare Edits

	Fac RVU	Non-Fac RVU	FUD	Status
51990	22.5	22.5	90	A
51992	25.39	25.39	90	A

	MUE		Modifiers	
51990	1	51	N/A 62*	80
51992	1	51	N/A 62*	80

* with documentation

Medicare References: 100-3,230.10

52000

52000 Cystourethroscopy (separate procedure)

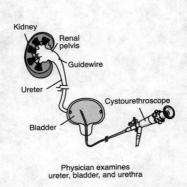

Kidney
Renal pelvis
Guidewire
Ureter
Bladder
Cystourethroscope

Physician examines ureter, bladder, and urethra

Explanation

The physician examines the urethra, bladder, and ureteric openings into the bladder with a cystourethroscope passed through the urethra and bladder. No other procedure is performed at this time. After examination, the physician removes the cystourethroscope.

Coding Tips

This separate procedure by definition is usually a component of a more complex service and is not identified separately. When performed alone or with other unrelated procedures/services it may be reported. If performed alone, list the code; if performed with other procedures/services, list the code and append modifier 59. When 52000 is performed with another separately identifiable procedure, the highest dollar value code is listed as the primary procedure and subsequent procedures are appended with modifier 51. If a microscope is attached to the cystourethroscope, it is not reported separately. Local anesthesia is included in this service. However, this procedure may be performed under general anesthesia, depending on the age and/or condition of the patient.

ICD-9-CM Procedural

57.32   Other cystoscopy

Anesthesia

52000   00910

ICD-9-CM Diagnostic

188.3   Malignant neoplasm of anterior wall of urinary bladder

188.4   Malignant neoplasm of posterior wall of urinary bladder

188.5   Malignant neoplasm of bladder neck

189.3   Malignant neoplasm of urethra

233.7   Carcinoma in situ of bladder

591   Hydronephrosis

595.0   Acute cystitis — (Use additional code to identify organism, such as E. coli: 041.41-041.49)

595.1   Chronic interstitial cystitis — (Use additional code to identify organism, such as E. coli: 041.41-041.49)

596.0   Bladder neck obstruction — (Use additional code to identify urinary incontinence: 625.6, 788.30-788.39)

596.1   Intestinovesical fistula — (Use additional code to identify urinary incontinence: 625.6, 788.30-788.39)

596.2   Vesical fistula, not elsewhere classified — (Use additional code to identify urinary incontinence: 625.6, 788.30-788.39)

596.3   Diverticulum of bladder — (Use additional code to identify urinary incontinence: 625.6, 788.30-788.39)

596.51   Hypertonicity of bladder — (Use additional code to identify urinary incontinence: 625.6, 788.30-788.39)

597.0   Urethral abscess

598.01   Urethral stricture due to infective diseases classified elsewhere — (Use additional code to identify urinary incontinence: 625.6, 788.30-788.39. Code first underlying disease: 095.8, 098.2, 120.0-120.9)

599.0   Urinary tract infection, site not specified — (Use additional code to identify organism, such as E. coli: 041.41-041.49)

599.1   Urethral fistula

599.2   Urethral diverticulum

599.5   Prolapsed urethral mucosa

599.71   Gross hematuria

599.72   Microscopic hematuria

599.81   Urethral hypermobility — (Use additional code to identify urinary incontinence: 625.6, 788.30-788.39)

599.82   Intrinsic (urethral) sphincter deficiency (ISD) — (Use additional code to identify urinary incontinence: 625.6, 788.30-788.39)

619.0   Urinary-genital tract fistula, female

625.6   Female stress incontinence

753.6   Congenital atresia and stenosis of urethra and bladder neck

788.0   Renal colic

788.1   Dysuria

788.21   Incomplete bladder emptying — (Code, if applicable, any causal condition first, such as: 600.0-600.9, with fifth digit 1)

788.31   Urge incontinence — (Code, if applicable, any causal condition first: 600.0-600.9, with fifth digit 1; 618.00-618.9; 753.23)

788.37   Continuous leakage — (Code, if applicable, any causal condition first: 600.0-600.9, with fifth digit 1; 618.00-618.9; 753.23)

788.5   Oliguria and anuria

788.7   Urethral discharge

793.5   Nonspecific (abnormal) findings on radiological and other examination of genitourinary organs

939.0   Foreign body in bladder and urethra

CCI Version 18.3

00910, 00916, 0213T, 0216T, 0228T, 0230T, 12001-12007, 12011-12057, 13100-13153, 36000, 36400-36410, 36420-36430, 36440, 36600, 36640, 37202, 43752, 51700-51703, 53000-53025, 53600-53621, 53660-53665, 57410, 62310-62319, 64400-64435, 64445-64450, 64479, 64483, 64490, 64493, 64505-64530, 69990, 76000-76001, 77001-77002, 93000-93010, 93040-93042, 93318, 94002, 94200, 94250, 94680-94690, 94770, 95812-95816, 95819, 95822, 95829, 95955, 96360, 96365, 96372, 96374-96376, 99148-99149, 99150, J2001, P9612

Note: These CCI edits are used for Medicare. Other payers may reimburse on codes listed above.

Medicare Edits

	Fac RVU	Non-Fac RVU	FUD	Status
52000	3.74	6.09	0	A

	MUE		Modifiers		
52000	1	51	N/A	N/A	N/A

* with documentation

Medicare References: None

Bladder

53060

53060 Drainage of Skene's gland abscess or cyst

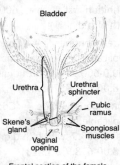

Frontal section of the female bladder and urethra showing Skene's (or paraurethral) gland

An abscess or cyst of the Skene's gland is drained

Explanation

The physician drains an abscess or a cyst of the Skene's gland, the paraurethral glands in the female. The physician makes an incision through the skin, subcutaneous tissue, and overlying layers of muscle, fat, and tissue (fascia) over the site of the abscess. By blunt or sharp dissection, the incision is carried into the abscessed area to provide drainage. Drains are inserted and the incision is closed in layers.

Coding Tips

For removal or destruction by electric current (fulguration) of Skene's glands, see 53270. Local anesthesia is included in this service. However, this procedure may be performed under general anesthesia, depending on the age and/or condition of the patient. For drainage of a subcutaneous abscess, see 10060–10061. Dilation or manipulation of the urethra is not separately identified. Surgical trays, A4550, are not separately reimbursed by Medicare; however, other third-party payers may cover them. Check with the specific payer to determine coverage.

ICD-9-CM Procedural

58.91 Incision of periurethral tissue
71.09 Other incision of vulva and perineum

Anesthesia

53060 00920, 00942

ICD-9-CM Diagnostic

597.0 Urethral abscess

599.89 Other specified disorders of urinary tract — (Use additional code to identify urinary incontinence: 625.6, 788.30-788.39)

Terms To Know

abscess. Circumscribed collection of pus resulting from bacteria, frequently associated with swelling and other signs of inflammation. Abscesses may be either punctured or aspirated or the physician may perform an incision and drainage. Diagnosis codes for abscesses are based upon anatomical location and type of tissue.

blunt dissection. Surgical technique used to expose an underlying area by separating along natural cleavage lines of tissue, without cutting. A blunt instrument or fingers are used to do this. This term is found in most surgery notes with no bearing on code selection.

cyst. Elevated encapsulated mass containing fluid, semisolid, or solid material with a membranous lining.

dissect. Cut apart or separate tissue for surgical purposes or for visual or microscopic study.

Skene's gland. Paraurethral ducts that drain a group of the female urethral glands into the vestibule.

vulva. Area on the female external genitalia that includes the labia majora and minora, mons pubis, clitoris, bulb of the vestibule, vaginal vestibule and orifice, and the greater and lesser vestibular glands.

CCI Version 18.3

0213T, 0216T, 0228T, 0230T, 12001-12007, 12011-12057, 13100-13153, 36000, 36400-36410, 36420-36430, 36440, 36600, 36640, 37202, 43752, 51701-51703, 53000-53025, 53080, 53270❖, 62310-62319, 64400-64435, 64445-64450, 64479, 64483, 64490, 64493, 64505-64530, 69990, 93000-93010, 93040-93042, 93318, 94002, 94200, 94250, 94680-94690, 94770, 95812-95816, 95819, 95822, 95829, 95955, 96360, 96365, 96372, 96374-96376, 99148-99149, 99150, J2001

Note: These CCI edits are used for Medicare. Other payers may reimburse on codes listed above.

Medicare Edits

	Fac RVU	Non-Fac RVU	FUD	Status
53060	4.99	5.56	10	A

	MUE		Modifiers		
53060	1	51	N/A	N/A	N/A

* with documentation

Medicare References: None

53230

53230 Excision of urethral diverticulum (separate procedure); female

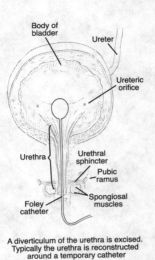

Body of bladder
Ureter
Ureteric orifice
Urethra
Urethral sphincter
Pubic ramus
Foley catheter
Spongiosal muscles

A diverticulum of the urethra is excised. Typically the urethra is reconstructed around a temporary catheter

Explanation

The physician removes a urethral diverticulum. A longitudinal incision is made in the anterior vaginal wall and the urethral diverticulum is separated from the vaginal wall by a combination of blunt and sharp dissection. The urethra may be opened back to the orifice of the diverticulum in order to facilitate identification. A balloon catheter may be inserted and inflated. Once the diverticulum has been excised, the urethra is closed over a catheter and the vaginal wall is repaired with a layered closure.

Coding Tips

This separate procedure by definition is usually a component of a more complex service and is not identified separately. When performed alone or with other unrelated procedures or services it may be reported. If performed alone, list the code; if performed with other procedures or services, list the code and append modifier 59. Dilation or manipulation of the urethra is not reported separately. For marsupialization of the urethral diverticulum, see 53240. For excision or fulguration of urethral polyps, see 53260. Surgical trays, A4550, are not separately reimbursed by Medicare; however, other third-party payers may cover them. Check with the specific payer to determine coverage.

ICD-9-CM Procedural

58.39   Other local excision or destruction of lesion or tissue of urethra

Anesthesia

53230   00942

ICD-9-CM Diagnostic

599.2   Urethral diverticulum

Terms To Know

diverticulum. Pouch or sac in the walls of an organ or canal.

excision. Surgical removal of an organ or tissue.

Foley catheter. Temporary indwelling urethral catheter held in place in the bladder by an inflated balloon containing fluid or air.

CCI Version 18.3

0213T, 0216T, 0228T, 0230T, 12001-12007, 12011-12057, 13100-13153, 36000, 36400-36410, 36420-36430, 36440, 36600, 36640, 37202, 43752, 51701-51703, 52301, 53000-53025, 62310-62319, 64400-64435, 64445-64450, 64479, 64483, 64490, 64493, 64505-64530, 69990, 93000-93010, 93040-93042, 93318, 94002, 94200, 94250, 94680-94690, 94770, 95812-95816, 95819, 95822, 95829, 95955, 96360, 96365, 96372, 96374-96376, 99148-99149, 99150

Note: These CCI edits are used for Medicare. Other payers may reimburse on codes listed above.

Medicare Edits

	Fac RVU	Non-Fac RVU	FUD	Status
53230	18.08	18.08	90	A

	MUE			Modifiers	
53230	1	51	N/A	62*	80

* with documentation

Medicare References: None

Coding Companion for Ob/Gyn

53240

53240 Marsupialization of urethral diverticulum, male or female

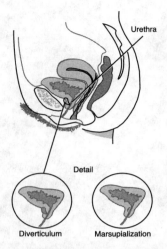

Detail

Diverticulum — Marsupialization

Physician converts the diverticulum into a depression (marsupialization)

Explanation

The physician repairs a urethral diverticulum by creating a pouch (marsupialization). A longitudinal incision is made in the anterior vaginal wall and the borders of the urethral diverticulum are raised and sutured to create a pouch. The interior of the sac separates and gradually closes by granulation. The urethra is closed over a catheter and the vaginal wall is repaired with a layered closure.

Coding Tips

Dilation or manipulation of the urethra and vagina is not reported separately. For excision of urethral diverticulum, see 53230. For excision or fulguration of urethral polyps, or urethral caruncle, see 53260 or 53265.

ICD-9-CM Procedural

58.39   Other local excision or destruction of lesion or tissue of urethra

Anesthesia

53240   00920, 00942

ICD-9-CM Diagnostic

599.2   Urethral diverticulum

Terms To Know

catheter. Flexible tube inserted into an area of the body for introducing or withdrawing fluid.

diverticulum. Pouch or sac in the walls of an organ or canal.

granulation. Formation of small, bead-like masses of cytoplasm or granules on the surface of healing wounds of an organ, membrane, or tissue.

marsupialization. Creation of a pouch in surgical treatment of a cyst in which one wall is resected and the remaining cut edges are sutured to adjacent tissue creating an open pouch of the previously enclosed cyst.

urethral diverticulum. Abnormal outpouching in the urethral wall that causes urinary urgency and frequency, persistent urinary tract infections, a weak stream with post-void dribbling, discomfort, or incontinence.

CCI Version 18.3

0213T, 0216T, 0228T, 0230T, 12001-12007, 12011-12057, 13100-13153, 36000, 36400-36410, 36420-36430, 36440, 36600, 36640, 37202, 43752, 51701-51703, 52301, 53000-53025, 53230, 62310-62319, 64400-64435, 64445-64450, 64479, 64483, 64490, 64493, 64505-64530, 69990, 93000-93010, 93040-93042, 93318, 94002, 94200, 94250, 94680-94690, 94770, 95812-95816, 95819, 95822, 95829, 95955, 96360, 96365, 96372, 96374-96376, 99148-99149, 99150

Note: These CCI edits are used for Medicare. Other payers may reimburse on codes listed above.

Medicare Edits

	Fac RVU	Non-Fac RVU	FUD	Status
53240	12.61	12.61	90	A

	MUE		Modifiers		
53240	1	51	N/A	N/A	N/A

* with documentation

Medicare References: None

53260-53275

53260 Excision or fulguration; urethral polyp(s), distal urethra
53265 urethral caruncle
53270 Skene's glands
53275 urethral prolapse

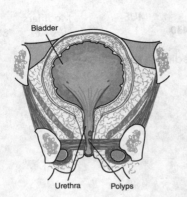

Physician fulgurates or excises polyp(s) in the distal urethra (53260), urethral caruncle (53265), Skene's gland (53270), and/or urethral prolapse (53275)

Explanation

The physician removes urethral polyps, caruncles, Skene's glands or treats urethral prolapse. The physician separates the urethra from the vaginal wall. The urethra is incised. A circular excision is made around the lesion and the targeted tissue is resected. The urethra and vaginal mucosa are reattached in layers. Report 53260 if removing distal urethral polyps; 53265 if removing a urethral caruncle; 53270 if removing the Skene's glands; or 53275 if treating urethral prolapse.

Coding Tips

Report 52285 if fulguration of urethral polyps is part of the treatment for female urethral syndrome. For drainage of an abscess or a cyst of the Skene's gland, see 53060.

ICD-9-CM Procedural

58.39 Other local excision or destruction of lesion or tissue of urethra
71.3 Other local excision or destruction of vulva and perineum

Anesthesia

00920, 00942

ICD-9-CM Diagnostic

597.89 Other urethritis
599.3 Urethral caruncle

599.5 Prolapsed urethral mucosa
599.81 Urethral hypermobility — (Use additional code to identify urinary incontinence: 625.6, 788.30-788.39)
599.89 Other specified disorders of urinary tract — (Use additional code to identify urinary incontinence: 625.6, 788.30-788.39)
599.9 Unspecified disorder of urethra and urinary tract
753.8 Other specified congenital anomaly of bladder and urethra

Terms To Know

anomaly. Irregularity in the structure or position of an organ or tissue.

congenital. Present at birth, occurring through heredity or an influence during gestation up to the moment of birth.

fulguration. Destruction of living tissue by using sparks from a high-frequency electric current.

polyp. Small growth on a stalk-like attachment projecting from a mucous membrane.

prolapse. Falling, sliding, or sinking of an organ from its normal location in the body.

resect. Cutting out or removing a portion or all of a bone, organ, or other structure.

simple polyp. Mucosal outgrowth of tissue that is hanging from a stalk and can easily be removed.

Skene's gland. Paraurethral ducts that drain a group of the female urethral glands into the vestibule.

urethral caruncle. Small, polyp-like growth of a deep red color found in women on the mucous membrane of the urethral opening.

CCI Version 18.3

0213T, 0216T, 0228T, 0230T, 12001-12007, 12011-12057, 13100-13153, 36000, 36400-36410, 36420-36430, 36440, 36600, 36640, 37202, 43752, 51701-51703, 53000-53025, 53080, 53230, 62310-62319, 64400-64435, 64445-64450, 64479, 64483, 64490, 64493, 64505-64530, 69990, 93000-93010, 93040-93042, 93318, 94002, 94200, 94250, 94680-94690, 94770, 95812-95816, 95819, 95822, 95829, 95955, 96360, 96365, 96372, 96374-96376, 99148-99149, 99150
Also not with 53260: J2001
Also not with 53265: J0670, J2001
Also not with 53270: J2001

Note: These CCI edits are used for Medicare. Other payers may reimburse on codes listed above.

Medicare Edits

	Fac RVU	Non-Fac RVU	FUD	Status
53260	5.36	6.0	10	A
53265	5.52	6.5	10	A
53270	5.61	6.26	10	A
53275	7.8	7.8	10	A

	MUE		Modifiers		
53260	1	51	N/A	N/A	N/A
53265	1	51	N/A	N/A	N/A
53270	1	51	N/A	N/A	N/A
53275	1	51	N/A	N/A	N/A

* with documentation

Medicare References: None

Coding Companion for Ob/Gyn

53430

53430 Urethroplasty, reconstruction of female urethra

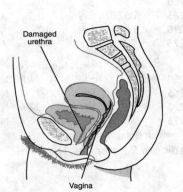

Damaged urethra

Vagina

A flap of vaginal tissue is used to construct a new urethra

Explanation

The physician uses perineal or vaginal tissue to reconstruct the urethra. With the patient in the lithotomy position and a catheter in the urethra, the physician cuts an inverted U-shaped flap above the urethral meatus and extending on the anterior vaginal wall. This flap is undermined with sharp dissection and spreading of the scissors around the upper portion of the urethral meatus, leaving a strip attached. The flap is sutured into a tube shape, reconstructing the distal urethra. The vaginal wall on each side is brought together in several layers to cover the new urethra. Small submucosal vessels are cauterized and a drain may be placed for one to two days.

Coding Tips

For suture of a urethral wound or injury, see 53502.

ICD-9-CM Procedural

58.46   Other reconstruction of urethra

Anesthesia

53430   00942

ICD-9-CM Diagnostic

188.5   Malignant neoplasm of bladder neck
189.3   Malignant neoplasm of urethra
598.01   Urethral stricture due to infective diseases classified elsewhere — (Use additional code to identify urinary incontinence: 625.6, 788.30-788.39.

Code first underlying disease: 095.8, 098.2, 120.0-120.9)
598.1   Traumatic urethral stricture — (Use additional code to identify urinary incontinence: 625.6, 788.30-788.39)
598.2   Postoperative urethral stricture — (Use additional code to identify urinary incontinence: 625.6, 788.30-788.39)
598.8   Other specified causes of urethral stricture — (Use additional code to identify urinary incontinence: 625.6, 788.30-788.39)
598.9   Unspecified urethral stricture — (Use additional code to identify urinary incontinence: 625.6, 788.30-788.39)
599.89   Other specified disorders of urinary tract — (Use additional code to identify urinary incontinence: 625.6, 788.30-788.39)
625.6   Female stress incontinence

Terms To Know

dissection. Separating by cutting tissue or body structures apart.

flap. Mass of flesh and skin partially excised from its location but retaining its blood supply that is moved to another site to repair adjacent or distant defects.

incontinence. Inability to control urination or defecation.

malignant. Any condition tending to progress toward death, specifically an invasive tumor with a loss of cellular differentiation that has the ability to spread or metastasize to other areas in the body.

reconstruction. Recreating, restoring, or rebuilding a body part or organ.

stricture. Narrowing of an anatomical structure.

urethroplasty. Surgical repair or reconstruction of the urethra to correct a stricture or problem caused congenitally, from previous surgical repair, trauma, or prolapse. There are many different types of urethroplasty performed on both males and females.

CCI Version 18.3

0213T, 0216T, 0228T, 0230T, 12001-12007, 12011-12057, 13100-13153, 36000, 36400-36410, 36420-36430, 36440, 36600, 36640, 37202, 43752, 51701-51703, 51990-51992, 52301, 53000-53025, 53080, 53502-53520, 53860❖, 62310-62319, 64400-64435, 64445-64450, 64479, 64483, 64490, 64493, 64505-64530, 69990, 93000-93010, 93040-93042, 93318, 94002, 94200, 94250, 94680-94690, 94770, 95812-95816, 95819, 95822, 95829, 95955,

96360, 96365, 96372, 96374-96376, 99148-99149, 99150

Note: These CCI edits are used for Medicare. Other payers may reimburse on codes listed above.

Medicare Edits

	Fac RVU	Non-Fac RVU	FUD	Status
53430	28.64	28.64	90	A

	MUE		Modifiers	
53430	1	51	N/A 62*	80

* with documentation

Medicare References: None

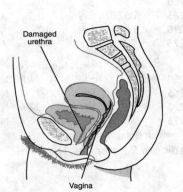

Coding Companion for Ob/Gyn

Urethra

53500

53500 Urethrolysis, transvaginal, secondary, open, including cystourethroscopy (eg, postsurgical obstruction, scarring)

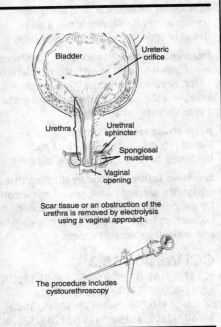

Scar tissue or an obstruction of the urethra is removed by electrolysis using a vaginal approach.

The procedure includes cystourethroscopy

Explanation

Transvaginal, secondary, open urethrolysis is performed in cases when voiding is obstructed due to excessive periurethral scarring caused by previous surgical repair of stress incontinence, procedures such as bladder neck suspension. Urethrolysis involves cutting obstructive adhesions or bands of fibrous tissue that have grown to fix the urethra to the pubic bone. An incision is made through the vagina. The adhering fibrous bands and periurethral scar tissue are visualized and dissected. Lysis and removal continues until the urethra is mobilized away from the surrounding fibrous tissue. Some correction to vaginal abnormalities may be accomplished before closure of the incision. Postsurgical cystourethroscopy is included in this procedure to examine the urethra following urethrolysis.

Coding Tips

Postsurgical diagnostic cystourethroscopy is included in this procedure to examine the urethra following urethrolysis. Urethrolysis performed by retropubic approach is reported with 53899. Do not report 53500 with 52000.

ICD-9-CM Procedural

58.5 Release of urethral stricture

Anesthesia

53500 00942

ICD-9-CM Diagnostic

597.81 Urethral syndrome NOS

598.00 Urethral stricture due to unspecified infection — (Use additional code to identify urinary incontinence: 625.6, 788.30-788.39)

598.01 Urethral stricture due to infective diseases classified elsewhere — (Use additional code to identify urinary incontinence: 625.6, 788.30-788.39. Code first underlying disease: 095.8, 098.2, 120.0-120.9)

598.1 Traumatic urethral stricture — (Use additional code to identify urinary incontinence: 625.6, 788.30-788.39)

598.2 Postoperative urethral stricture — (Use additional code to identify urinary incontinence: 625.6, 788.30-788.39)

598.8 Other specified causes of urethral stricture — (Use additional code to identify urinary incontinence: 625.6, 788.30-788.39)

598.9 Unspecified urethral stricture — (Use additional code to identify urinary incontinence: 625.6, 788.30-788.39)

Terms To Know

adhesion. Abnormal fibrous connection between two structures, soft tissue or bony structures, that may occur as the result of surgery, infection, or trauma.

lysis. Destruction, breakdown, dissolution, or decomposition of cells or substances by a specific catalyzing agent.

obstruction. Blockage that prevents normal function of the valve or structure.

scar tissue. Fibrous connective tissue that forms around a wounded area or injury, composed mainly of fibroblasts or collagenous fibers.

secondary. Second in order of occurrence or importance, or appearing during the course of another disease or condition.

stricture. Narrowing of an anatomical structure.

urethra. Small tube lined with mucous membrane that leads from the bladder to the exterior of the body.

CCI Version 18.3

00910, 0213T, 0216T, 0228T, 0230T, 12001-12007, 12011-12057, 13100-13153, 36000, 36400-36410, 36420-36430, 36440, 36600, 36640, 37202, 43752, 51700-51703, 52000, 52310-52315, 53000-53025, 53080, 53502-53510, 53520-53621❖, 53660-53665, 62310-62319, 64400-64435, 64445-64450,

64479, 64483, 64490, 64493, 64505-64530, 69990, 93000-93010, 93040-93042, 93318, 94002, 94200, 94250, 94680-94690, 94770, 95812-95816, 95819, 95822, 95829, 95955, 96360, 96365, 96372, 96374-96376, 99148-99149, 99150

Note: These CCI edits are used for Medicare. Other payers may reimburse on codes listed above.

Medicare Edits

	Fac RVU	Non-Fac RVU	FUD	Status
53500	22.3	22.3	90	A

	MUE		Modifiers		
53500	1	51	N/A	62*	80

* with documentation

Medicare References: None

Coding Companion for Ob/Gyn

53502

53502 Urethrorrhaphy, suture of urethral wound or injury, female

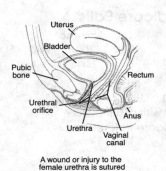

A wound or injury to the female urethra is sutured

Explanation

The physician repairs a urethral wound or injury, including the skin and even more traumatic wounds requiring more than a layered closure. Examples include debridement of cuts (lacerations) or tears (avulsion). Suturing of the urethra is done in layers to prevent later complications and fistula formations. The tissue can be constructed around a catheter.

Coding Tips

For plastic repair and reconstruction of the female urethra, see 53430. Use of an operating microscope is included in this procedure. Do not report 69990 separately.

ICD-9-CM Procedural

58.41   Suture of laceration of urethra
75.61   Repair of current obstetric laceration of bladder and urethra

Anesthesia

53502   00942

ICD-9-CM Diagnostic

599.84   Other specified disorders of urethra — (Use additional code to identify urinary incontinence: 625.6, 788.30-788.39)
634.22   Complete spontaneous abortion complicated by damage to pelvic organs or tissues

635.21   Legally induced abortion complicated by damage to pelvic organs or tissues, incomplete
635.22   Complete legally induced abortion complicated by damage to pelvic organs or tissues
636.21   Incomplete illegally induced abortion complicated by damage to pelvic organs or tissues
636.22   Complete illegally induced abortion complicated by damage to pelvic organs or tissues
637.21   Abortion, unspecified as to legality, incomplete, complicated by damage to pelvic organs or tissues
637.22   Abortion, unspecified as to legality, complete, complicated by damage to pelvic organs or tissues
638.2   Failed attempted abortion complicated by damage to pelvic organs or tissues
639.2   Damage to pelvic organs and tissues following abortion or ectopic and molar pregnancies
665.51   Other injury to pelvic organs, with delivery
665.54   Other injury to pelvic organs, postpartum condition or complication
867.0   Bladder and urethra injury without mention of open wound into cavity
867.1   Bladder and urethra injury with open wound into cavity
998.2   Accidental puncture or laceration during procedure

Terms To Know

avulsion. Forcible tearing away of a part, by surgical means or traumatic injury.

injury. Harm or damage sustained by the body.

laceration. Tearing injury; a torn, ragged-edged wound.

suture. Numerous stitching techniques employed in wound closure.

buried suture. Continuous or interrupted suture placed under the skin for a layered closure.

continuous suture. Running stitch with tension evenly distributed across a single strand to provide a leakproof closure line.

interrupted suture. Series of single stitches with tension isolated at each stitch, in which all stitches are not affected if one becomes loose, and the isolated sutures cannot act as a wick to transport an infection.

purse-string suture. Continuous suture placed around a tubular structure and tightened, to reduce or close the lumen.

retention suture. Secondary stitching that bridges the primary suture, providing support for the primary repair; a plastic or rubber bolster may be placed over the primary repair and under the retention sutures.

CCI Version 18.3

0213T, 0216T, 0228T, 0230T, 12001-12007, 12011-12057, 13100-13153, 36000, 36400-36410, 36420-36430, 36440, 36600, 36640, 37202, 43752, 51701-51703, 52301, 53000-53025, 53080, 62310-62319, 64400-64435, 64445-64450, 64479, 64483, 64490, 64493, 64505-64530, 69990, 93000-93010, 93040-93042, 93318, 94002, 94200, 94250, 94680-94690, 94770, 95812-95816, 95819, 95822, 95829, 95955, 96360, 96365, 96372, 96374-96376, 99148-99149, 99150

Note: These CCI edits are used for Medicare. Other payers may reimburse on codes listed above.

Medicare Edits

	Fac RVU	Non-Fac RVU	FUD	Status
53502	14.38	14.38	90	A

	MUE		Modifiers		
53502	1	51	N/A	N/A	N/A

* with documentation

Medicare References: None

53660-53665

53660 Dilation of female urethra including suppository and/or instillation; initial
53661 subsequent
53665 Dilation of female urethra, general or conduction (spinal) anesthesia

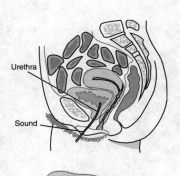

Urethra
Sound

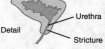

Detail

Urethra
Stricture

Physician passes a dilator through a stricture in the urethra

Explanation

The physician uses dilators of increasing size to widen the female urethra. A suppository or instillation of a saline solution may be used. Report 53660 for initial dilation, and 53661 for subsequent dilation. Use 53665 if general or spinal anesthesia is administered for dilation of female urethral stricture.

Coding Tips

These procedures include insertion of a suppository and/or instillation of a saline solution and are usually performed with local anesthesia. For urethral catheterization, see 51701–51703.

ICD-9-CM Procedural

58.6   Dilation of urethra
96.49   Other genitourinary instillation

Anesthesia

00910

ICD-9-CM Diagnostic

595.1   Chronic interstitial cystitis — (Use additional code to identify organism, such as E. coli: 041.41-041.49)

595.2   Other chronic cystitis — (Use additional code to identify organism, such as E. coli: 041.41-041.49)

595.3   Trigonitis — (Use additional code to identify organism, such as E. coli: 041.41-041.49)

597.80 Unspecified urethritis

597.81 Urethral syndrome NOS

597.89 Other urethritis

598.00 Urethral stricture due to unspecified infection — (Use additional code to identify urinary incontinence: 625.6, 788.30-788.39)

598.01 Urethral stricture due to infective diseases classified elsewhere — (Use additional code to identify urinary incontinence: 625.6, 788.30-788.39. Code first underlying disease: 095.8, 098.2, 120.0-120.9)

598.1   Traumatic urethral stricture — (Use additional code to identify urinary incontinence: 625.6, 788.30-788.39)

598.2   Postoperative urethral stricture — (Use additional code to identify urinary incontinence: 625.6, 788.30-788.39)

598.8   Other specified causes of urethral stricture — (Use additional code to identify urinary incontinence: 625.6, 788.30-788.39)

599.82 Intrinsic (urethral) sphincter deficiency (ISD) — (Use additional code to identify urinary incontinence: 625.6, 788.30-788.39)

599.83 Urethral instability — (Use additional code to identify urinary incontinence: 625.6, 788.30-788.39)

599.89 Other specified disorders of urinary tract — (Use additional code to identify urinary incontinence: 625.6, 788.30-788.39)

599.9   Unspecified disorder of urethra and urinary tract

625.6   Female stress incontinence

753.6   Congenital atresia and stenosis of urethra and bladder neck

788.1   Dysuria

788.20 Unspecified retention of urine — (Code, if applicable, any causal condition first, such as: 600.0-600.9, with fifth digit 1)

788.21 Incomplete bladder emptying — (Code, if applicable, any causal condition first, such as: 600.0-600.9, with fifth digit 1)

788.29 Other specified retention of urine — (Code, if applicable, any causal condition first, such as: 600.0-600.9, with fifth digit 1)

788.99 Other symptoms involving urinary system

Terms To Know

atresia. Congenital closure or absence of a tubular organ or an opening to the body surface.

cystitis. Inflammation of the urinary bladder. Symptoms include dysuria, frequency of urination, urgency, and hematuria.

dilation. Artificial increase in the diameter of an opening or lumen made by medication or by instrumentation.

stenosis. Narrowing or constriction of a passage.

suppository. Medication in the form of a solid mass at room temperature that dissolves at body temperature, for insertion into a body orifice such as the rectal, vaginal, or urethral opening.

trigonitis. Inflammation of the triangular area of mucous membrane at the base of the bladder, called the trigonum vesicae.

CCI Version 18.3

0213T, 0216T, 0228T, 0230T, 12001-12007, 12011-12057, 13100-13153, 36000, 36400-36410, 36420-36430, 36440, 36600, 36640, 37202, 43752, 53000-53025, 53080, 62310-62319, 64400-64435, 64445-64450, 64479, 64483, 64490, 64493, 64505-64530, 69990, 93000-93010, 93040-93042, 93318, 94002, 94200, 94250, 94680-94690, 94770, 95812-95816, 95819, 95822, 95829, 95955, 96360, 96365, 96372, 96374-96376, 99148-99149, 99150

Also not with 53660: 51701-51703, 53661❖, J0670, J2001, P9612

Also not with 53661: 51700-51703, J0670, J2001, P9612

Also not with 53665: 51701-51703, 53660-53661❖

Note: These CCI edits are used for Medicare. Other payers may reimburse on codes listed above.

Medicare Edits

	Fac RVU	Non-Fac RVU	FUD	Status
53660	1.23	2.12	0	A
53661	1.2	2.09	0	A
53665	1.14	1.14	0	A

	MUE		Modifiers		
53660	1	51	N/A	N/A	N/A
53661	1	51	N/A	N/A	N/A
53665	1	51	N/A	N/A	N/A

* with documentation

Medicare References: None

© 2012 OptumInsight, Inc.

53860

53860 Transurethral radiofrequency micro-remodeling of the female bladder neck and proximal urethra for stress urinary incontinence

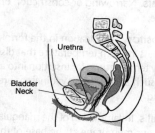

Urethra

Bladder Neck

Explanation

The physician uses radiofrequency energy to treat female stress urinary incontinence, the involuntary loss of urine from the urethra due to increased intra-abdominal pressure. Using a small transurethral probe, the physician applies low temperature radiofrequency energy to targeted submucosal areas of the bladder neck and urethra. This results in minute structural alterations to the collagen that, upon healing, makes the tissues firmer and increases the resistance to involuntary leakage.

Coding Tips

This procedure was formerly a CPT Category III code reported with 0193T.

ICD-9-CM Procedural

59.79   Other repair of urinary stress incontinence

Anesthesia

53860   00910

ICD-9-CM Diagnostic

625.6   Female stress incontinence

788.33 Mixed incontinence urge and stress (male)(female) — (Code, if applicable, any causal condition first: 600.0-600.9, with fifth digit 1; 618.00-618.9; 753.23)

Terms To Know

female stress incontinence. Involuntary escape of urine at times of minor stress against the female bladder, such as coughing, sneezing, or laughing.

urethra. Small tube lined with mucous membrane that leads from the bladder to the exterior of the body.

CCI Version 18.3

12001-12007, 12011-12057, 13100-13153, 36000, 36400-36410, 36420-36430, 36440, 36600, 36640, 37202, 43752, 51102, 51700-51703, 52000-52001, 52281, 52285❖, 52310-52315, 52500, 53000-53025, 53080, 53660-53665, 62310-62319, 64400-64435, 64445-64450, 64479, 64483, 64490, 64493, 64505-64530, 69990, 93000-93010, 93040-93042, 93318, 94002, 94200, 94250, 94680-94690, 94770, 95812-95816, 95819, 95822, 95829, 95955, 96360, 96365, 96372, 96374-96376, 99148-99149, 99150, J0670, J2001, P9612

Note: These CCI edits are used for Medicare. Other payers may reimburse on codes listed above.

Medicare Edits

	Fac RVU	Non-Fac RVU	FUD	Status
53860	6.88	44.8	90	A

	MUE		Modifiers		
53860	1	51	N/A	N/A	80*

* with documentation

Medicare References: None

55920

55920 Placement of needles or catheters into pelvic organs and/or genitalia (except prostate) for subsequent interstitial radioelement application

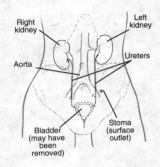

Needles or catheters are placed in the genitalia or pelvic organs

Explanation

The physician places needles or catheters into the pelvic organs and/or genitalia, excluding the prostate, for subsequent interstitial radioelement application. The radioactive isotopes that are introduced subsequently, such as iodine-125 or palladium-103, are contained within tiny seeds that are left in place to deliver radiation over a period of months. They do not cause any harm after becoming inert. This method provides radiation to the prescribed body area while minimizing exposure to normal tissue.

Coding Tips

For insertion of a uterine tandem and/or vaginal ovoids for clinical brachytherapy, see 57155. For insertion of Heyman capsules for clinical brachytherapy, see 58346.

ICD-9-CM Procedural

54.12 Reopening of recent laparotomy site
54.19 Other laparotomy
65.09 Other oophorotomy
68.0 Hysterotomy
69.95 Incision of cervix
70.12 Culdotomy
70.14 Other vaginotomy
71.09 Other incision of vulva and perineum
92.27 Implantation or insertion of radioactive elements

Anesthesia

55920 00940

ICD-9-CM Diagnostic

158.8 Malignant neoplasm of specified parts of peritoneum
158.9 Malignant neoplasm of peritoneum, unspecified
180.0 Malignant neoplasm of endocervix
180.1 Malignant neoplasm of exocervix
180.8 Malignant neoplasm of other specified sites of cervix
180.9 Malignant neoplasm of cervix uteri, unspecified site
183.0 Malignant neoplasm of ovary — (Use additional code to identify any functional activity)
183.8 Malignant neoplasm of other specified sites of uterine adnexa
196.6 Secondary and unspecified malignant neoplasm of intrapelvic lymph nodes
197.6 Secondary malignant neoplasm of retroperitoneum and peritoneum
198.6 Secondary malignant neoplasm of ovary
201.50 Hodgkin's disease, nodular sclerosis, unspecified site, extranodal and solid organ sites
201.60 Hodgkin's disease, mixed cellularity, unspecified site, extranodal and solid organ sites
201.70 Hodgkin's disease, lymphocytic depletion, unspecified site, extranodal and solid organ sites
209.74 Secondary neuroendocrine tumor of peritoneum
236.2 Neoplasm of uncertain behavior of ovary — (Use additional code to identify any functional activity)
785.6 Enlargement of lymph nodes
V10.43 Personal history of malignant neoplasm of ovary
V10.90 Personal history of unspecified malignant neoplasm
V84.02 Genetic susceptibility to malignant neoplasm of ovary — (Use additional code, if applicable, for any associated family history of the disease: V16-V19. Code first, if applicable, any current malignant neoplasms: 140.0-195.8, 200.0-208.9, 230.0-234.9. Use additional code, if applicable, for any personal history of malignant neoplasm: V10.0-V10.9)
V84.04 Genetic susceptibility to malignant neoplasm of endometrium — (Use additional code, if applicable, for any

associated family history of the disease: V16-V19. Code first, if applicable, any current malignant neoplasms: 140.0-195.8, 200.0-208.9, 230.0-234.9. Use additional code, if applicable, for any personal history of malignant neoplasm: V10.0-V10.9)
V84.09 Genetic susceptibility to other malignant neoplasm — (Use additional code, if applicable, for any associated family history of the disease: V16-V19. Code first, if applicable, any current malignant neoplasms: 140.0-195.8, 200.0-208.9, 230.0-234.9. Use additional code, if applicable, for any personal history of malignant neoplasm: V10.0-V10.9)
V87.41 Personal history of antineoplastic chemotherapy
V87.42 Personal history of monoclonal drug therapy
V88.01 Acquired absence of both cervix and uterus
V88.02 Acquired absence of uterus with remaining cervical stump
V88.03 Acquired absence of cervix with remaining uterus

CCI Version 18.3

0213T, 0216T, 0228T, 0230T, 12001-12007, 12011-12057, 13100-13153, 20555❖, 36000, 36400-36410, 36420-36430, 36440, 36600, 36640, 37202, 43752, 57155-57156, 58346, 62310-62319, 64400-64435, 64445-64450, 64479, 64483, 64490, 64493, 64505-64530, 69990, 93000-93010, 93040-93042, 93318, 94002, 94200, 94250, 94680-94690, 94770, 95812-95816, 95819, 95822, 95829, 95955, 96360, 96365, 96372, 96374-96376, 99148-99149, 99150

Note: These CCI edits are used for Medicare. Other payers may reimburse on codes listed above.

Medicare Edits

	Fac RVU	Non-Fac RVU	FUD	Status
55920	12.81	12.81	0	A

	MUE				Modifiers	
55920	1	51	N/A	N/A	80*

* with documentation

Medicare References: None

Reproductive

56405

56405 Incision and drainage of vulva or perineal abscess

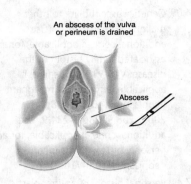
An abscess of the vulva or perineum is drained

Abscess

The wound may be packed with gauze

Explanation

The vulva includes the labia majora, labia minora, mons pubis, bulb of the vestibule, vestibule of the vagina, greater and lesser vestibular glands, and vaginal orifice. The perineum is the area between the vulva and the anus. The physician makes an incision into the abscess at its softest point and drains the purulent contents. The cavity of the abscess is flushed and often packed with medicated gauze to facilitate drainage.

Coding Tips

For incision and drainage of a cutaneous or subcutaneous cyst, furuncle, or abscess, see 10060 and 10061. For drainage of a Skene's gland abscess or cyst, see 53060.

ICD-9-CM Procedural

71.09   Other incision of vulva and perineum

Anesthesia

56405   00940

ICD-9-CM Diagnostic

597.0   Urethral abscess

614.4   Chronic or unspecified parametritis and pelvic cellulitis — (Use additional code to identify organism: 041.00-041.09, 041.10-041.19)

616.4   Other abscess of vulva — (Use additional code to identify organism: 041.00-041.09, 041.10-041.19)

616.9   Unspecified inflammatory disease of cervix, vagina, and vulva — (Use additional code to identify organism: 041.00-041.09, 041.10-041.19)

682.2   Cellulitis and abscess of trunk — (Use additional code to identify organism, such as 041.1, etc.)

752.49   Other congenital anomaly of cervix, vagina, and external female genitalia

Terms To Know

abscess. Circumscribed collection of pus resulting from bacteria, frequently associated with swelling and other signs of inflammation.

anomaly. Irregularity in the structure or position of an organ or tissue.

cellulitis. Sudden, severe, suppurative inflammation and edema in subcutaneous tissue or muscle, most often caused by bacterial infection secondary to a cutaneous lesion.

chronic. Persistent, continuing, or recurring.

congenital. Present at birth, occurring through heredity or an influence during gestation up to the moment of birth.

incision and drainage. Cutting open body tissue for the removal of tissue fluids or infected discharge from a wound or cavity.

parametritis. Inflammation and infection of the tissue in the structures around the uterus.

perineal. Pertaining to the pelvic floor area between the thighs; the diamond-shaped area bordered by the pubic symphysis in front, the ischial tuberosities on the sides, and the coccyx in back.

vulva. Area on the female external genitalia that includes the labia majora and minora, mons pubis, clitoris, bulb of the vestibule, vaginal vestibule and orifice, and the greater and lesser vestibular glands.

CCI Version 18.3

00940, 0213T, 0216T, 0228T, 0230T, 12001-12007, 12011-12057, 13100-13153, 36000, 36400-36410, 36420-36430, 36440, 36600, 36640, 37202, 43752, 51701-51703, 56440, 56605, 56820, 57100, 57180, 57500, 62310-62319, 64400-64435, 64445-64450, 64479, 64483, 64490, 64493, 64505-64530, 69990, 93000-93010, 93040-93042, 93318, 94002, 94200, 94250, 94680-94690, 94770, 95812-95816, 95819, 95822, 95829, 95955, 96360, 96365, 96372, 96374-96376, 99148-99149, 99150, J0670, J2001

Note: These CCI edits are used for Medicare. Other payers may reimburse on codes listed above.

Medicare Edits

	Fac RVU	Non-Fac RVU	FUD	Status
56405	3.23	3.27	10	A

	MUE		Modifiers		
56405	2	51	N/A	62	N/A

* with documentation

Medicare References: None

Vulva

56420

56420 Incision and drainage of Bartholin's gland abscess

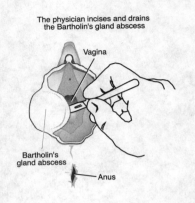

The physician incises and drains the Bartholin's gland abscess

Vagina

Bartholin's gland abscess

Anus

Explanation

The physician incises and drains a Bartholin's gland abscess. Bartholin's gland is at the end of the bulb of the vestibule of the vagina and is connected by a duct to the mucosa at the opening of the vagina. The physician makes an incision just inside the opening of the vagina through the mucosal surface into the cavity of the abscess to flush and drain it. A small wick or catheter may be left in the cavity to facilitate drainage.

Coding Tips

This is a unilateral procedure. If performed bilaterally, some payers require that the service be reported twice with modifier 50 appended to the second code while others require identification of the service only once with modifier 50 appended. Check with individual payers. Modifier 50 identifies a procedure performed identically on the opposite side of the body (mirror image). For marsupialization of Bartholin's gland, see 56440. For incision and drainage of a vulvar or perineal abscess, see 56405. For incision and drainage of a cutaneous or subcutaneous cyst, furuncle, or abscess, see 10060–10061. If a specimen is transported to an outside laboratory, report 99000 for conveyance.

ICD-9-CM Procedural

71.22   Incision of Bartholin's gland (cyst)

Anesthesia

56420   00940

ICD-9-CM Diagnostic

616.3   Abscess of Bartholin's gland — (Use additional code to identify organism: 041.00-041.09, 041.10-041.19)

Terms To Know

abscess. Circumscribed collection of pus resulting from bacteria, frequently associated with swelling and other signs of inflammation.

Bartholin's gland. Mucous-producing gland found in the vestibular bulbs on either side of the vaginal orifice and connected to the mucosal membrane at the opening by a duct.

Bartholin's gland abscess. Pocket of pus and surrounding cellulitis caused by infection of the Bartholin's gland and causing localized swelling and pain in the posterior labia majora that may extend into the lower vagina.

catheter. Flexible tube inserted into an area of the body for introducing or withdrawing fluid.

drain. Device that creates a channel to allow fluid from a cavity, wound, or infected area to exit the body.

incision and drainage. Cutting open body tissue for the removal of tissue fluids or infected discharge from a wound or cavity.

CCI Version 18.3

00940, 0213T, 0216T, 0228T, 0230T, 12001-12007, 12011-12057, 13100-13153, 36000, 36400-36410, 36420-36430, 36440, 36600, 36640, 37202, 43752, 51701-51703, 56405, 56440, 56605, 56820, 57100, 57180, 57500, 62310-62319, 64400-64435, 64445-64450, 64479, 64483, 64490, 64493, 64505-64530, 69990, 93000-93010, 93040-93042, 93318, 94002, 94200, 94250, 94680-94690, 94770, 95812-95816, 95819, 95822, 95829, 95955, 96360, 96365, 96372, 96374-96376, 99148-99149, 99150, J0670, J2001

Note: These CCI edits are used for Medicare. Other payers may reimburse on codes listed above.

Medicare Edits

	Fac RVU	Non-Fac RVU	FUD	Status
56420	2.73	3.65	10	A

	MUE		Modifiers		
56420	1	51	N/A	N/A	N/A

* with documentation

Medicare References: None

Coding Companion for Ob/Gyn

Vulva

56440

56440 Marsupialization of Bartholin's gland cyst

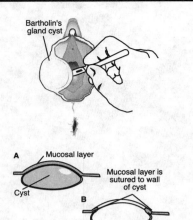

A   Mucosal layer

Cyst

Mucosal layer is sutured to wall of cyst

B

C   Cyst is deroofed   D   Site heals

The physician unroofs the Bartholin's gland cyst and sutures the edges of the gland site

Explanation

The physician treats a Bartholin's gland cyst with marsupialization. Bartholin's gland is at the end of the bulb of the vestibule of the vagina and is connected by a duct to the mucosa at the opening of the vagina. The physician makes an elliptical excision over the center of the Bartholin's gland cyst and then drains it. The lining of the cyst is everted and approximated to the vaginal mucosa with sutures creating a pouch. Marsupialization prevents recurrent cysts and infections.

Coding Tips

This is a unilateral procedure. If performed bilaterally, some payers require that the service be reported twice with modifier 50 appended to the second code while others require identification of the service only once with modifier 50 appended. Check with individual payers. Modifier 50 identifies a procedure performed identically on the opposite side of the body (mirror image). For incision and drainage of a Bartholin's gland abscess, see 56420.

ICD-9-CM Procedural

71.23   Marsupialization of Bartholin's gland (cyst)

Anesthesia

56440   00940

ICD-9-CM Diagnostic

616.2   Cyst of Bartholin's gland — (Use additional code to identify organism: 041.00-041.09, 041.10-041.19)

616.3   Abscess of Bartholin's gland — (Use additional code to identify organism: 041.00-041.09, 041.10-041.19)

Terms To Know

abscess. Circumscribed collection of pus resulting from bacteria, frequently associated with swelling and other signs of inflammation.

Bartholin's gland. Mucous-producing gland found in the vestibular bulbs on either side of the vaginal orifice and connected to the mucosal membrane at the opening by a duct.

cyst. Elevated encapsulated mass containing fluid, semisolid, or solid material with a membranous lining.

infection. Presence of microorganisms in body tissues that may result in cellular damage.

marsupialization. Creation of a pouch in surgical treatment of a cyst in which one wall is resected and the remaining cut edges are sutured to adjacent tissue creating an open pouch of the previously enclosed cyst.

CCI Version 18.3

00940, 0213T, 0216T, 0228T, 0230T, 12001-12007, 12011-12057, 13100-13153, 36000, 36400-36410, 36420-36430, 36440, 36600, 36640, 37202, 43752, 51701-51703, 56605, 56820, 57100, 57180, 57500, 62310-62319, 64400-64435, 64445-64450, 64479, 64483, 64490, 64493, 64505-64530, 69990, 93000-93010, 93040-93042, 93318, 94002, 94200, 94250, 94680-94690, 94770, 95812-95816, 95819, 95822, 95829, 95955, 96360, 96365, 96372, 96374-96376, 99148-99149, 99150, J2001

Note: These CCI edits are used for Medicare. Other payers may reimburse on codes listed above.

Medicare Edits

	Fac RVU	Non-Fac RVU	FUD	Status
56440	5.46	5.46	10	A

	MUE		Modifiers		
56440	1	51	N/A	N/A	N/A

* with documentation

Medicare References: None

Vulva

56441

56441 Lysis of labial adhesions

Adhesions between the labial folds are lysed

Explanation

The labia majora and minora are the greater and lesser folds of skin on the pudendum on either side of the vagina. The physician separates the labia majora from the labia minora, which are fused by fibrous bands of scar tissue. Using a blunt instrument and/or scissors, the labia are separated by breaking or cutting the fibrous tissue. The procedure is accomplished using general or local anesthesia.

Coding Tips

This is a bilateral procedure and as such is reported once even if the procedure is performed on both sides. For destruction of lesions of the vulva, see 56501–56515.

ICD-9-CM Procedural

71.01   Lysis of vulvar adhesions

Anesthesia

56441   00940

ICD-9-CM Diagnostic

624.4   Old laceration or scarring of vulva

629.29   Other female genital mutilation status

752.49   Other congenital anomaly of cervix, vagina, and external female genitalia

Terms To Know

adhesion. Abnormal fibrous connection between two structures, soft tissue or bony structures, that may occur as the result of surgery, infection, or trauma.

anomaly. Irregularity in the structure or position of an organ or tissue.

congenital. Present at birth, occurring through heredity or an influence during gestation up to the moment of birth.

fibrous tissue. Connective tissues.

lysis. Destruction, breakdown, dissolution, or decomposition of cells or substances by a specific catalyzing agent.

scar tissue. Fibrous connective tissue that forms around a wounded area or injury, composed mainly of fibroblasts or collagenous fibers.

vulva. Area on the female external genitalia that includes the labia majora and minora, mons pubis, clitoris, bulb of the vestibule, vaginal vestibule and orifice, and the greater and lesser vestibular glands.

CCI Version 18.3

00940, 0213T, 0216T, 0228T, 0230T, 12001-12007, 12011-12057, 13100-13153, 36000, 36400-36410, 36420-36430, 36440, 36600, 36640, 37202, 43752, 51701-51703, 56820, 57100, 57180, 57500, 62310-62319, 64400-64435, 64445-64450, 64479, 64483, 64490, 64493, 64505-64530, 69990, 93000-93010, 93040-93042, 93318, 94002, 94200, 94250, 94680-94690, 94770, 95812-95816, 95819, 95822, 95829, 95955, 96360, 96365, 96372, 96374-96376, 99148-99149, 99150, J0670, J2001

Note: These CCI edits are used for Medicare. Other payers may reimburse on codes listed above.

Medicare Edits

	Fac RVU	Non-Fac RVU	FUD	Status
56441	4.12	4.3	10	A

	MUE			Modifiers		
56441	1	51	N/A	N/A	80*

* with documentation

Medicare References: None

Coding Companion for Ob/Gyn

Vulva

56442

56442 Hymenotomy, simple incision

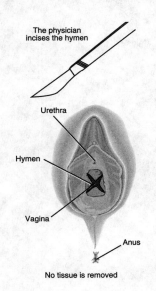

The physician incises the hymen

Urethra

Hymen

Vagina

Anus

No tissue is removed

Explanation

The physician performs a hymenotomy. A hymen is a membrane that partially or wholly occludes the vaginal opening. Following local injection of an anesthetic, the physician incises the hymenal membrane with a stellate (star-shaped) incision. This procedure is sometimes preceded by aspiration of the intact membrane with a needle and syringe.

Coding Tips

Local anesthesia is included in this service. However, this procedure may be performed under general anesthesia, depending on the age and/or condition of the patient. For partial hymenectomy or revision of the hymenal ring, see 56700. Surgical trays, A4550, are not separately reimbursed by Medicare; however, other third-party payers may cover them. Check with the specific payer to determine coverage.

ICD-9-CM Procedural

70.11   Hymenotomy

Anesthesia

56442   00940

ICD-9-CM Diagnostic

623.3   Tight hymenal ring

752.42   Imperforate hymen

752.49   Other congenital anomaly of cervix, vagina, and external female genitalia

Terms To Know

anomaly. Irregularity in the structure or position of an organ or tissue.

aspiration. Drawing fluid out by suction.

congenital. Present at birth, occurring through heredity or an influence during gestation up to the moment of birth.

incision. Act of cutting into tissue or an organ.

CCI Version 18.3

00940, 0213T, 0216T, 0228T, 0230T, 12001-12007, 12011-12057, 13100-13153, 36000, 36400-36410, 36420-36430, 36440, 36600, 36640, 37202, 43752, 51701-51703, 56605, 56820, 57100, 57180, 57410, 57500, 57800, 58100, 62310-62319, 64400-64435, 64445-64450, 64479, 64483, 64490, 64493, 64505-64530, 69990, 93000-93010, 93040-93042, 93318, 94002, 94200, 94250, 94680-94690, 94770, 95812-95816, 95819, 95822, 95829, 95955, 96360, 96365, 96372, 96374-96376, 99148-99149, 99150

Note: These CCI edits are used for Medicare. Other payers may reimburse on codes listed above.

Medicare Edits

	Fac RVU	Non-Fac RVU	FUD	Status
56442	1.44	1.44	0	A

	MUE		Modifiers		
56442	1	51	N/A	N/A	80*

* with documentation

Medicare References: None

Vulva

Coding Companion for Ob/Gyn

56501-56515

56501 Destruction of lesion(s), vulva; simple (eg, laser surgery, electrosurgery, cryosurgery, chemosurgery)

56515 extensive (eg, laser surgery, electrosurgery, cryosurgery, chemosurgery)

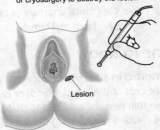

The physician may use laser, fulguration, or cryosurgery to destroy the lesion

Lesion

Report 56501 for simple or single lesions or 56515 for multiple or complicated lesions

Explanation

The vulva includes the labia majora, labia minora, mons pubis, bulb of the vestibule, vestibule of the vagina, greater and lesser vestibular glands, and vaginal orifice. The physician destroys one or more lesions of the vulva, After examining the lower genital tract and perianal area with a colposcope, the physician destroys any lesions of the vulva by any method including laser surgery, electrosurgery, chemosurgery, or cryosurgery.Use 56501 to report single, simple lesion destruction, or 56515 to report multiple or complicated destruction of extensive vulvar lesions.

Coding Tips

For removal or destruction by electric current (fulguration) of Skene's glands, see 53270. For destruction of vaginal lesions, see 57061–57065. For lysis of labial adhesions, see 56441.

ICD-9-CM Procedural

71.3 Other local excision or destruction of vulva and perineum

Anesthesia

00940

ICD-9-CM Diagnostic

054.11 Herpetic vulvovaginitis
054.12 Herpetic ulceration of vulva
078.11 Condyloma acuminatum
078.19 Other specified viral warts
184.4 Malignant neoplasm of vulva, unspecified site
198.82 Secondary malignant neoplasm of genital organs
221.2 Benign neoplasm of vulva
228.01 Hemangioma of skin and subcutaneous tissue
233.30 Carcinoma in situ, unspecified female genital organ
233.31 Carcinoma in situ, vagina
233.32 Carcinoma in situ, vulva
233.39 Carcinoma in situ, other female genital organ
236.3 Neoplasm of uncertain behavior of other and unspecified female genital organs
239.5 Neoplasm of unspecified nature of other genitourinary organs
456.6 Vulval varices
616.81 Mucositis (ulcerative) of cervix, vagina, and vulva — (Use additional code to identify organism: 041.00-041.09, 041.10-041.19) (Use additional E code to identify adverse effects of therapy: E879.2, E930.7, E933.1)
616.89 Other inflammatory disease of cervix, vagina and vulva — (Use additional code to identify organism: 041.00-041.09, 041.10-041.19)
624.01 Vulvar intraepithelial neoplasia I [VIN I]
624.02 Vulvar intraepithelial neoplasia II [VIN II]
624.09 Other dystrophy of vulva
624.6 Polyp of labia and vulva
624.8 Other specified noninflammatory disorder of vulva and perineum
625.8 Other specified symptom associated with female genital organs
698.1 Pruritus of genital organs
701.0 Circumscribed scleroderma
701.5 Other abnormal granulation tissue
709.9 Unspecified disorder of skin and subcutaneous tissue
752.49 Other congenital anomaly of cervix, vagina, and external female genitalia

Terms To Know

carcinoma in situ. Malignancy that arises from the cells of the vessel, gland, or organ of origin that remains confined to that site or has not invaded neighboring tissue.

condyloma. Infectious tumor-like growth caused by the human papilloma virus, with a branching connective tissue core and epithelial covering that occurs on the skin and mucous membranes of the perianal region and external genitalia.

cryosurgery. Application of intense cold, usually produced using liquid nitrogen, to locally freeze diseased or unwanted tissue and induce tissue necrosis without causing harm to adjacent tissue.

electrocautery. Division or cutting of tissue using high-frequency electrical current to produce heat, which destroys cells.

laser surgery. Use of concentrated, sharply defined light beams to cut, cauterize, coagulate, seal, or vaporize tissue.

varices. Enlarged, dilated, or twisted, turning veins.

CCI Version 18.3

00940, 0213T, 0216T, 0228T, 0230T, 12001-12007, 12011-12057, 13100-13153, 36000, 36400-36410, 36420-36430, 36440, 36600, 36640, 37202, 43752, 51701-51703, 56820, 57100, 57180, 57410, 57500, 57800, 58100, 62310-62319, 64400-64435, 64445-64450, 64479, 64483, 64490, 64493, 64505-64530, 69990, 93000-93010, 93040-93042, 93318, 94002, 94200, 94250, 94680-94690, 94770, 95812-95816, 95819, 95822, 95829, 95955, 96360, 96365, 96372, 96374-96376, 99148-99149, 99150, J0670, J2001

Also not with 56501: 55815❖, 56441❖

Also not with 56515: 53270, 56441, 56501, 56605

Note: These CCI edits are used for Medicare. Other payers may reimburse on codes listed above.

Medicare Edits

	Fac RVU	Non-Fac RVU	FUD	Status
56501	3.42	3.9	10	A
56515	5.93	6.68	10	A

	MUE		Modifiers		
56501	1	51	N/A	N/A	N/A
56515	1	51	N/A	N/A	N/A

* with documentation

Medicare References: 100-3,140.5

Vulva

Coding Companion for Ob/Gyn

© 2012 OptumInsight, Inc.

56605-56606

56605 Biopsy of vulva or perineum (separate procedure); 1 lesion

56606 each separate additional lesion (List separately in addition to code for primary procedure)

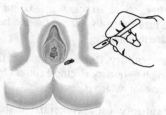

A portion of the vulvar or perineal lesion is excised for biopsy

Report 56605 for the first lesion and 56606 for each additional lesion

Explanation

The vulva includes the labia majora, labia minora, mons pubis, bulb of the vestibule, vestibule of the vagina, greater and lesser vestibular glands, and vaginal orifice. The perineum is the area between the vulva and the anus. The physician removes a sample of tissue from the vulva or perineum. After injecting a local anesthetic around the suspect tissue, the physician obtains a sample using a skin punch or sharp scalpel. A clip or suture can be used to control bleeding if pressure is not successful. Use 56605 for the biopsy of one lesion and 56606 for each additional lesion.

Coding Tips

Note that 56605, a separate procedure by definition, is usually a component of a more complex service and is not identified separately. When performed alone or with other unrelated procedures/services it may be reported. If performed alone, list the code; if performed with other procedures/services, list the code and append modifier 59. As an "add-on" code, 56606 is not subject to multiple procedure rules. No reimbursement reduction or modifier 51 is applied. "Add-on" codes describe additional intraservice work associated with the primary procedure. They are performed by the same physician on the same date of service as the primary

service/procedure, and must never be reported as a stand-alone code. These codes report the excision of a portion of a lesion for biopsy. If the entire lesion is excised, see 11420–11426 and 11620–11626. If a specimen is transported to an outside laboratory, report 99000 for conveyance.

ICD-9-CM Procedural

71.11 Biopsy of vulva

Anesthesia

56605 00940

56606 N/A

ICD-9-CM Diagnostic

054.11 Herpetic vulvovaginitis

054.12 Herpetic ulceration of vulva

078.11 Condyloma acuminatum

078.19 Other specified viral warts

184.4 Malignant neoplasm of vulva, unspecified site

198.2 Secondary malignant neoplasm of skin

198.82 Secondary malignant neoplasm of genital organs

214.9 Lipoma of unspecified site

221.2 Benign neoplasm of vulva

233.30 Carcinoma in situ, unspecified female genital organ

233.31 Carcinoma in situ, vagina

233.32 Carcinoma in situ, vulva

233.39 Carcinoma in situ, other female genital organ

234.8 Carcinoma in situ of other specified sites

236.3 Neoplasm of uncertain behavior of other and unspecified female genital organs

238.2 Neoplasm of uncertain behavior of skin

239.5 Neoplasm of unspecified nature of other genitourinary organs

616.10 Unspecified vaginitis and vulvovaginitis — (Use additional code to identify organism, such as: 041.00-041.09, 041.10-041.19, 041.41-041.49)

616.81 Mucositis (ulcerative) of cervix, vagina, and vulva — (Use additional code to identify organism: 041.00-041.09, 041.10-041.19) (Use additional E code to identify adverse effects of therapy: E879.2, E930.7, E933.1)

616.89 Other inflammatory disease of cervix, vagina and vulva — (Use additional

code to identify organism: 041.00-041.09, 041.10-041.19)

624.01 Vulvar intraepithelial neoplasia I [VIN I]

624.02 Vulvar intraepithelial neoplasia II [VIN II]

624.09 Other dystrophy of vulva

624.8 Other specified noninflammatory disorder of vulva and perineum

625.8 Other specified symptom associated with female genital organs

629.89 Other specified disorders of female genital organs

752.49 Other congenital anomaly of cervix, vagina, and external female genitalia

Terms To Know

carcinoma in situ. Malignancy that arises from the cells of the vessel, gland, or organ of origin that remains confined to that site or has not invaded neighboring tissue.

dystrophy of vulva. Abnormal cell growth of the fleshy external female genitalia.

neoplasm. New abnormal growth, tumor.

CCI Version 18.3

Also not with 56605: 00940, 0213T, 0216T, 0228T, 0230T, 10021-10022, 12001-12007, 12011-12057, 13100-13153, 36000, 36400-36410, 36420-36430, 36440, 36600, 36640, 37202, 43752, 51701-51703, 56820, 57100, 57180, 57410, 57500, 57800, 62310-62319, 64400-64435, 64445-64450, 64479, 64483, 64490, 64493, 64505-64530, 69990, 93000-93010, 93040-93042, 93318, 94002, 94200, 94250, 94680-94690, 94770, 95812-95816, 95819, 95822, 95829, 95955, 96360, 96365, 96372, 96374-96376, 99148-99149, 99150

Also not with 56606: 64430-64435

Note: These CCI edits are used for Medicare. Other payers may reimburse on codes listed above.

Medicare Edits

	Fac RVU	Non-Fac RVU	FUD	Status
56605	1.8	2.46	0	A
56606	0.87	1.11	N/A	A

	MUE		Modifiers		
56605	1	51	N/A	62	N/A
56606	-	N/A	N/A	62	N/A

* with documentation

Medicare References: None

Vulva

56620-56625

56620 Vulvectomy simple; partial
56625 complete

A partial vulvectomy involves removal of all or part of the labia on one side and the clitoris. A complete removal includes the labia, clitoris, and the urethral opening

Explanation

The physician removes part or all of the vulva to treat premalignant or malignant lesions. A simple complete vulvectomy includes removal of all of the labia majora, labia minora, and clitoris, while a simple, partial vulvectomy may include removal of part or all of the labia majora and labia minora on one side and the clitoris. The physician examines the lower genital tract and the perianal skin through a colposcope. In 56620, a wide semi-elliptical incision that contains the diseased area is made. In 56625, two wide elliptical incisions encompassing the vulvar area are made. One elliptical incision extends from well above the clitoris around both labia majora to a point just in front of the anus. The second elliptical incision starts at a point between the clitoris and the opening of the urethra and is carried around both sides of the opening of the vagina. The underlying subcutaneous fatty tissue is removed along with the large portion of excised skin. Vessels are clamped and tied off with sutures or are electrocoagulated to control bleeding. The considerable defect is usually closed in layers using separately reportable plastic techniques. Vaginal gauze packing may be placed in the vagina.

Coding Tips

Simple complete vulvectomy encompasses all of the labia majora and labia minora on both sides. Report any free grafts or flaps separately. If significant additional time and effort is documented, append modifier 22 and submit a cover letter and operative report.

ICD-9-CM Procedural
71.61   Unilateral vulvectomy
71.62   Bilateral vulvectomy

Anesthesia
00906

ICD-9-CM Diagnostic
171.6   Malignant neoplasm of connective and other soft tissue of pelvis
172.5   Malignant melanoma of skin of trunk, except scrotum
173.50 Unspecified malignant neoplasm of skin of trunk, except scrotum
173.51 Basal cell carcinoma of skin of trunk, except scrotum
173.52 Squamous cell carcinoma of skin of trunk, except scrotum
173.59 Other specified malignant neoplasm of skin of trunk, except scrotum
184.4   Malignant neoplasm of vulva, unspecified site
198.82 Secondary malignant neoplasm of genital organs
199.1   Other malignant neoplasm of unspecified site
221.2   Benign neoplasm of vulva
233.30 Carcinoma in situ, unspecified female genital organ
233.31 Carcinoma in situ, vagina
233.32 Carcinoma in situ, vulva
233.39 Carcinoma in situ, other female genital organ
236.3   Neoplasm of uncertain behavior of other and unspecified female genital organs
239.5   Neoplasm of unspecified nature of other genitourinary organs
616.4   Other abscess of vulva — (Use additional code to identify organism: 041.00-041.09, 041.10-041.19)
623.0   Dysplasia of vagina
623.8   Other specified noninflammatory disorder of vagina
624.3   Hypertrophy of labia
624.8   Other specified noninflammatory disorder of vulva and perineum
625.0   Dyspareunia
625.71 Vulvar vestibulitis
625.79 Other vulvodynia
698.1   Pruritus of genital organs
701.0   Circumscribed scleroderma
752.40 Unspecified congenital anomaly of cervix, vagina, and external female genitalia
752.41 Embryonic cyst of cervix, vagina, and external female genitalia
752.49 Other congenital anomaly of cervix, vagina, and external female genitalia
752.89 Other specified anomalies of genital organs
752.9   Unspecified congenital anomaly of genital organs
V50.1   Other plastic surgery for unacceptable cosmetic appearance
V50.8   Other elective surgery for purposes other than remedying health states
V84.09 Genetic susceptibility to other malignant neoplasm — (Use additional code, if applicable, for any associated family history of the disease: V16-V19. Code first, if applicable, any current malignant neoplasms: 140.0-195.8, 200.0-208.9, 230.0-234.9. Use additional code, if applicable, for any personal history of malignant neoplasm: V10.0-V10.9)

CCI Version 18.3
00940, 0213T, 0216T, 0228T, 0230T, 12001-12007, 12011-12057, 13100-13153, 36000, 36400-36410, 36420-36430, 36440, 36600, 36640, 37202, 43752, 51701-51703, 56820-56821, 57100, 57180, 57410, 57500, 58100, 62310-62319, 64400-64435, 64445-64450, 64479, 64483, 64490, 64493, 64505-64530, 69990, 93000-93010, 93040-93042, 93318, 94002, 94200, 94250, 94680-94690, 94770, 95812-95816, 95819, 95822, 95829, 95955, 96360, 96365, 96372, 96374-96376, 99148-99149, 99150

Also not with 56620: 56605-56606

Also not with 56625: 56605-56620, 57800

Note: These CCI edits are used for Medicare. Other payers may reimburse on codes listed above.

Medicare Edits

	Fac RVU	Non-Fac RVU	FUD	Status
56620	15.04	15.04	90	A
56625	17.99	17.99	90	A

	MUE			Modifiers	
56620	1	51	N/A	62*	80
56625	1	51	N/A	62*	80

* with documentation

Medicare References: None

Coding Companion for Ob/Gyn

56630

56630 Vulvectomy, radical, partial;

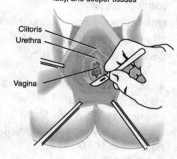

Up to 80 percent of the vulva is excised including the terminal portion of the urethra, vagina, skin, subcutaneous fatty, and deeper tissues

Clitoris
Urethra
Vagina

Explanation

The physician removes part of the vulva to treat malignancy. A partial radical vulvectomy includes partial or complete removal of a large, deep segment of skin from the following structures: abdomen and groin, labia majora, labia minora, clitoris, mons veneris, and terminal portions of the urethra, vagina, and other vulvar organs. Through incisions in the lower abdomen, thighs, and vulvar area, the physician removes skin, subcutaneous fatty tissue, and deeper tissue. Also included in the en bloc removal of tissue are portions of the saphenous veins and ligaments and the target lesion. The resulting large and disfiguring defect is usually closed using separately reported plastic surgical techniques, which may include pedicle flaps or free skin grafts. Subcutaneous rubber drains may be left in the surgical site, and vaginal gauze packing may be placed in the vagina.

Coding Tips

This procedure does not include removal of the inguinal and femoral lymph nodes. For a partial radical vulvectomy with unilateral inguinofemoral lymphadenectomy, see 56631. For a partial radical vulvectomy with bilateral inguinofemoral lymphadenectomy, see 56632. For a simple vulvectomy, see 56620 or 56625. Report any free grafts or flaps separately. If significant additional time and effort is documented, append modifier 22 and submit a cover letter and operative report.

ICD-9-CM Procedural

40.3 Regional lymph node excision
71.5 Radical vulvectomy

Anesthesia

56630 00904

ICD-9-CM Diagnostic

171.6 Malignant neoplasm of connective and other soft tissue of pelvis
172.5 Malignant melanoma of skin of trunk, except scrotum
173.50 Unspecified malignant neoplasm of skin of trunk, except scrotum
173.51 Basal cell carcinoma of skin of trunk, except scrotum
173.52 Squamous cell carcinoma of skin of trunk, except scrotum
173.59 Other specified malignant neoplasm of skin of trunk, except scrotum
184.4 Malignant neoplasm of vulva, unspecified site
196.5 Secondary and unspecified malignant neoplasm of lymph nodes of inguinal region and lower limb
198.82 Secondary malignant neoplasm of genital organs
209.36 Merkel cell carcinoma of other sites
209.71 Secondary neuroendocrine tumor of distant lymph nodes
209.79 Secondary neuroendocrine tumor of other sites
233.30 Carcinoma in situ, unspecified female genital organ
233.31 Carcinoma in situ, vagina
233.32 Carcinoma in situ, vulva
233.39 Carcinoma in situ, other female genital organ
236.3 Neoplasm of uncertain behavior of other and unspecified female genital organs
239.5 Neoplasm of unspecified nature of other genitourinary organs
239.89 Neoplasms of unspecified nature, other specified sites
278.1 Localized adiposity — (Use additional code to identify any associated intellectual disabilities.)
623.8 Other specified noninflammatory disorder of vagina
625.0 Dyspareunia
625.70 Vulvodynia, unspecified
625.71 Vulvar vestibulitis
625.79 Other vulvodynia

752.40 Unspecified congenital anomaly of cervix, vagina, and external female genitalia
752.41 Embryonic cyst of cervix, vagina, and external female genitalia
752.49 Other congenital anomaly of cervix, vagina, and external female genitalia
752.89 Other specified anomalies of genital organs
752.9 Unspecified congenital anomaly of genital organs
V84.09 Genetic susceptibility to other malignant neoplasm — (Use additional code, if applicable, for any associated family history of the disease: V16-V19. Code first, if applicable, any current malignant neoplasms: 140.0-195.8, 200.0-208.9, 230.0-234.9. Use additional code, if applicable, for any personal history of malignant neoplasm: V10.0-V10.9)

CCI Version 18.3

00940, 0213T, 0216T, 0228T, 0230T, 12001-12007, 12011-12057, 13100-13153, 36000, 36400-36410, 36420-36430, 36440, 36600, 36640, 37202, 43752, 51701-51703, 56605-56620, 56820-56821, 57100, 57180, 57410, 57500, 57800, 58100, 62310-62319, 64400-64435, 64445-64450, 64479, 64483, 64490, 64493, 64505-64530, 69990, 93000-93010, 93040-93042, 93318, 94002, 94200, 94250, 94680-94690, 94770, 95812-95816, 95819, 95822, 95829, 95955, 96360, 96365, 96372, 96374-96376, 99148-99149, 99150

Note: These CCI edits are used for Medicare. Other payers may reimburse on codes listed above.

Medicare Edits

	Fac RVU	Non-Fac RVU	FUD	Status
56630	26.49	26.49	90	A

	MUE		Modifiers		
56630	1	51	N/A	62*	80

* with documentation

Medicare References: None

Coding Companion for Ob/Gyn

Vulva

56631-56632

56631 Vulvectomy, radical, partial; with unilateral inguinofemoral lymphadenectomy

56632 with bilateral inguinofemoral lymphadenectomy

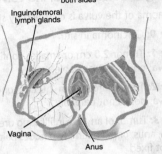

Up to 80 percent of the vulva is removed as well as inguinofemoral lymph glands. The lymph glands are removed from one or both sides.

Inguinofemoral lymph glands

Vagina

Anus

Reconstruction is reported separately

Explanation

The physician removes part of the vulva to treat malignancy. A partial radical vulvectomy includes the partial or complete removal of a large, deep segment of skin and tissue from the abdomen and groin, labia majora and minora, clitoris, mons veneris, and terminal portions of the urethra, vagina, and other vulvar organs. Through incisions in the lower abdomen, thighs, and vulvar area, the physician removes skin, subcutaneous fatty tissue, and deeper tissue. The physician also removes superficial and deep inguinal lymph nodes and adjacent femoral lymph nodes on one side in 56631 and on both sides in 56632. Also included in the en bloc removal of tissue are portions of the saphenous veins and ligaments and the target lesion. The resulting large and disfiguring defect is usually closed in layers using plastic surgical techniques, which may include pedicle flaps or free skin grafts. Subcutaneous rubber drains may be left in the surgical site, and vaginal gauze packing may be placed in the vagina.

Coding Tips

For a simple vulvectomy, see 56620 or 56625. For a partial radical vulvectomy without inguinofemoral lymphadenectomy, see 56630. For a complete radical vulvectomy with unilateral inguinofemoral lymphadenectomy, see 56634; for a complete radical vulvectomy with bilateral inguinofemoral

lymphadenectomy, see 56637. Report any free grafts or flaps separately.

ICD-9-CM Procedural

40.3 Regional lymph node excision

71.5 Radical vulvectomy

Anesthesia

00904

ICD-9-CM Diagnostic

171.6 Malignant neoplasm of connective and other soft tissue of pelvis

172.5 Malignant melanoma of skin of trunk, except scrotum

173.50 Unspecified malignant neoplasm of skin of trunk, except scrotum

173.51 Basal cell carcinoma of skin of trunk, except scrotum

173.52 Squamous cell carcinoma of skin of trunk, except scrotum

173.59 Other specified malignant neoplasm of skin of trunk, except scrotum

184.4 Malignant neoplasm of vulva, unspecified site

196.5 Secondary and unspecified malignant neoplasm of lymph nodes of inguinal region and lower limb

198.82 Secondary malignant neoplasm of genital organs

209.36 Merkel cell carcinoma of other sites

233.30 Carcinoma in situ, unspecified female genital organ

233.31 Carcinoma in situ, vagina

233.32 Carcinoma in situ, vulva

233.39 Carcinoma in situ, other female genital organ

236.3 Neoplasm of uncertain behavior of other and unspecified female genital organs

239.5 Neoplasm of unspecified nature of other genitourinary organs

623.8 Other specified noninflammatory disorder of vagina

624.9 Unspecified noninflammatory disorder of vulva and perineum

625.0 Dyspareunia

625.70 Vulvodynia, unspecified

625.71 Vulvar vestibulitis

625.79 Other vulvodynia

752.40 Unspecified congenital anomaly of cervix, vagina, and external female genitalia

752.41 Embryonic cyst of cervix, vagina, and external female genitalia

752.49 Other congenital anomaly of cervix, vagina, and external female genitalia

752.89 Other specified anomalies of genital organs

V84.09 Genetic susceptibility to other malignant neoplasm — (Use additional code, if applicable, for any associated family history of the disease: V16-V19. Code first, if applicable, any current malignant neoplasms: 140.0-195.8, 200.0-208.9, 230.0-234.9. Use additional code, if applicable, for any personal history of malignant neoplasm: V10.0-V10.9)

Terms To Know

lymphadenectomy. Dissection of lymph nodes free from the vessels and removal for examination by frozen section in a separate procedure to detect early-stage metastases.

CCI Version 18.3

00940, 0213T, 0216T, 0228T, 0230T, 12001-12007, 12011-12057, 13100-13153, 36000, 36400-36410, 36420-36430, 36440, 36600, 36640, 37202, 38760, 43752, 51701-51703, 56605-56606, 56630, 56820-56821, 57100, 57180, 57410, 57500, 57800, 58100, 62310-62319, 64400-64435, 64445-64450, 64479, 64483, 64490, 64493, 64505-64530, 69990, 93000-93010, 93040-93042, 93318, 94002, 94200, 94250, 94680-94690, 94770, 95812-95816, 95819, 95822, 95829, 95955, 96360, 96365, 96372, 96374-96376, 99148-99149, 99150

Also not with 56632: 38765

Note: These CCI edits are used for Medicare. Other payers may reimburse on codes listed above.

Medicare Edits

	Fac RVU	Non-Fac RVU	FUD	Status
56631	33.59	33.59	90	A
56632	39.04	39.04	90	A

	MUE		Modifiers		
56631	1	51	N/A	62	80
56632	1	51	N/A	62	80

* with documentation

Medicare References: None

Vulva

56633

56633 Vulvectomy, radical, complete;

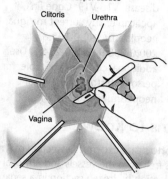

The distal portions of the urethra and vagina are excised with the labia. The physician may also remove skin, subcutaneous fatty tissue, and deeper tissues

Clitoris
Urethra
Vagina

More than 80 percent of the vulva is excised

Explanation

The physician removes the vulva to treat malignancy. A complete radical vulvectomy includes the removal of a large, deep segment of skin and tissue from the following structures: abdomen and groin, labia majora, labia minora, clitoris, mons veneris, and terminal portions of the urethra, vagina, and other vulvar organs. Deep tissue from more than 80 percent of the vulva is excised. Through incisions in the lower abdomen, thighs, and vulvar area, the physician removes skin, subcutaneous fatty tissue, and deeper tissues. Also included in the en bloc removal of tissue are portions of the saphenous veins and ligaments and the target lesion. The resulting large and disfiguring defect is usually closed in layers using separately reported plastic surgical techniques, which may include pedicle flaps or free skin grafts. Subcutaneous rubber drains may be used, and vaginal gauze packing may be placed in the vagina.

Coding Tips

This procedure does not include the removal of the inguinal and femoral lymph nodes. For a complete radical vulvectomy with unilateral inguinofemoral lymphadenectomy, see 56634. For a complete radical vulvectomy with bilateral inguinofemoral lymphadenectomy, see 56637. For a partial radical vulvectomy, see 56630–56632. For a simple vulvectomy, see 56620 and 56625. Report any free grafts or flaps separately.

ICD-9-CM Procedural

40.3   Regional lymph node excision
71.5   Radical vulvectomy

Anesthesia

56633   00904

ICD-9-CM Diagnostic

171.6   Malignant neoplasm of connective and other soft tissue of pelvis
172.5   Malignant melanoma of skin of trunk, except scrotum
173.50   Unspecified malignant neoplasm of skin of trunk, except scrotum
173.51   Basal cell carcinoma of skin of trunk, except scrotum
173.52   Squamous cell carcinoma of skin of trunk, except scrotum
173.59   Other specified malignant neoplasm of skin of trunk, except scrotum
184.4   Malignant neoplasm of vulva, unspecified site
196.5   Secondary and unspecified malignant neoplasm of lymph nodes of inguinal region and lower limb
198.82   Secondary malignant neoplasm of genital organs
209.36   Merkel cell carcinoma of other sites
209.71   Secondary neuroendocrine tumor of distant lymph nodes
209.79   Secondary neuroendocrine tumor of other sites
233.30   Carcinoma in situ, unspecified female genital organ
233.31   Carcinoma in situ, vagina
233.32   Carcinoma in situ, vulva
233.39   Carcinoma in situ, other female genital organ
236.3   Neoplasm of uncertain behavior of other and unspecified female genital organs
239.5   Neoplasm of unspecified nature of other genitourinary organs
239.89   Neoplasms of unspecified nature, other specified sites
752.40   Unspecified congenital anomaly of cervix, vagina, and external female genitalia
752.41   Embryonic cyst of cervix, vagina, and external female genitalia
752.49   Other congenital anomaly of cervix, vagina, and external female genitalia
752.89   Other specified anomalies of genital organs
V84.09   Genetic susceptibility to other malignant neoplasm — (Use

additional code, if applicable, for any associated family history of the disease: V16-V19. Code first, if applicable, any current malignant neoplasms: 140.0-195.8, 200.0-208.9, 230.0-234.9. Use additional code, if applicable, for any personal history of malignant neoplasm: V10.0-V10.9)

Terms To Know

staging of carcinoma of the vulva.

Carcinoma of the vulva is classified by stage:

Stage 0: Carcinoma in situ.

Stage 1: Tumor 2.0 cm or smaller confined to vulva; nodes not palpable.

Stage 2: Tumor larger than 2.0 cm confined to vulva; nodes not palpable.

Stage 3: Tumor of any size infiltrating urethra, vagina, anus, or perineum; two nodes palpable but not fixed.

Stage 4: Tumor of any size infiltrating anal or bladder mucosa; fixed to bone or metastases; fixed nodes.

Note: This staging does not apply to melanoma or secondary malignancies.

CCI Version 18.3

00940, 0213T, 0216T, 0228T, 0230T, 12001-12007, 12011-12057, 13100-13153, 36000, 36400-36410, 36420-36430, 36440, 36600, 36640, 37202, 43752, 51701-51703, 56605-56606, 56820-56821, 57100, 57180, 57410, 57500, 57800, 58100, 62310-62319, 64400-64435, 64445-64450, 64479, 64483, 64490, 64493, 64505-64530, 69990, 93000-93010, 93040-93042, 93318, 94002, 94200, 94250, 94680-94690, 94770, 95812-95816, 95819, 95822, 95829, 95955, 96360, 96365, 96372, 96374-96376, 99148-99149, 99150

Note: These CCI edits are used for Medicare. Other payers may reimburse on codes listed above.

Medicare Edits

	Fac RVU	Non-Fac RVU	FUD	Status
56633	34.42	34.42	90	A

	MUE		Modifiers		
56633	1	51	N/A	62	80

* with documentation

Medicare References: None

Coding Companion for Ob/Gyn

Vulva

56634-56637

56634 Vulvectomy, radical, complete; with unilateral inguinofemoral lymphadenectomy
56637 with bilateral inguinofemoral lymphadenectomy

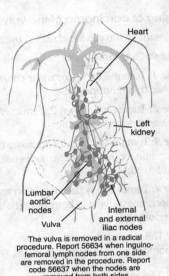

The vulva is removed in a radical procedure. Report 56634 when inguinofemoral lymph nodes from one side are removed in the procedure. Report code 56637 when the nodes are removed from both sides

Explanation

The physician removes the vulva to treat malignancy. A complete radical vulvectomy includes the removal of a large, deep segment of skin and tissue from the lower abdomen and groin, labia majora and minora, clitoris, mons veneris, and terminal portions of the urethra, vagina, and other vulvar organs. Deep tissue from more than 80 percent of the vulva is removed. Through incisions in the lower abdomen, thighs, and vulvar area, the physician removes skin, subcutaneous fatty tissue, and deeper tissues. The physician also removes the inguinal and femoral lymph nodes on one side in 56634 and on both sides in 56637. Also included in the en bloc removal of tissue are portions of the saphenous veins and ligaments and the target lesion. The resulting large and disfiguring defect is usually closed in layers using plastic surgical techniques, which may include pedicle flaps or free skin grafts. Subcutaneous rubber drains may be used, and vaginal gauze packing may be placed in the vagina.

Coding Tips

For a complete radical vulvectomy without inguinofemoral lymphadenectomy, see 56633. For a partial radical vulvectomy, see 56630–56632. Report any free grafts or flaps separately.

ICD-9-CM Procedural

40.3 Regional lymph node excision
71.5 Radical vulvectomy

Anesthesia

00904

ICD-9-CM Diagnostic

171.6 Malignant neoplasm of connective and other soft tissue of pelvis
172.5 Malignant melanoma of skin of trunk, except scrotum
173.50 Unspecified malignant neoplasm of skin of trunk, except scrotum
173.51 Basal cell carcinoma of skin of trunk, except scrotum
173.52 Squamous cell carcinoma of skin of trunk, except scrotum
173.59 Other specified malignant neoplasm of skin of trunk, except scrotum
184.4 Malignant neoplasm of vulva, unspecified site
196.5 Secondary and unspecified malignant neoplasm of lymph nodes of inguinal region and lower limb
198.82 Secondary malignant neoplasm of genital organs
209.36 Merkel cell carcinoma of other sites
209.71 Secondary neuroendocrine tumor of distant lymph nodes
209.79 Secondary neuroendocrine tumor of other sites
233.30 Carcinoma in situ, unspecified female genital organ
233.31 Carcinoma in situ, vagina
233.32 Carcinoma in situ, vulva
233.39 Carcinoma in situ, other female genital organ
236.3 Neoplasm of uncertain behavior of other and unspecified female genital organs
239.5 Neoplasm of unspecified nature of other genitourinary organs
239.89 Neoplasms of unspecified nature, other specified sites
752.40 Unspecified congenital anomaly of cervix, vagina, and external female genitalia
752.41 Embryonic cyst of cervix, vagina, and external female genitalia
752.49 Other congenital anomaly of cervix, vagina, and external female genitalia
752.89 Other specified anomalies of genital organs
V84.09 Genetic susceptibility to other malignant neoplasm — (Use

additional code, if applicable, for any associated family history of the disease: V16-V19. Code first, if applicable, any current malignant neoplasms: 140.0-195.8, 200.0-208.9, 230.0-234.9. Use additional code, if applicable, for any personal history of malignant neoplasm: V10.0-V10.9)

Terms To Know

lymphadenectomy. Dissection of lymph nodes free from the vessels and removal for examination by frozen section in a separate procedure to detect early-stage metastases.

CCI Version 18.3

00940, 0213T, 0216T, 0228T, 0230T, 12001-12007, 12011-12057, 13100-13153, 36000, 36400-36410, 36420-36430, 36440, 36600, 36640, 37202, 38760, 43752, 51701-51703, 56605-56606, 56633, 56820-56821, 57100, 57180, 57410, 57500, 57800, 58100, 62310-62319, 64400-64435, 64445-64450, 64479, 64483, 64490, 64493, 64505-64530, 69990, 93000-93010, 93040-93042, 93318, 94002, 94200, 94250, 94680-94690, 94770, 95812-95816, 95819, 95822, 95829, 95955, 96360, 96365, 96372, 96374-96376, 99148-99149, 99150

Also not with 56637: 38765

Note: These CCI edits are used for Medicare. Other payers may reimburse on codes listed above.

Medicare Edits

	Fac RVU	Non-Fac RVU	FUD	Status
56634	36.51	36.51	90	A
56637	42.78	42.78	90	A

	MUE		Modifiers		
56634	1	51	N/A	62	80
56637	1	51	N/A	62	80

* with documentation

Medicare References: None

Coding Companion for Ob/Gyn

Vulva

56640

56640 Vulvectomy, radical, complete, with inguinofemoral, iliac, and pelvic lymphadenectomy

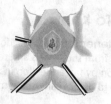

Physician removes the vulva and inguinofemoral, iliac, and pelvic lymph nodes from both sides

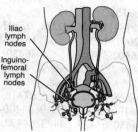

Iliac lymph nodes

Inguino-femoral lymph nodes

Explanation

The physician removes the vulva to treat malignancy. A complete radical vulvectomy includes the removal of a large, deep segment of skin and tissue from the following structures: lower abdomen and groin, labia majora, labia minora, clitoris, mons veneris, and terminal portions of the urethra, vagina, and other vulvar organs. Deep tissue from more than 80 percent of the vulva is removed. Through incisions in the lower abdomen, thighs, and vulvar area, the physician removes skin, subcutaneous fatty tissue, and deeper tissue. The physician also removes the inguinal and femoral lymph nodes on both sides as well as the iliac and pelvic lymph nodes in the pelvic cavity, which is entered through an abdominal incision. Also included in the en bloc removal of tissue are portions of the saphenous veins and ligaments and the target lesion. The resulting large and disfiguring defect is usually closed in layers using separately reported plastic surgical techniques, which may include pedicle flaps or free skin grafts. Subcutaneous rubber drains may be used, and vaginal gauze packing may be placed in the vagina.

Coding Tips

For a complete radical vulvectomy with bilateral inguinofemoral lymphadenectomy, see 56637. For a complete radical vulvectomy with unilateral inguinofemoral lymphadenectomy, see 56634. For a complete radical vulvectomy without inguinofemoral

lymphadenectomy, see 56633. For a partial radical vulvectomy, see 56630–56632. Report any free grafts or flaps separately. If plastic surgery techniques are used, they are separately reportable.

ICD-9-CM Procedural

40.59   Radical excision of other lymph nodes

71.5   Radical vulvectomy

Anesthesia

56640   00904

ICD-9-CM Diagnostic

171.6   Malignant neoplasm of connective and other soft tissue of pelvis

172.5   Malignant melanoma of skin of trunk, except scrotum

173.50   Unspecified malignant neoplasm of skin of trunk, except scrotum

173.51   Basal cell carcinoma of skin of trunk, except scrotum

173.52   Squamous cell carcinoma of skin of trunk, except scrotum

173.59   Other specified malignant neoplasm of skin of trunk, except scrotum

184.4   Malignant neoplasm of vulva, unspecified site

196.5   Secondary and unspecified malignant neoplasm of lymph nodes of inguinal region and lower limb

196.6   Secondary and unspecified malignant neoplasm of intrapelvic lymph nodes

198.82   Secondary malignant neoplasm of genital organs

209.36   Merkel cell carcinoma of other sites

209.71   Secondary neuroendocrine tumor of distant lymph nodes

209.79   Secondary neuroendocrine tumor of other sites

233.30   Carcinoma in situ, unspecified female genital organ

233.31   Carcinoma in situ, vagina

233.32   Carcinoma in situ, vulva

233.39   Carcinoma in situ, other female genital organ

236.3   Neoplasm of uncertain behavior of other and unspecified female genital organs

239.5   Neoplasm of unspecified nature of other genitourinary organs

239.89   Neoplasms of unspecified nature, other specified sites

V84.09   Genetic susceptibility to other malignant neoplasm — (Use additional code, if applicable, for any associated family history of the

disease: V16-V19. Code first, if applicable, any current malignant neoplasms: 140.0-195.8, 200.0-208.9, 230.0-234.9. Use additional code, if applicable, for any personal history of malignant neoplasm: V10.0-V10.9)

Terms To Know

staging of carcinoma of the vulva.

Carcinoma of the vulva is classified by stage:

Stage 0: Carcinoma in situ.

Stage 1: Tumor 2.0 cm or smaller confined to vulva; nodes not palpable.

Stage 2: Tumor larger than 2.0 cm confined to vulva; nodes not palpable.

Stage 3: Tumor of any size infiltrating urethra, vagina, anus, or perineum; two nodes palpable but not fixed.

Stage 4: Tumor of any size infiltrating anal or bladder mucosa; fixed to bone or metastases; fixed nodes.

Note: This staging does not apply to melanoma or secondary malignancies.

CCI Version 18.3

00940, 0213T, 0216T, 0228T, 0230T, 12001-12007, 12011-12057, 13100-13153, 36000, 36400-36410, 36420-36430, 36440, 36600, 36640, 37202, 38571-38572, 38765, 38770, 38780, 43752, 51701-51703, 56605-56606, 56820-56821, 57100, 57180, 57410, 57500, 57800, 58100, 62310-62319, 64400-64435, 64445-64450, 64479, 64483, 64490, 64493, 64505-64530, 69990, 93000-93010, 93040-93042, 93318, 94002, 94200, 94250, 94680-94690, 94770, 95812-95816, 95819, 95822, 95829, 95955, 96360, 96365, 96372, 96374-96376, 99148-99149, 99150

Note: These CCI edits are used for Medicare. Other payers may reimburse on codes listed above.

Medicare Edits

	Fac RVU	Non-Fac RVU	FUD	Status
56640	42.66	42.66	90	A

	MUE		Modifiers		
56640	1	51	50	62*	80

  * with documentation

Medicare References: None

Coding Companion for Ob/Gyn

Vulva

56700

56700 Partial hymenectomy or revision of hymenal ring

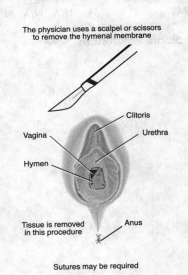

The physician uses a scalpel or scissors to remove the hymenal membrane

Clitoris
Vagina
Urethra
Hymen

Tissue is removed in this procedure
Anus

Sutures may be required

Explanation

A hymen is a membrane that partially or wholly occludes the vaginal opening. Following local injection of an anesthetic, the physician excises a portion of the hymenal membrane. Using a scalpel or scissors, the physician removes the membrane at its junction with the opening of the vagina. The cut margins of the vaginal mucosa are sutured with fine, absorbable material.

Coding Tips

Local anesthesia is included in this service. However, this procedure may be performed under general anesthesia, depending on the age and/or condition of the patient. If a specimen is transported to an outside laboratory, report 99000 for conveyance. For hymenotomy, see 56442. Surgical trays, A4550, are not separately reimbursed by Medicare; however, other third-party payers may cover them. Check with the specific payer to determine coverage.

ICD-9-CM Procedural

70.31 Hymenectomy
70.76 Hymenorrhaphy

Anesthesia

56700 00940

ICD-9-CM Diagnostic

184.0 Malignant neoplasm of vagina

198.82 Secondary malignant neoplasm of genital organs
221.1 Benign neoplasm of vagina
233.30 Carcinoma in situ, unspecified female genital organ
233.31 Carcinoma in situ, vagina
233.32 Carcinoma in situ, vulva
233.39 Carcinoma in situ, other female genital organ
236.3 Neoplasm of uncertain behavior of other and unspecified female genital organs
614.9 Unspecified inflammatory disease of female pelvic organs and tissues — (Use additional code to identify organism: 041.00-041.09, 041.10-041.19)
623.3 Tight hymenal ring
625.0 Dyspareunia
629.89 Other specified disorders of female genital organs
752.40 Unspecified congenital anomaly of cervix, vagina, and external female genitalia
752.41 Embryonic cyst of cervix, vagina, and external female genitalia
752.42 Imperforate hymen
752.49 Other congenital anomaly of cervix, vagina, and external female genitalia
752.89 Other specified anomalies of genital organs
752.9 Unspecified congenital anomaly of genital organs

Terms To Know

absorbable sutures. Strands prepared from collagen or a synthetic polymer and capable of being absorbed by tissue over time.

anomaly. Irregularity in the structure or position of an organ or tissue.

benign. Mild or nonmalignant in nature.

carcinoma in situ. Malignancy that arises from the cells of the vessel, gland, or organ of origin that remains confined to that site or has not invaded neighboring tissue.

congenital. Present at birth, occurring through heredity or an influence during gestation up to the moment of birth.

dyspareunia. Pain experienced during or after intercourse, commonly occurring in the clitoris, vagina, or labia.

malignant. Any condition tending to progress toward death, specifically an invasive tumor with a loss of cellular differentiation that has the ability to spread or metastasize to other areas in the body.

secondary. Second in order of occurrence or importance, or appearing during the course of another disease or condition.

CCI Version 18.3

00940, 0213T, 0216T, 0228T, 0230T, 12001-12007, 12011-12057, 13100-13153, 36000, 36400-36410, 36420-36430, 36440, 36600, 36640, 37202, 43752, 51701-51703, 56442, 56605-56606, 56820, 57100, 57180, 57410, 57500, 57800, 58100, 62310-62319, 64400-64435, 64445-64450, 64479, 64483, 64490, 64493, 64505-64530, 69990, 93000-93010, 93040-93042, 93318, 94002, 94200, 94250, 94680-94690, 94770, 95812-95816, 95819, 95822, 95829, 95955, 96360, 96365, 96372, 96374-96376, 99148-99149, 99150, J2001

Note: These CCI edits are used for Medicare. Other payers may reimburse on codes listed above.

Medicare Edits

	Fac RVU	Non-Fac RVU	FUD	Status
56700	5.6	5.6	10	A

	MUE		Modifiers		
56700	1	51	N/A	62*	80

* with documentation

Medicare References: None

Coding Companion for Ob/Gyn

Vulva

56740

56740 Excision of Bartholin's gland or cyst

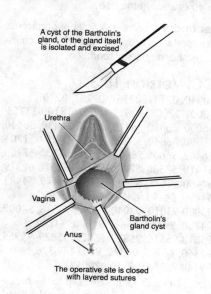

A cyst of the Bartholin's gland, or the gland itself, is isolated and excised

Urethra

Vagina

Anus

Bartholin's gland cyst

The operative site is closed with layered sutures

Explanation

The physician removes a cystic Bartholin's gland, which lies at the tail end of the bulb of the vestibular opening just inside of the vagina. The physician makes an incision through the vaginal mucosa. The cyst is isolated through the vaginal incision by dissecting the deeper fatty tissues and excised. The remaining cavity and skin are closed in layers using absorbable material.

Coding Tips

For excision of Skene's gland, see 53270. For marsupialization of Bartholin's gland, see 56440. For incision and drainage of Bartholin's gland abscess, see 56420. For excision of urethral caruncle, see 53265. For excision or marsupialization of urethral diverticulum, see 53230 and 53240. Surgical trays, A4550, are not separately reimbursed by Medicare; however, other third-party payers may cover them. Check with the specific payer to determine coverage.

ICD-9-CM Procedural

71.24   Excision or other destruction of Bartholin's gland (cyst)

Anesthesia

56740   00940

ICD-9-CM Diagnostic

616.2   Cyst of Bartholin's gland — (Use additional code to identify organism: 041.00-041.09, 041.10-041.19)

616.3   Abscess of Bartholin's gland — (Use additional code to identify organism: 041.00-041.09, 041.10-041.19)

Terms To Know

abscess. Circumscribed collection of pus resulting from bacteria, frequently associated with swelling and other signs of inflammation.

absorbable sutures. Strands prepared from collagen or a synthetic polymer and capable of being absorbed by tissue over time.

Bartholin's gland. Mucous-producing gland found in the vestibular bulbs on either side of the vaginal orifice and connected to the mucosal membrane at the opening by a duct.

Bartholin's gland abscess. Pocket of pus and surrounding cellulitis caused by infection of the Bartholin's gland and causing localized swelling and pain in the posterior labia majora that may extend into the lower vagina.

cyst. Elevated encapsulated mass containing fluid, semisolid, or solid material with a membranous lining.

dissect. Cut apart or separate tissue for surgical purposes or for visual or microscopic study.

excision. Surgical removal of an organ or tissue.

nonabsorbable sutures. Strands of natural or synthetic material that resist absorption into living tissue and are removed once healing is under way. Nonabsorbable sutures are commonly used to close skin wounds and repair tendons or collagenous tissue.

CCI Version 18.3

00940, 0213T, 0216T, 0228T, 0230T, 12001-12007, 12011-12057, 13100-13153, 36000, 36400-36410, 36420-36430, 36440, 36600, 36640, 37202, 43752, 51701-51703, 56420-56440, 56605-56606, 56820, 57100, 57180, 57410, 57500, 57800, 58100, 62310-62319, 64400-64435, 64445-64450, 64479, 64483, 64490, 64493, 64505-64530, 69990, 93000-93010, 93040-93042, 93318, 94002, 94200, 94250, 94680-94690, 94770, 95812-95816, 95819, 95822, 95829, 95955, 96360, 96365, 96372, 96374-96376, 99148-99149, 99150, J2001

Note: These CCI edits are used for Medicare. Other payers may reimburse on codes listed above.

Medicare Edits

	Fac RVU	Non-Fac RVU	FUD	Status
56740	8.88	8.88	10	A

	MUE		Modifiers		
56740	2	51	N/A	N/A	N/A

* with documentation

Medicare References: None

Vulva

56800

56800 Plastic repair of introitus

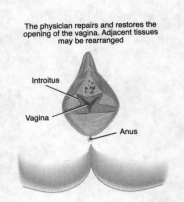

The physician repairs and restores the opening of the vagina. Adjacent tissues may be rearranged

Introitus

Vagina

Anus

The introitus is the entrance to the vagina

Explanation

The physician repairs and restores the anatomy of the opening of the vagina by excising scar tissue and strengthening the supporting tissues using tissue flaps and suturing techniques. This procedure varies greatly from patient to patient, depending on the defect to be corrected.

Coding Tips

This code is associated with congenital anomalies of the female genital system. For suture of a recent injury of the vagina or perineum, nonobstetrical, see 57200–57210.

ICD-9-CM Procedural

71.79   Other repair of vulva and perineum

Anesthesia

56800   00940

ICD-9-CM Diagnostic

623.2   Stricture or atresia of vagina — (Use additional E code to identify any external cause)

624.4   Old laceration or scarring of vulva

629.20   Female genital mutilation status, unspecified

629.21   Female genital mutilation, Type I status

629.22   Female genital mutilation, Type II status

629.23   Female genital mutilation, Type III status

629.29   Other female genital mutilation status

677   Late effect of complication of pregnancy, childbirth, and the puerperium — (Code first any sequelae)

752.40   Unspecified congenital anomaly of cervix, vagina, and external female genitalia

752.42   Imperforate hymen

752.49   Other congenital anomaly of cervix, vagina, and external female genitalia

759.9   Unspecified congenital anomaly

Terms To Know

anomaly. Irregularity in the structure or position of an organ or tissue.

atresia. Congenital closure or absence of a tubular organ or an opening to the body surface.

congenital. Present at birth, occurring through heredity or an influence during gestation up to the moment of birth.

defect. Imperfection, flaw, or absence.

excise. Remove or cut out.

genitalia. External organs related to reproduction.

introitus. Entrance into the vagina.

scar tissue. Fibrous connective tissue that forms around a wounded area or injury, composed mainly of fibroblasts or collagenous fibers.

stricture. Narrowing of an anatomical structure.

CCI Version 18.3

00940, 0213T, 0216T, 0228T, 0230T, 12001-12007, 12011-12057, 13100-13153, 36000, 36400-36410, 36420-36430, 36440, 36600, 36640, 37202, 43752, 51701-51703, 56605-56606, 56820, 57100, 57180, 57410, 57500, 57800, 58100, 62310-62319, 64400-64435, 64445-64450, 64479, 64483, 64490, 64493, 64505-64530, 69990, 93000-93010, 93040-93042, 93318, 94002, 94200, 94250, 94680-94690, 94770, 95812-95816, 95819, 95822, 95829, 95955, 96360, 96365, 96372, 96374-96376, 99148-99149, 99150

Note: These CCI edits are used for Medicare. Other payers may reimburse on codes listed above.

Medicare Edits

	Fac RVU	Non-Fac RVU	FUD	Status
56800	7.18	7.18	10	A

	MUE		Modifiers		
56800	1	51	N/A	62*	80

* with documentation

Medicare References: None

Vulva

Coding Companion for Ob/Gyn

56805

56805 Clitoroplasty for intersex state

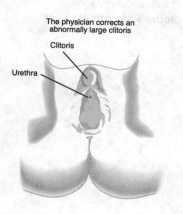

The physician corrects an abnormally large clitoris

Clitoris

Urethra

Explanation

The physician reduces the size of an enlarged clitoris, which has been masculinized by the production of male hormones from an abnormal adrenal gland. A portion of the body of the clitoris is resected with care to ensure preservation of vital nerves and blood vessels to the glans of the clitoris. The incisions are closed using plastic surgical techniques.

Coding Tips

To report the creation of a labia minora from excised clitoral tissue, report 58999 and include an operative report and cover letter.

ICD-9-CM Procedural

71.4 Operations on clitoris

Anesthesia

56805 00940

ICD-9-CM Diagnostic

255.2 Adrenogenital disorders

259.50 Androgen insensitivity, unspecified

259.51 Androgen insensitivity syndrome

259.52 Partial androgen insensitivity

752.49 Other congenital anomaly of cervix, vagina, and external female genitalia

752.7 Indeterminate sex and pseudohermaphroditism

Terms To Know

adrenal gland. Specialized group of secretory cells located above the kidneys that produce hormones that regulate the metabolism, maintain fluid balance, and control blood pressure. The adrenal glands also produce slight amounts of androgens, estrogens, and progesterone.

androgen. Male sex hormone. Testosterone is the primary androgen. In the fetus, androgens cause the formation of external male genitalia.

incision. Act of cutting into tissue or an organ.

pseudohermaphroditism-virilism-hirsutism syndrome. Possession of mature masculine somatic characteristics by a prepubescent male, girl, or woman. This syndrome may show at birth or develop later as result of adrenocortical dysfunction.

resect. Cutting out or removing a portion or all of a bone, organ, or other structure.

CCI Version 18.3

00940, 0213T, 0216T, 0228T, 0230T, 12001-12007, 12011-12057, 13100-13153, 36000, 36400-36410, 36420-36430, 36440, 36600, 36640, 37202, 43752, 51701-51703, 56605-56606, 56820, 57100, 57180, 57410, 57500, 58100, 62310-62319, 64400-64435, 64445-64450, 64479, 64483, 64490, 64493, 64505-64530, 69990, 93000-93010, 93040-93042, 93318, 94002, 94200, 94250, 94680-94690, 94770, 95812-95816, 95819, 95822, 95829, 95955, 96360, 96365, 96372, 96374-96376, 99148-99149, 99150

Note: These CCI edits are used for Medicare. Other payers may reimburse on codes listed above.

Medicare Edits

	Fac RVU	Non-Fac RVU	FUD	Status
56805	34.28	34.28	90	A

	MUE		Modifiers		
56805	1	51	N/A	62*	80

* with documentation

Medicare References: None

Coding Companion for Ob/Gyn

56810

56810 Perineoplasty, repair of perineum, nonobstetrical (separate procedure)

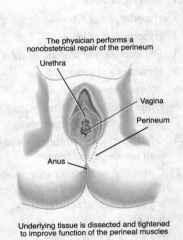

The physician performs a nonobstetrical repair of the perineum

Urethra
Vagina
Perineum
Anus

Underlying tissue is dissected and tightened to improve function of the perineal muscles

Explanation

With upward traction on the vagina, the physician makes an incision from the lower vaginal opening to a point just in front of the anus. The underlying weakened tissues are dissected and repaired and tightened by suturing. This restores strength to the pelvic floor, closes tissue defects, and improves function of the perineal muscles.

Coding Tips

This procedure is also known as perineorrhaphy. This separate procedure by definition is usually a component of a more complex service and is not identified separately. When performed alone or with other unrelated procedures/services it may be reported. If performed alone, list the code; if performed with other procedures/services, list the code and append modifier 59. For suture of a recent injury of the vagina or perineum, nonobstetrical, see 57200–57210. For plastic repair of introitus, see 56800.

ICD-9-CM Procedural

71.79   Other repair of vulva and perineum

Anesthesia

56810   00400

ICD-9-CM Diagnostic

184.8   Malignant neoplasm of other specified sites of female genital organs

195.3   Malignant neoplasm of pelvis

198.89   Secondary malignant neoplasm of other specified sites

229.8   Benign neoplasm of other specified sites

234.8   Carcinoma in situ of other specified sites

238.8   Neoplasm of uncertain behavior of other specified sites

239.89   Neoplasms of unspecified nature, other specified sites

618.05   Perineocele without mention of uterine prolapse — (Use additional code to identify urinary incontinence: 625.6, 788.31, 788.33-788.39)

618.7   Genital prolapse, old laceration of muscles of pelvic floor — (Use additional code to identify urinary incontinence: 625.6, 788.31, 788.33-788.39)

618.81   Incompetence or weakening of pubocervical tissue — (Use additional code to identify urinary incontinence: 625.6, 788.31, 788.33-788.39)

618.82   Incompetence or weakening of rectovaginal tissue — (Use additional code to identify urinary incontinence: 625.6, 788.31, 788.33-788.39)

618.83   Pelvic muscle wasting — (Use additional code to identify urinary incontinence: 625.6, 788.31, 788.33-788.39)

618.9   Unspecified genital prolapse — (Use additional code to identify urinary incontinence: 625.6, 788.31, 788.33-788.39)

625.0   Dyspareunia

625.6   Female stress incontinence

629.20   Female genital mutilation status, unspecified

629.21   Female genital mutilation, Type I status

629.22   Female genital mutilation, Type II status

629.23   Female genital mutilation, Type III status

629.29   Other female genital mutilation status

701.0   Circumscribed scleroderma

752.40   Unspecified congenital anomaly of cervix, vagina, and external female genitalia

752.41   Embryonic cyst of cervix, vagina, and external female genitalia

752.49   Other congenital anomaly of cervix, vagina, and external female genitalia

879.6   Open wound of other and unspecified parts of trunk, without mention of complication

879.7   Open wound of other and unspecified parts of trunk, complicated

959.14   Other injury of external genitals

959.19   Other injury of other sites of trunk

Terms To Know

dissect. Cut apart or separate tissue for surgical purposes or for visual or microscopic study.

dyspareunia. Pain experienced during or after intercourse, commonly occurring in the clitoris, vagina, or labia.

female stress incontinence. Involuntary escape of urine at times of minor stress against the female bladder, such as coughing, sneezing, or laughing.

incision. Act of cutting into tissue or an organ.

perineal. Pertaining to the pelvic floor area between the thighs; the diamond-shaped area bordered by the pubic symphysis in front, the ischial tuberosities on the sides, and the coccyx in back.

prolapse. Falling, sliding, or sinking of an organ from its normal location in the body.

CCI Version 18.3

00940, 0213T, 0216T, 0228T, 0230T, 12001-12007, 12011-12057, 13100-13153, 36000, 36400-36410, 36420-36430, 36440, 36600, 36640, 37202, 43752, 51701-51703, 56605-56606, 56820, 57100, 57180, 57410, 57500, 57800, 58100, 62310-62319, 64400-64435, 64445-64450, 64479, 64483, 64490, 64493, 64505-64530, 69990, 93000-93010, 93040-93042, 93318, 94002, 94200, 94250, 94680-94690, 94770, 95812-95816, 95819, 95822, 95829, 95955, 96360, 96365, 96372, 96374-96376, 99148-99149, 99150

Note: These CCI edits are used for Medicare. Other payers may reimburse on codes listed above.

Medicare Edits

	Fac RVU	Non-Fac RVU	FUD	Status
56810	7.74	7.74	10	A

	MUE		Modifiers		
56810	1	51	N/A	62	80

* with documentation

Medicare References: None

Vulva

Coding Companion for Ob/Gyn

© 2012 OptumInsight, Inc.

56820-56821

56820 Colposcopy of the vulva;
56821   with biopsy(s)

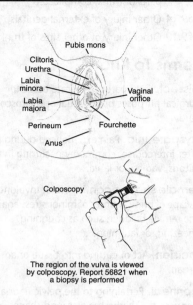

Colposcopy

The region of the vulva is viewed
by colposcopy. Report 56821 when
a biopsy is performed

Explanation

The physician performs a colposcopy of the vulva, the external genitalia region of the female that includes the labia, clitoris, mons pubis, vaginal vestibule, bulb and glands, and the vaginal orifice. The patient is placed in the lithotomy position and the vulva is inspected through the colposcope, a binocular microscope used for direct visualization of the vagina and cervix. The bright light of the colposcope is directed so as to inspect the vulva and perianal area for any lesions or ulceration. In 56821, a biopsy is taken of any vulvar tissue in question under direct vision. The number and size of the biopsy will depend on the lesions. Pressure is applied and hemostasis of the biopsy site is achieved.

Coding Tips

For colposcopy performed on the vagina, see 57420–57421. For colposcopy performed on the cervix, see 57452–57461.

ICD-9-CM Procedural

71.11 Biopsy of vulva
71.19 Other diagnostic procedures on vulva

Anesthesia

00940

ICD-9-CM Diagnostic

054.11 Herpetic vulvovaginitis
054.12 Herpetic ulceration of vulva
078.11 Condyloma acuminatum

078.19 Other specified viral warts
184.1 Malignant neoplasm of labia majora
184.2 Malignant neoplasm of labia minora
184.3 Malignant neoplasm of clitoris
184.4 Malignant neoplasm of vulva, unspecified site
198.82 Secondary malignant neoplasm of genital organs
221.2 Benign neoplasm of vulva
233.30 Carcinoma in situ, unspecified female genital organ
233.31 Carcinoma in situ, vagina
233.32 Carcinoma in situ, vulva
236.3 Neoplasm of uncertain behavior of other and unspecified female genital organs
456.6 Vulval varices
616.11 Vaginitis and vulvovaginitis in diseases classified elsewhere — (Use additional code to identify organism: 041.00-041.09, 041.10-041.19) (Code first underlying disease: 127.4)
616.2 Cyst of Bartholin's gland — (Use additional code to identify organism: 041.00-041.09, 041.10-041.19)
616.3 Abscess of Bartholin's gland — (Use additional code to identify organism: 041.00-041.09, 041.10-041.19)
616.4 Other abscess of vulva — (Use additional code to identify organism: 041.00-041.09, 041.10-041.19)
616.50 Unspecified ulceration of vulva — (Use additional code to identify organism: 041.00-041.09, 041.10-041.19)
616.51 Ulceration of vulva in disease classified elsewhere — (Use additional code to identify organism: 041.00-041.09, 041.10-041.19) (Code first underlying disease: 016.7, 136.1)
616.81 Mucositis (ulcerative) of cervix, vagina, and vulva — (Use additional code to identify organism: 041.00-041.09, 041.10-041.19) (Use additional E code to identify adverse effects of therapy: E879.2, E930.7, E933.1)
616.89 Other inflammatory disease of cervix, vagina and vulva — (Use additional code to identify organism: 041.00-041.09, 041.10-041.19)
616.9 Unspecified inflammatory disease of cervix, vagina, and vulva — (Use additional code to identify organism: 041.00-041.09, 041.10-041.19)
617.8 Endometriosis of other specified sites

624.01 Vulvar intraepithelial neoplasia I [VIN I]
624.02 Vulvar intraepithelial neoplasia II [VIN II]
624.09 Other dystrophy of vulva
624.1 Atrophy of vulva
624.2 Hypertrophy of clitoris
624.3 Hypertrophy of labia
624.4 Old laceration or scarring of vulva
624.5 Hematoma of vulva
624.6 Polyp of labia and vulva
624.8 Other specified noninflammatory disorder of vulva and perineum
625.8 Other specified symptom associated with female genital organs
654.81 Congenital or acquired abnormality of vulva, with delivery — (Code first any associated obstructed labor, 660.2)
698.1 Pruritus of genital organs
701.0 Circumscribed scleroderma
701.5 Other abnormal granulation tissue
752.41 Embryonic cyst of cervix, vagina, and external female genitalia
752.42 Imperforate hymen
V71.5 Observation following alleged rape or seduction

CCI Version 18.3

00940, 0213T, 0216T, 0228T, 0230T, 12001-12007, 12011-12057, 13100-13153, 36000, 36400-36410, 36420-36430, 36440, 36600, 36640, 37202, 43752, 51701-51703, 57410, 62310-62319, 64400-64435, 64445-64450, 64479, 64483, 64490, 64493, 64505-64530, 69990, 76000-76001, 77001-77002, 93000-93010, 93040-93042, 93318, 94002, 94200, 94250, 94680-94690, 94770, 95812-95816, 95819, 95822, 95829, 95955, 96360, 96365, 96372, 96374-96376, 99148-99149, 99150

Also not with 56821: 56605, 56820, J0670, J2001

Note: These CCI edits are used for Medicare. Other payers may reimburse on codes listed above.

Medicare Edits

	Fac RVU	Non-Fac RVU	FUD	Status
56820	2.55	3.3	0	A
56821	3.42	4.37	0	A

	MUE		Modifiers		
56820	1	51	N/A	N/A	N/A
56821	1	51	N/A	N/A	N/A

* with documentation

Medicare References: None

Vulva

57000

57000 Colpotomy; with exploration

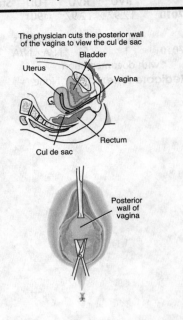

The physician cuts the posterior wall of the vagina to view the cul de sac

Bladder
Uterus
Vagina
Rectum
Cul de sac

Posterior wall of vagina

Explanation

Colpotomy is an incision in the wall of the vagina, usually to access a recess between the rectum and uterus formed by a fold in the peritoneum (cul de sac). Through a speculum inserted in the vagina, the physician grasps the posterior lip of the cervix with a toothed instrument called a tenaculum. The cervix is lifted up exposing the posterior vaginal pouch. An incision is made through the back wall of the vagina into the posterior pelvic cavity. Through this opening, the pelvic cavity can be explored using instruments. After exploration, the physician closes the incision with absorbable sutures.

Coding Tips

For colpotomy with drainage of a pelvic abscess, see 57010. Surgical trays, A4550, are not separately reimbursed by Medicare; however, other third-party payers may cover them. Check with the specific payer to determine coverage.

ICD-9-CM Procedural

70.12   Culdotomy

Anesthesia

57000   00942

ICD-9-CM Diagnostic

158.8   Malignant neoplasm of specified parts of peritoneum

184.0   Malignant neoplasm of vagina

197.6   Secondary malignant neoplasm of retroperitoneum and peritoneum

198.82   Secondary malignant neoplasm of genital organs

209.74   Secondary neuroendocrine tumor of peritoneum

209.79   Secondary neuroendocrine tumor of other sites

211.8   Benign neoplasm of retroperitoneum and peritoneum

221.1   Benign neoplasm of vagina

235.4   Neoplasm of uncertain behavior of retroperitoneum and peritoneum

236.3   Neoplasm of uncertain behavior of other and unspecified female genital organs

239.0   Neoplasm of unspecified nature of digestive system

239.5   Neoplasm of unspecified nature of other genitourinary organs

616.10   Unspecified vaginitis and vulvovaginitis — (Use additional code to identify organism, such as: 041.00-041.09, 041.10-041.19, 041.41-041.49)

623.8   Other specified noninflammatory disorder of vagina

623.9   Unspecified noninflammatory disorder of vagina

625.3   Dysmenorrhea

Terms To Know

absorbable sutures. Strands prepared from collagen or a synthetic polymer and capable of being absorbed by tissue over time.

benign. Mild or nonmalignant in nature.

culdotomy/colpotomy. Incision through the vaginal wall into the cul-de-sac of Douglas (retro uterine pouch).

dysmenorrhea. Painful menstruation that may be primary, or essential, due to prostaglandin production and the onset of menstruation; secondary due to uterine, tubal, or ovarian abnormality or disease; spasmodic arising uterine contractions; or obstructive due to some mechanical blockage or interference with the menstrual flow.

incision. Act of cutting into tissue or an organ.

malignant neoplasm. Any cancerous tumor or lesion exhibiting uncontrolled tissue growth that can progressively invade other parts of the body with its disease-generating cells.

peritoneum. Strong, continuous membrane that forms the lining of the abdominal and pelvic cavity. The parietal peritoneum, or outer layer, is attached to the abdominopelvic walls and the visceral peritoneum, or inner layer, surrounds the organs inside the abdominal cavity.

secondary. Second in order of occurrence or importance, or appearing during the course of another disease or condition.

speculum. Tool used to enlarge the opening of any canal or cavity.

CCI Version 18.3

00940, 0213T, 0216T, 0228T, 0230T, 12001-12007, 12011-12057, 13100-13153, 36000, 36400-36410, 36420-36430, 36440, 36600, 36640, 37202, 43752, 51701-51703, 57020, 57100, 57180, 57410-57420, 57452, 57500, 57800, 58100, 58800, 62310-62319, 64400-64435, 64445-64450, 64479, 64483, 64490, 64493, 64505-64530, 69990, 93000-93010, 93040-93042, 93318, 94002, 94200, 94250, 94680-94690, 94770, 95812-95816, 95819, 95822, 95829, 95955, 96360, 96365, 96372, 96374-96376, 99148-99149, 99150, P9612

Note: These CCI edits are used for Medicare. Other payers may reimburse on codes listed above.

Medicare Edits

	Fac RVU	Non-Fac RVU	FUD	Status
57000	5.51	5.51	10	A

	MUE			Modifiers	
57000	1	51	N/A	N/A	80*

* with documentation

Medicare References: None

Vagina

57010

57010 Colpotomy; with drainage of pelvic abscess

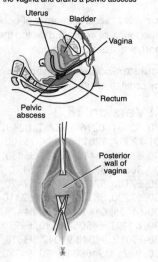

The physician cuts the posterior wall of the vagina and drains a pelvic abscess

Explanation

Colpotomy is an incision in the wall of the vagina, usually to access a recess between the rectum and uterus formed by a fold in the peritoneum (cul de sac). Through a speculum inserted in the vagina, the physician grasps the posterior lip of the cervix with a toothed instrument called a tenaculum. The cervix is lifted up exposing the posterior vaginal pouch. An incision is made through the back wall of the vagina into the posterior pelvic cavity. Through this opening, the pelvic cavity can be explored. The abscess in the cavity is located, entered, and drained through the vaginal incision. Rubber drains are often inserted and left in place for several days. The physician closes the incision with absorbable sutures.

Coding Tips

For a colpotomy with exploration, see 57000.

ICD-9-CM Procedural

70.14 Other vaginotomy

Anesthesia

57010 00942

ICD-9-CM Diagnostic

614.3 Acute parametritis and pelvic cellulitis — (Use additional code to identify organism: 041.00-041.09, 041.10-041.19)

614.4 Chronic or unspecified parametritis and pelvic cellulitis — (Use additional

code to identify organism: 041.00-041.09, 041.10-041.19)

616.10 Unspecified vaginitis and vulvovaginitis — (Use additional code to identify organism, such as: 041.00-041.09, 041.10-041.19, 041.41-041.49)

998.51 Infected postoperative seroma — (Use additional code to identify organism)

998.59 Other postoperative infection — (Use additional code to identify infection)

Terms To Know

abscess. Circumscribed collection of pus resulting from bacteria, frequently associated with swelling and other signs of inflammation.

absorbable sutures. Strands prepared from collagen or a synthetic polymer and capable of being absorbed by tissue over time.

acute. Sudden, severe. Documentation and reporting of an acute condition is important to establishing medical necessity.

cellulitis. Sudden, severe, suppurative inflammation and edema in subcutaneous tissue or muscle, most often caused by bacterial infection secondary to a cutaneous lesion.

chronic. Persistent, continuing, or recurring.

drain. Device that creates a channel to allow fluid from a cavity, wound, or infected area to exit the body.

incision. Act of cutting into tissue or an organ.

parametritis. Inflammation and infection of the tissue in the structures around the uterus.

seroma. Swelling caused by the collection of serum, or clear fluid, in the tissues.

CCI Version 18.3

00940, 0213T, 0216T, 0228T, 0230T, 12001-12007, 12011-12057, 13100-13153, 36000, 36400-36410, 36420-36430, 36440, 36600, 36640, 37202, 43752, 51701-51703, 57000, 57020, 57100, 57180, 57410-57420, 57452, 57500, 57800, 58100, 58800, 58820, 62310-62319, 64400-64435, 64445-64450, 64479, 64483, 64490, 64493, 64505-64530, 69990, 93000-93010, 93040-93042, 93318, 94002, 94200, 94250, 94680-94690, 94770, 95812-95816, 95819, 95822, 95829, 95955, 96360, 96365, 96372, 96374-96376, 99148-99149, 99150, P9612

Note: These CCI edits are used for Medicare. Other payers may reimburse on codes listed above.

Medicare Edits

	Fac RVU	Non-Fac RVU	FUD	Status
57010	12.97	12.97	90	A

	MUE		Modifiers		
57010	1	51	N/A	N/A	80*

* with documentation

Medicare References: None

Vagina

57020

57020 Colpocentesis (separate procedure)

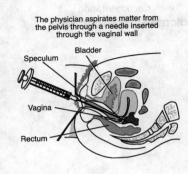

The physician aspirates matter from the pelvis through a needle inserted through the vaginal wall

Speculum
Bladder
Vagina
Rectum

Explanation

Colpocentesis is the aspiration of fluid in the peritoneum through the wall of the vagina. Through a speculum inserted in the vagina, the physician grasps the posterior lip of the cervix with a toothed instrument called a tenaculum. The cervix is lifted, exposing the posterior vaginal pouch and deep back wall of the vagina. A long needle attached to a syringe is inserted through the exposed vaginal wall and the posterior pelvic cavity is entered. Fluid is aspirated through the needle into the syringe.

Coding Tips

This separate procedure by definition is usually a component of a more complex service and is not identified separately. When performed alone or with other unrelated procedures or services it may be reported. If performed alone, list the code; if performed with other procedures or services, list the code and append modifier 59. If the aspirated fluid is transported to an outside laboratory, report 99000 for conveyance of the specimen.

ICD-9-CM Procedural

70.0   Culdocentesis

Anesthesia

57020   00940

ICD-9-CM Diagnostic

184.0   Malignant neoplasm of vagina

198.82 Secondary malignant neoplasm of genital organs

221.1   Benign neoplasm of vagina

233.30 Carcinoma in situ, unspecified female genital organ

233.31 Carcinoma in situ, vagina

233.32 Carcinoma in situ, vulva

233.39 Carcinoma in situ, other female genital organ

236.3   Neoplasm of uncertain behavior of other and unspecified female genital organs

239.5   Neoplasm of unspecified nature of other genitourinary organs

614.3   Acute parametritis and pelvic cellulitis — (Use additional code to identify organism: 041.00-041.09, 041.10-041.19)

614.4   Chronic or unspecified parametritis and pelvic cellulitis — (Use additional code to identify organism: 041.00-041.09, 041.10-041.19)

614.5   Acute or unspecified pelvic peritonitis, female — (Use additional code to identify organism: 041.00-041.09, 041.10-041.19)

614.7   Other chronic pelvic peritonitis, female — (Use additional code to identify organism: 041.00-041.09, 041.10-041.19)

614.8   Other specified inflammatory disease of female pelvic organs and tissues — (Use additional code to identify organism: 041.00-041.09, 041.10-041.19)

614.9   Unspecified inflammatory disease of female pelvic organs and tissues — (Use additional code to identify organism: 041.00-041.09, 041.10-041.19)

752.40 Unspecified congenital anomaly of cervix, vagina, and external female genitalia

752.41 Embryonic cyst of cervix, vagina, and external female genitalia

752.49 Other congenital anomaly of cervix, vagina, and external female genitalia

878.6   Open wound of vagina, without mention of complication

878.7   Open wound of vagina, complicated

Terms To Know

aspiration. Drawing fluid out by suction.

benign. Mild or nonmalignant in nature.

carcinoma in situ. Malignancy that arises from the cells of the vessel, gland, or organ of origin that remains confined to that site or has not invaded neighboring tissue.

malignant neoplasm. Any cancerous tumor or lesion exhibiting uncontrolled tissue growth that can progressively invade other parts of the body with its disease-generating cells.

peritoneum. Strong, continuous membrane that forms the lining of the abdominal and pelvic cavity. The parietal peritoneum, or outer layer, is attached to the abdominopelvic walls and the visceral peritoneum, or inner layer, surrounds the organs inside the abdominal cavity.

CCI Version 18.3

00940, 0213T, 0216T, 0228T, 0230T, 12001-12007, 12011-12057, 13100-13153, 36000, 36400-36410, 36420-36430, 36440, 36600, 36640, 37202, 43752, 51701-51703, 57100, 57180, 57410-57420, 57452, 57500, 57800, 58100, 58800, 62310-62319, 64400-64435, 64445-64450, 64479, 64483, 64490, 64493, 64505-64530, 69990, 93000-93010, 93040-93042, 93318, 94002, 94200, 94250, 94680-94690, 94770, 95812-95816, 95819, 95822, 95829, 95955, 96360, 96365, 96372, 96374-96376, 99148-99149, 99150

Note: These CCI edits are used for Medicare. Other payers may reimburse on codes listed above.

Medicare Edits

	Fac RVU	Non-Fac RVU	FUD	Status
57020	2.44	2.8	0	A

	MUE		Modifiers		
57020	1	51	N/A	N/A	80*

* with documentation

Medicare References: None

Vagina

57022-57023

57022 Incision and drainage of vaginal hematoma; obstetrical/postpartum

57023 non-obstetrical (eg, post-trauma, spontaneous bleeding)

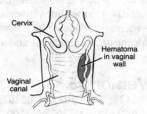

The hematoma may be post obstetrical or non-obstetrical

A vaginal hematoma is incised and drained. Report 57022 if the hematoma occurs in the post obstetrical period. Report 57023 if the hematoma is not associated with childbirth

Explanation

The physician incises and drains a vaginal hematoma in an obstetrical or postpartum patient. The patient is placed in a dorso-lithotomy position. The physician inserts a speculum into the vagina. The hematoma is visualized, and incised. Blood and clot are drained from the hematoma. Electrocautery or suture is used to control bleeding. When needed, a Hemovac drain is placed. The vagina is irrigated, and the area of hematoma is sponged with dressings. When hemostasis is achieved, the speculum is removed. Report 57022 when the procedure is performed on an obstetrical patient and 57023 when the procedure is performed on a non-obstetrical patient. Hemovac drains may be placed if the hematoma bed is still oozing.

Coding Tips

When either 57022 or 57023 is performed with another separately identifiable procedure, the highest dollar value code is listed as the primary procedure and subsequent procedures are appended with modifier 51. Surgical trays, A4550, are not separately reimbursed by Medicare; however, other third-party payers may cover them. Check with the specific payer to determine coverage.

ICD-9-CM Procedural

70.14   Other vaginotomy

75.91   Evacuation of obstetrical incisional hematoma of perineum

75.92   Evacuation of other hematoma of vulva or vagina

Anesthesia

00940

ICD-9-CM Diagnostic

623.6   Vaginal hematoma

665.70   Pelvic hematoma, unspecified as to episode of care

665.71   Pelvic hematoma, with delivery

665.72   Pelvic hematoma, delivered with postpartum complication

665.74   Pelvic hematoma, postpartum condition or complication

922.4   Contusion of genital organs

Terms To Know

contusion. Superficial injury (bruising) produced by impact without a break in the skin.

electrocautery. Division or cutting of tissue using high-frequency electrical current to produce heat, which destroys cells.

hematoma. Tumor-like collection of blood in some part of the body caused by a break in a blood vessel wall, usually as a result of trauma.

incision and drainage. Cutting open body tissue for the removal of tissue fluids or infected discharge from a wound or cavity.

seroma. Swelling caused by the collection of serum, or clear fluid, in the tissues.

CCI Version 18.3

00940, 0213T, 0216T, 0228T, 0230T, 12001-12007, 12011-12057, 13100-13153, 36000, 36400-36410, 36420-36430, 36440, 36600, 36640, 37202, 43752, 51701-51703, 57000-57020, 57100, 57180, 57400-57420, 57452, 57500, 57800, 58100, 58800, 62310-62319, 64400-64435, 64445-64450, 64479, 64483, 64490, 64493, 64505-64530, 69990, 93000-93010, 93040-93042, 93318, 94002, 94200, 94250, 94680-94690, 94770, 95812-95816, 95819, 95822, 95829, 95955, 96360, 96365, 96372, 96374-96376, 99148-99149, 99150, P9612

Note: These CCI edits are used for Medicare. Other payers may reimburse on codes listed above.

Medicare Edits

	Fac RVU	Non-Fac RVU	FUD	Status
57022	5.01	5.01	10	A
57023	9.29	9.29	10	A

	MUE		Modifiers		
57022	2	51	N/A	N/A	80*
57023	2	51	N/A	N/A	80*

* with documentation

Medicare References: None

Vagina

57061-57065

57061 Destruction of vaginal lesion(s); simple (eg, laser surgery, electrosurgery, cryosurgery, chemosurgery)

57065 extensive (eg, laser surgery, electrosurgery, cryosurgery, chemosurgery)

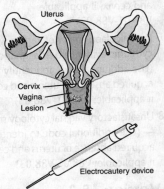

The physician destroys vaginal lesions with electrocautery, laser or cryoprobe

Uterus

Cervix
Vagina
Lesion

Electrocautery device

The lesions are few or small in 57061; the lesions are large or numerous in 57065

Explanation

Using a colposcope, a binocular microscope used for direct visualization of the vagina and cervix, the physician identifies lesion(s) in and/or around the vagina. The physician destroys the abnormal tissue by chemosurgery, electrosurgery, laser surgery, or cryotherapy. Use 57061 if the lesions are few in number, small, or simple. Use 57065 if the lesions are numerous, large, or difficult.

Coding Tips

For excision of a vaginal cyst or tumor, see 57135. For biopsy of a vaginal mucosa, see 57100–57105. Destruction of vulvar lesions is reported with 56501–56515.

ICD-9-CM Procedural

70.13 Lysis of intraluminal adhesions of vagina

70.32 Excision or destruction of lesion of cul-de-sac

70.33 Excision or destruction of lesion of vagina

Anesthesia
00940

ICD-9-CM Diagnostic

078.11 Condyloma acuminatum

078.19 Other specified viral warts

184.0 Malignant neoplasm of vagina

198.82 Secondary malignant neoplasm of genital organs

221.1 Benign neoplasm of vagina

236.3 Neoplasm of uncertain behavior of other and unspecified female genital organs

239.5 Neoplasm of unspecified nature of other genitourinary organs

616.81 Mucositis (ulcerative) of cervix, vagina, and vulva — (Use additional code to identify organism: 041.00-041.09, 041.10-041.19) (Use additional E code to identify adverse effects of therapy: E879.2, E930.7, E933.1)

616.89 Other inflammatory disease of cervix, vagina and vulva — (Use additional code to identify organism: 041.00-041.09, 041.10-041.19)

616.9 Unspecified inflammatory disease of cervix, vagina, and vulva — (Use additional code to identify organism: 041.00-041.09, 041.10-041.19)

623.0 Dysplasia of vagina

623.1 Leukoplakia of vagina

623.5 Leukorrhea, not specified as infective

623.7 Polyp of vagina

623.8 Other specified noninflammatory disorder of vagina

624.01 Vulvar intraepithelial neoplasia I [VIN I]

624.02 Vulvar intraepithelial neoplasia II [VIN II]

624.09 Other dystrophy of vulva

624.8 Other specified noninflammatory disorder of vulva and perineum

701.5 Other abnormal granulation tissue

795.05 Cervical high risk human papillomavirus (HPV) DNA test positive

Terms To Know

chemosurgery. Application of chemical agents to destroy tissue, originally referring to the in situ chemical fixation of premalignant or malignant lesions to facilitate surgical excision.

condyloma. Infectious tumor-like growth caused by the human papilloma virus, with a branching connective tissue core and epithelial covering that occurs on the skin and mucous membranes of the perianal region and external genitalia.

cryosurgery. Application of intense cold, usually produced using liquid nitrogen, to locally freeze diseased or unwanted tissue and induce tissue necrosis without causing harm to adjacent tissue.

destruction. Ablation or eradication of a structure or tissue.

electrocautery. Division or cutting of tissue using high-frequency electrical current to produce heat, which destroys cells.

laser surgery. Use of concentrated, sharply defined light beams to cut, cauterize, coagulate, seal, or vaporize tissue.

lesion. Area of damaged tissue that has lost continuity or function, due to disease or trauma.

polyp. Small growth on a stalk-like attachment projecting from a mucous membrane.

CCI Version 18.3

00940, 0213T, 0216T, 0228T, 0230T, 12001-12007, 12011-12057, 13100-13153, 36000, 36400-36410, 36420-36430, 36440, 36600, 36640, 37202, 43752, 51701-51703, 57100, 57180, 57452, 57500, 57800, 58100, 62310-62319, 64400-64435, 64445-64450, 64479, 64483, 64490, 64493, 64505-64530, 93000-93010, 93040-93042, 93318, 94002, 94200, 94250, 94680-94690, 94770, 95812-95816, 95819, 95822, 95829, 95955, 96360, 96365, 96372, 96374-96376, 99148-99149, 99150, J0670, J2001

Also not with 57061: 57410-57415, 69990

Also not with 57065: 57061, 57410-57420, P9612

Note: These CCI edits are used for Medicare. Other payers may reimburse on codes listed above.

Medicare Edits

	Fac RVU	Non-Fac RVU	FUD	Status
57061	2.93	3.4	10	A
57065	5.11	5.73	10	A

	MUE		Modifiers		
57061	1	51	N/A	N/A	N/A
57065	1	51	N/A	N/A	N/A

* with documentation

Medicare References: 100-3,140.5

Coding Companion for Ob/Gyn

© 2012 OptumInsight, Inc.

57100-57105

57100 Biopsy of vaginal mucosa; simple (separate procedure)

57105 extensive, requiring suture (including cysts)

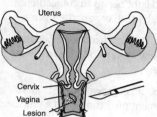

The physician removes a portion of a vaginal lesion for biopsy

Uterus

Cervix

Vagina

Lesion

The procedure is simple; no sutures are required in 57100; the excision site is extensive and requires sutures in 57105

Explanation

The physician takes a sample of vaginal mucosa for examination. After injecting a local anesthetic into the suspect area, the physician obtains a sample with a skin punch or sharp scalpel. In 57100, the biopsy is simple and no sutures are required. In 57105, sutures are required as the excision site is extensive and bleeding may need to be controlled.

Coding Tips

Note that 57100, a separate procedure by definition, is usually a component of a more complex service and is not identified separately. When performed alone or with other unrelated procedures/services it may be reported. If performed alone, list the code; if performed with other procedures/services, list the code and append modifier 59. If the excised tissue is transported to an outside laboratory, report 99000 for conveyance of the specimen. Any local or topical anesthetic is not reported separately.

ICD-9-CM Procedural

70.23 Biopsy of cul-de-sac
70.24 Vaginal biopsy

Anesthesia

00940

ICD-9-CM Diagnostic

054.11 Herpetic vulvovaginitis
078.11 Condyloma acuminatum
098.0 Gonococcal infection (acute) of lower genitourinary tract
184.0 Malignant neoplasm of vagina
221.1 Benign neoplasm of vagina
616.81 Mucositis (ulcerative) of cervix, vagina, and vulva — (Use additional code to identify organism: 041.00-041.09, 041.10-041.19) (Use additional E code to identify adverse effects of therapy: E879.2, E930.7, E933.1)
623.0 Dysplasia of vagina
623.1 Leukoplakia of vagina
795.00 Abnormal glandular Papanicolaou smear of cervix
795.01 Papanicolaou smear of cervix with atypical squamous cells of undetermined significance (ASC-US)
795.02 Papanicolaou smear of cervix with atypical squamous cells cannot exclude high grade squamous intraepithelial lesion (ASC-H)
795.03 Papanicolaou smear of cervix with low grade squamous intraepithelial lesion (LGSIL)
795.04 Papanicolaou smear of cervix with high grade squamous intraepithelial lesion (HGSIL)
795.05 Cervical high risk human papillomavirus (HPV) DNA test positive
795.08 Unsatisfactory cervical cytology smear
795.10 Abnormal glandular Papanicolaou smear of vagina — (Use additional code to identify acquired absence of uterus and cervix, if applicable: V88.01-V88.03)
795.11 Papanicolaou smear of vagina with atypical squamous cells of undetermined significance (ASC-US) — (Use additional code to identify acquired absence of uterus and cervix, if applicable: V88.01-V88.03)
795.12 Papanicolaou smear of vagina with atypical squamous cells cannot exclude high grade squamous intraepithelial lesion (ASC-H) — (Use additional code to identify acquired absence of uterus and cervix, if applicable: V88.01-V88.03)
795.13 Papanicolaou smear of vagina with low grade squamous intraepithelial lesion (LGSIL) — (Use additional code to identify acquired absence of uterus

and cervix, if applicable: V88.01-V88.03)
795.14 Papanicolaou smear of vagina with high grade squamous intraepithelial lesion (HGSIL) — (Use additional code to identify acquired absence of uterus and cervix, if applicable: V88.01-V88.03)
795.15 Vaginal high risk human papillomavirus (HPV) DNA test positive — (Use additional code to identify acquired absence of uterus and cervix, if applicable: V88.01-V88.03)
795.16 Papanicolaou smear of vagina with cytologic evidence of malignancy — (Use additional code to identify acquired absence of uterus and cervix, if applicable: V88.01-V88.03)
795.18 Unsatisfactory vaginal cytology smear — (Use additional code to identify acquired absence of uterus and cervix, if applicable: V88.01-V88.03)

CCI Version 18.3

00940, 0213T, 0216T, 0228T, 0230T, 10021-10022, 12001-12007, 12011-12057, 13100-13153, 36000, 36400-36410, 36420-36430, 36440, 36600, 36640, 37202, 43752, 51701-51703, 62310-62319, 64400-64435, 64445-64450, 64479, 64483, 64490, 64493, 64505-64530, 69990, 93000-93010, 93040-93042, 93318, 94002, 94200, 94250, 94680-94690, 94770, 95812-95816, 95819, 95822, 95829, 95955, 96360, 96365, 96372, 96374-96376, 99148-99149, 99150, J2001

Also not with 57100: 57415

Also not with 57105: 57061, 57100, 57180, 57410-57420, 57452, 57500, 57800, 58100

Note: These CCI edits are used for Medicare. Other payers may reimburse on codes listed above.

Medicare Edits

	Fac RVU	Non-Fac RVU	FUD	Status
57100	1.96	2.62	0	A
57105	3.73	4.03	10	A

	MUE		Modifiers		
57100	3		51	N/A N/A N/A
57105	2		51	N/A N/A N/A

* with documentation

Medicare References: None

Vagina

Coding Companion for Ob/Gyn

57106-57109

57106 Vaginectomy, partial removal of vaginal wall;

57107 with removal of paravaginal tissue (radical vaginectomy)

57109 with removal of paravaginal tissue (radical vaginectomy) with bilateral total pelvic lymphadenectomy and para-aortic lymph node sampling (biopsy)

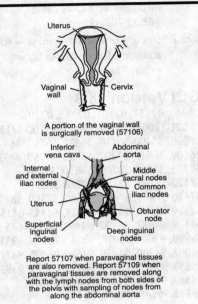

A portion of the vaginal wall is surgically removed (57106)

Report 57107 when paravaginal tissues are also removed. Report 57109 when paravaginal tissues are removed along with the lymph nodes from both sides of the pelvis with sampling of nodes from along the abdominal aorta

Explanation

The physician excises part of the vagina. This is sometimes preceded by injection of medication to constrict blood vessels to control bleeding. The vagina is everted and sizeable sections are removed by sharp and blunt dissection. In 57107, the physician removes surrounding diseased and/or damaged tissue. In 57109, the physician removes surrounding diseased and/or damaged tissue, in addition to removing the pelvic lymph nodes, and performing biopsy of the lymph nodes of the aorta to check for the extent of disease. Remaining vaginal and/or support tissue is inverted and sutured in place to obliterate some or all of the space formerly occupied by the vagina. The perineum is closed over the former vaginal opening.

Coding Tips

Lymph node removal is included in 57109 and should not be reported separately. For vaginectomy with complete removal of the vaginal wall, see 57110; with removal of paravaginal tissue (radical vaginectomy), see 57111; with removal of paravaginal tissue (radical vaginectomy) with bilateral total pelvic lymphadenectomy and para-aortic lymph node sampling, see 57112.

ICD-9-CM Procedural

40.3 Regional lymph node excision

70.4 Obliteration and total excision of vagina

Anesthesia

57106 00942
57107 00942
57109 00860, 00904, 00940, 00942

ICD-9-CM Diagnostic

184.0 Malignant neoplasm of vagina

184.1 Malignant neoplasm of labia majora

184.2 Malignant neoplasm of labia minora

184.4 Malignant neoplasm of vulva, unspecified site

184.8 Malignant neoplasm of other specified sites of female genital organs

184.9 Malignant neoplasm of female genital organ, site unspecified

196.2 Secondary and unspecified malignant neoplasm of intra-abdominal lymph nodes

198.82 Secondary malignant neoplasm of genital organs

221.1 Benign neoplasm of vagina

233.30 Carcinoma in situ, unspecified female genital organ

233.31 Carcinoma in situ, vagina

233.32 Carcinoma in situ, vulva

233.39 Carcinoma in situ, other female genital organ

236.3 Neoplasm of uncertain behavior of other and unspecified female genital organs

239.5 Neoplasm of unspecified nature of other genitourinary organs

616.89 Other inflammatory disease of cervix, vagina and vulva — (Use additional code to identify organism: 041.00-041.09, 041.10-041.19)

618.00 Unspecified prolapse of vaginal walls without mention of uterine prolapse — (Use additional code to identify urinary incontinence: 625.6, 788.31, 788.33-788.39)

618.09 Other prolapse of vaginal walls without mention of uterine prolapse — (Use additional code to identify urinary incontinence: 625.6, 788.31, 788.33-788.39)

618.84 Cervical stump prolapse — (Use additional code to identify urinary incontinence: 625.6, 788.31, 788.33-788.39)

618.89 Other specified genital prolapse — (Use additional code to identify urinary incontinence: 625.6, 788.31, 788.33-788.39)

623.2 Stricture or atresia of vagina — (Use additional E code to identify any external cause)

752.49 Other congenital anomaly of cervix, vagina, and external female genitalia

V84.02 Genetic susceptibility to malignant neoplasm of ovary — (Use additional code, if applicable, for any associated family history of the disease: V16-V19. Code first, if applicable, any current malignant neoplasms: 140.0-195.8, 200.0-208.9, 230.0-234.9. Use additional code, if applicable, for any personal history of malignant neoplasm: V10.0-V10.9)

CCI Version 18.3

00940, 0213T, 0216T, 0228T, 0230T, 12001-12007, 12011-12057, 13100-13153, 35840, 36000, 36400-36410, 36420-36430, 36440, 36600, 36640, 37202, 43752, 44950, 44970, 50715, 51701-51703, 56810, 57061, 57120-57135, 57180, 57268-57270, 57410-57421, 57452, 57800, 58100, 62310-62319, 64400-64435, 64445-64450, 64479, 64483, 64490, 64493, 64505-64530, 69990, 93000-93010, 93040-93042, 93318, 94002, 94200, 94250, 94680-94690, 94770, 95812-95816, 95819, 95822, 95829, 95955, 96360, 96365, 96372, 96374-96376, 99148-99149, 99150, P9612

Also not with 57106: 57065-57105, 57500

Also not with 57107: 57065-57106, 57111◊

Also not with 57109: 38570-38572, 38770, 38780, 57065-57107

Note: These CCI edits are used for Medicare. Other payers may reimburse on codes listed above.

Medicare Edits

	Fac RVU	Non-Fac RVU	FUD	Status
57106	14.37	14.37	90	A
57107	41.87	41.87	90	A
57109	47.88	47.88	90	A

	MUE		Modifiers		
57106	1	51	N/A	62*	80
57107	1	51	N/A	62*	80
57109	1	51	N/A	62*	80

* with documentation

Medicare References: None

Vagina

57110-57112

57110 Vaginectomy, complete removal of vaginal wall;
57111 with removal of paravaginal tissue (radical vaginectomy)
57112 with removal of paravaginal tissue (radical vaginectomy) with bilateral total pelvic lymphadenectomy and para-aortic lymph node sampling (biopsy)

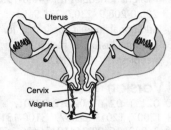

The physician excises the entire vagina

The perineum is closed over the operative wound

Explanation

The physician performs a complete removal of the vaginal wall. This is sometimes proceeded by injection of medication to constrict blood vessels to control bleeding. The vagina is everted. An incision circumscribes the hymen, and the vagina is marked into four quadrants. Each quadrant of vaginal wall is removed by sharp and blunt dissection. In 57111, the physician removes surrounding diseased and/or damaged tissue. In 57112, the physician removes surrounding diseased and/or damaged tissue, in addition to removing the pelvic lymph nodes, and performs biopsy of the lymph nodes of the aorta to check for the extent of disease. The remaining support tissues are inverted and sutured in place obliterating the space formerly occupied by the vagina. The perineum is closed over the former vaginal opening.

Coding Tips

Lymph node removal is included in 57112 and should not be reported separately. For vaginectomy with partial removal of the vaginal wall, see 57106; with removal of paravaginal tissue (radical vaginectomy), see

57107; with removal of paravaginal tissue (radical vaginectomy) with bilateral total pelvic lymphadenectomy and para-aortic lymph node sampling, see 57109.

ICD-9-CM Procedural

40.3 Regional lymph node excision
70.4 Obliteration and total excision of vagina

Anesthesia

57110 00942
57111 00904, 00942
57112 00860, 00904, 00940, 00942

ICD-9-CM Diagnostic

184.0 Malignant neoplasm of vagina
184.1 Malignant neoplasm of labia majora
184.2 Malignant neoplasm of labia minora
184.4 Malignant neoplasm of vulva, unspecified site
184.8 Malignant neoplasm of other specified sites of female genital organs
196.2 Secondary and unspecified malignant neoplasm of intra-abdominal lymph nodes
198.82 Secondary malignant neoplasm of genital organs
221.1 Benign neoplasm of vagina
233.30 Carcinoma in situ, unspecified female genital organ
233.31 Carcinoma in situ, vagina
233.32 Carcinoma in situ, vulva
233.39 Carcinoma in situ, other female genital organ
236.3 Neoplasm of uncertain behavior of other and unspecified female genital organs
616.10 Unspecified vaginitis and vulvovaginitis — (Use additional code to identify organism, such as: 041.00-041.09, 041.10-041.19, 041.41-041.49)
616.11 Vaginitis and vulvovaginitis in diseases classified elsewhere — (Use additional code to identify organism: 041.00-041.09, 041.10-041.19) (Code first underlying disease: 127.4)
616.89 Other inflammatory disease of cervix, vagina and vulva — (Use additional code to identify organism: 041.00-041.09, 041.10-041.19)
618.00 Unspecified prolapse of vaginal walls without mention of uterine prolapse — (Use additional code to identify urinary incontinence: 625.6, 788.31, 788.33-788.39)

618.05 Perineocele without mention of uterine prolapse — (Use additional code to identify urinary incontinence: 625.6, 788.31, 788.33-788.39)
618.09 Other prolapse of vaginal walls without mention of uterine prolapse — (Use additional code to identify urinary incontinence: 625.6, 788.31, 788.33-788.39)
618.84 Cervical stump prolapse — (Use additional code to identify urinary incontinence: 625.6, 788.31, 788.33-788.39)
623.2 Stricture or atresia of vagina — (Use additional E code to identify any external cause)

CCI Version 18.3

00940, 0213T, 0216T, 0228T, 0230T, 12001-12007, 12011-12057, 13100-13153, 36000, 36400-36410, 36420-36430, 36440, 36600, 36640, 37202, 43752, 44950, 44970, 50715, 51701-51703, 56810, 57061, 57120-57135, 57180, 57268-57270, 57410-57421, 57452, 57500, 57800, 58100, 62310-62319, 64400-64435, 64445-64450, 64479, 64483, 64490, 64493, 64505-64530, 69990, 93000-93010, 93040-93042, 93318, 94002, 94200, 94250, 94680-94690, 94770, 95812-95816, 95819, 95822, 95829, 95955, 96360, 96365, 96372, 96374-96376, 99148-99149, 99150, P9612

Also not with 57110: 57065-57107, 57109

Also not with 57111: 35840, 57065-57106, 57109-57110

Also not with 57112: 35840, 38570-38572, 38770, 38780, 57065-57107, 57109-57111

Note: These CCI edits are used for Medicare. Other payers may reimburse on codes listed above.

Medicare Edits

	Fac RVU	Non-Fac RVU	FUD	Status
57110	26.79	26.79	90	A
57111	48.02	48.02	90	A
57112	48.62	48.62	90	A

	MUE		Modifiers		
57110	1	51	N/A	62*	80
57111	1	51	N/A	62*	80
57112	1	51	N/A	62*	80

* with documentation

Medicare References: None

Coding Companion for Ob/Gyn

Vagina

57120

57120 Colpocleisis (Le Fort type)

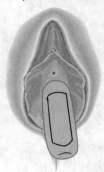

The vagina is surgically obliterated. The vagina is everted and a strip is removed from the posterior and anterior walls

The vagina is again inverted and the vaginal opening permanently closed

Explanation

The physician grasps the deepest portion of the vaginal vault and everts the vagina. Two large flaps of vaginal wall are removed from opposite sides of the prolapsed vagina. The vaginal walls are sutured to one another and this structure is inverted back inside the body. The former vaginal opening is closed with sutures obliterating the vagina and preventing uterine prolapse.

Coding Tips

This procedure is rarely used: code with caution. For vaginectomy other than Le Fort, see 57106–57109 and 57110–57112.

ICD-9-CM Procedural

70.8   Obliteration of vaginal vault

Anesthesia

57120   00942

ICD-9-CM Diagnostic

184.0   Malignant neoplasm of vagina
198.82   Secondary malignant neoplasm of genital organs
221.1   Benign neoplasm of vagina
233.30   Carcinoma in situ, unspecified female genital organ
233.31   Carcinoma in situ, vagina
233.32   Carcinoma in situ, vulva
233.39   Carcinoma in situ, other female genital organ

236.3   Neoplasm of uncertain behavior of other and unspecified female genital organs
239.5   Neoplasm of unspecified nature of other genitourinary organs
618.00   Unspecified prolapse of vaginal walls without mention of uterine prolapse — (Use additional code to identify urinary incontinence: 625.6, 788.31, 788.33-788.39)
618.01   Cystocele without mention of uterine prolapse, midline — (Use additional code to identify urinary incontinence: 625.6, 788.31, 788.33-788.39)
618.02   Cystocele without mention of uterine prolapse, lateral — (Use additional code to identify urinary incontinence: 625.6, 788.31, 788.33-788.39)
618.05   Perineocele without mention of uterine prolapse — (Use additional code to identify urinary incontinence: 625.6, 788.31, 788.33-788.39)
618.09   Other prolapse of vaginal walls without mention of uterine prolapse — (Use additional code to identify urinary incontinence: 625.6, 788.31, 788.33-788.39)
618.4   Uterovaginal prolapse, unspecified — (Use additional code to identify urinary incontinence: 625.6, 788.31, 788.33-788.39)
618.84   Cervical stump prolapse — (Use additional code to identify urinary incontinence: 625.6, 788.31, 788.33-788.39)
752.49   Other congenital anomaly of cervix, vagina, and external female genitalia

Terms To Know

anomaly. Irregularity in the structure or position of an organ or tissue.

benign. Mild or nonmalignant in nature.

carcinoma in situ. Malignancy that arises from the cells of the vessel, gland, or organ of origin that remains confined to that site or has not invaded neighboring tissue.

congenital. Present at birth, occurring through heredity or an influence during gestation up to the moment of birth.

malignant neoplasm. Any cancerous tumor or lesion exhibiting uncontrolled tissue growth that can progressively invade other parts of the body with its disease-generating cells.

prolapse. Falling, sliding, or sinking of an organ from its normal location in the body.

CCI Version 18.3

00940, 0213T, 0216T, 0228T, 0230T, 12001-12007, 12011-12057, 13100-13153, 36000, 36400-36410, 36420-36430, 36440, 36600, 36640, 37202, 43752, 50715, 51701-51703, 56810, 57061, 57065-57105, 57135, 57180, 57268-57270, 57410-57420, 57452, 57500, 57800, 58100, 62310-62319, 64400-64435, 64445-64450, 64479, 64483, 64490, 64493, 64505-64530, 69990, 93000-93010, 93040-93042, 93318, 94002, 94200, 94250, 94680-94690, 94770, 95812-95816, 95819, 95822, 95829, 95955, 96360, 96365, 96372, 96374-96376, 99148-99149, 99150, P9612

Note: These CCI edits are used for Medicare. Other payers may reimburse on codes listed above.

Medicare Edits

	Fac RVU	Non-Fac RVU	FUD	Status
57120	15.24	15.24	90	A

	MUE		Modifiers		
57120	1	51	N/A	62*	80

* with documentation

Medicare References: None

Coding Companion for Ob/Gyn

Vagina

57130

57130 Excision of vaginal septum

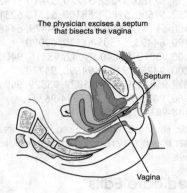

The physician excises a septum
that bisects the vagina

Septum

Vagina

The septum may be medial or transverse.
Sutures may be required

Explanation

The physician excises a vaginal septum, an anomaly that separates the vagina into two portions. The septum can be longitudinal, creating two vaginal canals, or transverse, blocking the vagina and preventing menstrual flow. For a small, thin septum, the procedure is often done by injecting a local anesthetic in the tissues around the septum and making an incision through the narrowest portion of the septum. The divided tissue is tied off with suture material and the tissue is excised. For a thicker and more extensive septum, the procedure may be done under general anesthesia. The tissue is excised, and the resulting vaginal lining defects are closed. The vagina is packed with medicated gauze or a support device.

Coding Tips

Local anesthesia is included in this service. However, this procedure may be performed under general anesthesia, depending on the age and/or condition of the patient. Report any free grafts or flaps separately. For excision of a vaginal cyst or tumor, see 57135.

ICD-9-CM Procedural

70.33 Excision or destruction of lesion of vagina

Anesthesia

57130 00940

ICD-9-CM Diagnostic

752.49 Other congenital anomaly of cervix, vagina, and external female genitalia

Terms To Know

anomaly. Irregularity in the structure or position of an organ or tissue.

congenital. Present at birth, occurring through heredity or an influence during gestation up to the moment of birth.

excision. Surgical removal of an organ or tissue.

genitalia. External organs related to reproduction.

septum. Anatomical partition or dividing wall.

CCI Version 18.3

00940, 0213T, 0216T, 0228T, 0230T, 12001-12007, 12011-12057, 13100-13153, 36000, 36400-36410, 36420-36430, 36440, 36600, 36640, 37202, 43752, 50715, 51701-51703, 56810, 57022, 57100, 57180, 57410-57420, 57452, 57500, 57800, 58100, 62310-62319, 64400-64435, 64445-64450, 64479, 64483, 64490, 64493, 64505-64530, 69990, 93000-93010, 93040-93042, 93318, 94002, 94200, 94250, 94680-94690, 94770, 95812-95816, 95819, 95822, 95829, 95955, 96360, 96365, 96372, 96374-96376, 99148-99149, 99150, J0670, J2001

Note: These CCI edits are used for Medicare. Other payers may reimburse on codes listed above.

Medicare Edits

	Fac RVU	Non-Fac RVU	FUD	Status
57130	4.77	5.32	10	A

	MUE		Modifiers		
57130	1	51	N/A	62*	80

* with documentation

Medicare References: None

Vagina

57135

57135 Excision of vaginal cyst or tumor

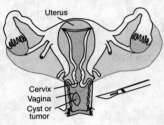

The physician removes a vaginal cyst or tumor

Uterus

Cervix
Vagina
Cyst or
tumor

Sutures are required

Explanation

Through a speculum inserted in the vagina, the physician uses a forceps or hemostat clamp to grasp and elongate the vaginal tissue containing the cyst or tumor, causing the mucosa to tent. With a scalpel or scissors, the physician excises an ellipse of tissue containing the lesion. The defect is closed with absorbable sutures.

Coding Tips

If the excised tissue is transported to an outside laboratory, report 99000 for conveyance of the specimen. For excision of a vaginal septum, see 57130. For destruction of vaginal lesion(s), see 57061–57065. For excision with partial or complete removal of the vagina, see 57106–57112.

ICD-9-CM Procedural

70.33   Excision or destruction of lesion of vagina

Anesthesia

57135   00940

ICD-9-CM Diagnostic

184.0   Malignant neoplasm of vagina
198.82 Secondary malignant neoplasm of genital organs
221.1   Benign neoplasm of vagina
233.30 Carcinoma in situ, unspecified female genital organ
233.31 Carcinoma in situ, vagina

233.32 Carcinoma in situ, vulva
233.39 Carcinoma in situ, other female genital organ
236.3   Neoplasm of uncertain behavior of other and unspecified female genital organs
239.5   Neoplasm of unspecified nature of other genitourinary organs
623.7   Polyp of vagina
623.8   Other specified noninflammatory disorder of vagina
752.41 Embryonic cyst of cervix, vagina, and external female genitalia

Terms To Know

absorbable sutures. Strands prepared from collagen or a synthetic polymer and capable of being absorbed by tissue over time.

benign. Mild or nonmalignant in nature.

carcinoma in situ. Malignancy that arises from the cells of the vessel, gland, or organ of origin that remains confined to that site or has not invaded neighboring tissue. Carcinoma in situ codes are found in their own subchapter of neoplasms according to site.

cyst. Elevated encapsulated mass containing fluid, semisolid, or solid material with a membranous lining.

excision. Surgical removal of an organ or tissue.

forceps. Tool used for grasping or compressing tissue.

hemostat. Tool for clamping vessels and arresting hemorrhaging.

malignant neoplasm. Any cancerous tumor or lesion exhibiting uncontrolled tissue growth that can progressively invade other parts of the body with its disease-generating cells.

polyp. Small growth on a stalk-like attachment projecting from a mucous membrane.

simple polyp. Mucosal outgrowth of tissue that is hanging from a stalk and can easily be removed.

speculum. Tool used to enlarge the opening of any canal or cavity.

tumor. Pathological swelling or enlargement; a neoplastic growth of uncontrolled, abnormal multiplication of cells.

CCI Version 18.3

00940, 0213T, 0216T, 0228T, 0230T, 12001-12007, 12011-12057, 13100-13153, 36000, 36400-36410, 36420-36430, 36440, 36600, 36640, 37202, 43752, 50715,

51701-51703, 56810, 57061, 57065-57105, 57180, 57410-57421, 57452, 57500, 57800, 58100, 62310-62319, 64400-64435, 64445-64450, 64479, 64483, 64490, 64493, 64505-64530, 69990, 93000-93010, 93040-93042, 93318, 94002, 94200, 94250, 94680-94690, 94770, 95812-95816, 95819, 95822, 95829, 95955, 96360, 96365, 96372, 96374-96376, 99148-99149, 99150, J0670, J2001, P9612

Note: These CCI edits are used for Medicare. Other payers may reimburse on codes listed above.

Medicare Edits

	Fac RVU	Non-Fac RVU	FUD	Status
57135	5.14	5.71	10	A

	MUE		Modifiers		
57135	2	51	N/A	N/A	N/A

* with documentation

Medicare References: None

Vagina

57150

57150 Irrigation of vagina and/or application of medicament for treatment of bacterial, parasitic, or fungoid disease

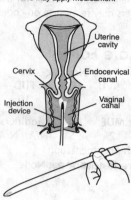

The physician irrigates the vagina and may apply medicament

Explanation

The physician passes a catheter or similar tube high into the vaginal canal and flushes the canal with medicated solution from a large syringe. The physician also paints infected areas with medication using a cotton-tipped applicator or similar device.

Coding Tips

For clinical brachytherapy to treat cancerous conditions via insertion of vaginal ovoids and/or uterine tandems, see 57155. For introduction of packing or hemostatic agent to stop nonobstetrical vaginal hemorrhaging, see 57180. Surgical trays, A4550, are not separately reimbursed by Medicare; however, other third-party payers may cover them. Check with the specific payer to determine coverage.

ICD-9-CM Procedural

96.44 Vaginal douche
96.49 Other genitourinary instillation

Anesthesia

57150 00940

ICD-9-CM Diagnostic

054.11 Herpetic vulvovaginitis
112.1 Candidiasis of vulva and vagina — (Use additional code to identify

manifestation: 321.0-321.1, 380.15, 711.6)
127.4 Enterobiasis
131.01 Trichomonal vulvovaginitis
616.0 Cervicitis and endocervicitis — (Use additional code to identify organism: 041.00-041.09, 041.10-041.19)
616.10 Unspecified vaginitis and vulvovaginitis — (Use additional code to identify organism, such as: 041.00-041.09, 041.10-041.19, 041.41-041.49)
616.11 Vaginitis and vulvovaginitis in diseases classified elsewhere — (Use additional code to identify organism: 041.00-041.09, 041.10-041.19) (Code first underlying disease: 127.4)
616.81 Mucositis (ulcerative) of cervix, vagina, and vulva — (Use additional code to identify organism: 041.00-041.09, 041.10-041.19) (Use additional E code to identify adverse effects of therapy: E879.2, E930.7, E933.1)
623.5 Leukorrhea, not specified as infective

Terms To Know

candida. Yeast-like fungi causing itching and white, cheesy vaginal discharge.

catheter. Flexible tube inserted into an area of the body for introducing or withdrawing fluid.

enterobiasis. Infection with pinworms, especially nematodes of the genus E. vermicularis, usually located in portions of the intestine.

irrigation. To wash out or cleanse a body cavity, wound, or tissue with water or other fluid.

leukorrhea. White mucousy vaginal discharge.

trichomonas vaginalis. Vaginal infection by a single-celled, flagellate protozoan causing discharge, inflammation, and itching.

CCI Version 18.3

00940, 0213T, 0216T, 0228T, 0230T, 12001-12007, 12011-12057, 13100-13153, 36000, 36400-36410, 36420-36430, 36440, 36600, 36640, 37202, 43752, 50715, 51701-51703, 57100, 57410, 57420, 57452, 57500, 57800, 58100, 62310-62319, 64400-64435, 64445-64450, 64479, 64483, 64490, 64493, 64505-64530, 69990, 93000-93010, 93040-93042, 93318, 94002, 94200, 94250, 94680-94690, 94770, 95812-95816, 95819, 95822, 95829, 95955,

96360, 96365, 96372, 96374-96376, 99148-99149, 99150

Note: These CCI edits are used for Medicare. Other payers may reimburse on codes listed above.

Medicare Edits

	Fac RVU	Non-Fac RVU	FUD	Status
57150	0.87	1.38	0	A

	MUE		Modifiers		
57150	1	51	N/A	N/A	N/A

* with documentation

Medicare References: None

Coding Companion for Ob/Gyn

Vagina

57155

57155 Insertion of uterine tandem and/or vaginal ovoids for clinical brachytherapy

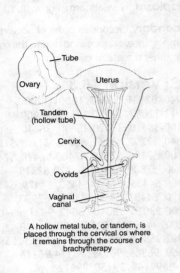

A hollow metal tube, or tandem, is placed through the cervical os where it remains through the course of brachytherapy

Explanation

The physician places a brachytherapy applicator (also called a tandem and ovoids) prior to the first brachytherapy treatment for cervical cancer. Under appropriate anesthesia, a hollow plastic sleeve that has been custom fitted to the uterine cavity is inserted into the uterus through the cervical opening and sutured into place onto the cervix. This sleeve remains in the uterus for the duration of the brachytherapy treatments, keeping the cervix open to allow for comfortable positioning of the tandem (a hollow metal tube that is inserted into the sleeve). Two ovoids, containing small radiation shields that reduce radiation doses to the bladder and rectum, are then positioned on either side of the cervix. Separately reportable brachytherapy follows, after which the tandem and ovoids are removed.

Coding Tips

The tandem holds radiotherapy doses. Additionally, in some instances, ovoids are placed high in the vaginal cavity and around the cervix. Any insertions may have shields to protect the bladder and/or rectum. For insertion of radioelement sources or ribbons, see 77761–77763 or 77776–77778.

ICD-9-CM Procedural

92.27 Implantation or insertion of radioactive elements

Anesthesia

57155 00940

ICD-9-CM Diagnostic

179 Malignant neoplasm of uterus, part unspecified

180.0 Malignant neoplasm of endocervix

180.1 Malignant neoplasm of exocervix

180.8 Malignant neoplasm of other specified sites of cervix

180.9 Malignant neoplasm of cervix uteri, unspecified site

182.0 Malignant neoplasm of corpus uteri, except isthmus

182.1 Malignant neoplasm of isthmus

182.8 Malignant neoplasm of other specified sites of body of uterus

184.0 Malignant neoplasm of vagina

184.8 Malignant neoplasm of other specified sites of female genital organs

184.9 Malignant neoplasm of female genital organ, site unspecified

198.82 Secondary malignant neoplasm of genital organs

233.1 Carcinoma in situ of cervix uteri

233.2 Carcinoma in situ of other and unspecified parts of uterus

233.30 Carcinoma in situ, unspecified female genital organ

233.31 Carcinoma in situ, vagina

233.32 Carcinoma in situ, vulva

233.39 Carcinoma in situ, other female genital organ

236.0 Neoplasm of uncertain behavior of uterus

236.3 Neoplasm of uncertain behavior of other and unspecified female genital organs

Terms To Know

brachytherapy. Form of radiation therapy in which radioactive pellets or seeds are implanted directly into the tissue being treated to deliver their dose of radiation in a more directed fashion. Brachytherapy provides radiation to the prescribed body area while minimizing exposure to normal tissue.

carcinoma in situ. Malignancy that arises from the cells of the vessel, gland, or organ of origin that remains confined to that site or has not invaded neighboring tissue.

endometrial carcinoma. Cancer of the inner lining of the uterine wall.

insertion. Placement or implantation into a body part.

malignant. Any condition tending to progress toward death, specifically an invasive tumor with a loss of cellular differentiation that has the ability to spread or metastasize to other areas in the body.

neoplasm. New abnormal growth, tumor.

secondary. Second in order of occurrence or importance, or appearing during the course of another disease or condition.

CCI Version 18.3

00940, 0213T, 0216T, 0228T, 0230T, 12001-12007, 12011-12057, 13100-13153, 36000, 36400-36410, 36420-36430, 36440, 36600, 36640, 37202, 43752, 50715, 51701-51703, 57100, 57150, 57156❖, 57180, 57400-57420, 57452, 57530, 57800, 58100, 62310-62319, 64400-64435, 64445-64450, 64479, 64483, 64490, 64493, 64505-64530, 69990, 93000-93010, 93040-93042, 93318, 94002, 94200, 94250, 94680-94690, 94770, 95812-95816, 95819, 95822, 95829, 95955, 96360, 96365, 96372, 96374-96376, 99143-99149, 99150, P9612

Note: These CCI edits are used for Medicare. Other payers may reimburse on codes listed above.

Medicare Edits

	Fac RVU	Non-Fac RVU	FUD	Status
57155	8.2	12.65	0	A

	MUE			Modifiers	
57155	1	51	N/A	62	N/A

* with documentation

Medicare References: None

© 2012 OptumInsight, Inc.

57156

57156 Insertion of a vaginal radiation afterloading apparatus for clinical brachytherapy

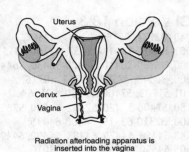

Radiation afterloading apparatus is inserted into the vagina

(left margin) Vagina

Explanation

A non-radioactive applicator or cylinder is placed into the uterine cavity and vagina in preparation for clinical brachytherapy. Under appropriate anesthesia, the physician inserts the applicator/cylinder and secures it into position, often using radiological guidance. The applicator is subsequently loaded with the radiation sources, often using a remote system in which the applicators are connected to an "afterloader" machine via a series of guide tubes. Remote afterloading systems provide radiation exposure protection to health care professionals by delivering radiation sources along the guide tubes into the prespecified positions within the applicator without staff presence in the treatment room. Separately reportable vaginal brachytherapy is then administered using low-dose rate (LDR) or high-dose rate (HDR) radiotherapy. Code 57156 reports insertion of the afterloading apparatus only.

Coding Tips

For insertion of a uterine tandem and/or vaginal ovoids, see 57155.

ICD-9-CM Procedural

92.27 Implantation or insertion of radioactive elements

Anesthesia

57156 00940

ICD-9-CM Diagnostic

179	Malignant neoplasm of uterus, part unspecified
180.0	Malignant neoplasm of endocervix
180.1	Malignant neoplasm of exocervix
180.8	Malignant neoplasm of other specified sites of cervix
180.9	Malignant neoplasm of cervix uteri, unspecified site
182.0	Malignant neoplasm of corpus uteri, except isthmus
182.1	Malignant neoplasm of isthmus
182.8	Malignant neoplasm of other specified sites of body of uterus
184.0	Malignant neoplasm of vagina
184.8	Malignant neoplasm of other specified sites of female genital organs
184.9	Malignant neoplasm of female genital organ, site unspecified
198.82	Secondary malignant neoplasm of genital organs
233.1	Carcinoma in situ of cervix uteri
233.2	Carcinoma in situ of other and unspecified parts of uterus
233.30	Carcinoma in situ, unspecified female genital organ
233.31	Carcinoma in situ, vagina
233.32	Carcinoma in situ, vulva
233.39	Carcinoma in situ, other female genital organ
236.0	Neoplasm of uncertain behavior of uterus
236.3	Neoplasm of uncertain behavior of other and unspecified female genital organs

Terms To Know

brachytherapy. Form of radiation therapy in which radioactive pellets or seeds are implanted directly into the tissue being treated to deliver their dose of radiation in a more directed fashion. Brachytherapy provides radiation to the prescribed body area while minimizing exposure to normal tissue.

carcinoma in situ. Malignancy that arises from the cells of the vessel, gland, or organ of origin that remains confined to that site or has not invaded neighboring tissue.

endometrial carcinoma. Cancer of the inner lining of the uterine wall.

insertion. Placement or implantation into a body part.

malignant. Any condition tending to progress toward death, specifically an invasive tumor with a loss of cellular differentiation that has the ability to spread or metastasize to other areas in the body.

neoplasm. New abnormal growth, tumor.

secondary. Second in order of occurrence or importance, or appearing during the course of another disease or condition.

CCI Version 18.3

00940, 0213T, 0216T, 12001-12007, 12011-12057, 13100-13153, 36000, 36400-36410, 36420-36430, 36440, 36600, 36640, 37202, 43752, 50715, 51701-51703, 57100, 57150, 57180, 57400-57420, 57452, 57530, 57800, 58100, 62310-62319, 64400-64435, 64445-64450, 64479, 64483, 64490, 64493, 64505-64530, 69990, 93000-93010, 93040-93042, 93318, 94002, 94200, 94250, 94680-94690, 94770, 95812-95816, 95819, 95822, 95829, 95955, 96360, 96365, 96372, 96374-96376, 99148-99149, 99150, P9612

Note: These CCI edits are used for Medicare. Other payers may reimburse on codes listed above.

Medicare Edits

	Fac RVU	Non-Fac RVU	FUD	Status
57156	4.16	5.59	0	A

	MUE			Modifiers	
57156	1	51	N/A	N/A	80*

* with documentation

Medicare References: None

57160

57160 Fitting and insertion of pessary or other intravaginal support device

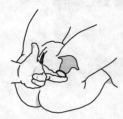
The physician inserts a pessary or other support device

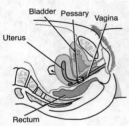
Bladder Pessary Vagina
Uterus
Rectum

Explanation
The physician fits a pessary to a patient, provides instructions for its use, and inserts it into the vagina. A pessary is a prosthesis that comes in different shapes and styles and is used to support the uterus, cervical stump, or hernias of the pelvic floor. The pessary selection and fitting will depend on the patient's symptoms and anatomy.

Coding Tips
Supplies used when providing this service may be reported with 99070 or with the appropriate HCPCS Level II code. Check with the specific payer to determine coverage.

ICD-9-CM Procedural
96.18   Insertion of other vaginal pessary
97.25   Replacement of other vaginal pessary

Anesthesia
57160   00940

ICD-9-CM Diagnostic
618.00 Unspecified prolapse of vaginal walls without mention of uterine prolapse — (Use additional code to identify urinary incontinence: 625.6, 788.31, 788.33-788.39)
618.01 Cystocele without mention of uterine prolapse, midline — (Use additional code to identify urinary incontinence: 625.6, 788.31, 788.33-788.39)

618.02 Cystocele without mention of uterine prolapse, lateral — (Use additional code to identify urinary incontinence: 625.6, 788.31, 788.33-788.39)
618.03 Urethrocele without mention of uterine prolapse — (Use additional code to identify urinary incontinence: 625.6, 788.31, 788.33-788.39)
618.04 Rectocele without mention of uterine prolapse — (Use additional code to identify urinary incontinence: 625.6, 788.31, 788.33-788.39) (Use additional code for any associated fecal incontinence: 787.60-787.63)
618.05 Perineocele without mention of uterine prolapse — (Use additional code to identify urinary incontinence: 625.6, 788.31, 788.33-788.39)
618.09 Other prolapse of vaginal walls without mention of uterine prolapse — (Use additional code to identify urinary incontinence: 625.6, 788.31, 788.33-788.39)
618.1   Uterine prolapse without mention of vaginal wall prolapse — (Use additional code to identify urinary incontinence: 625.6, 788.31, 788.33-788.39)
618.2   Uterovaginal prolapse, incomplete — (Use additional code to identify urinary incontinence: 625.6, 788.31, 788.33-788.39)
618.3   Uterovaginal prolapse, complete — (Use additional code to identify urinary incontinence: 625.6, 788.31, 788.33-788.39)
618.4   Uterovaginal prolapse, unspecified — (Use additional code to identify urinary incontinence: 625.6, 788.31, 788.33-788.39)
618.5   Prolapse of vaginal vault after hysterectomy — (Use additional code to identify urinary incontinence: 625.6, 788.31, 788.33-788.39)
618.6   Vaginal enterocele, congenital or acquired — (Use additional code to identify urinary incontinence: 625.6, 788.31, 788.33-788.39)
618.81 Incompetence or weakening of pubocervical tissue — (Use additional code to identify urinary incontinence: 625.6, 788.31, 788.33-788.39)
618.82 Incompetence or weakening of rectovaginal tissue — (Use additional code to identify urinary incontinence: 625.6, 788.31, 788.33-788.39)
618.83 Pelvic muscle wasting — (Use additional code to identify urinary

incontinence: 625.6, 788.31, 788.33-788.39)
618.84 Cervical stump prolapse — (Use additional code to identify urinary incontinence: 625.6, 788.31, 788.33-788.39)
618.89 Other specified genital prolapse — (Use additional code to identify urinary incontinence: 625.6, 788.31, 788.33-788.39)
618.9   Unspecified genital prolapse — (Use additional code to identify urinary incontinence: 625.6, 788.31, 788.33-788.39)
625.6   Female stress incontinence
878.6   Open wound of vagina, without mention of complication
878.7   Open wound of vagina, complicated

Terms To Know

insertion. Placement or implantation into a body part.

prolapse. Falling, sliding, or sinking of an organ from its normal location in the body.

prosthetic. Device that replaces all or part of an internal body organ or body part, or that replaces part of the function of a permanently inoperable or malfunctioning internal body organ or body part.

CCI Version 18.3
00940, 0213T, 0216T, 0228T, 0230T, 12001-12007, 12011-12057, 13100-13153, 36000, 36400-36410, 36420-36430, 36440, 36600, 36640, 37202, 43752, 50715, 51701-51703, 57100, 57150, 57180, 57410, 57420, 57452, 57500, 57800, 62310-62319, 64400-64435, 64445-64450, 64479, 64483, 64490, 64493, 64505-64530, 69990, 93000-93010, 93040-93042, 93318, 94002, 94200, 94250, 94680-94690, 94770, 95812-95816, 95819, 95822, 95829, 95955, 96360, 96365, 96372, 96374-96376, 99148-99149, 99150

Note: These CCI edits are used for Medicare. Other payers may reimburse on codes listed above.

Medicare Edits

	Fac RVU	Non-Fac RVU	FUD	Status
57160	1.41	2.28	0	A

	MUE		Modifiers		
57160	1	51	N/A	N/A	N/A

* with documentation

Medicare References: None

Vagina

57170

57170 Diaphragm or cervical cap fitting with instructions

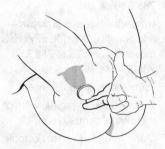
Fitting of cervical cap or diaphragm

Explanation

The physician fits a diaphragm or cervical cap and provides instructions for use. A diaphragm is a device that acts as a mechanical barrier between the vagina and the cervical canal. Cervical caps are larger, cup-like diaphragms placed over the cervix and held in place by suction. Either device can be used to prevent pregnancy.

Coding Tips

This procedure may also be performed by a registered nurse, physician assistant, nurse practitioner, or other trained paramedical person under the supervision of a physician. Because this procedure is usually not done out of medical necessity, the patient may be responsible for charges. Verify with the insurance carrier for coverage. Supplies used when providing this service may be reported with the appropriate HCPCS Level II code. Check with the specific payer to determine coverage.

ICD-9-CM Procedural

96.17 Insertion of vaginal diaphragm
97.24 Replacement and refitting of vaginal diaphragm

Anesthesia

57170 00940

ICD-9-CM Diagnostic

V24.2 Routine postpartum follow-up

V25.02 General counseling for initiation of other contraceptive measures
V25.09 Other general counseling and advice for contraceptive management
V25.49 Surveillance of other previously prescribed contraceptive method

Terms To Know

cervical cap. Contraceptive device similar in form and function to the diaphragm but that can be left in place for 48 hours.

diaphragm. Flexible disk inserted into the vagina and against the cervix as a method of birth control.

CCI Version 18.3

00940, 0213T, 0216T, 0228T, 0230T, 12001-12007, 12011-12057, 13100-13153, 36000, 36400-36410, 36420-36430, 36440, 36600, 36640, 37202, 43752, 50715, 51701-51703, 57100, 57150, 57410, 57420, 57452, 57500, 57800, 58100, 62310-62319, 64400-64435, 64445-64450, 64479, 64483, 64490, 64493, 64505-64530, 69990, 93000-93010, 93040-93042, 93318, 94002, 94200, 94250, 94680-94690, 94770, 95812-95816, 95819, 95822, 95829, 95955, 96360, 96365, 96372, 96374-96376, 99148-99149, 99150, J2001

Note: These CCI edits are used for Medicare. Other payers may reimburse on codes listed above.

Medicare Edits

	Fac RVU	Non-Fac RVU	FUD	Status
57170	1.44	1.86	0	A

	MUE		Modifiers		
57170	1	51	N/A	N/A	80*

* with documentation

Medicare References: None

Coding Companion for Ob/Gyn

Vagina

57180

57180 Introduction of any hemostatic agent or pack for spontaneous or traumatic nonobstetrical vaginal hemorrhage (separate procedure)

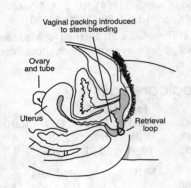

Vaginal packing introduced to stem bleeding

Ovary and tube

Uterus

Retrieval loop

Explanation

The physician pushes gauze packing into the vagina to put pressure on bleeding that is not related to childbirth or pregnancy. The packing may be coated with a chemical to make the blood clot and stop hemorrhaging.

Coding Tips

This separate procedure by definition is usually a component of a more complex service and is not identified separately. When performed alone or with other unrelated procedures/services it may be reported. If performed alone, list the code; if performed with other procedures/services, list the code and append modifier 59. When 57180 is performed with another separately identifiable procedure, the highest dollar value code is listed as the primary procedure and subsequent procedures are appended with modifier 51. This procedure might be performed by a registered nurse, physician assistant, nurse practitioner, or other trained paramedical person under the supervision of a physician. The removal of packing is not identified separately. If ablation or cauterization is necessary to stop vaginal hemorrhage, it is identified separately. Surgical trays, A4550, are not separately reimbursed by Medicare; however, other third-party payers may cover them. Check with the specific payer to determine coverage.

ICD-9-CM Procedural

96.14 Vaginal packing

97.26 Replacement of vaginal or vulvar packing or drain

Anesthesia

57180 00940

ICD-9-CM Diagnostic

623.8 Other specified noninflammatory disorder of vagina

626.9 Unspecified disorder of menstruation and other abnormal bleeding from female genital tract

867.4 Uterus injury without mention of open wound into cavity

878.6 Open wound of vagina, without mention of complication

878.7 Open wound of vagina, complicated

996.32 Mechanical complication due to intrauterine contraceptive device

996.76 Other complications due to genitourinary device, implant, and graft — (Use additional code to identify complication: 338.18-338.19, 338.28-338.29)

998.11 Hemorrhage complicating a procedure

Terms To Know

complication. Condition arising after the beginning of observation and treatment that modifies the course of the patient's illness or the medical care required, or an undesired result or misadventure in medical care.

hemorrhage. Internal or external bleeding with loss of significant amounts of blood.

hemostasis. Interruption of blood flow or the cessation or arrest of bleeding.

introduction. Induction of an instrument, such as a catheter, needle, or endotracheal tube.

packing. Material placed into a cavity or wound, such as gels, gauze, pads, and sponges.

CCI Version 18.3

00940, 0213T, 0216T, 0228T, 0230T, 12001-12007, 12011-12057, 13100-13153, 36000, 36400-36410, 36420-36430, 36440, 36600, 36640, 37202, 43752, 50715, 51701-51703, 57100, 57800, 62310-62319, 64400-64435, 64445-64450, 64479, 64483, 64490, 64493, 64505-64530, 69990, 93000-93010, 93040-93042, 93318, 94002, 94200, 94250, 94680-94690, 94770, 95812-95816, 95819, 95822, 95829, 95955,

96360, 96365, 96372, 96374-96376, 99148-99149, 99150, J0670, J2001

Note: These CCI edits are used for Medicare. Other payers may reimburse on codes listed above.

Medicare Edits

	Fac RVU	Non-Fac RVU	FUD	Status
57180	3.16	4.21	10	A

	MUE		Modifiers		
57180	1	51	N/A	N/A	N/A

* with documentation

Medicare References: None

Vagina

57200-57210

57200 Colporrhaphy, suture of injury of vagina (nonobstetrical)

57210 Colpoperineorrhaphy, suture of injury of vagina and/or perineum (nonobstetrical)

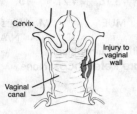

The laceration or injury is non-obstetrical in nature. Report 57210 when the injury involves or is limited to the perineum

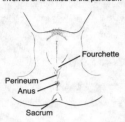

Explanation

The physician inserts a speculum into the vagina and identifies the extent of the vaginal laceration or wound that is not related to childbirth or pregnancy. Usually a local anesthetic is used; however, some instances may require general anesthesia. The wound is closed with absorbable sutures. In 57210, after the speculum is removed, the perineal laceration is closed in layers with sutures.

Coding Tips

These are nonobstetrical procedures and should not be used if the injury is a result of delivery. Local anesthesia is included in this service. However, these procedures may be performed under general anesthesia, depending on the age and/or condition of the patient. For episiotomy or vaginal repair following delivery, see 59300.

ICD-9-CM Procedural

70.71 Suture of laceration of vagina

Anesthesia

00942

ICD-9-CM Diagnostic

629.20 Female genital mutilation status, unspecified

629.21 Female genital mutilation, Type I status

629.22 Female genital mutilation, Type II status

629.23 Female genital mutilation, Type III status

629.29 Other female genital mutilation status

878.4 Open wound of vulva, without mention of complication

878.5 Open wound of vulva, complicated

878.6 Open wound of vagina, without mention of complication

878.7 Open wound of vagina, complicated

878.8 Open wound of other and unspecified parts of genital organs, without mention of complication

878.9 Open wound of other and unspecified parts of genital organs, complicated

911.6 Trunk, superficial foreign body (splinter), without major open wound and without mention of infection

911.7 Trunk, superficial foreign body (splinter), without major open wound, infected

926.0 Crushing injury of external genitalia — (Use additional code to identify any associated injuries: 800-829, 850.0-854.1, 860.0-869.1)

939.2 Foreign body in vulva and vagina

939.9 Foreign body in unspecified site in genitourinary tract

959.14 Other injury of external genitals

995.53 Child sexual abuse — (Use additional code, if applicable, to identify any associated injuries. Use additional E code to identify nature of abuse, E960-E968, and perpetrator, E967.0-E967.9)

995.83 Adult sexual abuse — (Use additional code to identify any associated injury and perpetrator, E967.0-E967.9)

Terms To Know

absorbable sutures. Strands prepared from collagen or a synthetic polymer and capable of being absorbed by tissue over time.

foreign body. Any object or substance found in an organ and tissue that does not belong under normal circumstances.

perineal. Pertaining to the pelvic floor area between the thighs; the diamond-shaped area bordered by the pubic symphysis in front, the ischial tuberosities on the sides, and the coccyx in back.

CCI Version 18.3

00940, 0213T, 0216T, 0228T, 0230T, 12001-12007, 12011-12057, 13100-13153, 36000, 36400-36410, 36420-36430, 36440, 36600, 36640, 37202, 43752, 44950, 44970, 50715, 51701-51703, 57100-57105, 57410, 57420, 57452, 57500, 57800, 58100, 62310-62319, 64400-64435, 64445-64450, 64479, 64483, 64490, 64493, 64505-64530, 69990, 93000-93010, 93040-93042, 93318, 94002, 94200, 94250, 94680-94690, 94770, 95812-95816, 95819, 95822, 95829, 95955, 96360, 96365, 96372, 96374-96376, 99148-99149, 99150, P9612

Also not with 57200: 57180

Also not with 57210: 45560, 56605-56606, 56800, 56810, 57180-57200, 59300

Note: These CCI edits are used for Medicare. Other payers may reimburse on codes listed above.

Medicare Edits

	Fac RVU	Non-Fac RVU	FUD	Status
57200	8.88	8.88	90	A
57210	10.91	10.91	90	A

	MUE			Modifiers	
57200	1	51	N/A	62*	80
57210	1	51	N/A	62*	80

* with documentation

Medicare References: None

Vagina

57220

57220 Plastic operation on urethral sphincter, vaginal approach (eg, Kelly urethral plication)

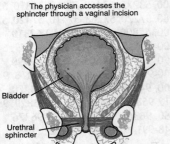

The physician accesses the sphincter through a vaginal incision

Bladder

Urethral sphincter

Cross section of female bladder

Sutures at the junction of the bladder and urethra support the urethral sphincter

Explanation

The physician accesses the urethral sphincter from the vagina. With a catheter in the urethra, the physician dissects the midline vaginal wall separating it from the bladder and the proximal urethra. Sutures are placed at the junction of the bladder and urethra on each side of the urethra. This supports the area. Excess vaginal tissue is excised and the vaginal wall is closed.

Coding Tips

For a Marshall-Marchetti-Krantz urethral suspension, abdominal approach, see 51840 and 51841. For laparoscopic repair of stress incontinence only, see 51990 and 51992.

ICD-9-CM Procedural

59.3   Plication of urethrovesical junction

Anesthesia

57220   00940

ICD-9-CM Diagnostic

599.81 Urethral hypermobility — (Use additional code to identify urinary incontinence: 625.6, 788.30-788.39)

599.82 Intrinsic (urethral) sphincter deficiency (ISD) — (Use additional code to identify urinary incontinence: 625.6, 788.30-788.39)

599.83 Urethral instability — (Use additional code to identify urinary incontinence: 625.6, 788.30-788.39)

599.84 Other specified disorders of urethra — (Use additional code to identify urinary incontinence: 625.6, 788.30-788.39)

599.89 Other specified disorders of urinary tract — (Use additional code to identify urinary incontinence: 625.6, 788.30-788.39)

625.6   Female stress incontinence

Terms To Know

catheter. Flexible tube inserted into an area of the body for introducing or withdrawing fluid.

dissect. Cut apart or separate tissue for surgical purposes or for visual or microscopic study.

excision. Surgical removal of an organ or tissue.

female stress incontinence. Involuntary escape of urine at times of minor stress against the female bladder, such as coughing, sneezing, or laughing.

plication. Surgical technique involving folding, tucking, or pleating to reduce the size of a hollow structure or organ.

proximal. Located closest to a specified reference point, usually the midline.

sphincter. Ring-like band of muscle that surrounds a bodily opening, constricting and relaxing as required for normal physiological functioning.

CCI Version 18.3

00940, 0213T, 0216T, 0228T, 0230T, 12001-12007, 12011-12057, 13100-13153, 36000, 36400-36410, 36420-36430, 36440, 36600, 36640, 37202, 43752, 44950, 44970, 45560, 50715, 51701-51703, 53000-53025, 53200, 56810, 57061, 57065-57105, 57180, 57268, 57410, 57420, 57452, 57500, 57800, 58100, 62310-62319, 64400-64435, 64445-64450, 64479, 64483, 64490, 64493, 64505-64530, 69990, 93000-93010, 93040-93042, 93318, 94002, 94200, 94250, 94680-94690, 94770, 95812-95816, 95819, 95822, 95829, 95955, 96360, 96365, 96372, 96374-96376, 99148-99149, 99150, P9612

Note: These CCI edits are used for Medicare. Other payers may reimburse on codes listed above.

Medicare Edits

	Fac RVU	Non-Fac RVU	FUD	Status
57220	9.53	9.53	90	A

	MUE		Modifiers		
57220	1	51	N/A	62*	80

* with documentation

Medicare References: None

Coding Companion for Ob/Gyn

Vagina

57230

57230   Plastic repair of urethrocele

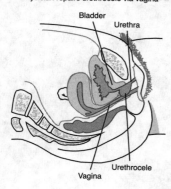

Physician repairs urethrocele via vagina

Bladder
Urethra
Vagina
Urethrocele

Explanation

The physician repairs a urethrocele, which is a sagging or prolapse of the urethra through its opening or a bulging of the posterior wall of the urethra against the vaginal canal. The prolapsed urethral tissue is excised from the meatus in a circular manner. The cut edges of urethral mucosa and vaginal mucosa are sutured.

Coding Tips

For a Marshall-Marchetti-Krantz urethral suspension, abdominal approach, see 51840 and 51841. For laparoscopic repair of stress incontinence only, see 51990 and 51992.

ICD-9-CM Procedural

70.51   Repair of cystocele

Anesthesia

57230   00940, 00942

ICD-9-CM Diagnostic

618.00   Unspecified prolapse of vaginal walls without mention of uterine prolapse — (Use additional code to identify urinary incontinence: 625.6, 788.31, 788.33-788.39)

618.01   Cystocele without mention of uterine prolapse, midline — (Use additional code to identify urinary incontinence: 625.6, 788.31, 788.33-788.39)

618.02   Cystocele without mention of uterine prolapse, lateral — (Use additional

code to identify urinary incontinence: 625.6, 788.31, 788.33-788.39)

618.03   Urethrocele without mention of uterine prolapse — (Use additional code to identify urinary incontinence: 625.6, 788.31, 788.33-788.39)

618.09   Other prolapse of vaginal walls without mention of uterine prolapse — (Use additional code to identify urinary incontinence: 625.6, 788.31, 788.33-788.39)

618.2   Uterovaginal prolapse, incomplete — (Use additional code to identify urinary incontinence: 625.6, 788.31, 788.33-788.39)

618.3   Uterovaginal prolapse, complete — (Use additional code to identify urinary incontinence: 625.6, 788.31, 788.33-788.39)

618.4   Uterovaginal prolapse, unspecified — (Use additional code to identify urinary incontinence: 625.6, 788.31, 788.33-788.39)

Terms To Know

cystocele. Herniation of the bladder into the vagina.

excise. Remove or cut out.

meatus. Opening or passage into the body.

prolapse. Falling, sliding, or sinking of an organ from its normal location in the body.

suture. Numerous stitching techniques employed in wound closure.

buried suture. Continuous or interrupted suture placed under the skin for a layered closure.

continuous suture. Running stitch with tension evenly distributed across a single strand to provide a leakproof closure line.

interrupted suture. Series of single stitches with tension isolated at each stitch, in which all stitches are not affected if one becomes loose, and the isolated sutures cannot act as a wick to transport an infection.

purse-string suture. Continuous suture placed around a tubular structure and tightened, to reduce or close the lumen.

retention suture. Secondary stitching that bridges the primary suture, providing support for the primary repair; a plastic or rubber bolster may be placed over the primary repair and under the retention sutures.

urethrocele. Urethral herniation into the vaginal wall.

uterovaginal prolapse. Uterus displaces downward and is exposed in the external genitalia.

CCI Version 18.3

00940, 0213T, 0216T, 0228T, 0230T, 12001-12007, 12011-12057, 13100-13153, 36000, 36400-36410, 36420-36430, 36440, 36600, 36640, 37202, 43752, 44950, 44970, 45560, 50715, 51701-51703, 53000-53025, 53200, 53275, 53450-53460, 56810, 57100, 57180, 57220, 57268, 57410, 57420, 57452, 57500, 57800, 58100, 62310-62319, 64400-64435, 64445-64450, 64479, 64483, 64490, 64493, 64505-64530, 69990, 93000-93010, 93040-93042, 93318, 94002, 94200, 94250, 94680-94690, 94770, 95812-95816, 95819, 95822, 95829, 95955, 96360, 96365, 96372, 96374-96376, 99148-99149, 99150, P9612

Note: These CCI edits are used for Medicare. Other payers may reimburse on codes listed above.

Medicare Edits

	Fac RVU	Non-Fac RVU	FUD	Status
57230	11.88	11.88	90	A

	MUE		Modifiers		
57230	1	51	N/A	62*	80

* with documentation

Medicare References: None

57240

57240 Anterior colporrhaphy, repair of cystocele with or without repair of urethrocele

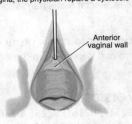

Through an incision in the anterior wall of the vagina, the physician repairs a cystocele

Anterior vaginal wall

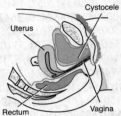

Cystocele

Uterus

Rectum

Vagina

Any urethrocele may also be repaired

Explanation

The physician repairs a cystocele, which is a herniation of the bladder through its support tissues and against the anterior vaginal wall causing it to bulge downward. The physician may also repair a urethrocele, which is a prolapse of the urethra. An incision is made from the apex of the vagina to within 1 cm of the urethral meatus. Plication sutures are placed along the urethral course from the meatus to the bladder neck. A suture is placed through the pubourethral ligament to the posterior symphysis pubis on each side of the urethra. The sutures are tied (ligated) and the posterior urethra is pulled upward to a retropubic position. If a cystocele is repaired, mattress sutures are placed in the mobilized paravesical tissue. The vaginal mucosa is closed.

Coding Tips

This procedure includes any repair of a urethrocele the physician may perform together with the cystocele repair. For a Marshall-Marchetti-Krantz urethral suspension, abdominal approach, see 51840 and 51841. For plastic repair of a urethrocele, see 57230.

ICD-9-CM Procedural

70.51   Repair of cystocele

Anesthesia

57240   00942

ICD-9-CM Diagnostic

618.00   Unspecified prolapse of vaginal walls without mention of uterine prolapse — (Use additional code to identify urinary incontinence: 625.6, 788.31, 788.33-788.39)

618.01   Cystocele without mention of uterine prolapse, midline — (Use additional code to identify urinary incontinence: 625.6, 788.31, 788.33-788.39)

618.02   Cystocele without mention of uterine prolapse, lateral — (Use additional code to identify urinary incontinence: 625.6, 788.31, 788.33-788.39)

618.03   Urethrocele without mention of uterine prolapse — (Use additional code to identify urinary incontinence: 625.6, 788.31, 788.33-788.39)

618.09   Other prolapse of vaginal walls without mention of uterine prolapse — (Use additional code to identify urinary incontinence: 625.6, 788.31, 788.33-788.39)

618.2   Uterovaginal prolapse, incomplete — (Use additional code to identify urinary incontinence: 625.6, 788.31, 788.33-788.39)

618.3   Uterovaginal prolapse, complete — (Use additional code to identify urinary incontinence: 625.6, 788.31, 788.33-788.39)

618.4   Uterovaginal prolapse, unspecified — (Use additional code to identify urinary incontinence: 625.6, 788.31, 788.33-788.39)

618.81   Incompetence or weakening of pubocervical tissue — (Use additional code to identify urinary incontinence: 625.6, 788.31, 788.33-788.39)

618.82   Incompetence or weakening of rectovaginal tissue — (Use additional code to identify urinary incontinence: 625.6, 788.31, 788.33-788.39)

618.83   Pelvic muscle wasting — (Use additional code to identify urinary incontinence: 625.6, 788.31, 788.33-788.39)

618.89   Other specified genital prolapse — (Use additional code to identify urinary incontinence: 625.6, 788.31, 788.33-788.39)

625.6   Female stress incontinence

Terms To Know

colporrhaphy. Plastic repair or reconstruction of the vagina by suturing the vaginal wall and surrounding fibrous tissue.

cystocele. Herniation of the bladder into the vagina.

meatus. Opening or passage into the body.

plication. Surgical technique involving folding, tucking, or pleating to reduce the size of a hollow structure or organ.

prolapse. Falling, sliding, or sinking of an organ from its normal location in the body.

urethrocele. Urethral herniation into the vaginal wall.

uterovaginal prolapse. Uterus displaces downward and is exposed in the external genitalia.

CCI Version 18.3

00940, 0213T, 0216T, 0228T, 0230T, 12001-12007, 12011-12057, 13100-13153, 15777, 36000, 36400-36410, 36420-36430, 36440, 36600, 36640, 37202, 43752, 44950, 44970, 50715, 51701-51703, 53000-53025, 56810, 57065-57105, 57180, 57220-57230, 57250, 57285, 57410, 57420, 57452, 57500, 57800, 58100, 62310-62319, 64400-64435, 64445-64450, 64479, 64483, 64490, 64493, 64505-64530, 69990, 93000-93010, 93040-93042, 93318, 94002, 94200, 94250, 94680-94690, 94770, 95812-95816, 95819, 95822, 95829, 95955, 96360, 96365, 96372, 96374-96376, 99148-99149, 99150, P9612

Note: These CCI edits are used for Medicare. Other payers may reimburse on codes listed above.

Medicare Edits

	Fac RVU	Non-Fac RVU	FUD	Status
57240	19.8	19.8	90	A

	MUE		Modifiers		
57240	1	51	N/A	62*	80

* with documentation

Medicare References: None

Vagina

Coding Companion for Ob/Gyn

57250

57250 Posterior colporrhaphy, repair of rectocele with or without perineorrhaphy

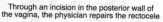
Through an incision in the posterior wall of the vagina, the physician repairs the rectocele

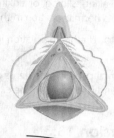

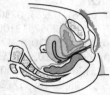
The perineum may also be repaired

Explanation

The physician repairs a rectocele by colporrhaphy. A rectocele is a protrusion of part of the rectum through its supporting tissues against the vagina causing a bulging in the vagina. Colporrhaphy involves a plastic repair of the vagina and the fibrous tissue separating the vagina and rectum. The physician makes a posterior midline incision that includes the perineum and posterior vaginal wall. In order to strengthen the area, the rectovaginal fascia is plicated by folding and tacking, and it is closed with layered sutures. The physician may also perform a perineorrhaphy, which is a plastic repair of the perineum, including midline approximation of the levator and perineal muscles. Excess fascia in the posterior vaginal wall is excised. The incisions are closed with sutures.

Coding Tips

This procedure includes any perineorrhaphy the physician may perform. For repair of a rectocele (separate procedure) without posterior colporrhaphy, see 45560. For combined anteroposterior colporrhaphy, see 57260–57265.

ICD-9-CM Procedural

70.52   Repair of rectocele

Anesthesia

57250   00942

ICD-9-CM Diagnostic

618.00   Unspecified prolapse of vaginal walls without mention of uterine prolapse — (Use additional code to identify urinary incontinence: 625.6, 788.31, 788.33-788.39)

618.04   Rectocele without mention of uterine prolapse — (Use additional code to identify urinary incontinence: 625.6, 788.31, 788.33-788.39) (Use additional code for any associated fecal incontinence: 787.60-787.63)

618.05   Perineocele without mention of uterine prolapse — (Use additional code to identify urinary incontinence: 625.6, 788.31, 788.33-788.39)

618.2   Uterovaginal prolapse, incomplete — (Use additional code to identify urinary incontinence: 625.6, 788.31, 788.33-788.39)

618.3   Uterovaginal prolapse, complete — (Use additional code to identify urinary incontinence: 625.6, 788.31, 788.33-788.39)

618.4   Uterovaginal prolapse, unspecified — (Use additional code to identify urinary incontinence: 625.6, 788.31, 788.33-788.39)

618.5   Prolapse of vaginal vault after hysterectomy — (Use additional code to identify urinary incontinence: 625.6, 788.31, 788.33-788.39)

618.6   Vaginal enterocele, congenital or acquired — (Use additional code to identify urinary incontinence: 625.6, 788.31, 788.33-788.39)

618.7   Genital prolapse, old laceration of muscles of pelvic floor — (Use additional code to identify urinary incontinence: 625.6, 788.31, 788.33-788.39)

618.82   Incompetence or weakening of rectovaginal tissue — (Use additional code to identify urinary incontinence: 625.6, 788.31, 788.33-788.39)

625.6   Female stress incontinence

788.33   Mixed incontinence urge and stress (male)(female) — (Code, if applicable, any causal condition first: 600.0-600.9, with fifth digit 1; 618.00-618.9; 753.23)

Terms To Know

colporrhaphy. Plastic repair or reconstruction of the vagina by suturing the vaginal wall and surrounding fibrous tissue.

enterocele. Intestinal herniation into the vaginal wall.

female stress incontinence. Involuntary escape of urine at times of minor stress against the female bladder, such as coughing, sneezing, or laughing.

rectocele. Rectal tissue herniation into the vaginal wall.

uterovaginal prolapse. Uterus displaces downward and is exposed in the external genitalia.

CCI Version 18.3

00940, 0213T, 0216T, 0228T, 0230T, 12001-12007, 12011-12057, 13100-13153, 15777, 36000, 36400-36410, 36420-36430, 36440, 36600, 36640, 37202, 43752, 44950, 44970, 45560, 50715, 51701-51703, 56810, 57061, 57100, 57106, 57135, 57180, 57289❖, 57410, 57420, 57452, 57500, 57800, 58100, 62310-62319, 64400-64435, 64445-64450, 64479, 64483, 64490, 64493, 64505-64530, 69990, 93000-93010, 93040-93042, 93318, 94002, 94200, 94250, 94680-94690, 94770, 95812-95816, 95819, 95822, 95829, 95955, 96360, 96365, 96372, 96374-96376, 99148-99149, 99150, P9612

Note: These CCI edits are used for Medicare. Other payers may reimburse on codes listed above.

Medicare Edits

	Fac RVU	Non-Fac RVU	FUD	Status
57250	20.05	20.05	90	A

	MUE		Modifiers		
57250	1	51	N/A	62*	80

* with documentation

Medicare References: None

Vagina

© 2012 OptumInsight, Inc.

138 — Vagina

CPT only © 2012 American Medical Association. All Rights Reserved.

Coding Companion for Ob/Gyn

57260-57265

57260 Combined anteroposterior colporrhaphy;
57265 with enterocele repair

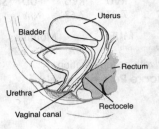

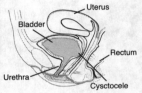

A plastic repair of the vaginal canal is performed, often to correct herniation of bladder (cystocele). Report code 57265 when an enterocele (herniation of the intestine) is repaired during the procedure

Explanation

The physician repairs both a cystocele and rectocele by colporrhaphy. Colporrhaphy involves a plastic repair of the vagina and the fibrous tissue separating the bladder, vagina, and rectum. A cystocele is a herniation of the bladder through its support tissues causing the anterior vaginal wall to bulge downward. A rectocele is a protrusion of part of the rectum through its support tissues causing the posterior vaginal wall to bulge. Using a combined vaginal approach and a posterior midline incision that includes the perineum and posterior vaginal wall, the physician dissects the tissues between the bladder, urethra, vagina, and rectum. The specific tissue weaknesses are repaired and strengthened using tissue transfer techniques and layered and plication suturing. The physician may also repair a urethrocele, which is a prolapse of the urethra, and perform a perineorrhaphy, which is a plastic repair of the perineum, including midline approximation of the levator and perineal muscles. The incisions are closed with sutures.

Coding Tips

For a vaginal repair of an enterocele without anteroposterior repair, see 57268. For a Marshall-Marchetti-Krantz urethral suspension, abdominal approach, see 51840 and 51841. For laparoscopic repair of stress incontinence only, see 51990 and 51992.

ICD-9-CM Procedural

70.50   Repair of cystocele and rectocele
70.92   Other operations on cul-de-sac

Anesthesia

00942

ICD-9-CM Diagnostic

618.00   Unspecified prolapse of vaginal walls without mention of uterine prolapse — (Use additional code to identify urinary incontinence: 625.6, 788.31, 788.33-788.39)

618.03   Urethrocele without mention of uterine prolapse — (Use additional code to identify urinary incontinence: 625.6, 788.31, 788.33-788.39)

618.04   Rectocele without mention of uterine prolapse — (Use additional code to identify urinary incontinence: 625.6, 788.31, 788.33-788.39) (Use additional code for any associated fecal incontinence: 787.60-787.63)

618.05   Perineocele without mention of uterine prolapse — (Use additional code to identify urinary incontinence: 625.6, 788.31, 788.33-788.39)

618.09   Other prolapse of vaginal walls without mention of uterine prolapse — (Use additional code to identify urinary incontinence: 625.6, 788.31, 788.33-788.39)

618.2   Uterovaginal prolapse, incomplete — (Use additional code to identify urinary incontinence: 625.6, 788.31, 788.33-788.39)

618.3   Uterovaginal prolapse, complete — (Use additional code to identify urinary incontinence: 625.6, 788.31, 788.33-788.39)

618.4   Uterovaginal prolapse, unspecified — (Use additional code to identify urinary incontinence: 625.6, 788.31, 788.33-788.39)

618.5   Prolapse of vaginal vault after hysterectomy — (Use additional code to identify urinary incontinence: 625.6, 788.31, 788.33-788.39)

618.6   Vaginal enterocele, congenital or acquired — (Use additional code to identify urinary incontinence: 625.6, 788.31, 788.33-788.39)

618.7   Genital prolapse, old laceration of muscles of pelvic floor — (Use additional code to identify urinary incontinence: 625.6, 788.31, 788.33-788.39)

618.81   Incompetence or weakening of pubocervical tissue — (Use additional code to identify urinary incontinence: 625.6, 788.31, 788.33-788.39)

618.82   Incompetence or weakening of rectovaginal tissue — (Use additional code to identify urinary incontinence: 625.6, 788.31, 788.33-788.39)

618.84   Cervical stump prolapse — (Use additional code to identify urinary incontinence: 625.6, 788.31, 788.33-788.39)

618.89   Other specified genital prolapse — (Use additional code to identify urinary incontinence: 625.6, 788.31, 788.33-788.39)

625.6   Female stress incontinence

788.33   Mixed incontinence urge and stress (male)(female) — (Code, if applicable, any causal condition first: 600.0-600.9, with fifth digit 1; 618.00-618.9; 753.23)

CCI Version 18.3

00940, 0213T, 0216T, 0228T, 0230T, 12001-12007, 12011-12057, 13100-13153, 15777, 36000, 36400-36410, 36420-36430, 36440, 36600, 36640, 37202, 43752, 44950, 44970, 45560, 50715, 51701-51703, 56800, 56810, 57061, 57100, 57180, 57268-57270, 57410, 57420, 57452, 57500, 57800, 58100, 62310-62319, 64400-64435, 64445-64450, 64479, 64483, 64490, 64493, 64505-64530, 69990, 93000-93010, 93040-93042, 93318, 94002, 94200, 94250, 94680-94690, 94770, 95812-95816, 95819, 95822, 95829, 95955, 96360, 96365, 96372, 96374-96376, 99148-99149, 99150, P9612

Also not with 57260: 53620❖, 53660, 57120, 57220-57250, 57285

Also not with 57265: 57220-57260, 57284-57285, 58800

Note: These CCI edits are used for Medicare. Other payers may reimburse on codes listed above.

Medicare Edits

	Fac RVU	Non-Fac RVU	FUD	Status
57260	24.72	24.72	90	A
57265	27.15	27.15	90	A

	MUE		Modifiers		
57260	1	51	N/A	62*	80
57265	1	51	N/A	62*	80

* with documentation

Medicare References: None

Vagina

57267

57267 Insertion of mesh or other prosthesis for repair of pelvic floor defect, each site (anterior, posterior compartment), vaginal approach (List separately in addition to code for primary procedure)

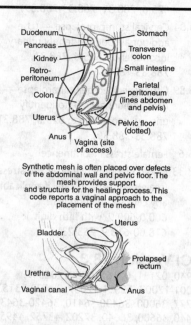

Synthetic mesh is often placed over defects of the abdominal wall and pelvic floor. The mesh provides support and structure for the healing process. This code reports a vaginal approach to the placement of the mesh

Explanation

The physician inserts mesh or other prosthetic support material to repair a pelvic floor defect using a vaginal approach. Pelvic floor defects resulting in prolapse of the pelvic viscera occur when the pelvic fascia weakens or is damaged. The physician selects the appropriate type of prosthetic support material. Some mesh supports, such as horseshoe shaped mesh, are purchased preformed in the desired configuration. Other types of mesh supports, such as tension free tapes, are cut and fashioned by the physician during surgery into the required shapes and sizes. The mesh is inserted through the vagina and placed at the site requiring support. The exact placement of the mesh is determined by the type of pelvic floor defect being repaired. For example, horseshoe mesh is placed between the pubis and sacrum to close the area between the pelvic viscera and the inferior pelvic hiatus. Report 57267 in addition to the primary procedure for each site requiring insertion of mesh or other prosthesis, such as an anterior repair for cystocele or a posterior repair for a rectocele.

Coding Tips

As an "add-on" code, 57267 is not subject to multiple procedure rules. No reimbursement reduction or modifier 51 is applied. "Add-on" codes describe additional intra-service work associated with the primary procedure. They are performed by the same physician on the same date of service as the primary service/procedure, and must never be reported as a stand-alone code. 57267 is reported together with codes for the primary vaginal or rectocele repair, 45560 or 57240–57265.

ICD-9-CM Procedural

The ICD-9-CM procedural code(s) would be the same as the actual procedure performed because these are in-addition-to codes.

Anesthesia

57267 N/A

ICD-9-CM Diagnostic

This is an add-on code. Refer to the corresponding primary procedure code for ICD-9-CM diagnosis code links.

Terms To Know

anterior. Situated in the front area or toward the belly surface of the body.

approach. Method or anatomical location used to gain access to a body organ or specific area for procedures. The approach is not coded separately although it may be a specified component of the procedure, such as laparoscopic vs. incisional, or spinal procedures in which the amount of dissection required to expose the spine significantly alters with the site of approach.

cystocele. Herniation of the bladder into the vagina.

fascia. Fibrous sheet or band of tissue that envelops organs, muscles, and groupings of muscles.

insertion. Placement or implantation into a body part.

pelvis. Distal anterior portion of the trunk that lies between the hipbones, sacrum, and coccyx bones; the inferior portion of the abdominal cavity.

posterior. Located in the back part or caudal end of the body.

prolapse. Falling, sliding, or sinking of an organ from its normal location in the body.

prosthesis. Man-made substitute for a missing body part.

rectocele. Rectal tissue herniation into the vaginal wall.

viscera. Large interior organs enclosed within a cavity, generally referring to the abdominal organs.

Vagina

57268-57270

57268 Repair of enterocele, vaginal approach (separate procedure)

57270 Repair of enterocele, abdominal approach (separate procedure)

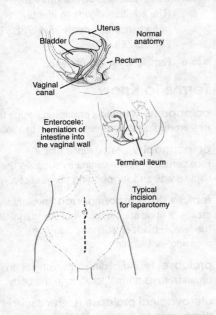

Uterus
Bladder
Normal anatomy
Rectum
Vaginal canal

Enterocele: herniation of intestine into the vaginal wall

Terminal ileum

Typical incision for laparotomy

Explanation

The physician repairs an enterocele, which is a herniation of the bowel contents of the rectouterine pouch that protrudes into the septum of tissue between the bladder and vagina or between the vagina and rectum. Through the vaginal approach in 57268, the physician incises and ligates the enterocele sac and approximates the uterosacral ligaments and endopelvic fascia anterior to the rectum. In 57270, the approach is made through an incision in the lower abdominal wall. A vaginal hysterectomy, anterior (cystocele) and posterior (rectocele) colporrhaphy, and perineorrhaphy may also be performed to augment the support.

Coding Tips

These separate procedures by definition are usually a component of a more complex service and are not identified separately. When performed alone or with other unrelated procedures/services they may be reported. If performed alone, list the code; if performed with other procedures/services, list the code and append modifier 59. If anteroposterior colporrhaphy is performed with enterocele repair, report 57265. For laparoscopic repair of stress incontinence only, see 51990 and 51992.

ICD-9-CM Procedural

70.92   Other operations on cul-de-sac

Anesthesia

57268   00942
57270   00840

ICD-9-CM Diagnostic

618.6   Vaginal enterocele, congenital or acquired — (Use additional code to identify urinary incontinence: 625.6, 788.31, 788.33-788.39)

625.6   Female stress incontinence

Terms To Know

anterior. Situated in the front area or toward the belly surface of the body.

approach. Method or anatomical location used to gain access to a body organ or specific area for procedures. The approach is not coded separately although it may be a specified component of the procedure, such as laparoscopic vs. incisional, or spinal procedures in which the amount of dissection required to expose the spine significantly alters with the site of approach.

enterocele. Intestinal herniation into the vaginal wall.

fascia. Fibrous sheet or band of tissue that envelops organs, muscles, and groupings of muscles.

female stress incontinence. Involuntary escape of urine at times of minor stress against the female bladder, such as coughing, sneezing, or laughing.

incise. To cut open or into.

ligate. To tie off a blood vessel or duct with a suture or a soft, thin wire (ligature wire).

posterior. Located in the back part or caudal end of the body.

CCI Version 18.3

00940, 0213T, 0216T, 0228T, 0230T, 12001-12007, 12011-12057, 13100-13153, 36000, 36400-36410, 36420-36430, 36440, 36600, 36640, 37202, 43752, 44950, 44970, 50715, 51701-51703, 56810, 57100, 57180, 57410, 57420, 57452, 57500, 57800, 58100, 62310-62319, 64400-64435, 64445-64450, 64479, 64483, 64490, 64493, 64505-64530, 93000-93010, 93040-93042, 93318, 94002, 94200, 94250, 94680-94690, 94770, 95812-95816, 95819, 95822, 95829, 95955, 96360, 96365, 96372, 96374-96376, 99148-99149, 99150, P9612

Also not with 57268: 45560, 57061, 57135, 57270, 58800, 69990

Also not with 57270: 44005, 44180, 44602-44605, 44850, 49000-49010, 49255, 49320

Note: These CCI edits are used for Medicare. Other payers may reimburse on codes listed above.

Medicare Edits

	Fac RVU	Non-Fac RVU	FUD	Status
57268	14.38	14.38	90	A
57270	23.8	23.8	90	A

	MUE			Modifiers	
57268	1	51	N/A	62*	80
57270	1	51	N/A	62*	80

* with documentation

Medicare References: None

Vagina

57280

57280 Colpopexy, abdominal approach

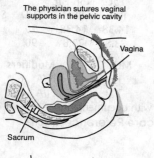

The physician sutures vaginal supports in the pelvic cavity

Vagina

Sacrum

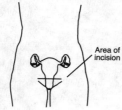

Area of incision

Explanation

Through a lower abdominal incision, the physician attaches the vault of the vagina to the prominent point of the sacrum. This is accomplished by suturing surgical fabric or a strip of abdominal wall fascia to the tissue in front of the internal sacral wall inside the pelvic cavity forming a bridge. The apex of the vagina is firmly sutured to this bridge. This stabilizes the vaginal vault and prevents prolapse of the vagina. The abdominal incision is closed with sutures.

Coding Tips

Transvaginal colporrhaphy often accompanies this procedure and should not be reported separately. For laparoscopic repair of stress incontinence only, see 51990 and 51992. For colpopexy by extra-peritoneal approach, see 57282. For colpopexy by intra-peritoneal approach, see 57283.

ICD-9-CM Procedural

70.77 Vaginal suspension and fixation

Anesthesia

57280 00840

ICD-9-CM Diagnostic

618.00 Unspecified prolapse of vaginal walls without mention of uterine prolapse — (Use additional code to identify urinary incontinence: 625.6, 788.31, 788.33-788.39)

618.01 Cystocele without mention of uterine prolapse, midline — (Use additional code to identify urinary incontinence: 625.6, 788.31, 788.33-788.39)

618.02 Cystocele without mention of uterine prolapse, lateral — (Use additional code to identify urinary incontinence: 625.6, 788.31, 788.33-788.39)

618.03 Urethrocele without mention of uterine prolapse — (Use additional code to identify urinary incontinence: 625.6, 788.31, 788.33-788.39)

618.04 Rectocele without mention of uterine prolapse — (Use additional code to identify urinary incontinence: 625.6, 788.31, 788.33-788.39) (Use additional code for any associated fecal incontinence: 787.60-787.63)

618.05 Perineocele without mention of uterine prolapse — (Use additional code to identify urinary incontinence: 625.6, 788.31, 788.33-788.39)

618.09 Other prolapse of vaginal walls without mention of uterine prolapse — (Use additional code to identify urinary incontinence: 625.6, 788.31, 788.33-788.39)

618.1 Uterine prolapse without mention of vaginal wall prolapse — (Use additional code to identify urinary incontinence: 625.6, 788.31, 788.33-788.39)

618.2 Uterovaginal prolapse, incomplete — (Use additional code to identify urinary incontinence: 625.6, 788.31, 788.33-788.39)

618.3 Uterovaginal prolapse, complete — (Use additional code to identify urinary incontinence: 625.6, 788.31, 788.33-788.39)

618.4 Uterovaginal prolapse, unspecified — (Use additional code to identify urinary incontinence: 625.6, 788.31, 788.33-788.39)

618.5 Prolapse of vaginal vault after hysterectomy — (Use additional code to identify urinary incontinence: 625.6, 788.31, 788.33-788.39)

618.81 Incompetence or weakening of pubocervical tissue — (Use additional code to identify urinary incontinence: 625.6, 788.31, 788.33-788.39)

618.82 Incompetence or weakening of rectovaginal tissue — (Use additional code to identify urinary incontinence: 625.6, 788.31, 788.33-788.39)

618.83 Pelvic muscle wasting — (Use additional code to identify urinary

incontinence: 625.6, 788.31, 788.33-788.39)

618.84 Cervical stump prolapse — (Use additional code to identify urinary incontinence: 625.6, 788.31, 788.33-788.39)

618.89 Other specified genital prolapse — (Use additional code to identify urinary incontinence: 625.6, 788.31, 788.33-788.39)

625.6 Female stress incontinence

Terms To Know

colpopexy. Suturing a prolapsed vagina to its surrounding structures for vaginal fixation.

colporrhaphy. Plastic repair or reconstruction of the vagina by suturing the vaginal wall and surrounding fibrous tissue.

female stress incontinence. Involuntary escape of urine at times of minor stress against the female bladder, such as coughing, sneezing, or laughing.

prolapse. Falling, sliding, or sinking of an organ from its normal location in the body.

uterovaginal prolapse. Uterus displaces downward and is exposed in the external genitalia.

CCI Version 18.3

00940, 0213T, 0216T, 0228T, 0230T, 12001-12007, 12011-12057, 13100-13153, 36000, 36400-36410, 36420-36430, 36440, 36600, 36640, 37202, 43752, 44005, 44180, 44602-44605, 44850, 44950, 44970, 49000-49010, 49255, 49320, 49570, 50715, 51701-51703, 57100, 57180, 57268-57270, 57282-57283❖, 57410, 57420, 57425, 57452, 57500, 57800, 62310-62319, 64400-64435, 64445-64450, 64479, 64483, 64490, 64493, 64505-64530, 69990, 93000-93010, 93040-93042, 93318, 94002, 94200, 94250, 94680-94690, 94770, 95812-95816, 95819, 95822, 95829, 95955, 96360, 96365, 96372, 96374-96376, 99148-99149, 99150, P9612

Note: These CCI edits are used for Medicare. Other payers may reimburse on codes listed above.

Medicare Edits

	Fac RVU	Non-Fac RVU	FUD	Status
57280	28.43	28.43	90	A

	MUE			Modifiers	
57280	1	51	N/A	62*	80

* with documentation

Medicare References: None

Coding Companion for Ob/Gyn

Vagina

57282

57282 Colpopexy, vaginal; extra-peritoneal approach (sacrospinous, iliococcygeus)

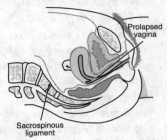

The physician accesses the ligament through an incision in the posterior vaginal wall

Prolapsed vagina

Sacrospinous ligament

The incision is closed with sutures. The physician uses sutures to fix the vagina to the sacrospinous ligament

Explanation

Colpopexy is performed by transvaginal, extraperitoneal approach to restore the apex or vault of the vagina to its anatomic position in cases of prolapse. Extraperitoneal transvaginal approach is used to perform a sacrospinous ligament fixation or iliococcygeus fascial suspension. Sacrospinous ligament fixation is performed using an anterior transvaginal approach through the paravaginal space or a posterior transvaginal approach by perforation of the rectal pillar. A pair of sutures are placed approximately 1 to 2 cm apart in the sacrospinous ligaments. After placing the sutures in the sacrospinous ligaments, the apex of the vagina is identified and the sutures in the sacrospinal ligaments are incorporated into the apex of the vagina allowing for maximal suspension of the vaginal vault. Iliococcygeus fascial suspension is performed by extraperitoneal transvaginal approach. The rectum is first retracted medially. The iliococcygeus muscle is located lateral to the rectum and anterior to the ischial spine. A single suture is placed in both sides of the apex of the vaginal vault to provide bilateral fixation of the vault to the iliococcygeus fascia.

Coding Tips

Transvaginal colporrhaphy performed at the same surgical session may be reported separately. For colpopexy by abdominal approach, see 57280. For colpopexy by intra-peritoneal approach, see 57283.

ICD-9-CM Procedural

70.77 Vaginal suspension and fixation

Anesthesia

57282 00840, 00940

ICD-9-CM Diagnostic

618.00 Unspecified prolapse of vaginal walls without mention of uterine prolapse — (Use additional code to identify urinary incontinence: 625.6, 788.31, 788.33-788.39)

618.01 Cystocele without mention of uterine prolapse, midline — (Use additional code to identify urinary incontinence: 625.6, 788.31, 788.33-788.39)

618.02 Cystocele without mention of uterine prolapse, lateral — (Use additional code to identify urinary incontinence: 625.6, 788.31, 788.33-788.39)

618.03 Urethrocele without mention of uterine prolapse — (Use additional code to identify urinary incontinence: 625.6, 788.31, 788.33-788.39)

618.04 Rectocele without mention of uterine prolapse — (Use additional code to identify urinary incontinence: 625.6, 788.31, 788.33-788.39) (Use additional code for any associated fecal incontinence: 787.60-787.63)

618.05 Perineocele without mention of uterine prolapse — (Use additional code to identify urinary incontinence: 625.6, 788.31, 788.33-788.39)

618.09 Other prolapse of vaginal walls without mention of uterine prolapse — (Use additional code to identify urinary incontinence: 625.6, 788.31, 788.33-788.39)

618.1 Uterine prolapse without mention of vaginal wall prolapse — (Use additional code to identify urinary incontinence: 625.6, 788.31, 788.33-788.39)

618.2 Uterovaginal prolapse, incomplete — (Use additional code to identify urinary incontinence: 625.6, 788.31, 788.33-788.39)

618.3 Uterovaginal prolapse, complete — (Use additional code to identify urinary incontinence: 625.6, 788.31, 788.33-788.39)

618.4 Uterovaginal prolapse, unspecified — (Use additional code to identify urinary incontinence: 625.6, 788.31, 788.33-788.39)

618.5 Prolapse of vaginal vault after hysterectomy — (Use additional code to identify urinary incontinence: 625.6, 788.31, 788.33-788.39)

618.7 Genital prolapse, old laceration of muscles of pelvic floor — (Use additional code to identify urinary incontinence: 625.6, 788.31, 788.33-788.39)

618.81 Incompetence or weakening of pubocervical tissue — (Use additional code to identify urinary incontinence: 625.6, 788.31, 788.33-788.39)

618.82 Incompetence or weakening of rectovaginal tissue — (Use additional code to identify urinary incontinence: 625.6, 788.31, 788.33-788.39)

618.83 Pelvic muscle wasting — (Use additional code to identify urinary incontinence: 625.6, 788.31, 788.33-788.39)

618.84 Cervical stump prolapse — (Use additional code to identify urinary incontinence: 625.6, 788.31, 788.33-788.39)

618.89 Other specified genital prolapse — (Use additional code to identify urinary incontinence: 625.6, 788.31, 788.33-788.39)

625.6 Female stress incontinence

CCI Version 18.3

00940, 0213T, 0216T, 0228T, 0230T, 12001-12007, 12011-12057, 13100-13153, 36000, 36400-36410, 36420-36430, 36440, 36600, 36640, 37202, 43752, 44005, 44180, 44602-44605, 44850, 44950, 44970, 49000-49010, 50715, 51701-51703, 57100, 57180, 57268-57270, 57410, 57420, 57452, 57500, 57800, 58100, 62310-62319, 64400-64435, 64445-64450, 64479, 64483, 64490, 64493, 64505-64530, 69990, 93000-93010, 93040-93042, 93318, 94002, 94200, 94250, 94680-94690, 94770, 95812-95816, 95819, 95822, 95829, 95955, 96360, 96365, 96372, 96374-96376, 99148-99149, 99150

Note: These CCI edits are used for Medicare. Other payers may reimburse on codes listed above.

Medicare Edits

	Fac RVU	Non-Fac RVU	FUD	Status
57282	14.93	14.93	90	A

	MUE		Modifiers		
57282	1	51	N/A	62*	80

* with documentation

Medicare References: None

Vagina

Coding Companion for Ob/Gyn

57283

57283 Colpopexy, vaginal; intra-peritoneal approach (uterosacral, levator myorrhaphy)

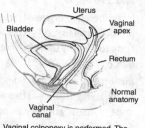

Vaginal colpopexy is performed. The approach is vaginal.

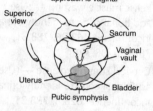

The vaginal column may be attached to ligaments of the sacral spine or other areas to support it anatomically

Explanation

Colpopexy is performed by transvaginal, intraperitoneal approach to restore the apex or vault of the vagina to its anatomic position in cases of prolapse. Intraperitoneal technique is used to perform a uterosacral ligament suspension or a levator myorrhaphy, which are performed using a posterior transvaginal approach. Uterosacral ligament suspension is performed by first locating the uterosacral ligament remnant with the use of Allis clamps posterior and medial to the ischial spine. Prior to placement of sutures in the ligaments, the ureters are located by palpation. Two to three nonabsorbable sutures are placed in each ligament and tied together. The ligaments are placated and brought together in the midline. Sutures are placed in the apical portion of the anterior and posterior vaginal walls to secure and anchor the vaginal walls to the plicated uterosacral ligaments. Levator myorrhaphy uses the levator musculature to repair the vaginal vault prolapse. The levator musculature is brought together and a high levator shelf created. The shelf is created by tagging and tying together the levator muscles at a site slightly above the junction of the levator and rectum. The vaginal vault is anchored to the shelf.

Coding Tips

This approach requires a different level of intra-service physician work than the extra-peritoneal approach and is often performed in conjunction with a hysterectomy.

ICD-9-CM Procedural

70.77 Vaginal suspension and fixation

Anesthesia

57283 00840

ICD-9-CM Diagnostic

618.00 Unspecified prolapse of vaginal walls without mention of uterine prolapse — (Use additional code to identify urinary incontinence: 625.6, 788.31, 788.33-788.39)

618.01 Cystocele without mention of uterine prolapse, midline — (Use additional code to identify urinary incontinence: 625.6, 788.31, 788.33-788.39)

618.02 Cystocele without mention of uterine prolapse, lateral — (Use additional code to identify urinary incontinence: 625.6, 788.31, 788.33-788.39)

618.03 Urethrocele without mention of uterine prolapse — (Use additional code to identify urinary incontinence: 625.6, 788.31, 788.33-788.39)

618.04 Rectocele without mention of uterine prolapse — (Use additional code to identify urinary incontinence: 625.6, 788.31, 788.33-788.39) (Use additional code for any associated fecal incontinence: 787.60-787.63)

618.05 Perineocele without mention of uterine prolapse — (Use additional code to identify urinary incontinence: 625.6, 788.31, 788.33-788.39)

618.09 Other prolapse of vaginal walls without mention of uterine prolapse — (Use additional code to identify urinary incontinence: 625.6, 788.31, 788.33-788.39)

618.1 Uterine prolapse without mention of vaginal wall prolapse — (Use additional code to identify urinary incontinence: 625.6, 788.31, 788.33-788.39)

618.2 Uterovaginal prolapse, incomplete — (Use additional code to identify urinary incontinence: 625.6, 788.31, 788.33-788.39)

618.3 Uterovaginal prolapse, complete — (Use additional code to identify urinary incontinence: 625.6, 788.31, 788.33-788.39)

618.4 Uterovaginal prolapse, unspecified — (Use additional code to identify

urinary incontinence: 625.6, 788.31, 788.33-788.39)

618.5 Prolapse of vaginal vault after hysterectomy — (Use additional code to identify urinary incontinence: 625.6, 788.31, 788.33-788.39)

618.7 Genital prolapse, old laceration of muscles of pelvic floor — (Use additional code to identify urinary incontinence: 625.6, 788.31, 788.33-788.39)

618.81 Incompetence or weakening of pubocervical tissue — (Use additional code to identify urinary incontinence: 625.6, 788.31, 788.33-788.39)

618.82 Incompetence or weakening of rectovaginal tissue — (Use additional code to identify urinary incontinence: 625.6, 788.31, 788.33-788.39)

618.83 Pelvic muscle wasting — (Use additional code to identify urinary incontinence: 625.6, 788.31, 788.33-788.39)

618.84 Cervical stump prolapse — (Use additional code to identify urinary incontinence: 625.6, 788.31, 788.33-788.39)

618.89 Other specified genital prolapse — (Use additional code to identify urinary incontinence: 625.6, 788.31, 788.33-788.39)

625.6 Female stress incontinence

CCI Version 18.3

00940, 0213T, 0216T, 0228T, 0230T, 12001-12007, 12011-12057, 13100-13153, 36000, 36400-36410, 36420-36430, 36440, 36600, 36640, 37202, 43752, 44005, 44180, 44950, 44970, 50715, 51701-51703, 57100, 57180, 57268-57270, 57282❖, 57410, 57420, 57452, 57500, 57800, 58100, 62310-62319, 64400-64435, 64445-64450, 64479, 64483, 64490, 64493, 64505-64530, 69990, 93000-93010, 93040-93042, 93318, 94002, 94200, 94250, 94680-94690, 94770, 95812-95816, 95819, 95822, 95829, 95955, 96360, 96365, 96372, 96374-96376, 99148-99149, 99150

Note: These CCI edits are used for Medicare. Other payers may reimburse on codes listed above.

Medicare Edits

	Fac RVU	Non-Fac RVU	FUD	Status
57283	20.59	20.59	90	A

	MUE		Modifiers	
57283	1	51	N/A	62*	80

* with documentation

Medicare References: None

Vagina

57284-57285

57284 Paravaginal defect repair (including repair of cystocele, if performed); open abdominal approach

57285 vaginal approach

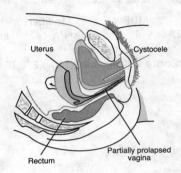

The physician repairs paravaginal defects

Uterus
Cystocele
Rectum
Partially prolapsed vagina

Explanation

The physician repairs a paravaginal defect, in which there is loss of the lateral vaginal attachment to the pelvic sidewall, by dissecting the tissues between the vagina and the bladder and urethra. The specific tissue weaknesses are found, repaired, and strengthened using tissue transfer techniques and plication suturing. The paravaginal repair may be performed alone or in conjunction with cystocele repair, in which a herniation of the bladder through its support tissues into the anterior vaginal wall causes it to bulge downward. These procedures help restore the normal anatomic relationships of the urethra, bladder, and vagina. Report 57284 if access is achieved via laparotomy (open abdominal approach) and 57285 if a vaginal approach is utilized.

Coding Tips

If only one of the components of these procedures is performed, see other codes in this section of CPT. For example, if repair of cystocele with anterior colporrhaphy is performed by itself, report 57240. For a Marshall-Marchetti-Krantz urethral suspension, abdominal approach, see 51840 and 51841. For laparoscopic repair of stress incontinence, see 51990 and 51992. For sling operation for stress incontinence, see 57288.

ICD-9-CM Procedural

70.51 Repair of cystocele

70.54 Repair of cystocele with graft or prosthesis

70.77 Vaginal suspension and fixation

70.78 Vaginal suspension and fixation with graft or prosthesis

Anesthesia

57284 00840, 00860, 00942
57285 00942

ICD-9-CM Diagnostic

618.00 Unspecified prolapse of vaginal walls without mention of uterine prolapse — (Use additional code to identify urinary incontinence: 625.6, 788.31, 788.33-788.39)

618.01 Cystocele without mention of uterine prolapse, midline — (Use additional code to identify urinary incontinence: 625.6, 788.31, 788.33-788.39)

618.02 Cystocele without mention of uterine prolapse, lateral — (Use additional code to identify urinary incontinence: 625.6, 788.31, 788.33-788.39)

618.03 Urethrocele without mention of uterine prolapse — (Use additional code to identify urinary incontinence: 625.6, 788.31, 788.33-788.39)

618.04 Rectocele without mention of uterine prolapse — (Use additional code to identify urinary incontinence: 625.6, 788.31, 788.33-788.39) (Use additional code for any associated fecal incontinence: 787.60-787.63)

618.05 Perineocele without mention of uterine prolapse — (Use additional code to identify urinary incontinence: 625.6, 788.31, 788.33-788.39)

618.09 Other prolapse of vaginal walls without mention of uterine prolapse — (Use additional code to identify urinary incontinence: 625.6, 788.31, 788.33-788.39)

618.1 Uterine prolapse without mention of vaginal wall prolapse — (Use additional code to identify urinary incontinence: 625.6, 788.31, 788.33-788.39)

618.2 Uterovaginal prolapse, incomplete — (Use additional code to identify urinary incontinence: 625.6, 788.31, 788.33-788.39)

618.3 Uterovaginal prolapse, complete — (Use additional code to identify urinary incontinence: 625.6, 788.31, 788.33-788.39)

618.4 Uterovaginal prolapse, unspecified — (Use additional code to identify urinary incontinence: 625.6, 788.31, 788.33-788.39)

618.5 Prolapse of vaginal vault after hysterectomy — (Use additional code to identify urinary incontinence: 625.6, 788.31, 788.33-788.39)

618.82 Incompetence or weakening of rectovaginal tissue — (Use additional code to identify urinary incontinence: 625.6, 788.31, 788.33-788.39)

618.83 Pelvic muscle wasting — (Use additional code to identify urinary incontinence: 625.6, 788.31, 788.33-788.39)

618.84 Cervical stump prolapse — (Use additional code to identify urinary incontinence: 625.6, 788.31, 788.33-788.39)

618.89 Other specified genital prolapse — (Use additional code to identify urinary incontinence: 625.6, 788.31, 788.33-788.39)

625.6 Female stress incontinence

CCI Version 18.3

00940, 0213T, 0216T, 0228T, 0230T, 12001-12007, 12011-12057, 13100-13153, 36000, 36400-36410, 36420-36430, 36440, 36600, 36640, 37202, 43752, 51701-51703, 57100, 57423, 57452, 57500, 57800, 58100, 62310-62319, 64400-64435, 64445-64450, 64479, 64483, 64490, 64493, 64505-64530, 69990, 93000-93010, 93040-93042, 93318, 94002, 94200, 94250, 94680-94690, 94770, 95812-95816, 95819, 95822, 95829, 95955, 96360, 96365, 96372, 96374-96376, 99148-99149, 99150, P9612

Also not with 57284: 43653, 44005, 44180, 44602-44605, 44820-44850, 44950, 44970, 49000-49010, 49255, 49320, 49570, 50715, 51715, 51840-51841, 51990, 57240, 57260, 57268-57270, 57285❖, 57410, 57420, 58660

Also not with 57285: 15777, 51840❖, 57020, 57180, 57268, 57400-57420, 57530

Note: These CCI edits are used for Medicare. Other payers may reimburse on codes listed above.

Medicare Edits

	Fac RVU	Non-Fac RVU	FUD	Status
57284	24.35	24.35	90	A
57285	20.08	20.08	90	A

	MUE		Modifiers		
57284	1	51	N/A	62	80
57285	1	51	N/A	62	80

* with documentation

Medicare References: 100-3,230.10

57287

57287 Removal or revision of sling for stress incontinence (eg, fascia or synthetic)

Pubic bone
Urethra
Bladder
Suspending suture

Overhead schematic showing suspension sutures (fascial suspension may also be found)

A synthetic or fascial sling for stress incontinence is revisited and either revised or removed

Bladder
Urethra
Synthetic sling

Explanation

The physician removes or revises a fascial or synthetic sling previously placed to correct urinary stress incontinence. To remove a sling, the physician makes a small abdominal skin incision to the level of the rectus fascia and releases the arm of the sling from the rectus abdominis. The physician releases the sling's attachment to the junction of the urethra via canals or tunnels formed by an instrument or a finger placed through a vertical or flap incision in the vaginal wall. In revision of a sling the physician may remove and partially or completely replace the sling using fascia or a synthetic graft through an abdominal and vaginal approach. The sling may be revised by increasing the tension on the sling using suture at one or both of the attachment sites at the junction of the urethra and/or to the rectus abdominis muscle. At the end of the procedure the area is irrigated, and hemostasis is achieved. The abdominal and/or vaginal incisions are closed with layered sutures.

Coding Tips

When 57287 is performed with another separately identifiable procedure, the highest dollar value code is listed as the primary procedure and subsequent procedures are appended with modifier 51. For initial sling operation, see 57288. For laparoscopic sling operation for stress incontinence, see 51992.

ICD-9-CM Procedural

59.79 Other repair of urinary stress incontinence

Anesthesia

57287 00860, 00942

ICD-9-CM Diagnostic

625.6 Female stress incontinence

996.39 Mechanical complication of genitourinary device, implant, and graft, other

996.65 Infection and inflammatory reaction due to other genitourinary device, implant, and graft — (Use additional code to identify specified infections)

996.76 Other complications due to genitourinary device, implant, and graft — (Use additional code to identify complication: 338.18-338.19, 338.28-338.29)

V53.6 Fitting and adjustment of urinary device

Terms To Know

complication. Condition arising after the beginning of observation and treatment that modifies the course of the patient's illness or the medical care required, or an undesired result or misadventure in medical care.

fascia. Fibrous sheet or band of tissue that envelops organs, muscles, and groupings of muscles.

female stress incontinence. Involuntary escape of urine at times of minor stress against the female bladder, such as coughing, sneezing, or laughing.

hemostasis. Interruption of blood flow or the cessation or arrest of bleeding.

infection. Presence of microorganisms in body tissues that may result in cellular damage.

removal. Process of moving out of or away from, or the fact of being removed.

revision. Reordering or rearrangement of tissue to suit a particular need or function.

CCI Version 18.3

00940, 0213T, 0216T, 0228T, 0230T, 12001-12007, 12011-12057, 13100-13153, 36000, 36400-36410, 36420-36430, 36440, 36600, 36640, 37202, 43752, 44950, 44970, 50715, 51701-51703, 51992❖, 53000-53025, 57020, 57100, 57180, 57220, 57268, 57288-57289, 57410, 57420, 57452, 57500, 57800, 58100, 58267❖, 58293❖, 62310-62319, 64400-64435, 64445-64450, 64479, 64483, 64490, 64493, 64505-64530,

69990, 93000-93010, 93040-93042, 93318, 94002, 94200, 94250, 94680-94690, 94770, 95812-95816, 95819, 95822, 95829, 95955, 96360, 96365, 96372, 96374-96376, 99148-99149, 99150, P9612

Note: These CCI edits are used for Medicare. Other payers may reimburse on codes listed above.

Medicare Edits

	Fac RVU	Non-Fac RVU	FUD	Status
57287	20.23	20.23	90	A

	MUE			Modifiers	
57287	1		51	N/A	62*	80

* with documentation

Medicare References: 100-3,230.10

Coding Companion for Ob/Gyn

Vagina

57288

57288 Sling operation for stress incontinence (eg, fascia or synthetic)

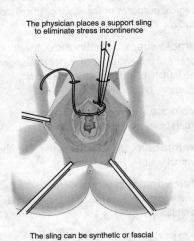

The physician places a support sling to eliminate stress incontinence

The sling can be synthetic or fascial

Explanation

Through vaginal and abdominal incisions, the physician places a sling under the junction of the urethra and bladder. The physician places a catheter in the bladder, makes an incision in the anterior wall of the vagina, and folds and tacks the tissues around the urethra. A sling is formed out of synthetic material or from fascia harvested from the sheath of the rectus abdominis muscle. The loop end of the sling is sutured around the junction of the urethra. An incision is made in the lower abdomen and the ends of the sling are grasped with a clamp and pulled into the incision and sutured to the rectus abdominis sheath. The abdominal and vaginal incisions are closed in layers by suturing.

Coding Tips

For removal or revision of a sling, see 57287. For a Marshall-Marchetti-Krantz urethral suspension, abdominal approach, see 51840 and 51841. For laparoscopic sling operation for stress incontinence, see 51992. Supplies used when providing this procedure may be reported with the appropriate HCPCS Level II code. Check with the specific payer to determine coverage.

ICD-9-CM Procedural

59.4   Suprapubic sling operation

59.71   Levator muscle operation for urethrovesical suspension

70.77   Vaginal suspension and fixation

Anesthesia

57288   00860, 00940, 00942

ICD-9-CM Diagnostic

625.6   Female stress incontinence

Terms To Know

anterior. Situated in the front area or toward the belly surface of the body.

fascia. Fibrous sheet or band of tissue that envelops organs, muscles, and groupings of muscles.

female stress incontinence. Involuntary escape of urine at times of minor stress against the female bladder, such as coughing, sneezing, or laughing.

incision. Act of cutting into tissue or an organ.

CCI Version 18.3

00940, 0213T, 0216T, 0228T, 0230T, 12001-12007, 12011-12057, 13100-13153, 36000, 36400-36410, 36420-36430, 36440, 36600, 36640, 37202, 43752, 44950, 44970, 50715, 51701-51703, 51992, 52000, 53000-53025, 56810, 57100, 57180, 57220, 57268, 57289, 57410, 57420, 57452, 57500, 57800, 58100, 58267❖, 58293❖, 62310-62319, 64400-64435, 64445-64450, 64479, 64483, 64490, 64493, 64505-64530, 93000-93010, 93040-93042, 93318, 94002, 94200, 94250, 94680-94690, 94770, 95812-95816, 95819, 95822, 95829, 95955, 96360, 96365, 96372, 96374-96376, 99148-99149, 99150, P9612

Note: These CCI edits are used for Medicare. Other payers may reimburse on codes listed above.

Medicare Edits

	Fac RVU	Non-Fac RVU	FUD	Status
57288	21.16	21.16	90	A

	MUE		Modifiers		
57288	1	51	N/A	62*	80

* with documentation

Medicare References: None

Vagina

57289

57289 Pereyra procedure, including anterior colporrhaphy

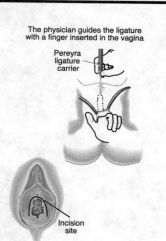

The physician guides the ligature with a finger inserted in the vagina

Pereyra ligature carrier

Incision site

A cystocele is also repaired

The proximal urethra is sutured to the rectus abdominus muscle

Explanation

The physician makes an inverted U-shaped incision in the area between the vagina and the urethra. By blunt and sharp dissection, the physician creates an opening in the space on each side of the urethra as it passes into the bladder. Using a continuous suture for each side, the physician stitches the fascial tissues along the urethra to the urethrovesical junction. The physician makes an incision in the abdomen above the pubis and, doing each side in turn, drives a Pereyra ligature carrier through the tissues just lateral to the midline and takes it down to the sutured tissue. The sutures are threaded into the instrument and brought back through the abdominal incision. The urethrovesical junction is elevated by pulling on the sutures and fixing them around the rectus abdominis muscle. In addition, the physician performs an anterior colporrhaphy using a vaginal approach, which corrects a cystocele and repairs the tissues between the vagina, bladder, and urethra.

Coding Tips

For a Marshall-Marchetti-Krantz urethral suspension, abdominal approach, see 51840 and 51841. For laparoscopic repair of stress incontinence, see 51990 and 51992. For anterior colporrhaphy with repair of cystocele, see 57240.

ICD-9-CM Procedural

59.6   Paraurethral suspension

70.51   Repair of cystocele

Anesthesia

57289   00942

ICD-9-CM Diagnostic

618.00 Unspecified prolapse of vaginal walls without mention of uterine prolapse — (Use additional code to identify urinary incontinence: 625.6, 788.31, 788.33-788.39)

618.01 Cystocele without mention of uterine prolapse, midline — (Use additional code to identify urinary incontinence: 625.6, 788.31, 788.33-788.39)

618.02 Cystocele without mention of uterine prolapse, lateral — (Use additional code to identify urinary incontinence: 625.6, 788.31, 788.33-788.39)

618.03 Urethrocele without mention of uterine prolapse — (Use additional code to identify urinary incontinence: 625.6, 788.31, 788.33-788.39)

618.05 Perineocele without mention of uterine prolapse — (Use additional code to identify urinary incontinence: 625.6, 788.31, 788.33-788.39)

618.09 Other prolapse of vaginal walls without mention of uterine prolapse — (Use additional code to identify urinary incontinence: 625.6, 788.31, 788.33-788.39)

618.1   Uterine prolapse without mention of vaginal wall prolapse — (Use additional code to identify urinary incontinence: 625.6, 788.31, 788.33-788.39)

618.2   Uterovaginal prolapse, incomplete — (Use additional code to identify urinary incontinence: 625.6, 788.31, 788.33-788.39)

618.3   Uterovaginal prolapse, complete — (Use additional code to identify urinary incontinence: 625.6, 788.31, 788.33-788.39)

618.4   Uterovaginal prolapse, unspecified — (Use additional code to identify urinary incontinence: 625.6, 788.31, 788.33-788.39)

618.84 Cervical stump prolapse — (Use additional code to identify urinary incontinence: 625.6, 788.31, 788.33-788.39)

625.6   Female stress incontinence

Terms To Know

anterior. Situated in the front area or toward the belly surface of the body.

colporrhaphy. Plastic repair or reconstruction of the vagina by suturing the vaginal wall and surrounding fibrous tissue.

cystocele. Herniation of the bladder into the vagina.

dissect. Cut apart or separate tissue for surgical purposes or for visual or microscopic study.

female stress incontinence. Involuntary escape of urine at times of minor stress against the female bladder, such as coughing, sneezing, or laughing.

prolapse. Falling, sliding, or sinking of an organ from its normal location in the body.

urethrocele. Urethral herniation into the vaginal wall.

uterovaginal prolapse. Uterus displaces downward and is exposed in the external genitalia.

CCI Version 18.3

00940, 0213T, 0216T, 0228T, 0230T, 12001-12007, 12011-12057, 13100-13153, 36000, 36400-36410, 36420-36430, 36440, 36600, 36640, 37202, 43752, 44950, 44970, 50715, 51701-51703, 51840❖, 56810, 57100, 57180-57200, 57230-57240, 57260, 57268, 57410, 57420, 57452, 57500, 57800, 58100, 62310-62319, 64400-64435, 64445-64450, 64479, 64483, 64490, 64493, 64505-64530, 69990, 93000-93010, 93040-93042, 93318, 94002, 94200, 94250, 94680-94690, 94770, 95812-95816, 95819, 95822, 95829, 95955, 96360, 96365, 96372, 96374-96376, 99148-99149, 99150, P9612

Note: These CCI edits are used for Medicare. Other payers may reimburse on codes listed above.

Medicare Edits

	Fac RVU	Non-Fac RVU	FUD	Status
57289	21.36	21.36	90	A

	MUE		Modifiers	
57289	1	51	N/A 62*	80

* with documentation

Medicare References: None

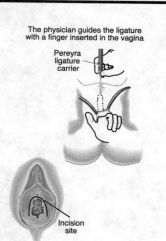

Vagina

57291-57292

57291 Construction of artificial vagina; without graft
57292 with graft

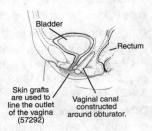

An artificial vagina is constructed. Report 57291 when no graft is used. Report 57292 when a skin graft is used in the procedure.

Explanation

For construction of an artificial vagina without graft, the physician develops a vagina by a program of perineal pressure using progressively longer and wider firm obturators. Pressure is applied to the soft area between the urethra and rectum with an obturator. Over several months of consistent, daily use by the patient, a sexually functional vagina can be created. In 57292, the physician creates or enlarges the vagina using one or more skin grafts. Through a midline episiotomy incision, the physician creates a space between the urethra and rectum. Using split thickness or full thickness skin grafts, the space is lined and the vagina created. An obturator or mold is inserted into the vagina and a catheter is passed into the bladder and left for several days. The full thickness skin donor sites are closed using plastic surgical techniques. The split thickness sites are dressed with medicated gauze.

Coding Tips

For repair of an injury of the vagina and perineum, see 57210. For vaginoplasty, see 57335.

ICD-9-CM Procedural

70.61 Vaginal construction
70.63 Vaginal construction with graft or prosthesis
86.63 Full-thickness skin graft to other sites
86.69 Other skin graft to other sites

Anesthesia

00904

ICD-9-CM Diagnostic

184.0 Malignant neoplasm of vagina
198.82 Secondary malignant neoplasm of genital organs
221.1 Benign neoplasm of vagina
233.30 Carcinoma in situ, unspecified female genital organ
233.31 Carcinoma in situ, vagina
233.32 Carcinoma in situ, vulva
233.39 Carcinoma in situ, other female genital organ
236.3 Neoplasm of uncertain behavior of other and unspecified female genital organs
239.5 Neoplasm of unspecified nature of other genitourinary organs
752.49 Other congenital anomaly of cervix, vagina, and external female genitalia
959.12 Other injury of abdomen
959.19 Other injury of other sites of trunk
V51.8 Other aftercare involving the use of plastic surgery

Terms To Know

anomaly. Irregularity in the structure or position of an organ or tissue.

benign. Mild or nonmalignant in nature.

carcinoma in situ. Malignancy that arises from the cells of the vessel, gland, or organ of origin that remains confined to that site or has not invaded neighboring tissue.

catheter. Flexible tube inserted into an area of the body for introducing or withdrawing fluid.

congenital. Present at birth, occurring through heredity or an influence during gestation up to the moment of birth.

episiotomy. Deliberate incision in the perineal tissue to facilitate delivery of the fetus and avoid traumatic tearing. In a midline or median episiotomy, the incision is made from the vagina straight down toward the anus. In a mediolateral episiotomy, the incision slants to one side.

free graft. Unattached piece of skin and tissue moved to another part of the body and sutured into place to repair a defect.

genitalia. External organs related to reproduction.

incision. Act of cutting into tissue or an organ.

malignant neoplasm. Any cancerous tumor or lesion exhibiting uncontrolled tissue growth that can progressively invade other parts of the body with its disease-generating cells.

perineal. Pertaining to the pelvic floor area between the thighs; the diamond-shaped area bordered by the pubic symphysis in front, the ischial tuberosities on the sides, and the coccyx in back.

CCI Version 18.3

00940, 0213T, 0216T, 0228T, 0230T, 12001-12007, 12011-12057, 13100-13153, 36000, 36400-36410, 36420-36430, 36440, 36600, 36640, 37202, 43752, 44950, 44970, 50715, 51701-51703, 56810, 57100, 57180, 57295❖, 57410, 57420, 57452, 57500, 57800, 58100, 62310-62319, 64400-64435, 64445-64450, 64479, 64483, 64490, 64493, 64505-64530, 69990, 93000-93010, 93040-93042, 93318, 94002, 94200, 94250, 94680-94690, 94770, 95812-95816, 95819, 95822, 95829, 95955, 96360, 96365, 96372, 96374-96376, 99148-99149, 99150

Also not with 57292: 57291

Note: These CCI edits are used for Medicare. Other payers may reimburse on codes listed above.

Medicare Edits

	Fac RVU	Non-Fac RVU	FUD	Status
57291	18.3	18.3	90	A
57292	24.49	24.49	90	A

	MUE			Modifiers	
57291	1	51	N/A	N/A	80
57292	1	51	N/A	62*	80

* with documentation

Medicare References: None

Coding Companion for Ob/Gyn

57295

57295 Revision (including removal) of prosthetic vaginal graft; vaginal approach

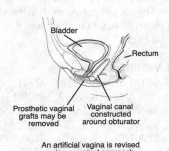

Bladder

Rectum

Prosthetic vaginal grafts may be removed

Vaginal canal constructed around obturator

An artificial vagina is revised using a vaginal approach

Explanation

The physician revises or removes a previously placed prosthetic vaginal graft via a vaginal approach. The patient is placed in the lithotomy position and a speculum is inserted. The physician visualizes the vagina. The apex of the vagina is accessed with deep retractors. Dissection is carried out to reach the affected graft material. Depending upon the type of complication (i.e., stricture or infection), the vaginal graft may be completely or partially excised to remove eroding mesh or revisions may be made in the graft and surrounding tissue. The vaginal epithelial layers and pelvic fascia are rearranged or reapproximated and closed. Vaginal packing is put in place.

Coding Tips

Revision of prosthetic vaginal graft is done for complications, such as infection, that require surgical intervention. Complete removal of the graft is included. For initial construction of an artificial vagina using a graft, see 57292.

ICD-9-CM Procedural

70.14   Other vaginotomy
70.62   Vaginal reconstruction
70.64   Vaginal reconstruction with graft or prosthesis
70.79   Other repair of vagina
70.91   Other operations on vagina

Anesthesia

57295   00940

ICD-9-CM Diagnostic

054.11   Herpetic vulvovaginitis
098.0   Gonococcal infection (acute) of lower genitourinary tract
098.2   Gonococcal infections, chronic, of lower genitourinary tract
099.53   Chlamydia trachomatis infection of lower genitourinary sites — (Use additional code to specify site of infection: 595.4, 616.0, 616.11)
112.1   Candidiasis of vulva and vagina — (Use additional code to identify manifestation: 321.0-321.1, 380.15, 711.6)
184.0   Malignant neoplasm of vagina
198.82   Secondary malignant neoplasm of genital organs
221.1   Benign neoplasm of vagina
233.30   Carcinoma in situ, unspecified female genital organ
233.31   Carcinoma in situ, vagina
233.32   Carcinoma in situ, vulva
233.39   Carcinoma in situ, other female genital organ
236.3   Neoplasm of uncertain behavior of other and unspecified female genital organs
239.5   Neoplasm of unspecified nature of other genitourinary organs
616.10   Unspecified vaginitis and vulvovaginitis — (Use additional code to identify organism, such as: 041.00-041.09, 041.10-041.19, 041.41-041.49)
616.11   Vaginitis and vulvovaginitis in diseases classified elsewhere — (Use additional code to identify organism: 041.00-041.09, 041.10-041.19) (Code first underlying disease: 127.4)
629.31   Erosion of implanted vaginal mesh and other prosthetic materials to surrounding organ or tissue
629.32   Exposure of implanted vaginal mesh and other prosthetic materials into vagina
752.49   Other congenital anomaly of cervix, vagina, and external female genitalia
996.30   Mechanical complication of unspecified genitourinary device, implant, and graft
996.39   Mechanical complication of genitourinary device, implant, and graft, other
996.52   Mechanical complication due to other tissue graft, not elsewhere classified

996.59   Mechanical complication due to other implant and internal device, not elsewhere classified
996.60   Infection and inflammatory reaction due to unspecified device, implant, and graft — (Use additional code to identify specified infections)
996.65   Infection and inflammatory reaction due to other genitourinary device, implant, and graft — (Use additional code to identify specified infections)
996.70   Other complications due to unspecified device, implant, and graft — (Use additional code to identify complication: 338.18-338.19, 338.28-338.29)
996.76   Other complications due to genitourinary device, implant, and graft — (Use additional code to identify complication: 338.18-338.19, 338.28-338.29)
V51.8   Other aftercare involving the use of plastic surgery

CCI Version 18.3

00940, 0213T, 0216T, 0228T, 0230T, 12001-12007, 12011-12057, 13100-13153, 36000, 36400-36410, 36420-36430, 36440, 36600, 36640, 37202, 43752, 51701-51703, 56810, 57100, 57180, 57400-57420, 57452, 57500, 57800, 58100, 62310-62319, 64400-64435, 64445-64450, 64479, 64483, 64490, 64493, 64505-64530, 69990, 93000-93010, 93040-93042, 93318, 94002, 94200, 94250, 94680-94690, 94770, 95812-95816, 95819, 95822, 95829, 95955, 96360, 96365, 96372, 96374-96376, 99148-99149, 99150

Note: These CCI edits are used for Medicare. Other payers may reimburse on codes listed above.

Medicare Edits

	Fac RVU	Non-Fac RVU	FUD	Status
57295	14.29	14.29	90	A

	MUE		Modifiers	
57295	1	51	N/A 62*	80

* with documentation

Medicare References: None

Vagina

57296

57296 Revision (including removal) of prosthetic vaginal graft; open abdominal approach

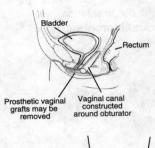

Bladder
Rectum
Prosthetic vaginal grafts may be removed
Vaginal canal constructed around obturator

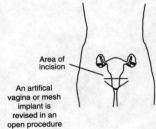

Area of incision

An artifical vagina or mesh implant is revised in an open procedure

Explanation

The physician revises or removes a previously placed prosthetic vaginal graft using an open abdominal approach in conjunction with a vaginal approach. A laparotomy incision is made and the physician dissects into the pelvis. The vagina is elevated with tools or with the physician's hand. The graft is located, the peritoneum is opened over it, and the graft is dissected free and removed. Depending upon the type of complication (i.e., stricture or infection), the vaginal graft may be completely or partially excised to remove eroding mesh or revisions may be made in the graft and surrounding tissue. Endopelvic fascia is reapproximated and the vaginal epithelial layers and pelvic fascia are rearranged or reapproximated and closed. The abdominal incision is repaired in layers. Vaginal packing is put in place.

Coding Tips

Revision of prosthetic vaginal graft is done for complications, such as infection, that require surgical intervention. 57296 is performed by open abdominal approach. Complete removal of the graft is included. For vaginal approach, see 57295.

ICD-9-CM Procedural

70.79   Other repair of vagina
70.91   Other operations on vagina

Anesthesia

57296   00840, 00940

ICD-9-CM Diagnostic

054.11   Herpetic vulvovaginitis
098.0   Gonococcal infection (acute) of lower genitourinary tract
098.2   Gonococcal infections, chronic, of lower genitourinary tract
099.53   Chlamydia trachomatis infection of lower genitourinary sites — (Use additional code to specify site of infection: 595.4, 616.0, 616.11)
112.1   Candidiasis of vulva and vagina — (Use additional code to identify manifestation: 321.0-321.1, 380.15, 711.6)
616.10   Unspecified vaginitis and vulvovaginitis — (Use additional code to identify organism, such as: 041.00-041.09, 041.10-041.19, 041.41-041.49)
616.11   Vaginitis and vulvovaginitis in diseases classified elsewhere — (Use additional code to identify organism: 041.00-041.09, 041.10-041.19) (Code first underlying disease: 127.4)
629.31   Erosion of implanted vaginal mesh and other prosthetic materials to surrounding organ or tissue
629.32   Exposure of implanted vaginal mesh and other prosthetic materials into vagina
752.49   Other congenital anomaly of cervix, vagina, and external female genitalia
996.30   Mechanical complication of unspecified genitourinary device, implant, and graft
996.39   Mechanical complication of genitourinary device, implant, and graft, other
996.52   Mechanical complication due to other tissue graft, not elsewhere classified
996.59   Mechanical complication due to other implant and internal device, not elsewhere classified
996.60   Infection and inflammatory reaction due to unspecified device, implant, and graft — (Use additional code to identify specified infections)
996.65   Infection and inflammatory reaction due to other genitourinary device, implant, and graft — (Use additional code to identify specified infections)
996.70   Other complications due to unspecified device, implant, and graft — (Use additional code to identify complication: 338.18-338.19, 338.28-338.29)

996.76   Other complications due to genitourinary device, implant, and graft — (Use additional code to identify complication: 338.18-338.19, 338.28-338.29)
V51.8   Other aftercare involving the use of plastic surgery

Terms To Know

infection. Presence of microorganisms in body tissues that may result in cellular damage.

prosthetic. Device that replaces all or part of an internal body organ or body part, or that replaces part of the function of a permanently inoperable or malfunctioning internal body organ or body part.

revision. Reordering or rearrangement of tissue to suit a particular need or function.

stricture. Narrowing of an anatomical structure.

CCI Version 18.3

00940, 0213T, 0216T, 0228T, 0230T, 12001-12007, 12011-12057, 13100-13153, 36000, 36400-36410, 36420-36430, 36440, 36600, 36640, 37202, 43752, 44005, 44180, 44602-44605, 44820-44850, 44950, 44970, 49000-49010, 49255, 49320, 49570, 51701-51703, 56810, 57100, 57180, 57291-57295❖, 57400-57420, 57426, 57452, 57500, 62310-62319, 64400-64435, 64445-64450, 64479, 64483, 64490, 64493, 64505-64530, 69990, 93000-93010, 93040-93042, 93318, 94002, 94200, 94250, 94680-94690, 94770, 95812-95816, 95819, 95822, 95829, 95955, 96360, 96365, 96372, 96374-96376, 99148-99149, 99150

Note: These CCI edits are used for Medicare. Other payers may reimburse on codes listed above.

Medicare Edits

	Fac RVU	Non-Fac RVU	FUD	Status
57296	28.39	28.39	90	A

	MUE		Modifiers		
57296	1	51	N/A	62*	80

* with documentation

Medicare References: None

Vagina

57300

57300 Closure of rectovaginal fistula; vaginal or transanal approach

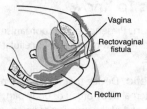

The physician closes a fistula between the vagina and rectum. The repair is made transvaginally or transanally.

Vagina

Rectovaginal fistula

Rectum

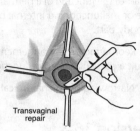

Transvaginal repair

Explanation

The physician closes a rectovaginal fistula, which is an abnormal passage between the rectum and the vagina. The physician also repairs the perineum, fascia, and muscle-supporting structures between the rectum and vagina. The scar tissue and tract between the rectum and vagina are excised and the clean edges sutured together. Often a flap of tissue is transplanted between the vagina and the rectum and the area is closed in layers. The rectal wall opening is closed by inverting the mucosa into the rectal canal. The vaginal wall opening is closed by inverting the mucosal layer into the vaginal wall. Sometimes the vaginal side is left open for drainage.

Coding Tips

For closure of a rectovaginal fistula, abdominal approach, see 57305. For closure of a rectovaginal fistula, abdominal approach with concomitant colostomy, see 57307. To report closure of a urethrovaginal fistula, see 57310 and 57311. To report vaginal closure of a vesicovaginal fistula, see 57320 and 57330; abdominal closure, see 51900.

ICD-9-CM Procedural

70.73   Repair of rectovaginal fistula

Anesthesia

57300   00902

ICD-9-CM Diagnostic

619.1   Digestive-genital tract fistula, female

677   Late effect of complication of pregnancy, childbirth, and the puerperium — (Code first any sequelae)

Terms To Know

approach. Method or anatomical location used to gain access to a body organ or specific area for procedures. The approach is not coded separately although it may be a specified component of the procedure, such as laparoscopic vs. incisional, or spinal procedures in which the amount of dissection required to expose the spine significantly alters with the site of approach.

closure. Repairing an incision or wound by suture or other means.

excise. Remove or cut out.

flap. Mass of flesh and skin partially excised from its location but retaining its blood supply that is moved to another site to repair adjacent or distant defects.

free flap. Tissue that is completely detached from the donor site and transplanted to the recipient site, receiving its blood supply from capillary ingrowth at the recipient site.

late effect. Abnormality, dysfunction, or other residual condition produced after the acute phase of an illness, injury, or disease is over. There is no time limit on when late effects can appear.

rectovaginal fistula. Abnormal communication between the rectum and the vagina that may follow obstetrical laceration repair, vaginal or rectal surgery, radiation therapy, trauma, or infection with fecal incontinence or leakage into the vaginal canal.

CCI Version 18.3

00940, 0213T, 0216T, 0228T, 0230T, 12001-12007, 12011-12057, 13100-13153, 36000, 36400-36410, 36420-36430, 36440, 36600, 36640, 37202, 43752, 44950, 44970, 45560, 50715, 51701-51703, 56810, 57100, 57180-57210, 57250, 57305❖, 57410, 57420, 57452, 57500, 57800, 58100, 62310-62319, 64400-64435, 64445-64450, 64479, 64483, 64490, 64493, 64505-64530, 69990, 93000-93010, 93040-93042, 93318, 94002, 94200, 94250, 94680-94690, 94770, 95812-95816, 95819, 95822, 95829, 95955, 96360, 96365, 96372, 96374-96376, 99148-99149, 99150, P9612

Note: These CCI edits are used for Medicare. Other payers may reimburse on codes listed above.

Medicare Edits

	Fac RVU	Non-Fac RVU	FUD	Status
57300	16.44	16.44	90	A

	MUE		Modifiers		
57300	1	51	N/A	62*	80

* with documentation

Medicare References: None

Vagina

57305

57305 Closure of rectovaginal fistula; abdominal approach

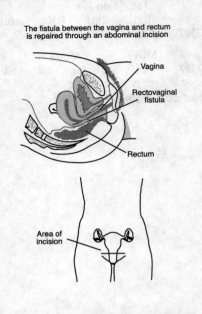

The fistula between the vagina and rectum is repaired through an abdominal incision

Vagina

Rectovaginal fistula

Rectum

Area of incision

Explanation

Through a lower abdominal incision, the physician closes a rectovaginal fistula, which is an abnormal passage between the rectum and the vagina. The physician also repairs the perineum, fascia, and muscle-supporting structures between the rectum and vagina. The scar tissue and tract between the rectum and vagina are excised and the clean edges sutured together. Often a flap of tissue is transplanted in between the vagina and the rectum and the area is closed in multiple layers. The rectal wall opening is closed by inverting the mucosa into the rectal canal. The vaginal wall opening is closed by inverting the mucosal layer into the vaginal wall. Sometimes the vaginal side is left open for drainage. The abdominal incision is closed with sutures.

Coding Tips

For closure of a rectovaginal fistula, vaginal or transanal approach, see 57300. For closure of a rectovaginal fistula, abdominal approach with concomitant colostomy, see 57307. To report closure of a urethrovaginal fistula, see 57310 and 57311. To report vaginal closure of a vesicovaginal fistula, see 57320 and 57330; abdominal closure, see 51900.

ICD-9-CM Procedural

46.10 Colostomy, not otherwise specified

70.73 Repair of rectovaginal fistula

Anesthesia

57305 00840

ICD-9-CM Diagnostic

619.1 Digestive-genital tract fistula, female

677 Late effect of complication of pregnancy, childbirth, and the puerperium — (Code first any sequelae)

Terms To Know

approach. Method or anatomical location used to gain access to a body organ or specific area for procedures. The approach is not coded separately although it may be a specified component of the procedure, such as laparoscopic vs. incisional, or spinal procedures in which the amount of dissection required to expose the spine significantly alters with the site of approach.

closure. Repairing an incision or wound by suture or other means.

concomitant. Occurring at the same time, accompanying.

fascia. Fibrous sheet or band of tissue that envelops organs, muscles, and groupings of muscles.

late effect. Abnormality, dysfunction, or other residual condition produced after the acute phase of an illness, injury, or disease is over. There is no time limit on when late effects can appear.

mucosa. Moist tissue lining the mouth (buccal mucosa), stomach (gastric mucosa), intestines, and respiratory tract.

rectovaginal fistula. Abnormal communication between the rectum and the vagina that may follow obstetrical laceration repair, vaginal or rectal surgery, radiation therapy, trauma, or infection with fecal incontinence or leakage into the vaginal canal.

scar tissue. Fibrous connective tissue that forms around a wounded area or injury, composed mainly of fibroblasts or collagenous fibers.

CCI Version 18.3

00940, 0213T, 0216T, 0228T, 0230T, 12001-12007, 12011-12057, 13100-13153, 36000, 36400-36410, 36420-36430, 36440, 36600, 36640, 37202, 43752, 44005, 44180, 44602-44605, 44850, 44950, 44970, 49000-49010, 49255, 49320, 49570, 50715, 51701-51703, 56810, 57100, 57180, 57410, 57500, 57800, 58100, 62310-62319, 64400-64435, 64445-64450, 64479, 64483, 64490, 64493, 64505-64530, 69990, 93000-93010, 93040-93042, 93318, 94002, 94200, 94250, 94680-94690, 94770, 95812-95816, 95819, 95822, 95829, 95955, 96360, 96365, 96372, 96374-96376, 99148-99149, 99150, P9612

Note: These CCI edits are used for Medicare. Other payers may reimburse on codes listed above.

Medicare Edits

	Fac RVU	Non-Fac RVU	FUD	Status
57305	27.31	27.31	90	A

	MUE		Modifiers	
57305	1	51	N/A 62*	80

* with documentation

Medicare References: None

Vagina

57307

57307 Closure of rectovaginal fistula; abdominal approach, with concomitant colostomy

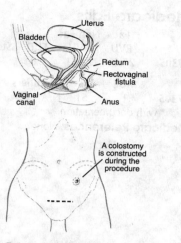

Typical incision for abdominal approach

Explanation

Through a lower abdominal incision, the physician closes a rectovaginal fistula, which is an abnormal passage between the rectum and vagina. The scar tissue and tract between the rectum and vagina are excised and the clean edges sutured together. The rectal wall opening created during the excision is closed by inverting the mucosa into the rectal canal. The vaginal wall opening is closed by inverting the mucosal layer into the vaginal canal. Sometimes the vaginal side is left open for drainage. A transverse colostomy is also done to divert the flow of feces and to allow healing of the rectal colon repair. The abdominal incision is closed with sutures.

Coding Tips

After the fistula repair has healed, a second operation is done to take down the colostomy and re-establish normal function of the bowel. For closure of a rectovaginal fistula, vaginal or transanal approach, see 57300. For closure of a rectovaginal fistula, abdominal approach, without colostomy, see 57305. To report closure of a urethrovaginal fistula, see 57310 and 57311. To report vaginal closure of a vesicovaginal fistula, see 57320 and 57330; abdominal closure, see 51900.

ICD-9-CM Procedural

46.10   Colostomy, not otherwise specified
70.73   Repair of rectovaginal fistula

Anesthesia

57307   00840

ICD-9-CM Diagnostic

619.1   Digestive-genital tract fistula, female
677   Late effect of complication of pregnancy, childbirth, and the puerperium — (Code first any sequelae)

Terms To Know

approach. Method or anatomical location used to gain access to a body organ or specific area for procedures. The approach is not coded separately although it may be a specified component of the procedure, such as laparoscopic vs. incisional, or spinal procedures in which the amount of dissection required to expose the spine significantly alters with the site of approach.

colostomy. Artificial surgical opening anywhere along the length of the colon to the skin surface for the diversion of feces.

concomitant. Occurring at the same time, accompanying.

late effect. Abnormality, dysfunction, or other residual condition produced after the acute phase of an illness, injury, or disease is over. There is no time limit on when late effects can appear.

rectovaginal fistula. Abnormal communication between the rectum and the vagina that may follow obstetrical laceration repair, vaginal or rectal surgery, radiation therapy, trauma, or infection with fecal incontinence or leakage into the vaginal canal.

scar tissue. Fibrous connective tissue that forms around a wounded area or injury, composed mainly of fibroblasts or collagenous fibers.

transverse. Crosswise at right angles to the long axis of a structure or part.

CCI Version 18.3

00940, 0213T, 0216T, 0228T, 0230T, 12001-12007, 12011-12057, 13100-13153, 36000, 36400-36410, 36420-36430, 36440, 36600, 36640, 37202, 43752, 44005, 44180, 44320, 44602-44605, 44820-44850, 44950, 44970, 49000-49010, 49255, 49320, 49570, 50715, 51701-51703, 56810, 57100, 57180, 57305, 57410, 57420, 57452, 57500, 57800, 58100, 62310-62319, 64400-64435, 64445-64450, 64479, 64483, 64490, 64493, 64505-64530, 69990, 93000-93010, 93040-93042, 93318, 94002, 94200, 94250, 94680-94690, 94770, 95812-95816, 95819, 95822, 95829, 95955, 96360, 96365, 96372, 96374-96376, 99148-99149, 99150, P9612

Note: These CCI edits are used for Medicare. Other payers may reimburse on codes listed above.

Medicare Edits

	Fac RVU	Non-Fac RVU	FUD	Status
57307	31.15	31.15	90	A

	MUE		Modifiers		
57307	1	51	N/A	62*	80

* with documentation

Medicare References: None

Vagina

57308

57308 Closure of rectovaginal fistula; transperineal approach, with perineal body reconstruction, with or without levator plication

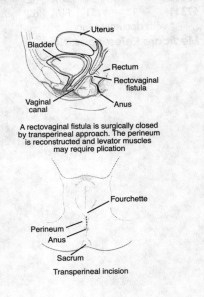

A rectovaginal fistula is surgically closed by transperineal approach. The perineum is reconstructed and levator muscles may require plication

Explanation

Through a perineal incision, the physician closes a rectovaginal fistula, which is an abnormal passage between the rectum and vagina. The physician also repairs the perineum, fascia, and muscle-supporting structures between the rectum and vagina. The scar tissue and tract between the rectum and vagina are excised and the clean edges sutured together. Often a flap of tissue is transplanted in between the vagina and rectum and the area is closed in multiple layers. The rectal wall opening created during the excision is closed by inverting the mucosa into the rectal canal. The vaginal wall opening is closed by inverting the mucosal layer into the vaginal canal. Sometimes the vaginal side is left open for drainage. The perineal area is reconstructed, sometimes with tucks or folds sutured in the levator muscles to maintain support.

Coding Tips

For closure of a rectovaginal fistula, abdominal approach, with concomitant colostomy, see 57307; without colostomy, see 57305. For closure of a rectovaginal fistula, vaginal or transanal approach, see 57300. To report closure of a urethrovaginal fistula, see 57310 and 57311. To report vaginal closure of a vesicovaginal fistula, see 57320 and 57330; abdominal closure, see 51900.

ICD-9-CM Procedural

70.73   Repair of rectovaginal fistula

Anesthesia

57308   00860, 00904

ICD-9-CM Diagnostic

619.1   Digestive-genital tract fistula, female

677   Late effect of complication of pregnancy, childbirth, and the puerperium — (Code first any sequelae)

Terms To Know

approach. Method or anatomical location used to gain access to a body organ or specific area for procedures. The approach is not coded separately although it may be a specified component of the procedure, such as laparoscopic vs. incisional, or spinal procedures in which the amount of dissection required to expose the spine significantly alters with the site of approach.

late effect. Abnormality, dysfunction, or other residual condition produced after the acute phase of an illness, injury, or disease is over. There is no time limit on when late effects can appear.

perineal. Pertaining to the pelvic floor area between the thighs; the diamond-shaped area bordered by the pubic symphysis in front, the ischial tuberosities on the sides, and the coccyx in back.

plication. Surgical technique involving folding, tucking, or pleating to reduce the size of a hollow structure or organ.

reconstruction. Recreating, restoring, or rebuilding a body part or organ.

rectovaginal fistula. Abnormal communication between the rectum and the vagina that may follow obstetrical laceration repair, vaginal or rectal surgery, radiation therapy, trauma, or infection with fecal incontinence or leakage into the vaginal canal.

scar tissue. Fibrous connective tissue that forms around a wounded area or injury, composed mainly of fibroblasts or collagenous fibers.

CCI Version 18.3

00940, 0213T, 0216T, 0228T, 0230T, 12001-12007, 12011-12057, 13100-13153, 36000, 36400-36410, 36420-36430, 36440, 36600, 36640, 37202, 43752, 44950, 44970, 50715, 51701-51703, 57410, 57420, 57452, 62310-62319, 64400-64435, 64445-64450, 64479, 64483, 64490, 64493, 64505-64530, 69990, 93000-93010, 93040-93042, 93318, 94002, 94200, 94250, 94680-94690, 94770,

95812-95816, 95819, 95822, 95829, 95955, 96360, 96365, 96372, 96374-96376, 99148-99149, 99150

Note: These CCI edits are used for Medicare. Other payers may reimburse on codes listed above.

Medicare Edits

	Fac RVU	Non-Fac RVU	FUD	Status
57308	19.1	19.1	90	A

	MUE		Modifiers		
57308	1	51	N/A	62*	80

* with documentation

Medicare References: None

Coding Companion for Ob/Gyn

Vagina

57310-57311

57310 Closure of urethrovaginal fistula;
57311   with bulbocavernosus transplant

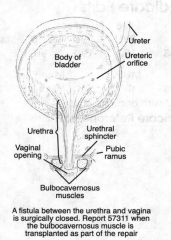

A fistula between the urethra and vagina is surgically closed. Report 57311 when the bulbocavernosus muscle is transplanted as part of the repair

Explanation

The physician closes a urethrovaginal fistula, which is an abnormal passage between the urethra and vagina. With a catheter in the urethra, the fistula tract is excised and the defect in the urethra is sutured closed. A pad of fatty tissue is sutured between the repaired urethral defect and the vaginal defect in 57310. In 57311, a pad of fatty tissue and a strip of the bulbocavernosus muscle are brought through a tunnel created between the vagina and one labium. The fat and muscle flap are sutured between the repaired urethral defect and the vaginal defect. In either case, the involved area in the vagina is excised and the defect is sutured closed. The catheter is left in place for several days to allow healing of the urethra.

Coding Tips

For closure of a rectovaginal fistula, vaginal or transanal approach, see 57300. For closure of a rectovaginal fistula, abdominal approach, see 57305. For closure of a rectovaginal fistula, abdominal approach, with concomitant colostomy, see 57307. To report vaginal closure of a vesicovaginal fistula, see 57320 and 57330; abdominal closure, see 51900.

ICD-9-CM Procedural

58.43   Closure of other fistula of urethra

Anesthesia

00940, 00942

ICD-9-CM Diagnostic

619.0   Urinary-genital tract fistula, female
677   Late effect of complication of pregnancy, childbirth, and the puerperium — (Code first any sequelae)

Terms To Know

absorbable sutures. Strands prepared from collagen or a synthetic polymer and capable of being absorbed by tissue over time.

closure. Repairing an incision or wound by suture or other means.

complication. Condition arising after the beginning of observation and treatment that modifies the course of the patient's illness or the medical care required, or an undesired result or misadventure in medical care.

defect. Imperfection, flaw, or absence.

excise. Remove or cut out.

late effect. Abnormality, dysfunction, or other residual condition produced after the acute phase of an illness, injury, or disease is over. There is no time limit on when late effects can appear.

transplant. Insertion of an organ or tissue from one person or site into another.

urethrovaginal fistula. Abnormal communication between the urethra and the vagina resulting in urinary leakage from the vagina.

CCI Version 18.3

00940, 0213T, 0216T, 0228T, 0230T, 12001-12007, 12011-12057, 13100-13153, 36000, 36400-36410, 36420-36430, 36440, 36600, 36640, 37202, 43752, 44950, 44970, 50715, 51701-51703, 56810, 57100, 57410, 57420, 57452, 57500, 57800, 58100, 62310-62319, 64400-64435, 64445-64450, 64479, 64483, 64490, 64493, 64505-64530, 69990, 93000-93010, 93040-93042, 93318, 94002, 94200, 94250, 94680-94690, 94770, 95812-95816, 95819, 95822, 95829, 95955, 96360, 96365, 96372, 96374-96376, 99148-99149, 99150

Also not with 57310: 53200, 53275, 53502, 53520, 57180-57200, 57220-57230, P9612

Also not with 57311: 57180, 57310

Note: These CCI edits are used for Medicare. Other payers may reimburse on codes listed above.

Medicare Edits

	Fac RVU	Non-Fac RVU	FUD	Status
57310	13.57	13.57	90	A
57311	15.44	15.44	90	A

	MUE		Modifiers		
57310	1	51	N/A	62*	80
57311	1	51	N/A	62*	80

* with documentation

Medicare References: None

Vagina

57320-57330

57320 Closure of vesicovaginal fistula; vaginal approach

57330 transvesical and vaginal approach

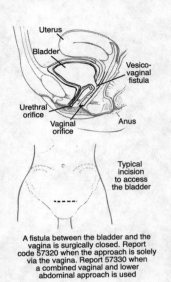

A fistula between the bladder and the vagina is surgically closed. Report code 57320 when the approach is solely via the vagina. Report 57330 when a combined vaginal and lower abdominal approach is used

Explanation

The physician closes a vesicovaginal fistula, which is an abnormal passage between the bladder and the vagina. In 57320, the procedure is done through the vagina with catheters via the urethra into both ureters. The fistula and surrounding scar tissue of the vaginal wall are usually excised. The bladder wall is opened and the bladder interior is explored. The fistula is excised along with the surrounding tissue to assure preservation of only healthy tissue. The resulting defect is closed with sutures in layers, starting with the bladder wall and ending with the vaginal mucosa. In 57330, the procedure is done through the vagina and through the lower abdomen, with catheters through the urethra into both ureters. The physician opens the bladder wall through the lower abdominal incision and excises the fistula. The resulting defect is closed with sutures in layers, starting with the bladder wall and ending with the abdominal wall. Through the vagina, the physician excises the fistula and surrounding scar tissue of the vaginal wall. In some cases, a pedicle graft of tissue may be sutured in between the bladder and the vagina. A urethral or suprapubic catheter is left in the bladder to prevent distension of the bladder and tension to the sutured areas.

Coding Tips

For closure of a vesicovaginal fistula, abdominal approach, see 51900. For closure of a urethrovaginal fistula, see 57310 and 57311. For closure of a rectovaginal fistula, vaginal or transanal approach, see 57300. For closure of a rectovaginal fistula, abdominal approach, see 57305. For closure of a rectovaginal fistula, abdominal approach with colostomy, see 57307.

ICD-9-CM Procedural

57.84 Repair of other fistula of bladder

Anesthesia

57320 00940

57330 00860

ICD-9-CM Diagnostic

619.0 Urinary-genital tract fistula, female

677 Late effect of complication of pregnancy, childbirth, and the puerperium — (Code first any sequelae)

Terms To Know

approach. Method or anatomical location used to gain access to a body organ or specific area for procedures. The approach is not coded separately although it may be a specified component of the procedure, such as laparoscopic vs. incisional, or spinal procedures in which the amount of dissection required to expose the spine significantly alters with the site of approach.

closure. Repairing an incision or wound by suture or other means.

complication. Condition arising after the beginning of observation and treatment that modifies the course of the patient's illness or the medical care required, or an undesired result or misadventure in medical care.

late effect. Abnormality, dysfunction, or other residual condition produced after the acute phase of an illness, injury, or disease is over. There is no time limit on when late effects can appear.

scar tissue. Fibrous connective tissue that forms around a wounded area or injury, composed mainly of fibroblasts or collagenous fibers.

vesicovaginal fistula. Abnormal communication between the bladder and the vagina that is the most common genital fistula, often with urinary leakage causing skin irritation of the vulva and thighs, or total incontinence.

CCI Version 18.3

00940, 0213T, 0216T, 0228T, 0230T, 12001-12007, 12011-12057, 13100-13153, 36000, 36400-36410, 36420-36430, 36440, 36600, 36640, 37202, 43752, 44950, 44970, 50715, 51701-51703, 56810, 57100, 57180, 57410, 57420, 57452, 57500, 57800, 58100, 62310-62319, 64400-64435, 64445-64450, 64479, 64483, 64490, 64493, 64505-64530, 69990, 93000-93010, 93040-93042, 93318, 94002, 94200, 94250, 94680-94690, 94770, 95812-95816, 95819, 95822, 95829, 95955, 96360, 96365, 96372, 96374-96376, 99148-99149, 99150

Also not with 57330: 57320

Note: These CCI edits are used for Medicare. Other payers may reimburse on codes listed above.

Medicare Edits

	Fac RVU	Non-Fac RVU	FUD	Status
57320	15.78	15.78	90	A
57330	21.74	21.74	90	A

	MUE		Modifiers		
57320	1	51	N/A	62*	80
57330	1	51	N/A	62*	80

* with documentation

Medicare References: None

Coding Companion for Ob/Gyn

© 2012 OptumInsight, Inc.

Vagina

57335

57335 Vaginoplasty for intersex state

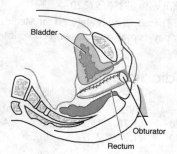

This is for congenital absence of a vagina. The physician creates a vagina using split-thickness or full-thickness grafts

Bladder

Obturator

Rectum

The vagina is created between the urethra and rectum. An obturator mold is placed in the newly created vagina

Explanation

The physician uses various plastic surgical techniques to correct a small, underdeveloped vagina due to the overproduction of male hormones. The physician constructs a larger and more functional vagina using carefully placed incisions and skin grafts.

Coding Tips

For construction of an artificial vagina without graft, see 57291; with graft, see 57292. For clitoroplasty, see 56805.

ICD-9-CM Procedural

70.79   Other repair of vagina

Anesthesia

57335   00940

ICD-9-CM Diagnostic

255.2   Adrenogenital disorders

259.50 Androgen insensitivity, unspecified

259.51 Androgen insensitivity syndrome

259.52 Partial androgen insensitivity

752.40 Unspecified congenital anomaly of cervix, vagina, and external female genitalia

752.49 Other congenital anomaly of cervix, vagina, and external female genitalia

Terms To Know

androgen. Male sex hormone. Testosterone is the primary androgen. In the fetus, androgens cause the formation of external male genitalia.

anomaly. Irregularity in the structure or position of an organ or tissue.

congenital. Present at birth, occurring through heredity or an influence during gestation up to the moment of birth.

full thickness skin graft. Graft consisting of skin and subcutaneous tissue.

hormone. Chemical substance produced by the body that has a regulatory effect on the function of its specific target organ(s).

split thickness skin graft. Graft using the epidermis and part of the dermis.

CCI Version 18.3

00940, 0213T, 0216T, 0228T, 0230T, 12001-12007, 12011-12057, 13100-13153, 36000, 36400-36410, 36420-36430, 36440, 36600, 36640, 37202, 43752, 44950, 44970, 50715, 51701-51703, 56810, 57100, 57180, 57410, 57420, 57452, 57500, 57800, 58100, 62310-62319, 64400-64435, 64445-64450, 64479, 64483, 64490, 64493, 64505-64530, 69990, 93000-93010, 93040-93042, 93318, 94002, 94200, 94250, 94680-94690, 94770, 95812-95816, 95819, 95822, 95829, 95955, 96360, 96365, 96372, 96374-96376, 99148-99149, 99150

Note: These CCI edits are used for Medicare. Other payers may reimburse on codes listed above.

Medicare Edits

	Fac RVU	Non-Fac RVU	FUD	Status
57335	33.57	33.57	90	A

	MUE		Modifiers		
57335	1	51	N/A	62*	80

* with documentation

Medicare References: None

Coding Companion for Ob/Gyn

57400

57400 Dilation of vagina under anesthesia (other than local)

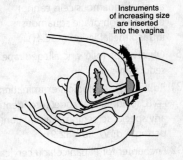

The physician dilates the vagina with obturator dilators. The patient is under general anesthesia

Instruments of increasing size are inserted into the vagina

Explanation

The physician enlarges the vagina by using a set of progressively longer and wider vaginal obturator dilators. The physician inserts the vaginal dilators sequentially from smaller to larger with firm and gentle pressure while the patient is under anesthesia (other than local).

Coding Tips

For pelvic exam under anesthesia, see 57410. For removal of an impacted foreign body of the vagina, under anesthesia, see 57415.

ICD-9-CM Procedural

96.16   Other vaginal dilation

Anesthesia

57400   00940

ICD-9-CM Diagnostic

616.81   Mucositis (ulcerative) of cervix, vagina, and vulva — (Use additional code to identify organism: 041.00-041.09, 041.10-041.19) (Use additional E code to identify adverse effects of therapy: E879.2, E930.7, E933.1)

616.89   Other inflammatory disease of cervix, vagina and vulva — (Use additional code to identify organism: 041.00-041.09, 041.10-041.19)

623.2   Stricture or atresia of vagina — (Use additional E code to identify any external cause)

752.49   Other congenital anomaly of cervix, vagina, and external female genitalia

Terms To Know

anomaly. Irregularity in the structure or position of an organ or tissue.

atresia. Congenital closure or absence of a tubular organ or an opening to the body surface.

colpalgia. Pain in the vagina.

congenital. Present at birth, occurring through heredity or an influence during gestation up to the moment of birth.

dilation. Artificial increase in the diameter of an opening or lumen made by medication or by instrumentation.

stricture. Narrowing of an anatomical structure.

CCI Version 18.3

00940, 0213T, 0216T, 0228T, 0230T, 12001-12007, 12011-12057, 13100-13153, 36000, 36400-36410, 36420-36430, 36440, 36600, 36640, 37202, 43752, 51701-51703, 57100, 57180, 57410-57421, 57452-57500, 57530, 57800, 58100, 62310-62319, 64400-64435, 64445-64450, 64479, 64483, 64490, 64493, 64505-64530, 69990, 93000-93010, 93040-93042, 93318, 94002, 94200, 94250, 94680-94690, 94770, 95812-95816, 95819, 95822, 95829, 95955, 96360, 96365, 96372, 96374-96376, 99148-99149, 99150

Note: These CCI edits are used for Medicare. Other payers may reimburse on codes listed above.

Medicare Edits

	Fac RVU	Non-Fac RVU	FUD	Status
57400	3.98	3.98	0	A

	MUE		Modifiers		
57400	1	51	N/A	N/A	80*

* with documentation

Medicare References: None

57410

57410 Pelvic examination under anesthesia (other than local)

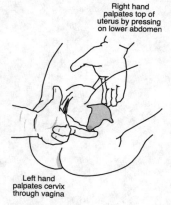

The pelvic exam is performed while the patient is under anesthesia

Right hand palpates top of uterus by pressing on lower abdomen

Left hand palpates cervix through vagina

Explanation

The physician performs a manual examination of the vagina, including the cervix, uterus, tubes, and ovaries. During the examination, the patient is under anesthesia (other than local) because of the patient's inability to tolerate the procedure while fully alert or awake.

Coding Tips

When 57410 is performed with another separately identifiable procedure, the highest dollar value code is listed as the primary procedure and subsequent procedures are appended with modifier 51. A pelvic exam under anesthesia done with other gynecological surgical procedures is generally an integral portion of the surgical procedure and is not identified separately. For removal of an impacted foreign body of the vagina, under anesthesia, see 57415.

ICD-9-CM Procedural

70.29 Other diagnostic procedures on vagina and cul-de-sac
89.26 Gynecological examination

Anesthesia

57410 00940

ICD-9-CM Diagnostic

180.0 Malignant neoplasm of endocervix
180.1 Malignant neoplasm of exocervix

182.0 Malignant neoplasm of corpus uteri, except isthmus
182.1 Malignant neoplasm of isthmus
233.1 Carcinoma in situ of cervix uteri
256.0 Hyperestrogenism
614.1 Chronic salpingitis and oophoritis — (Use additional code to identify organism: 041.00-041.09, 041.10-041.19)
614.6 Pelvic peritoneal adhesions, female (postoperative) (postinfection) — (Use additional code to identify organism: 041.00-041.09, 041.10-041.19) (Use additional code to identify any associated infertility: 628.2)
616.0 Cervicitis and endocervicitis — (Use additional code to identify organism: 041.00-041.09, 041.10-041.19)
617.0 Endometriosis of uterus
617.1 Endometriosis of ovary
617.3 Endometriosis of pelvic peritoneum
617.4 Endometriosis of rectovaginal septum and vagina
618.00 Unspecified prolapse of vaginal walls without mention of uterine prolapse — (Use additional code to identify urinary incontinence: 625.6, 788.31, 788.33-788.39)
618.1 Uterine prolapse without mention of vaginal wall prolapse — (Use additional code to identify urinary incontinence: 625.6, 788.31, 788.33-788.39)
620.0 Follicular cyst of ovary
620.1 Corpus luteum cyst or hematoma
620.4 Prolapse or hernia of ovary and fallopian tube
620.5 Torsion of ovary, ovarian pedicle, or fallopian tube
621.0 Polyp of corpus uteri
621.1 Chronic subinvolution of uterus
621.2 Hypertrophy of uterus
621.5 Intrauterine synechiae
621.6 Malposition of uterus
621.7 Chronic inversion of uterus
622.11 Mild dysplasia of cervix
622.12 Moderate dysplasia of cervix
622.4 Stricture and stenosis of cervix
622.7 Mucous polyp of cervix
623.7 Polyp of vagina
625.0 Dyspareunia
625.3 Dysmenorrhea
625.5 Pelvic congestion syndrome
625.6 Female stress incontinence
626.0 Absence of menstruation

626.4 Irregular menstrual cycle
626.6 Metrorrhagia
627.1 Postmenopausal bleeding
633.10 Tubal pregnancy without intrauterine pregnancy — (Use additional code from category 639 to identify any associated complications)
752.11 Embryonic cyst of fallopian tubes and broad ligaments
795.02 Papanicolaou smear of cervix with atypical squamous cells cannot exclude high grade squamous intraepithelial lesion (ASC-H)
V71.5 Observation following alleged rape or seduction
V72.31 Routine gynecological examination — (Use additional code(s) to identify any special screening examination(s) performed: V73.0-V82.9)
V72.32 Encounter for Papanicolaou cervical smear to confirm findings of recent normal smear following initial abnormal smear — (Use additional code(s) to identify any special screening examination(s) performed: V73.0-V82.9)

CCI Version 18.3

00940, 0213T, 0216T, 0228T, 0230T, 12001-12007, 12011-12057, 13100-13153, 36000, 36400-36410, 36420-36430, 36440, 36600, 36640, 37202, 43752, 51701-51703, 57100, 57180, 57500, 57800, 58100, 62310-62319, 64400-64435, 64445-64450, 64479, 64483, 64490, 64493, 64505-64530, 69990, 93000-93010, 93040-93042, 93318, 94002, 94200, 94250, 94680-94690, 94770, 95812-95816, 95819, 95822, 95829, 95955, 96360, 96365, 96372, 96374-96376, 99148-99149, 99150

Note: These CCI edits are used for Medicare. Other payers may reimburse on codes listed above.

Medicare Edits

	Fac RVU	Non-Fac RVU	FUD	Status
57410	3.19	3.19	0	A

	MUE		Modifiers		
57410	1	51	N/A	N/A	N/A

* with documentation

Medicare References: None

Coding Companion for Ob/Gyn

Vagina

57415

57415 Removal of impacted vaginal foreign body (separate procedure) under anesthesia (other than local)

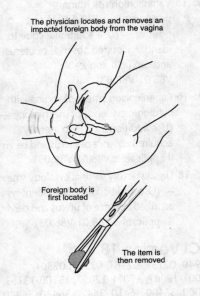

The physician locates and removes an impacted foreign body from the vagina

Foreign body is first located

The item is then removed

Explanation

Using a vaginal speculum, the physician removes a foreign body lodged in the vagina. During the procedure, the patient is under anesthesia (other than local) because of the patient's inability to tolerate the procedure while fully alert or awake, as in the case of a young child or due to the type or size of the object being removed.

Coding Tips

This separate procedure by definition is usually a component of a more complex service and is not identified separately. When performed alone or with other unrelated procedures or services it may be reported. If performed alone, list the code; if performed with other procedures or services, list the code and append modifier 59. For removal of an impacted vaginal foreign body without anesthesia, see the appropriate evaluation and management code.

ICD-9-CM Procedural

98.17 Removal of intraluminal foreign body from vagina without incision

Anesthesia

57415 00940

ICD-9-CM Diagnostic

939.2 Foreign body in vulva and vagina

Terms To Know

foreign body. Any object or substance found in an organ and tissue that does not belong under normal circumstances.

impaction. State of being tightly wedged or lodged into or between something.

removal. Process of moving out of or away from, or the fact of being removed.

separate procedures. Services commonly carried out as a fundamental part of a total service and, as such, do not usually warrant separate identification. These services are identified in CPT with the parenthetical phrase (separate procedure) at the end of the description and are payable only when performed alone.

speculum. Tool used to enlarge the opening of any canal or cavity.

CCI Version 18.3

00940, 0213T, 0216T, 0228T, 0230T, 12001-12007, 12011-12057, 13100-13153, 36000, 36400-36410, 36420-36430, 36440, 36600, 36640, 37202, 43752, 51701-51703, 57180, 57410, 57420, 57452, 57500, 57800, 58100, 62310-62319, 64400-64435, 64445-64450, 64479, 64483, 64490, 64493, 64505-64530, 69990, 93000-93010, 93040-93042, 93318, 94002, 94200, 94250, 94680-94690, 94770, 95812-95816, 95819, 95822, 95829, 95955, 96360, 96365, 96372, 96374-96376, 99148-99149, 99150

Note: These CCI edits are used for Medicare. Other payers may reimburse on codes listed above.

Medicare Edits

	Fac RVU	Non-Fac RVU	FUD	Status
57415	4.75	4.75	10	A

	MUE		Modifiers		
57415	1	51	N/A	N/A	80*

* with documentation

Medicare References: None

Coding Companion for Ob/Gyn

Vagina

57420-57421

57420 Colposcopy of the entire vagina, with cervix if present;

57421 with biopsy(s) of vagina/cervix

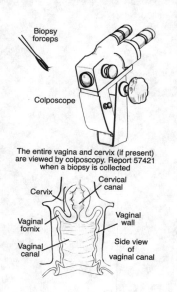

The entire vagina and cervix (if present) are viewed by colposcopy. Report 57421 when a biopsy is collected

Labels: Biopsy forceps, Colposcope, Cervical canal, Cervix, Vaginal fornix, Vaginal canal, Vaginal wall, Side view of vaginal canal

Explanation

The physician performs a colposcopy of the vagina and the cervix, if present. The patient is placed in the lithotomy position and a speculum is inserted into the vagina. The vagina is inspected through the colposcope, a binocular microscope providing direct, magnified visualization of the vagina and cervix. The physician examines the tissue for discharge, inflammation, ulceration, and lesions. The cervix is exposed, cleansed, and inspected for any ulceration or lesions. Acetic acid may be applied to help enhance visualization of the columnar villi and any lesions. In 57241, the area is examined and questionable tissue is removed from the vagina and/or cervix under direct visualization. The number and size of the biopsy(ies) is variable; multiple biopsies may be taken. Pressure is applied with a cotton swab as silver nitrate or other solution is applied with another applicator directly onto the biopsy site(s) for hemostasis. The instruments are removed.

Coding Tips

For colposcopy performed on the vulva, see 56820–56821. Surgical trays, A4550, are not separately reimbursed by Medicare; however, other third-party payers may cover them. Check with the specific payer to determine coverage.

ICD-9-CM Procedural

70.21 Vaginoscopy

70.23 Biopsy of cul-de-sac

70.24 Vaginal biopsy

Anesthesia

00940

ICD-9-CM Diagnostic

180.0 Malignant neoplasm of endocervix

180.1 Malignant neoplasm of exocervix

180.8 Malignant neoplasm of other specified sites of cervix

184.0 Malignant neoplasm of vagina

233.31 Carcinoma in situ, vagina

616.0 Cervicitis and endocervicitis — (Use additional code to identify organism: 041.00-041.09, 041.10-041.19)

617.4 Endometriosis of rectovaginal septum and vagina

623.0 Dysplasia of vagina

623.1 Leukoplakia of vagina

623.5 Leukorrhea, not specified as infective

623.6 Vaginal hematoma

623.7 Polyp of vagina

626.7 Postcoital bleeding

627.0 Premenopausal menorrhagia

627.1 Postmenopausal bleeding

795.04 Papanicolaou smear of cervix with high grade squamous intraepithelial lesion (HGSIL)

795.06 Papanicolaou smear of cervix with cytologic evidence of malignancy

795.10 Abnormal glandular Papanicolaou smear of vagina — (Use additional code to identify acquired absence of uterus and cervix, if applicable: V88.01-V88.03)

795.11 Papanicolaou smear of vagina with atypical squamous cells of undetermined significance (ASC-US) — (Use additional code to identify acquired absence of uterus and cervix, if applicable: V88.01-V88.03)

795.12 Papanicolaou smear of vagina with atypical squamous cells cannot exclude high grade squamous intraepithelial lesion (ASC-H) — (Use additional code to identify acquired absence of uterus and cervix, if applicable: V88.01-V88.03)

795.13 Papanicolaou smear of vagina with low grade squamous intraepithelial lesion (LGSIL) — (Use additional code to identify acquired absence of uterus and cervix, if applicable: V88.01-V88.03)

795.14 Papanicolaou smear of vagina with high grade squamous intraepithelial lesion (HGSIL) — (Use additional code to identify acquired absence of uterus and cervix, if applicable: V88.01-V88.03)

795.15 Vaginal high risk human papillomavirus (HPV) DNA test positive — (Use additional code to identify acquired absence of uterus and cervix, if applicable: V88.01-V88.03)

795.16 Papanicolaou smear of vagina with cytologic evidence of malignancy — (Use additional code to identify acquired absence of uterus and cervix, if applicable: V88.01-V88.03)

795.18 Unsatisfactory vaginal cytology smear — (Use additional code to identify acquired absence of uterus and cervix, if applicable: V88.01-V88.03)

CCI Version 18.3

00940, 0213T, 0216T, 0228T, 0230T, 12001-12007, 12011-12057, 13100-13153, 36000, 36400-36410, 36420-36430, 36440, 36600, 36640, 37202, 43752, 51701-51703, 57061, 57100, 57180, 57410, 57452, 62310-62319, 64400-64435, 64445-64450, 64479, 64483, 64490, 64493, 64505-64530, 69990, 76000-76001, 77001-77002, 93000-93010, 93040-93042, 93318, 94002, 94200, 94250, 94680-94690, 94770, 95812-95816, 95819, 95822, 95829, 95955, 96360, 96365, 96372, 96374-96376, 99148-99149, 99150

Also not with 57421: 57420, 57455-57456, 57500-57505, 57800, 58100, J0670, J2001

Note: These CCI edits are used for Medicare. Other payers may reimburse on codes listed above.

Medicare Edits

	Fac RVU	Non-Fac RVU	FUD	Status
57420	2.68	3.45	0	A
57421	3.66	4.64	0	A

	MUE		Modifiers		
57420	1	51	N/A	N/A	N/A
57421	1	51	N/A	N/A	N/A

* with documentation

Medicare References: None

Vagina

57423

57423 Paravaginal defect repair (including repair of cystocele, if performed), laparoscopic approach

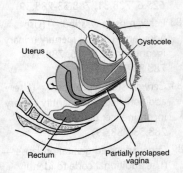

The physician repairs paravaginal defects

Explanation

The physician performs laparoscopic repair of a paravaginal defect, in which there is loss of the lateral vaginal attachment to the pelvic sidewall. Through small stab incisions in the abdomen, a fiberoptic laparoscope and trocars are inserted into the abdominal/pelvic space and the abdomen is insufflated. The bladder may be filled with sterile water to allow the surgeon to identify the superior border of the bladder's edge and then drained to prevent injury after the space of Retzius has been entered and the pubic ramus visualized. Following identification of the defect, the surgeon inserts the nondominant hand into the vagina in order to elevate the anterior vaginal wall and pubocervical fascia to their normal positions. Nonabsorbable sutures with attached needles are introduced through the laparoscopy port and grasped using a laparoscopic needle driver. A series of four to six sutures are placed and tied sequentially along the defects from the ischial spine toward the urethra. The procedure is repeated on the opposite side if a bilateral defect is present. The paravaginal defect repair may be performed alone or in conjunction with cystocele repair, in which a herniation of the bladder through its support tissues into the anterior vaginal wall causes it to bulge downward. These procedures help restore the normal anatomic relationships of the urethra, bladder, and vagina. At completion of the procedure, laparoscopic tools are removed,

excess gas expelled, and fascial defects and skin edges are sutured.

Coding Tips

If only one of the components of this procedure is performed, see other codes in this section of CPT. For example, if repair of cystocele with anterior colporrhaphy is performed by itself, report 57240. For a Marshall-Marchetti-Krantz urethral suspension, abdominal approach, see 51840 and 51841. For laparoscopic repair of stress incontinence, see 51990 and 51992. For sling operation for stress incontinence, see 57288.

ICD-9-CM Procedural

70.51 Repair of cystocele
70.54 Repair of cystocele with graft or prosthesis
70.77 Vaginal suspension and fixation
70.78 Vaginal suspension and fixation with graft or prosthesis

Anesthesia

57423 00840, 00860

ICD-9-CM Diagnostic

618.00 Unspecified prolapse of vaginal walls without mention of uterine prolapse — (Use additional code to identify urinary incontinence: 625.6, 788.31, 788.33-788.39)

618.01 Cystocele without mention of uterine prolapse, midline — (Use additional code to identify urinary incontinence: 625.6, 788.31, 788.33-788.39)

618.02 Cystocele without mention of uterine prolapse, lateral — (Use additional code to identify urinary incontinence: 625.6, 788.31, 788.33-788.39)

618.03 Urethrocele without mention of uterine prolapse — (Use additional code to identify urinary incontinence: 625.6, 788.31, 788.33-788.39)

618.04 Rectocele without mention of uterine prolapse — (Use additional code to identify urinary incontinence: 625.6, 788.31, 788.33-788.39) (Use additional code for any associated fecal incontinence: 787.60-787.63)

618.05 Perineocele without mention of uterine prolapse — (Use additional code to identify urinary incontinence: 625.6, 788.31, 788.33-788.39)

618.1 Uterine prolapse without mention of vaginal wall prolapse — (Use additional code to identify urinary incontinence: 625.6, 788.31, 788.33-788.39)

618.2 Uterovaginal prolapse, incomplete — (Use additional code to identify urinary incontinence: 625.6, 788.31, 788.33-788.39)

618.3 Uterovaginal prolapse, complete — (Use additional code to identify urinary incontinence: 625.6, 788.31, 788.33-788.39)

618.4 Uterovaginal prolapse, unspecified — (Use additional code to identify urinary incontinence: 625.6, 788.31, 788.33-788.39)

618.5 Prolapse of vaginal vault after hysterectomy — (Use additional code to identify urinary incontinence: 625.6, 788.31, 788.33-788.39)

618.82 Incompetence or weakening of rectovaginal tissue — (Use additional code to identify urinary incontinence: 625.6, 788.31, 788.33-788.39)

618.83 Pelvic muscle wasting — (Use additional code to identify urinary incontinence: 625.6, 788.31, 788.33-788.39)

618.84 Cervical stump prolapse — (Use additional code to identify urinary incontinence: 625.6, 788.31, 788.33-788.39)

625.6 Female stress incontinence

CCI Version 18.3

0213T, 0216T, 0228T, 0230T, 12001-12007, 12011-12057, 13100-13153, 36000, 36400-36410, 36420-36430, 36440, 36600, 36640, 37202, 43752, 44180, 44602-44605, 49320, 51701-51702, 51840-51841, 51990, 57240, 57260, 57410, 58660, 62310-62319, 64400-64435, 64445-64450, 64479, 64483, 64490, 64493, 64505-64530, 69990, 76000-76001, 77001-77002, 93000-93010, 93040-93042, 93318, 94002, 94200, 94250, 94680-94690, 94770, 95812-95816, 95819, 95822, 95829, 95955, 96360, 96365, 96372, 96374-96376, 99148-99149, 99150

Note: These CCI edits are used for Medicare. Other payers may reimburse on codes listed above.

Medicare Edits

	Fac RVU	Non-Fac RVU	FUD	Status
57423	27.46	27.46	90	A

	MUE			Modifiers	
57423	1	51	N/A	62	80

* with documentation

Medicare References: None

Coding Companion for Ob/Gyn

57425

57425 Laparoscopy, surgical, colpopexy (suspension of vaginal apex)

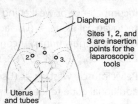

The top of the vagina is surgically suspended, often from tissues surrounding the sacrum. The procedure is performed laparoscopically

Sites 1, 2, and 3 are insertion points for the laparoscopic tools

Explanation

The physician performs a laparoscopic colpopexy and suspends or reattaches the apex of the vagina to the uterosacral ligaments to correct a uterovaginal prolapse and restore the vaginal apex to its normal anatomic position, often post-hysterectomy. Through small stab incisions in the abdomen, a fiberoptic laparoscope and trocars are inserted into the abdominal/pelvic space. The bowel is mobilized or moved aside to provide a better view and easier access to the uterosacral ligaments. A vaginal probe is placed for manipulation and to help ensure the cul-de-sac is properly closed. The peritoneum is incised over the vaginal apex. After the vaginal vault is elevated into its normal position, and the cul-de-sac is obliterated, if necessary, a suture is placed through the base of the right uterosacral ligament and through the apex of the vagina-securing it posteriorly to the top of the rectovaginal fascia and anteriorly to the pubocervical fascia (to a dermal or mesh graft, if placed) and secured. Four total sutures are used to elevate the vagina, this being done twice through each ligament and the vaginal apex on each side.

Coding Tips

A surgical laparoscopy always includes a diagnostic laparoscopy; the diagnostic laparoscopy should not be reported separately. For open colpopexy by abdominal approach, see 57280. For colposcopic diagnostic visualization of the vagina, see 57420.

ICD-9-CM Procedural

70.77   Vaginal suspension and fixation

Anesthesia

57425   00840, 00860

ICD-9-CM Diagnostic

618.00   Unspecified prolapse of vaginal walls without mention of uterine prolapse — (Use additional code to identify urinary incontinence: 625.6, 788.31, 788.33-788.39)

618.01   Cystocele without mention of uterine prolapse, midline — (Use additional code to identify urinary incontinence: 625.6, 788.31, 788.33-788.39)

618.02   Cystocele without mention of uterine prolapse, lateral — (Use additional code to identify urinary incontinence: 625.6, 788.31, 788.33-788.39)

618.03   Urethrocele without mention of uterine prolapse — (Use additional code to identify urinary incontinence: 625.6, 788.31, 788.33-788.39)

618.04   Rectocele without mention of uterine prolapse — (Use additional code to identify urinary incontinence: 625.6, 788.31, 788.33-788.39) (Use additional code for any associated fecal incontinence: 787.60-787.63)

618.05   Perineocele without mention of uterine prolapse — (Use additional code to identify urinary incontinence: 625.6, 788.31, 788.33-788.39)

618.09   Other prolapse of vaginal walls without mention of uterine prolapse — (Use additional code to identify urinary incontinence: 625.6, 788.31, 788.33-788.39)

618.1   Uterine prolapse without mention of vaginal wall prolapse — (Use additional code to identify urinary incontinence: 625.6, 788.31, 788.33-788.39)

618.2   Uterovaginal prolapse, incomplete — (Use additional code to identify urinary incontinence: 625.6, 788.31, 788.33-788.39)

618.3   Uterovaginal prolapse, complete — (Use additional code to identify urinary incontinence: 625.6, 788.31, 788.33-788.39)

618.4   Uterovaginal prolapse, unspecified — (Use additional code to identify urinary incontinence: 625.6, 788.31, 788.33-788.39)

618.5   Prolapse of vaginal vault after hysterectomy — (Use additional code

to identify urinary incontinence: 625.6, 788.31, 788.33-788.39)

618.81   Incompetence or weakening of pubocervical tissue — (Use additional code to identify urinary incontinence: 625.6, 788.31, 788.33-788.39)

618.82   Incompetence or weakening of rectovaginal tissue — (Use additional code to identify urinary incontinence: 625.6, 788.31, 788.33-788.39)

618.83   Pelvic muscle wasting — (Use additional code to identify urinary incontinence: 625.6, 788.31, 788.33-788.39)

618.84   Cervical stump prolapse — (Use additional code to identify urinary incontinence: 625.6, 788.31, 788.33-788.39)

618.89   Other specified genital prolapse — (Use additional code to identify urinary incontinence: 625.6, 788.31, 788.33-788.39)

625.6   Female stress incontinence

Terms To Know

fascia. Fibrous sheet or band of tissue that envelops organs, muscles, and groupings of muscles.

female stress incontinence. Involuntary escape of urine at times of minor stress against the female bladder, such as coughing, sneezing, or laughing.

CCI Version 18.3

0213T, 0216T, 0228T, 0230T, 12001-12007, 12011-12057, 13100-13153, 36000, 36400-36410, 36420-36430, 36440, 36600, 36640, 37202, 43752, 44180, 44602-44605, 44950, 44970, 49320, 50715, 51701-51703, 57282, 57410, 58660, 62310-62319, 64400-64435, 64445-64450, 64479, 64483, 64490, 64493, 64505-64530, 69990, 76000-76001, 77001-77002, 93000-93010, 93040-93042, 93318, 94002, 94200, 94250, 94680-94690, 94770, 95812-95816, 95819, 95822, 95829, 95955, 96360, 96365, 96372, 96374-96376, 99148-99149, 99150

Note: These CCI edits are used for Medicare. Other payers may reimburse on codes listed above.

Medicare Edits

	Fac RVU	Non-Fac RVU	FUD	Status
57425	28.91	28.91	90	A

	MUE			Modifiers	
57425	1		51	N/A	62*	80

* with documentation

Medicare References: None

Vagina

57426

57426 Revision (including removal) of prosthetic vaginal graft, laparoscopic approach

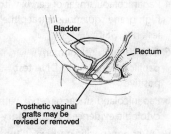

Bladder

Rectum

Prosthetic vaginal grafts may be revised or removed

Explanation

The physician revises or removes a previously placed prosthetic vaginal graft via a laparoscopic approach. Through small stab incisions in the umbilicus and/or abdomen, a fiberoptic laparoscope and trocars are inserted into the peritoneal cavity. Depending upon the type of complication (e.g., mesh erosion into the bladder or persistent vaginal/pelvic pain), the vaginal graft may be completely or partially excised to remove eroding mesh or revisions may be made in the graft and surrounding tissue.

Coding Tips

For revision, including removal, of a prosthetic vaginal graft, vaginal approach, see 57295; abdominal approach, see 57296.

ICD-9-CM Procedural

70.62 Vaginal reconstruction
70.79 Other repair of vagina
70.91 Other operations on vagina

Anesthesia

57426 00840, 00940

ICD-9-CM Diagnostic

054.11 Herpetic vulvovaginitis
098.0 Gonococcal infection (acute) of lower genitourinary tract
098.2 Gonococcal infections, chronic, of lower genitourinary tract

099.53 Chlamydia trachomatis infection of lower genitourinary sites — (Use additional code to specify site of infection: 595.4, 616.0, 616.11)

112.1 Candidiasis of vulva and vagina — (Use additional code to identify manifestation: 321.0-321.1, 380.15, 711.6)

616.10 Unspecified vaginitis and vulvovaginitis — (Use additional code to identify organism, such as: 041.00-041.09, 041.10-041.19, 041.41-041.49)

616.11 Vaginitis and vulvovaginitis in diseases classified elsewhere — (Use additional code to identify organism: 041.00-041.09, 041.10-041.19) (Code first underlying disease: 127.4)

629.31 Erosion of implanted vaginal mesh and other prosthetic materials to surrounding organ or tissue

629.32 Exposure of implanted vaginal mesh and other prosthetic materials into vagina

752.49 Other congenital anomaly of cervix, vagina, and external female genitalia

996.30 Mechanical complication of unspecified genitourinary device, implant, and graft

996.39 Mechanical complication of genitourinary device, implant, and graft, other

996.52 Mechanical complication due to other tissue graft, not elsewhere classified

996.59 Mechanical complication due to other implant and internal device, not elsewhere classified

996.60 Infection and inflammatory reaction due to unspecified device, implant, and graft — (Use additional code to identify specified infections)

996.65 Infection and inflammatory reaction due to other genitourinary device, implant, and graft — (Use additional code to identify specified infections)

996.70 Other complications due to unspecified device, implant, and graft — (Use additional code to identify complication: 338.18-338.19, 338.28-338.29)

996.76 Other complications due to genitourinary device, implant, and graft — (Use additional code to identify complication: 338.18-338.19, 338.28-338.29)

V51.8 Other aftercare involving the use of plastic surgery

Terms To Know

approach. Method or anatomical location used to gain access to a body organ or specific area for procedures. The approach is not coded separately although it may be a specified component of the procedure, such as laparoscopic vs. incisional, or spinal procedures in which the amount of dissection required to expose the spine significantly alters with the site of approach.

graft. Tissue implant from another part of the body or another person.

revision. Reordering or rearrangement of tissue to suit a particular need or function.

CCI Version 18.3

0213T, 0216T, 0228T, 0230T, 12001-12007, 12011-12057, 13100-13153, 36000, 36400-36410, 36420-36430, 36440, 36600, 36640, 37202, 43752, 44005, 44180, 44602-44605, 49320, 50715, 51701-51703, 57100, 57180, 57295, 57400-57415, 57500, 57800, 58100, 58660, 62310-62319, 64400-64435, 64445-64450, 64479, 64483, 64490, 64493, 64505-64530, 69990, 93000-93010, 93040-93042, 93318, 94002, 94200, 94250, 94680-94690, 94770, 95812-95816, 95819, 95822, 95829, 95955, 96360, 96365, 96372, 96374-96376, 99148-99149, 99150

Note: These CCI edits are used for Medicare. Other payers may reimburse on codes listed above.

Medicare Edits

	Fac RVU	Non-Fac RVU	FUD	Status
57426	25.44	25.44	90	A

	MUE		Modifiers		
57426	1	51	N/A	62*	80

* with documentation

Medicare References: None

Vagina

57452-57454

57452 Colposcopy of the cervix including upper/adjacent vagina;

57454 with biopsy(s) of the cervix and endocervical curettage

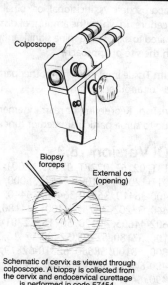

Colposcope

Biopsy forceps

External os (opening)

Schematic of cervix as viewed through colposcope. A biopsy is collected from the cervix and endocervical curettage is performed in code 57454.

Explanation

The physician examines the cervix, including the upper/adjacent portion of the vagina through a colposcope, a binocular microscope used for direct visualization of the vagina, ectocervix, and endocervix. The physician may insert a speculum into the vagina to fully expose the cervix as part of this procedure. In 57454, both a biopsy and an endocervical curettage are performed. For biopsy, an instrument is inserted in the vagina and used to take one or more small tissue samples of the cervix. For endocervical curettage, a small curette is passed into the endocervical canal, which is the passage between the external cervical os and the uterine cavity. A specimen is obtained by scraping in the canal with the curette. The instrument is removed.

Coding Tips

Note that 57452, a separate procedure by definition, is usually a component of a more complex service and is not identified separately. When performed alone or with other unrelated procedures/services it may be reported. If performed alone, list the code; if performed with other procedures/services, list the code and append modifier 59. Local anesthesia is included in 57454. However, this procedure may be performed under general anesthesia, depending on the age and/or condition of the patient. If a specimen is transported to an outside laboratory, report 99000 for handling or conveyance. For

colposcopy with loop electrode biopsy(s) of the cervix, report 57460. For colposcopy with loop electrode conization of the cervix, report 57461.

ICD-9-CM Procedural

67.11	Endocervical biopsy
67.12	Other cervical biopsy
67.19	Other diagnostic procedures on cervix
67.32	Destruction of lesion of cervix by cauterization
70.21	Vaginoscopy

Anesthesia
00940

ICD-9-CM Diagnostic

079.4	Human papilloma virus in conditions classified elsewhere and of unspecified site — (Note: This code is to be used as an additional code to identify the viral agent in diseases classifiable elsewhere and viral infection of unspecified nature or site)
180.0	Malignant neoplasm of endocervix
180.1	Malignant neoplasm of exocervix
182.0	Malignant neoplasm of corpus uteri, except isthmus
182.1	Malignant neoplasm of isthmus
184.0	Malignant neoplasm of vagina
198.82	Secondary malignant neoplasm of genital organs
219.0	Benign neoplasm of cervix uteri
233.1	Carcinoma in situ of cervix uteri
616.0	Cervicitis and endocervicitis — (Use additional code to identify organism: 041.00-041.09, 041.10-041.19)
616.11	Vaginitis and vulvovaginitis in diseases classified elsewhere — (Use additional code to identify organism: 041.00-041.09, 041.10-041.19) (Code first underlying disease: 127.4)
617.4	Endometriosis of rectovaginal septum and vagina
622.0	Erosion and ectropion of cervix
622.10	Dysplasia of cervix, unspecified
622.11	Mild dysplasia of cervix
622.12	Moderate dysplasia of cervix
622.2	Leukoplakia of cervix (uteri)
622.3	Old laceration of cervix
622.4	Stricture and stenosis of cervix
622.5	Incompetence of cervix
622.7	Mucous polyp of cervix
626.7	Postcoital bleeding
795.00	Abnormal glandular Papanicolaou smear of cervix

795.01	Papanicolaou smear of cervix with atypical squamous cells of undetermined significance (ASC-US)
795.02	Papanicolaou smear of cervix with atypical squamous cells cannot exclude high grade squamous intraepithelial lesion (ASC-H)
795.03	Papanicolaou smear of cervix with low grade squamous intraepithelial lesion (LGSIL)
795.04	Papanicolaou smear of cervix with high grade squamous intraepithelial lesion (HGSIL)
795.05	Cervical high risk human papillomavirus (HPV) DNA test positive
795.06	Papanicolaou smear of cervix with cytologic evidence of malignancy
795.39	Other nonspecific positive culture findings
V10.41	Personal history of malignant neoplasm of cervix uteri
V67.09	Follow-up examination, following other surgery
V71.5	Observation following alleged rape or seduction
V71.6	Observation following other inflicted injury

CCI Version 18.3

00940, 0213T, 0216T, 0228T, 0230T, 12001-12007, 12011-12057, 13100-13153, 36000, 36400-36410, 36420-36430, 36440, 36600, 36640, 37202, 43752, 51701-51703, 57100, 57180, 57410, 62310-62319, 64400-64435, 64445-64450, 64479, 64483, 64490, 64493, 64505-64530, 69990, 76000-76001, 77001-77002, 93000-93010, 93040-93042, 93318, 94002, 94200, 94250, 94680-94690, 94770, 95812-95816, 95819, 95822, 95829, 95955, 96360, 96365, 96372, 96374-96376, 99148-99149, 99150

Also not with 57454: 57420-57421, 57452, 57455-57456, 57500-57505, 57800, 58100

Note: These CCI edits are used for Medicare. Other payers may reimburse on codes listed above.

Medicare Edits

	Fac RVU	Non-Fac RVU	FUD	Status
57452	2.73	3.23	0	A
57454	4.06	4.57	0	A

	MUE		Modifiers		
57452	1		51	N/A	N/A	N/A
57454	1		51	N/A	N/A	N/A

* with documentation

Medicare References: None

Coding Companion for Ob/Gyn

Cervix Uteri

57455-57456

57455 Colposcopy of the cervix including upper/adjacent vagina; with biopsy(s) of the cervix

57456 with endocervical curettage

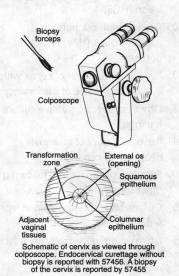

Biopsy forceps
Colposcope

Transformation zone
External os (opening)
Squamous epithelium
Adjacent vaginal tissues
Columnar epithelium

Schematic of cervix as viewed through colposcope. Endocervical curettage without biopsy is reported with 57456. A biopsy of the cervix is reported by 57455

Explanation

The physician views the cervix, including the upper/adjacent portion of the vagina through a colposcope, a binocular microscope used for direct visualization of the vagina, ectocervix, and endocervix. The physician may insert a speculum into the vagina to fully expose the cervix as part of this procedure. The physician removes tissue for a biopsy of the cervix in 57455 and performs endocervical curettage in 57456. For biopsy, an instrument is inserted in the vagina and used to take one or more small tissue samples of the cervix. For endocervical curettage, a small curette is passed into the endocervical canal, which is the passage between the external cervical os and the uterine cavity. A specimen is obtained by scraping in the canal with the curette. The instrument is removed.

Coding Tips

For colposcopy performed on the vulva, see 56820–56821. For colposcopy performed on the vagina, see 57420–57421. For colposcopy of the cervix with a biopsy of the cervix and endocervical curettage, see 57454.

ICD-9-CM Procedural

67.11 Endocervical biopsy
67.12 Other cervical biopsy
67.19 Other diagnostic procedures on cervix
67.32 Destruction of lesion of cervix by cauterization
70.21 Vaginoscopy

Anesthesia

00940

ICD-9-CM Diagnostic

079.4 Human papilloma virus in conditions classified elsewhere and of unspecified site — (Note: This code is to be used as an additional code to identify the viral agent in diseases classifiable elsewhere and viral infection of unspecified nature or site)
180.0 Malignant neoplasm of endocervix
180.1 Malignant neoplasm of exocervix
182.0 Malignant neoplasm of corpus uteri, except isthmus
182.1 Malignant neoplasm of isthmus
184.0 Malignant neoplasm of vagina
198.82 Secondary malignant neoplasm of genital organs
219.0 Benign neoplasm of cervix uteri
233.1 Carcinoma in situ of cervix uteri
233.30 Carcinoma in situ, unspecified female genital organ
233.31 Carcinoma in situ, vagina
616.0 Cervicitis and endocervicitis — (Use additional code to identify organism: 041.00-041.09, 041.10-041.19)
616.11 Vaginitis and vulvovaginitis in diseases classified elsewhere — (Use additional code to identify organism: 041.00-041.09, 041.10-041.19) (Code first underlying disease: 127.4)
617.4 Endometriosis of rectovaginal septum and vagina
622.0 Erosion and ectropion of cervix
622.10 Dysplasia of cervix, unspecified
622.11 Mild dysplasia of cervix
622.12 Moderate dysplasia of cervix
622.2 Leukoplakia of cervix (uteri)
622.3 Old laceration of cervix
622.4 Stricture and stenosis of cervix
622.5 Incompetence of cervix
622.6 Hypertrophic elongation of cervix
622.7 Mucous polyp of cervix
626.7 Postcoital bleeding
752.49 Other congenital anomaly of cervix, vagina, and external female genitalia
795.00 Abnormal glandular Papanicolaou smear of cervix
795.01 Papanicolaou smear of cervix with atypical squamous cells of undetermined significance (ASC-US)
795.02 Papanicolaou smear of cervix with atypical squamous cells cannot exclude high grade squamous intraepithelial lesion (ASC-H)
795.03 Papanicolaou smear of cervix with low grade squamous intraepithelial lesion (LGSIL)
795.04 Papanicolaou smear of cervix with high grade squamous intraepithelial lesion (HGSIL)
795.05 Cervical high risk human papillomavirus (HPV) DNA test positive
795.06 Papanicolaou smear of cervix with cytologic evidence of malignancy
795.09 Other abnormal Papanicolaou smear of cervix and cervical HPV — (Use additional code for associated human papillomavirus: 079.4)
795.39 Other nonspecific positive culture findings
V10.41 Personal history of malignant neoplasm of cervix uteri

CCI Version 18.3

00940, 0213T, 0216T, 0228T, 0230T, 12001-12007, 12011-12057, 13100-13153, 36000, 36400-36410, 36420-36430, 36440, 36600, 36640, 37202, 43752, 51701-51703, 57100, 57180, 57410, 57420, 57452, 57500-57505, 57800, 58100, 62310-62319, 64400-64435, 64445-64450, 64479, 64483, 64490, 64493, 64505-64530, 69990, 76000-76001, 77001-77002, 93000-93010, 93040-93042, 93318, 94002, 94200, 94250, 94680-94690, 94770, 95812-95816, 95819, 95822, 95829, 95955, 96360, 96365, 96372, 96374-96376, 99148-99149, 99150

Note: These CCI edits are used for Medicare. Other payers may reimburse on codes listed above.

Medicare Edits

	Fac RVU	Non-Fac RVU	FUD	Status
57455	3.31	4.26	0	A
57456	3.09	4.03	0	A

	MUE		Modifiers		
57455	1	51	N/A	N/A	N/A
57456	1	51	N/A	N/A	N/A

* with documentation

Medicare References: None

Cervix Uteri

57460

57460 Colposcopy of the cervix including upper/adjacent vagina; with loop electrode biopsy(s) of the cervix

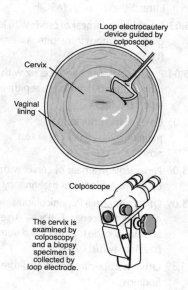

Loop electrocautery device guided by colposcope

Cervix

Vaginal lining

Colposcope

The cervix is examined by colposcopy and a biopsy specimen is collected by loop electrode.

Explanation

The physician views the cervix, including the upper/adjacent portion of the vagina through a colposcope, a binocular microscope used for direct visualization of the vagina, ectocervix, and endocervix. The physician inserts a speculum into the vagina to fully expose the cervix. A biopsy specimen of cervical tissue is removed by the loop electrode excision procedure (LEEP). LEEP uses a hot cautery wire containing an electrical cutting current as a cutting instrument. Due to the electrical current, a grounding pad is attached to the patient's leg during the procedure.

Coding Tips

When 57460 is performed with another separately identifiable procedure, the highest dollar value code is listed as the primary procedure and subsequent procedures are appended with modifier 51. For cauterization of the cervix, see 57510–57513. If conization of the cervix is performed, see 57520–57522. For loop electrode conization of the cervix by colposcopy, report 57461. Local anesthesia is included in the service. However, this procedure may be performed under general anesthesia, depending on the age and/or condition of the patient.

ICD-9-CM Procedural

67.11 Endocervical biopsy
67.12 Other cervical biopsy
67.19 Other diagnostic procedures on cervix
70.21 Vaginoscopy

Anesthesia

57460 00940

ICD-9-CM Diagnostic

180.0 Malignant neoplasm of endocervix
180.1 Malignant neoplasm of exocervix
180.8 Malignant neoplasm of other specified sites of cervix
182.0 Malignant neoplasm of corpus uteri, except isthmus
182.1 Malignant neoplasm of isthmus
182.8 Malignant neoplasm of other specified sites of body of uterus
184.0 Malignant neoplasm of vagina
198.82 Secondary malignant neoplasm of genital organs
219.0 Benign neoplasm of cervix uteri
221.2 Benign neoplasm of vulva
233.1 Carcinoma in situ of cervix uteri
233.30 Carcinoma in situ, unspecified female genital organ
233.31 Carcinoma in situ, vagina
233.32 Carcinoma in situ, vulva
233.39 Carcinoma in situ, other female genital organ
236.0 Neoplasm of uncertain behavior of uterus
239.5 Neoplasm of unspecified nature of other genitourinary organs
616.0 Cervicitis and endocervicitis — (Use additional code to identify organism: 041.00-041.09, 041.10-041.19)
616.81 Mucositis (ulcerative) of cervix, vagina, and vulva — (Use additional code to identify organism: 041.00-041.09, 041.10-041.19) (Use additional E code to identify adverse effects of therapy: E879.2, E930.7, E933.1)
616.89 Other inflammatory disease of cervix, vagina and vulva — (Use additional code to identify organism: 041.00-041.09, 041.10-041.19)
617.4 Endometriosis of rectovaginal septum and vagina
622.0 Erosion and ectropion of cervix
622.10 Dysplasia of cervix, unspecified
622.12 Moderate dysplasia of cervix
622.2 Leukoplakia of cervix (uteri)
622.7 Mucous polyp of cervix
795.02 Papanicolaou smear of cervix with atypical squamous cells cannot exclude high grade squamous intraepithelial lesion (ASC-H)
795.03 Papanicolaou smear of cervix with low grade squamous intraepithelial lesion (LGSIL)
795.04 Papanicolaou smear of cervix with high grade squamous intraepithelial lesion (HGSIL)
795.05 Cervical high risk human papillomavirus (HPV) DNA test positive
795.06 Papanicolaou smear of cervix with cytologic evidence of malignancy
795.39 Other nonspecific positive culture findings
V10.41 Personal history of malignant neoplasm of cervix uteri
V67.09 Follow-up examination, following other surgery
V71.5 Observation following alleged rape or seduction
V71.6 Observation following other inflicted injury

CCI Version 18.3

00940, 0213T, 0216T, 0228T, 0230T, 12001-12007, 12011-12057, 13100-13153, 36000, 36400-36410, 36420-36430, 36440, 36600, 36640, 37202, 43752, 51701-51703, 57100, 57180, 57410, 57420-57421, 57452-57455, 57500, 57800, 58100, 62310-62319, 64400-64435, 64445-64450, 64479, 64483, 64490, 64493, 64505-64530, 69990, 76000-76001, 77001-77002, 93000-93010, 93040-93042, 93318, 94002, 94200, 94250, 94680-94690, 94770, 95812-95816, 95819, 95822, 95829, 95955, 96360, 96365, 96372, 96374-96376, 99148-99149, 99150, J0670, J2001

Note: These CCI edits are used for Medicare. Other payers may reimburse on codes listed above.

Medicare Edits

	Fac RVU	Non-Fac RVU	FUD	Status
57460	4.88	8.58	0	A

	MUE		Modifiers		
57460	1	51	N/A	N/A	N/A

* with documentation

Medicare References: None

Cervix Uteri

57461

57461 Colposcopy of the cervix including upper/adjacent vagina; with loop electrode conization of the cervix

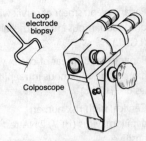

Report 57461 when a loop electrode is used for conization of the cervix

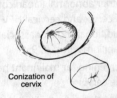

Conization of cervix

Explanation

The physician views the cervix, including the upper/adjacent portion of the vagina, through a colposcope, a binocular microscope used for direct visualization of the vagina, ectocervix, and endocervix, and performs a loop electrode excision procedure (LEEP). The physician inserts a speculum into the vagina to fully expose the cervix. The electric grounding pad is placed on the patient's leg and safety checks are run. The cutting current is set. Using a loop, the lesion is removed as one specimen. If the lesion is large and another pass is required, two equal specimens are removed and labeled for the axis of orientation. The same procedure is done again with a smaller loop if an endocervical excision is necessary. The bleeding vessels are cauterized, the vagina is inspected for any accidental injury, and the instruments are removed.

Coding Tips

For colposcopy performed on the vulva, see 56820–56821. For colposcopy performed on the vagina, see 57420–57421. For colposcopy of the cervix with a biopsy of the cervix and endocervical curettage, see 57454. For a loop electrode biopsy of the cervix by colposcopy, see 57460.

ICD-9-CM Procedural

67.32   Destruction of lesion of cervix by cauterization

70.21   Vaginoscopy

Anesthesia
57461   00940

ICD-9-CM Diagnostic

180.0   Malignant neoplasm of endocervix

180.1   Malignant neoplasm of exocervix

182.0   Malignant neoplasm of corpus uteri, except isthmus

182.1   Malignant neoplasm of isthmus

184.0   Malignant neoplasm of vagina

198.82   Secondary malignant neoplasm of genital organs

219.0   Benign neoplasm of cervix uteri

233.1   Carcinoma in situ of cervix uteri

233.30   Carcinoma in situ, unspecified female genital organ

233.31   Carcinoma in situ, vagina

233.39   Carcinoma in situ, other female genital organ

616.0   Cervicitis and endocervicitis — (Use additional code to identify organism: 041.00-041.09, 041.10-041.19)

616.11   Vaginitis and vulvovaginitis in diseases classified elsewhere — (Use additional code to identify organism: 041.00-041.09, 041.10-041.19) (Code first underlying disease: 127.4)

617.4   Endometriosis of rectovaginal septum and vagina

622.0   Erosion and ectropion of cervix

622.10   Dysplasia of cervix, unspecified

622.12   Moderate dysplasia of cervix

622.2   Leukoplakia of cervix (uteri)

622.3   Old laceration of cervix

622.4   Stricture and stenosis of cervix

622.5   Incompetence of cervix

622.6   Hypertrophic elongation of cervix

622.7   Mucous polyp of cervix

752.49   Other congenital anomaly of cervix, vagina, and external female genitalia

795.00   Abnormal glandular Papanicolaou smear of cervix

795.02   Papanicolaou smear of cervix with atypical squamous cells cannot exclude high grade squamous intraepithelial lesion (ASC-H)

795.03   Papanicolaou smear of cervix with low grade squamous intraepithelial lesion (LGSIL)

795.04   Papanicolaou smear of cervix with high grade squamous intraepithelial lesion (HGSIL)

795.05   Cervical high risk human papillomavirus (HPV) DNA test positive

795.06   Papanicolaou smear of cervix with cytologic evidence of malignancy

795.39   Other nonspecific positive culture findings

V10.41   Personal history of malignant neoplasm of cervix uteri

V67.09   Follow-up examination, following other surgery

V71.5   Observation following alleged rape or seduction

V71.6   Observation following other inflicted injury

CCI Version 18.3

00940, 0213T, 0216T, 0228T, 0230T, 12001-12007, 12011-12057, 13100-13153, 36000, 36400-36410, 36420-36430, 36440, 36600, 36640, 37202, 43752, 51701-51703, 57100, 57180, 57410, 57420-57421, 57452-57460, 57500, 57800, 58100, 62310-62319, 64400-64435, 64445-64450, 64479, 64483, 64490, 64493, 64505-64530, 69990, 76000-76001, 77001-77002, 93000-93010, 93040-93042, 93318, 94002, 94200, 94250, 94680-94690, 94770, 95812-95816, 95819, 95822, 95829, 95955, 96360, 96365, 96372, 96374-96376, 99148-99149, 99150, J0670, J2001

Note: These CCI edits are used for Medicare. Other payers may reimburse on codes listed above.

Medicare Edits

	Fac RVU	Non-Fac RVU	FUD	Status
57461	5.63	9.67	0	A

	MUE		Modifiers		
57461	1	51	N/A	N/A	N/A

* with documentation

Medicare References: None

Coding Companion for Ob/Gyn

© 2012 OptumInsight, Inc.

57500

57500 Biopsy of cervix, single or multiple, or local excision of lesion, with or without fulguration (separate procedure)

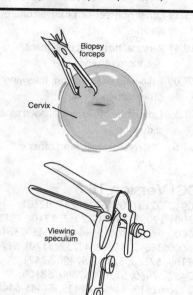

Biopsy forceps

Cervix

Viewing speculum

Explanation

The physician inserts a speculum into the vagina to view the cervix. A small cut is made in the cervix and biopsy forceps are used to remove a piece or multiple pieces of tissue, or to completely remove a lesion. Bleeding, usually minimal, may be stopped by electric current (fulguration).

Coding Tips

This separate procedure by definition is usually a component of a more complex service and is not identified separately. When performed alone or with other unrelated procedures/services it may be reported. If performed alone, list the code; if performed with other procedures/services, list the code and append modifier 59. When 57500 is performed with another separately identifiable procedure, the highest dollar value code is listed as the primary procedure and subsequent procedures are appended with modifier 51. Local anesthesia is included in the service. However, this procedure may be performed under general anesthesia, depending on the age and/or condition of the patient.

ICD-9-CM Procedural

67.11	Endocervical biopsy
67.12	Other cervical biopsy
67.31	Marsupialization of cervical cyst
67.39	Other excision or destruction of lesion or tissue of cervix

Anesthesia

57500 00940

ICD-9-CM Diagnostic

180.0	Malignant neoplasm of endocervix
180.1	Malignant neoplasm of exocervix
180.8	Malignant neoplasm of other specified sites of cervix
180.9	Malignant neoplasm of cervix uteri, unspecified site
182.0	Malignant neoplasm of corpus uteri, except isthmus
198.82	Secondary malignant neoplasm of genital organs
219.0	Benign neoplasm of cervix uteri
221.8	Benign neoplasm of other specified sites of female genital organs
221.9	Benign neoplasm of female genital organ, site unspecified
228.00	Hemangioma of unspecified site
229.8	Benign neoplasm of other specified sites
233.1	Carcinoma in situ of cervix uteri
616.0	Cervicitis and endocervicitis — (Use additional code to identify organism: 041.00-041.09, 041.10-041.19)
616.81	Mucositis (ulcerative) of cervix, vagina, and vulva — (Use additional code to identify organism: 041.00-041.09, 041.10-041.19) (Use additional E code to identify adverse effects of therapy: E879.2, E930.7, E933.1)
622.0	Erosion and ectropion of cervix
622.10	Dysplasia of cervix, unspecified
622.11	Mild dysplasia of cervix
622.12	Moderate dysplasia of cervix
622.2	Leukoplakia of cervix (uteri)
622.7	Mucous polyp of cervix
622.8	Other specified noninflammatory disorder of cervix
623.5	Leukorrhea, not specified as infective
623.8	Other specified noninflammatory disorder of vagina
625.3	Dysmenorrhea
625.8	Other specified symptom associated with female genital organs
626.2	Excessive or frequent menstruation
626.4	Irregular menstrual cycle
626.6	Metrorrhagia
626.8	Other disorder of menstruation and other abnormal bleeding from female genital tract
795.00	Abnormal glandular Papanicolaou smear of cervix
795.01	Papanicolaou smear of cervix with atypical squamous cells of undetermined significance (ASC-US)
795.02	Papanicolaou smear of cervix with atypical squamous cells cannot exclude high grade squamous intraepithelial lesion (ASC-H)
795.03	Papanicolaou smear of cervix with low grade squamous intraepithelial lesion (LGSIL)
795.04	Papanicolaou smear of cervix with high grade squamous intraepithelial lesion (HGSIL)
795.05	Cervical high risk human papillomavirus (HPV) DNA test positive
795.08	Unsatisfactory cervical cytology smear
795.09	Other abnormal Papanicolaou smear of cervix and cervical HPV — (Use additional code for associated human papillomavirus: 079.4)
V76.2	Screening for malignant neoplasm of the cervix
V84.09	Genetic susceptibility to other malignant neoplasm — (Use additional code, if applicable, for any associated family history of the disease: V16-V19. Code first, if applicable, any current malignant neoplasms: 140.0-195.8, 200.0-208.9, 230.0-234.9. Use additional code, if applicable, for any personal history of malignant neoplasm: V10.0-V10.9)

CCI Version 18.3

0213T, 0216T, 0228T, 0230T, 10021-10022, 12001-12007, 12011-12057, 13100-13153, 36000, 36400-36410, 36420-36430, 36440, 36600, 36640, 37202, 43752, 51701-51703, 57100, 57180, 57420, 57452, 62310-62319, 64400-64435, 64445-64450, 64479, 64483, 64490, 64493, 64505-64530, 69990, 93000-93010, 93040-93042, 93318, 94002, 94200, 94250, 94680-94690, 94770, 95812-95816, 95819, 95822, 95829, 95955, 96360, 96365, 96372, 96374-96376, 99148-99149, 99150, J0670, J2001

Note: These CCI edits are used for Medicare. Other payers may reimburse on codes listed above.

Medicare Edits

	Fac RVU	Non-Fac RVU	FUD	Status
57500	2.26	3.85	0	A

	MUE		Modifiers		
57500	1	51	N/A	N/A	N/A

* with documentation

Medicare References: None

Cervix Uteri

Coding Companion for Ob/Gyn

57505

57505 Endocervical curettage (not done as part of a dilation and curettage)

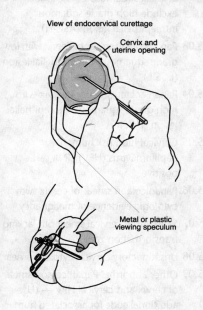

View of endocervical curettage

Cervix and uterine opening

Metal or plastic viewing speculum

Explanation

The physician inserts a speculum into the vagina to view the cervix. A small curette is used to scrape tissue from the endocervix, which is the region of the opening of the cervix into the uterine cavity.

Coding Tips

When 57505 is performed with another separately identifiable procedure, the highest dollar value code is listed as the primary procedure and subsequent procedures are appended with modifier 51. This procedure is usually performed with a local anesthesia. A paracervical anesthetic block is considered an inherent part of the surgical package.

ICD-9-CM Procedural

69.09   Other dilation and curettage of uterus

Anesthesia

57505   00940

ICD-9-CM Diagnostic

180.0   Malignant neoplasm of endocervix

180.8   Malignant neoplasm of other specified sites of cervix

218.0   Submucous leiomyoma of uterus

218.2   Subserous leiomyoma of uterus

219.0   Benign neoplasm of cervix uteri

233.1   Carcinoma in situ of cervix uteri

236.0   Neoplasm of uncertain behavior of uterus

616.0   Cervicitis and endocervicitis — (Use additional code to identify organism: 041.00-041.09, 041.10-041.19)

616.81   Mucositis (ulcerative) of cervix, vagina, and vulva — (Use additional code to identify organism: 041.00-041.09, 041.10-041.19) (Use additional E code to identify adverse effects of therapy: E879.2, E930.7, E933.1)

616.89   Other inflammatory disease of cervix, vagina and vulva — (Use additional code to identify organism: 041.00-041.09, 041.10-041.19)

617.0   Endometriosis of uterus

622.0   Erosion and ectropion of cervix

622.10   Dysplasia of cervix, unspecified

622.11   Mild dysplasia of cervix

622.12   Moderate dysplasia of cervix

622.2   Leukoplakia of cervix (uteri)

622.7   Mucous polyp of cervix

623.0   Dysplasia of vagina

623.1   Leukoplakia of vagina

623.8   Other specified noninflammatory disorder of vagina

625.3   Dysmenorrhea

626.0   Absence of menstruation

626.2   Excessive or frequent menstruation

626.4   Irregular menstrual cycle

626.6   Metrorrhagia

627.1   Postmenopausal bleeding

795.00   Abnormal glandular Papanicolaou smear of cervix

795.01   Papanicolaou smear of cervix with atypical squamous cells of undetermined significance (ASC-US)

795.02   Papanicolaou smear of cervix with atypical squamous cells cannot exclude high grade squamous intraepithelial lesion (ASC-H)

795.03   Papanicolaou smear of cervix with low grade squamous intraepithelial lesion (LGSIL)

795.04   Papanicolaou smear of cervix with high grade squamous intraepithelial lesion (HGSIL)

795.05   Cervical high risk human papillomavirus (HPV) DNA test positive

795.07   Satisfactory cervical smear but lacking transformation zone

795.08   Unsatisfactory cervical cytology smear

795.11   Papanicolaou smear of vagina with atypical squamous cells of undetermined significance (ASC-US) — (Use additional code to identify

acquired absence of uterus and cervix, if applicable: V88.01-V88.03)

795.12   Papanicolaou smear of vagina with atypical squamous cells cannot exclude high grade squamous intraepithelial lesion (ASC-H) — (Use additional code to identify acquired absence of uterus and cervix, if applicable: V88.01-V88.03)

795.13   Papanicolaou smear of vagina with low grade squamous intraepithelial lesion (LGSIL) — (Use additional code to identify acquired absence of uterus and cervix, if applicable: V88.01-V88.03)

795.14   Papanicolaou smear of vagina with high grade squamous intraepithelial lesion (HGSIL) — (Use additional code to identify acquired absence of uterus and cervix, if applicable: V88.01-V88.03)

795.15   Vaginal high risk human papillomavirus (HPV) DNA test positive — (Use additional code to identify acquired absence of uterus and cervix, if applicable: V88.01-V88.03)

795.16   Papanicolaou smear of vagina with cytologic evidence of malignancy — (Use additional code to identify acquired absence of uterus and cervix, if applicable: V88.01-V88.03)

CCI Version 18.3

0213T, 0216T, 0228T, 0230T, 12001-12007, 12011-12057, 13100-13153, 36000, 36400-36410, 36420-36430, 36440, 36600, 36640, 37202, 43752, 51701-51703, 57100, 57180, 57410, 57420, 57452, 57520❖, 57530, 57800, 58100, 58120❖, 62310-62319, 64400-64435, 64445-64450, 64479, 64483, 64490, 64493, 64505-64530, 69990, 93000-93010, 93040-93042, 93318, 94002, 94200, 94250, 94680-94690, 94770, 95812-95816, 95819, 95822, 95829, 95955, 96360, 96365, 96372, 96374-96376, 99148-99149, 99150, J0670, J2001

Note: These CCI edits are used for Medicare. Other payers may reimburse on codes listed above.

Medicare Edits

	Fac RVU	Non-Fac RVU	FUD	Status
57505	2.74	3.04	10	A

	MUE		Modifiers		
57505	1	51	N/A	N/A	N/A

* with documentation

Medicare References: None

57510-57513

57510 Cautery of cervix; electro or thermal
57511   cryocautery, initial or repeat
57513   laser ablation

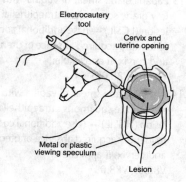

Electrocautery tool

Cervix and uterine opening

Metal or plastic viewing speculum

Lesion

Explanation

The physician inserts a speculum into the vagina to view the cervix. In 57510, electric current or heat is used to destroy the outer layers of the cervix causing them to slough off. In 57511, the outer layers of the cervix are destroyed by freezing using a liquid such as carbon dioxide, freon, nitrous oxide, or nitrogen, or a low temperature instrument. The outer layers of the cervix slough off. This code can be used for a first-time or repeat procedure. In 57513, a laser is directed at the cervix to vaporize the outer cells.

Coding Tips

The code choice for cauterization is determined by the equipment/method of cautery used. When 57510, 57511, or 57513 is performed with another separately identifiable procedure, the highest dollar value code is listed as the primary procedure and subsequent procedures are appended with modifier 51. Local anesthesia is included in the service.

ICD-9-CM Procedural

67.32 Destruction of lesion of cervix by cauterization
67.33 Destruction of lesion of cervix by cryosurgery
67.39 Other excision or destruction of lesion or tissue of cervix

Anesthesia
00940

ICD-9-CM Diagnostic

180.1 Malignant neoplasm of exocervix
180.8 Malignant neoplasm of other specified sites of cervix
219.0 Benign neoplasm of cervix uteri
233.1 Carcinoma in situ of cervix uteri
236.0 Neoplasm of uncertain behavior of uterus
239.5 Neoplasm of unspecified nature of other genitourinary organs
616.0 Cervicitis and endocervicitis — (Use additional code to identify organism: 041.00-041.09, 041.10-041.19)
616.81 Mucositis (ulcerative) of cervix, vagina, and vulva — (Use additional code to identify organism: 041.00-041.09, 041.10-041.19) (Use additional E code to identify adverse effects of therapy: E879.2, E930.7, E933.1)
616.89 Other inflammatory disease of cervix, vagina and vulva — (Use additional code to identify organism: 041.00-041.09, 041.10-041.19)
617.0 Endometriosis of uterus
622.0 Erosion and ectropion of cervix
622.10 Dysplasia of cervix, unspecified
622.11 Mild dysplasia of cervix
622.12 Moderate dysplasia of cervix
622.2 Leukoplakia of cervix (uteri)
622.6 Hypertrophic elongation of cervix
622.7 Mucous polyp of cervix
622.8 Other specified noninflammatory disorder of cervix
625.0 Dyspareunia
625.3 Dysmenorrhea
626.2 Excessive or frequent menstruation
626.6 Metrorrhagia
626.7 Postcoital bleeding
626.8 Other disorder of menstruation and other abnormal bleeding from female genital tract
627.1 Postmenopausal bleeding
752.40 Unspecified congenital anomaly of cervix, vagina, and external female genitalia
752.49 Other congenital anomaly of cervix, vagina, and external female genitalia
795.00 Abnormal glandular Papanicolaou smear of cervix

795.01 Papanicolaou smear of cervix with atypical squamous cells of undetermined significance (ASC-US)
795.02 Papanicolaou smear of cervix with atypical squamous cells cannot exclude high grade squamous intraepithelial lesion (ASC-H)
795.03 Papanicolaou smear of cervix with low grade squamous intraepithelial lesion (LGSIL)
795.04 Papanicolaou smear of cervix with high grade squamous intraepithelial lesion (HGSIL)
795.05 Cervical high risk human papillomavirus (HPV) DNA test positive
795.06 Papanicolaou smear of cervix with cytologic evidence of malignancy
795.07 Satisfactory cervical smear but lacking transformation zone
795.08 Unsatisfactory cervical cytology smear
795.09 Other abnormal Papanicolaou smear of cervix and cervical HPV — (Use additional code for associated human papillomavirus: 079.4)

CCI Version 18.3

0213T, 0216T, 0228T, 0230T, 12001-12007, 12011-12057, 13100-13153, 36000, 36400-36410, 36420-36430, 36440, 36600, 36640, 37202, 43752, 51701-51703, 57100, 57180, 57410, 57420, 57452, 57500, 57800, 58100, 62310-62319, 64400-64435, 64445-64450, 64479, 64483, 64490, 64493, 64505-64530, 69990, 93000-93010, 93040-93042, 93318, 94002, 94200, 94250, 94680-94690, 94770, 95812-95816, 95819, 95822, 95829, 95955, 96360, 96365, 96372, 96374-96376, 99148-99149, 99150, J0670, J2001

Also not with 57510: 57530

Also not with 57511: 57510❖, 57522-57530

Also not with 57513: 57510-57511❖, 57522-57530

Note: These CCI edits are used for Medicare. Other payers may reimburse on codes listed above.

Medicare Edits

	Fac RVU	Non-Fac RVU	FUD	Status
57510	3.44	3.91	10	A
57511	3.95	4.34	10	A
57513	3.97	4.29	10	A

	MUE		Modifiers		
57510	1	51	N/A	N/A	N/A
57511	1	51	N/A	N/A	N/A
57513	1	51	N/A	N/A	N/A

    * with documentation

Medicare References: None

Cervix Uteri

Coding Companion for Ob/Gyn

57520-57522

57520 Conization of cervix, with or without fulguration, with or without dilation and curettage, with or without repair; cold knife or laser

57522 loop electrode excision

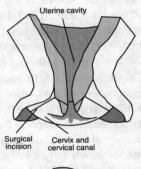

Cone-shaped portion of cervix is removed

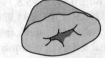

Explanation

The physician performs a conization of the cervix, with or without fulguration, with or without dilation and curettage, with or without repair by using the cold knife or laser technique in 57520 and loop electrode excision (LEEP technique) in 57522. The physician inserts a speculum into the vagina to view and fully expose the cervix. For most cases, the appropriate local anesthesia is administered as opposed to forms of premedication. Using a scalpel or laser instrument, a cone or slice of tissue including about 1-2 cm of the endocervix, as well as exocervical cells, is cut from the end of the cervix with the axis of the cone parallel to the axis of the cervix. Bleeding may be stopped by electric current. The cervix may need to be dilated and a curette used directly after conization to scrape tissue that is to be taken from further inside the uterus. The physician also may need to place interrupted figure-of-eight sutures to incorporate the bleeding site if direct cautery does not achieve hemostasis. For the LEEP procedure, the electric grounding pad is placed and safety checks are run. The cutting current is set. Using a loop that encompasses the entire lesion, an excision of the ectocervix is done with every effort made to remove the entire lesion in one specimen. If the lesion is large and another pass is required, two equal specimens are removed and labeled for the axis of orientation. The same procedure is done again with a smaller loop if an endocervical excision is necessary. The cervix may be dilated and an endocervical curettage collected. When all specimens have been collected, the bleeding vessels are cauterized, the vagina is inspected for any accidental injury, and the speculum is removed.

Coding Tips

If the cervical stump is excised (following supracervical hysterectomy), see 57540 and 57550. When 57520 is performed with another separately identifiable procedure, the highest dollar value code is listed as the primary procedure and subsequent procedures are appended with modifier 51. Local anesthesia is included in the service. However, this procedure may be performed under general anesthesia, depending on the age and/or condition of the patient. For dilation and curettage only, see 58120.

ICD-9-CM Procedural

67.2	Conization of cervix
67.32	Destruction of lesion of cervix by cauterization
67.39	Other excision or destruction of lesion or tissue of cervix
69.09	Other dilation and curettage of uterus

Anesthesia
00940

ICD-9-CM Diagnostic

180.0	Malignant neoplasm of endocervix
180.1	Malignant neoplasm of exocervix
180.8	Malignant neoplasm of other specified sites of cervix
198.82	Secondary malignant neoplasm of genital organs
219.0	Benign neoplasm of cervix uteri
233.1	Carcinoma in situ of cervix uteri
233.30	Carcinoma in situ, unspecified female genital organ
233.31	Carcinoma in situ, vagina
233.32	Carcinoma in situ, vulva
233.39	Carcinoma in situ, other female genital organ
236.0	Neoplasm of uncertain behavior of uterus
616.0	Cervicitis and endocervicitis — (Use additional code to identify organism: 041.00-041.09, 041.10-041.19)
622.0	Erosion and ectropion of cervix
622.10	Dysplasia of cervix, unspecified
622.6	Hypertrophic elongation of cervix
622.7	Mucous polyp of cervix
622.8	Other specified noninflammatory disorder of cervix
623.0	Dysplasia of vagina
625.3	Dysmenorrhea
626.2	Excessive or frequent menstruation
626.4	Irregular menstrual cycle
626.6	Metrorrhagia
626.8	Other disorder of menstruation and other abnormal bleeding from female genital tract
627.1	Postmenopausal bleeding
795.00	Abnormal glandular Papanicolaou smear of cervix
795.01	Papanicolaou smear of cervix with atypical squamous cells of undetermined significance (ASC-US)
795.02	Papanicolaou smear of cervix with atypical squamous cells cannot exclude high grade squamous intraepithelial lesion (ASC-H)
795.09	Other abnormal Papanicolaou smear of cervix and cervical HPV — (Use additional code for associated human papillomavirus: 079.4)

CCI Version 18.3

0213T, 0216T, 0228T, 0230T, 12001-12007, 12011-12057, 13100-13153, 36000, 36400-36410, 36420-36430, 36440, 36600, 36640, 37202, 43752, 51701-51703, 57100, 57180, 57410, 57452-57455, 57460-57500, 58100, 58120, 62310-62319, 64400-64435, 64445-64450, 64479, 64483, 64490, 64493, 64505-64530, 69990, 93000-93010, 93040-93042, 93318, 94002, 94200, 94250, 94680-94690, 94770, 95812-95816, 95819, 95822, 95829, 95955, 96360, 96365, 96372, 96374-96376, 99148-99149, 99150, J0670, J2001, P9612

Also not with 57520: 57420, 57510-57513, 57522-57530, 57720-57800

Also not with 57522: 57420-57421, 57510❖, 57530, 57800

Note: These CCI edits are used for Medicare. Other payers may reimburse on codes listed above.

Medicare Edits

	Fac RVU	Non-Fac RVU	FUD	Status
57520	8.13	9.12	90	A
57522	7.27	7.86	90	A

	MUE		Modifiers		
57520	1	51	N/A	N/A	N/A
57522	1	51	N/A	N/A	N/A

* with documentation

Medicare References: None

Coding Companion for Ob/Gyn

Cervix Uteri

57530

57530 Trachelectomy (cervicectomy), amputation of cervix (separate procedure)

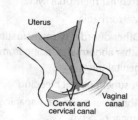

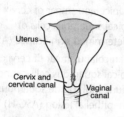

The cervix is surgically removed

Explanation

The physician inserts a speculum into the vagina to view the cervix and perform an amputation of the cervix. A tool is used to pull down the cervix. A scalpel is then used to divide the cervix from the uterus just after it enters the vagina. The physician removes the cervix through the vagina and stops the bleeding with cautery and sutures.

Coding Tips

This separate procedure by definition is usually a component of a more complex service and is not identified separately. When performed alone or with other unrelated procedures/services it may be reported. If performed alone, list the code; if performed with other procedures/services, list the code and append modifier 59. When 57530 is performed with another separately identifiable procedure, the highest dollar value code is listed as the primary procedure and subsequent procedures are appended with modifier 51. Local anesthesia is included in the service. For radical trachelectomy with lymphadenectomy, with or without the removal of a tube and/or ovary, see 57531. For radical abdominal hysterectomy, see 58210.

ICD-9-CM Procedural

67.4 Amputation of cervix

Anesthesia

57530 00940

ICD-9-CM Diagnostic

180.0 Malignant neoplasm of endocervix

180.1 Malignant neoplasm of exocervix

180.8 Malignant neoplasm of other specified sites of cervix

196.2 Secondary and unspecified malignant neoplasm of intra-abdominal lymph nodes

196.6 Secondary and unspecified malignant neoplasm of intrapelvic lymph nodes

219.0 Benign neoplasm of cervix uteri

233.1 Carcinoma in situ of cervix uteri

236.0 Neoplasm of uncertain behavior of uterus

239.5 Neoplasm of unspecified nature of other genitourinary organs

622.10 Dysplasia of cervix, unspecified

622.11 Mild dysplasia of cervix

622.12 Moderate dysplasia of cervix

795.00 Abnormal glandular Papanicolaou smear of cervix

795.01 Papanicolaou smear of cervix with atypical squamous cells of undetermined significance (ASC-US)

795.02 Papanicolaou smear of cervix with atypical squamous cells cannot exclude high grade squamous intraepithelial lesion (ASC-H)

795.03 Papanicolaou smear of cervix with low grade squamous intraepithelial lesion (LGSIL)

795.07 Satisfactory cervical smear but lacking transformation zone

795.09 Other abnormal Papanicolaou smear of cervix and cervical HPV — (Use additional code for associated human papillomavirus: 079.4)

V10.42 Personal history of malignant neoplasm of other parts of uterus

V84.01 Genetic susceptibility to malignant neoplasm of breast — (Use additional code, if applicable, for any associated family history of the disease: V16-V19. Code first, if applicable, any current malignant neoplasms: 140.0-195.8, 200.0-208.9, 230.0-234.9. Use additional code, if applicable, for any personal history of malignant neoplasm: V10.0-V10.9)

V84.02 Genetic susceptibility to malignant neoplasm of ovary — (Use additional code, if applicable, for any associated family history of the disease: V16-V19. Code first, if applicable, any current malignant neoplasms: 140.0-195.8, 200.0-208.9, 230.0-234.9. Use additional code, if applicable, for any personal history of malignant neoplasm: V10.0-V10.9)

V84.04 Genetic susceptibility to malignant neoplasm of endometrium — (Use additional code, if applicable, for any associated family history of the disease: V16-V19. Code first, if applicable, any current malignant neoplasms: 140.0-195.8, 200.0-208.9, 230.0-234.9. Use additional code, if applicable, for any personal history of malignant neoplasm: V10.0-V10.9)

V84.09 Genetic susceptibility to other malignant neoplasm — (Use additional code, if applicable, for any associated family history of the disease: V16-V19. Code first, if applicable, any current malignant neoplasms: 140.0-195.8, 200.0-208.9, 230.0-234.9. Use additional code, if applicable, for any personal history of malignant neoplasm: V10.0-V10.9)

CCI Version 18.3

0213T, 0216T, 0228T, 0230T, 12001-12007, 12011-12057, 13100-13153, 36000, 36400-36410, 36420-36430, 36440, 36600, 36640, 37202, 43752, 44950, 44970, 50715, 51701-51703, 57100, 57160-57180, 57410, 57420-57421, 57452-57500, 58100, 62310-62319, 64400-64435, 64445-64450, 64479, 64483, 64490, 64493, 64505-64530, 69990, 93000-93010, 93040-93042, 93318, 94002, 94200, 94250, 94680-94690, 94770, 95812-95816, 95819, 95822, 95829, 95955, 96360, 96365, 96372, 96374-96376, 99148-99149, 99150, P9612

Note: These CCI edits are used for Medicare. Other payers may reimburse on codes listed above.

Medicare Edits

	Fac RVU	Non-Fac RVU	FUD	Status
57530	10.28	10.28	90	A

	MUE		Modifiers		
57530	1	51	N/A	62*	80

* with documentation

Medicare References: None

Coding Companion for Ob/Gyn

Cervix Uteri

57531

57531 Radical trachelectomy, with bilateral total pelvic lymphadenectomy and para-aortic lymph node sampling biopsy, with or without removal of tube(s), with or without removal of ovary(s)

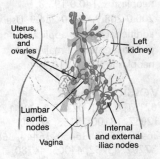

Uterus, tubes, and ovaries
Left kidney
Lumbar aortic nodes
Vagina
Internal and external iliac nodes

The cervix is removed in a radical procedure that includes removal of lymph nodes from the pelvic region and biopsy sampling of nodes from along the aorta. The uterine tubes and/or ovaries may also be removed during the procedure

Explanation

The physician inserts a speculum into the vagina to view the cervix and perform a radical excision of the cervix, including removal of local lymph nodes. A tool is used to pull down the cervix. A scalpel is used to divide the cervix from the uterus just after it enters the vagina. The physician removes the cervix through the vagina, stops the bleeding with cautery, and also removes the pelvic lymph nodes bilaterally, performs a para-aortic lymph node biopsy, and may remove one or both tubes and/or ovaries.

Coding Tips

This procedure includes bilateral total pelvic lymphadenectomy, para-aortic lymph node sampling biopsy, and removal of a tube(s), with removal of an ovary(s). For trachelectomy (cervicectomy), amputation of the cervix alone, see 57530. For radical vaginal hysterectomy, see 58285. For radical abdominal hysterectomy, see 58210.

ICD-9-CM Procedural

40.53 Radical excision of iliac lymph nodes
40.59 Radical excision of other lymph nodes
65.39 Other unilateral oophorectomy
65.49 Other unilateral salpingo-oophorectomy

65.51 Other removal of both ovaries at same operative episode
65.61 Other removal of both ovaries and tubes at same operative episode
65.62 Other removal of remaining ovary and tube
66.4 Total unilateral salpingectomy
66.51 Removal of both fallopian tubes at same operative episode
66.52 Removal of remaining fallopian tube
67.4 Amputation of cervix

Anesthesia

57531 00846

ICD-9-CM Diagnostic

180.0 Malignant neoplasm of endocervix
180.1 Malignant neoplasm of exocervix
180.8 Malignant neoplasm of other specified sites of cervix
196.2 Secondary and unspecified malignant neoplasm of intra-abdominal lymph nodes
196.6 Secondary and unspecified malignant neoplasm of intrapelvic lymph nodes
219.0 Benign neoplasm of cervix uteri
233.1 Carcinoma in situ of cervix uteri
236.0 Neoplasm of uncertain behavior of uterus
239.5 Neoplasm of unspecified nature of other genitourinary organs
622.10 Dysplasia of cervix, unspecified
622.11 Mild dysplasia of cervix
622.12 Moderate dysplasia of cervix
795.00 Abnormal glandular Papanicolaou smear of cervix
795.01 Papanicolaou smear of cervix with atypical squamous cells of undetermined significance (ASC-US)
795.02 Papanicolaou smear of cervix with atypical squamous cells cannot exclude high grade squamous intraepithelial lesion (ASC-H)
795.03 Papanicolaou smear of cervix with low grade squamous intraepithelial lesion (LGSIL)
795.07 Satisfactory cervical smear but lacking transformation zone
795.09 Other abnormal Papanicolaou smear of cervix and cervical HPV — (Use additional code for associated human papillomavirus: 079.4)
V10.42 Personal history of malignant neoplasm of other parts of uterus
V84.02 Genetic susceptibility to malignant neoplasm of ovary — (Use additional

code, if applicable, for any associated family history of the disease: V16-V19. Code first, if applicable, any current malignant neoplasms: 140.0-195.8, 200.0-208.9, 230.0-234.9. Use additional code, if applicable, for any personal history of malignant neoplasm: V10.0-V10.9)

V84.04 Genetic susceptibility to malignant neoplasm of endometrium — (Use additional code, if applicable, for any associated family history of the disease: V16-V19. Code first, if applicable, any current malignant neoplasms: 140.0-195.8, 200.0-208.9, 230.0-234.9. Use additional code, if applicable, for any personal history of malignant neoplasm: V10.0-V10.9)

V84.09 Genetic susceptibility to other malignant neoplasm — (Use additional code, if applicable, for any associated family history of the disease: V16-V19. Code first, if applicable, any current malignant neoplasms: 140.0-195.8, 200.0-208.9, 230.0-234.9. Use additional code, if applicable, for any personal history of malignant neoplasm: V10.0-V10.9)

CCI Version 18.3

0213T, 0216T, 0228T, 0230T, 12001-12007, 12011-12057, 13100-13153, 36000, 36400-36410, 36420-36430, 36440, 36600, 36640, 37202, 38571-38572, 38770, 38780, 43752, 44950, 44970, 49002, 50715, 51701-51703, 57410, 57420-57421, 57452, 57530, 58150, 58700-58720, 58940, 58960, 62310-62319, 64400-64435, 64445-64450, 64479, 64483, 64490, 64493, 64505-64530, 69990, 93000-93010, 93040-93042, 93318, 94002, 94200, 94250, 94680-94690, 94770, 95812-95816, 95819, 95822, 95829, 95955, 96360, 96365, 96372, 96374-96376, 99148-99149, 99150

Note: These CCI edits are used for Medicare. Other payers may reimburse on codes listed above.

Medicare Edits

	Fac RVU	Non-Fac RVU	FUD	Status
57531	51.57	51.57	90	A

	MUE			Modifiers	
57531	1	51	N/A	62*	80

* with documentation

Medicare References: None

57540-57545

57540 Excision of cervical stump, abdominal approach;
57545 with pelvic floor repair

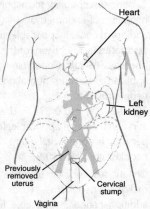

A cervical stump (remnant from a previous hysterectomy) is excised. Report 57540 for an abdominal approach. Code 57545 reports repair to the pelvic floor during the same operative session

Explanation

The physician makes an incision horizontally just within the pubic hairline. For 57540, the physician removes the cervical stump, which is the part of the cervix left after the supracervical uterus has been removed. The incision is closed by suturing. For 57545, the physician removes the cervical stump and repairs the muscular floor of the pelvis where the cervix rests using suture plication. This involves folding the tissues on top of each other and suturing. The incision is sutured.

Coding Tips

This service is performed on patients who have had a supracervical abdominal hysterectomy. When either of these procedures are performed with another separately identifiable procedure, the highest dollar value code is listed as the primary procedure and subsequent procedures are appended with modifier 51. For the initial supracervical abdominal hysterectomy, report 58180. For excision of a cervical stump, vaginal approach, report 57550.

ICD-9-CM Procedural

67.4 Amputation of cervix
70.79 Other repair of vagina

Anesthesia

00840

ICD-9-CM Diagnostic

180.0 Malignant neoplasm of endocervix
180.1 Malignant neoplasm of exocervix
180.8 Malignant neoplasm of other specified sites of cervix
219.0 Benign neoplasm of cervix uteri
233.1 Carcinoma in situ of cervix uteri
236.0 Neoplasm of uncertain behavior of uterus
239.5 Neoplasm of unspecified nature of other genitourinary organs
618.7 Genital prolapse, old laceration of muscles of pelvic floor — (Use additional code to identify urinary incontinence: 625.6, 788.31, 788.33-788.39)
618.81 Incompetence or weakening of pubocervical tissue — (Use additional code to identify urinary incontinence: 625.6, 788.31, 788.33-788.39)
618.82 Incompetence or weakening of rectovaginal tissue — (Use additional code to identify urinary incontinence: 625.6, 788.31, 788.33-788.39)
618.83 Pelvic muscle wasting — (Use additional code to identify urinary incontinence: 625.6, 788.31, 788.33-788.39)
618.84 Cervical stump prolapse — (Use additional code to identify urinary incontinence: 625.6, 788.31, 788.33-788.39)
622.0 Erosion and ectropion of cervix
622.10 Dysplasia of cervix, unspecified
622.11 Mild dysplasia of cervix
622.12 Moderate dysplasia of cervix
625.6 Female stress incontinence
795.00 Abnormal glandular Papanicolaou smear of cervix
795.01 Papanicolaou smear of cervix with atypical squamous cells of undetermined significance (ASC-US)
795.02 Papanicolaou smear of cervix with atypical squamous cells cannot exclude high grade squamous intraepithelial lesion (ASC-H)
795.04 Papanicolaou smear of cervix with high grade squamous intraepithelial lesion (HGSIL)
795.05 Cervical high risk human papillomavirus (HPV) DNA test positive
795.07 Satisfactory cervical smear but lacking transformation zone
795.08 Unsatisfactory cervical cytology smear

795.09 Other abnormal Papanicolaou smear of cervix and cervical HPV — (Use additional code for associated human papillomavirus: 079.4)
V84.04 Genetic susceptibility to malignant neoplasm of endometrium — (Use additional code, if applicable, for any associated family history of the disease: V16-V19. Code first, if applicable, any current malignant neoplasms: 140.0-195.8, 200.0-208.9, 230.0-234.9. Use additional code, if applicable, for any personal history of malignant neoplasm: V10.0-V10.9)

CCI Version 18.3

0213T, 0216T, 0228T, 0230T, 12001-12007, 12011-12057, 13100-13153, 36000, 36400-36410, 36420-36430, 36440, 36600, 36640, 37202, 43752, 44005, 44180, 44602-44605, 44850, 44950, 44970, 49000-49010, 49255, 49320, 49570, 50715, 51701-51703, 57100, 57410, 57420-57421, 57452, 57500, 57522-57530, 57800, 58100❖, 62310-62319, 64400-64435, 64445-64450, 64479, 64483, 64490, 64493, 64505-64530, 69990, 93000-93010, 93040-93042, 93318, 94002, 94200, 94250, 94680-94690, 94770, 95812-95816, 95819, 95822, 95829, 95955, 96360, 96365, 96372, 96374-96376, 99148-99149, 99150, P9612

Also not with 57540: 57180

Also not with 57545: 57180-57200, 57540

Note: These CCI edits are used for Medicare. Other payers may reimburse on codes listed above.

Medicare Edits

	Fac RVU	Non-Fac RVU	FUD	Status
57540	23.26	23.26	90	A
57545	24.54	24.54	90	A

	MUE			Modifiers		
57540	1		51	N/A	62*	80
57545	1		51	N/A	62*	80

* with documentation

Medicare References: None

Cervix Uteri

Coding Companion for Ob/Gyn

57550

57550 Excision of cervical stump, vaginal approach;

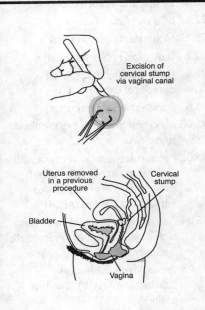

Excision of cervical stump via vaginal canal

Uterus removed in a previous procedure

Cervical stump

Bladder

Vagina

Explanation

Through an incision at the apex of the vagina, the physician removes the cervical stump, which is the part of the cervix left after the supracervical uterus has been removed. The vaginal incision is closed with sutures.

Coding Tips

This service is performed on patients who have had a supracervical abdominal hysterectomy. In some cases, scar tissue is an additional complication. Any manipulation or dilation of the vagina is not reported separately. When 57550 is performed with another separately identifiable procedure, the highest dollar value code is listed as the primary procedure and subsequent procedures are appended with modifier 51. For the initial supracervical abdominal hysterectomy, report 58180. For excision of a cervical stump, vaginal approach, with anterior and/or posterior repair, see 57555; with repair of endocele, see 57556. For excision of a cervical stump, abdominal approach, see 57540–57545.

ICD-9-CM Procedural

67.4   Amputation of cervix

Anesthesia

57550   00940

ICD-9-CM Diagnostic

180.0   Malignant neoplasm of endocervix

180.1   Malignant neoplasm of exocervix

180.8   Malignant neoplasm of other specified sites of cervix

219.0   Benign neoplasm of cervix uteri

233.1   Carcinoma in situ of cervix uteri

236.0   Neoplasm of uncertain behavior of uterus

239.5   Neoplasm of unspecified nature of other genitourinary organs

618.84   Cervical stump prolapse — (Use additional code to identify urinary incontinence: 625.6, 788.31, 788.33-788.39)

622.0   Erosion and ectropion of cervix

622.10   Dysplasia of cervix, unspecified

622.11   Mild dysplasia of cervix

622.12   Moderate dysplasia of cervix

795.00   Abnormal glandular Papanicolaou smear of cervix

795.01   Papanicolaou smear of cervix with atypical squamous cells of undetermined significance (ASC-US)

795.02   Papanicolaou smear of cervix with atypical squamous cells cannot exclude high grade squamous intraepithelial lesion (ASC-H)

795.03   Papanicolaou smear of cervix with low grade squamous intraepithelial lesion (LGSIL)

795.04   Papanicolaou smear of cervix with high grade squamous intraepithelial lesion (HGSIL)

795.05   Cervical high risk human papillomavirus (HPV) DNA test positive

795.07   Satisfactory cervical smear but lacking transformation zone

795.08   Unsatisfactory cervical cytology smear

795.09   Other abnormal Papanicolaou smear of cervix and cervical HPV — (Use additional code for associated human papillomavirus: 079.4)

V84.02   Genetic susceptibility to malignant neoplasm of ovary — (Use additional code, if applicable, for any associated family history of the disease: V16-V19. Code first, if applicable, any current malignant neoplasms: 140.0-195.8, 200.0-208.9, 230.0-234.9. Use additional code, if applicable, for any personal history of malignant neoplasm: V10.0-V10.9)

V84.04   Genetic susceptibility to malignant neoplasm of endometrium — (Use additional code, if applicable, for any associated family history of the disease: V16-V19. Code first, if applicable, any current malignant

neoplasms: 140.0-195.8, 200.0-208.9, 230.0-234.9. Use additional code, if applicable, for any personal history of malignant neoplasm: V10.0-V10.9)

V84.09   Genetic susceptibility to other malignant neoplasm — (Use additional code, if applicable, for any associated family history of the disease: V16-V19. Code first, if applicable, any current malignant neoplasms: 140.0-195.8, 200.0-208.9, 230.0-234.9. Use additional code, if applicable, for any personal history of malignant neoplasm: V10.0-V10.9)

Terms To Know

cervical ectropion. Eversion or turning outward of the cervical canal with epithelium extending further out of the external os of the cervix.

cervical intraepithelial neoplasia. Classification system used to report abnormalities in the epithelial cells of the cervix uteri: *1)* CIN I: Cervical intraepithelial neoplasia I, low-grade abnormality, mild dysplasia. *2)* CIN II: Cervical intraepithelial neoplasia II, high-grade abnormality, moderate dysplasia. *3)* CIN III: Cervical intraepithelial neoplasia III, carcinoma in situ, severe dysplasia.

CCI Version 18.3

0213T, 0216T, 0228T, 0230T, 12001-12007, 12011-12057, 13100-13153, 36000, 36400-36410, 36420-36430, 36440, 36600, 36640, 37202, 43752, 50715, 51701-51703, 57100, 57180-57200, 57410, 57420-57421, 57452, 57500, 57522-57530, 57545❖, 57800, 58100❖, 62310-62319, 64400-64435, 64445-64450, 64479, 64483, 64490, 64493, 64505-64530, 69990, 93000-93010, 93040-93042, 93318, 94002, 94200, 94250, 94680-94690, 94770, 95812-95816, 95819, 95822, 95829, 95955, 96360, 96365, 96372, 96374-96376, 99148-99149, 99150, P9612

Note: These CCI edits are used for Medicare. Other payers may reimburse on codes listed above.

Medicare Edits

	Fac RVU	Non-Fac RVU	FUD	Status
57550	12.2	12.2	90	A

	MUE		Modifiers		
57550	1	51	N/A	62*	80

* with documentation

Medicare References: None

Coding Companion for Ob/Gyn

Cervix Uteri

57555-57556

57555 Excision of cervical stump, vaginal approach; with anterior and/or posterior repair

57556 with repair of enterocele

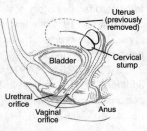

A cervical stump is excised by vaginal approach and anterior and/or posterior repair is performed at the same session

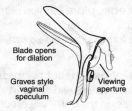

Explanation

Through an incision in the apex of the vagina, the physician removes the cervical stump. In 57555, the physician also repairs the relaxed or herniated tissues in the front or back wall of the vagina. Through the vaginal incision, the physician dissects the tissues between the bladder, urethra, vagina, and rectum. The specific tissue weaknesses are repaired and strengthened using tissue transfer techniques and layered and plication suturing. The incisions are closed with sutures. In 57556, the physician also repairs an enterocele, which is a herniation of the bowel against the rectouterine pouch. Through the vaginal incision, the physician incises and ligates the enterocele sac and approximates the uterosacral ligaments and endopelvic fascia anterior to the rectum. The incisions are closed with sutures.

Coding Tips

This service is performed on patients who have had a supracervical abdominal hysterectomy. When either of these procedures are performed with another separately identifiable procedure, the highest dollar value code is listed as the primary procedure and subsequent procedures are appended with modifier 51. For the initial supracervical abdominal hysterectomy, report 58180. For excision of cervical stump only, vaginal approach, see 57550. If performing a repair of the vagina without surgical excision of the cervical stump, see 57200–57210 and 57240–57265.

ICD-9-CM Procedural

67.4 Amputation of cervix

70.50 Repair of cystocele and rectocele

70.92 Other operations on cul-de-sac

Anesthesia

00940, 00942

ICD-9-CM Diagnostic

180.0 Malignant neoplasm of endocervix

180.1 Malignant neoplasm of exocervix

219.0 Benign neoplasm of cervix uteri

233.1 Carcinoma in situ of cervix uteri

617.0 Endometriosis of uterus

618.03 Urethrocele without mention of uterine prolapse — (Use additional code to identify urinary incontinence: 625.6, 788.31, 788.33-788.39)

618.04 Rectocele without mention of uterine prolapse — (Use additional code to identify urinary incontinence: 625.6, 788.31, 788.33-788.39) (Use additional code for any associated fecal incontinence: 787.60-787.63)

618.05 Perineocele without mention of uterine prolapse — (Use additional code to identify urinary incontinence: 625.6, 788.31, 788.33-788.39)

618.1 Uterine prolapse without mention of vaginal wall prolapse — (Use additional code to identify urinary incontinence: 625.6, 788.31, 788.33-788.39)

618.2 Uterovaginal prolapse, incomplete — (Use additional code to identify urinary incontinence: 625.6, 788.31, 788.33-788.39)

618.5 Prolapse of vaginal vault after hysterectomy — (Use additional code to identify urinary incontinence: 625.6, 788.31, 788.33-788.39)

618.6 Vaginal enterocele, congenital or acquired — (Use additional code to identify urinary incontinence: 625.6, 788.31, 788.33-788.39)

618.81 Incompetence or weakening of pubocervical tissue — (Use additional code to identify urinary incontinence: 625.6, 788.31, 788.33-788.39)

618.82 Incompetence or weakening of rectovaginal tissue — (Use additional code to identify urinary incontinence: 625.6, 788.31, 788.33-788.39)

618.84 Cervical stump prolapse — (Use additional code to identify urinary incontinence: 625.6, 788.31, 788.33-788.39)

622.0 Erosion and ectropion of cervix

622.11 Mild dysplasia of cervix

622.12 Moderate dysplasia of cervix

622.2 Leukoplakia of cervix (uteri)

622.8 Other specified noninflammatory disorder of cervix

625.6 Female stress incontinence

795.00 Abnormal glandular Papanicolaou smear of cervix

795.02 Papanicolaou smear of cervix with atypical squamous cells cannot exclude high grade squamous intraepithelial lesion (ASC-H)

795.04 Papanicolaou smear of cervix with high grade squamous intraepithelial lesion (HGSIL)

795.05 Cervical high risk human papillomavirus (HPV) DNA test positive

CCI Version 18.3

0213T, 0216T, 0228T, 0230T, 12001-12007, 12011-12057, 13100-13153, 36000, 36400-36410, 36420-36430, 36440, 36600, 36640, 37202, 43752, 50715, 51701-51703, 57100, 57180-57200, 57400-57410, 57420-57421, 57452, 57500, 57522-57530, 57550, 57800, 58100❖, 62310-62319, 64400-64435, 64445-64450, 64479, 64483, 64490, 64493, 64505-64530, 69990, 93000-93010, 93040-93042, 93318, 94002, 94200, 94250, 94680-94690, 94770, 95812-95816, 95819, 95822, 95829, 95955, 96360, 96365, 96372, 96374-96376, 99148-99149, 99150, P9612

Also not with 57555: 57240-57260, 57556

Also not with 57556: 57260-57265, 57268, 57283

Note: These CCI edits are used for Medicare. Other payers may reimburse on codes listed above.

Medicare Edits

	Fac RVU	Non-Fac RVU	FUD	Status
57555	17.94	17.94	90	A
57556	16.86	16.86	90	A

	MUE		Modifiers		
57555	1	51	N/A	62*	80
57556	1	51	N/A	62*	80

* with documentation

Medicare References: None

Cervix Uteri

57558

57558 Dilation and curettage of cervical stump

Uterus removed in an earlier procedure

Cervical stump and canal

Vaginal canal

Curette

Explanation

The physician performs a dilation and curettage of the cervical stump. The physician inserts a speculum into the vagina to view the cervix. The physician enlarges the cervix using a dilator and scrapes tissue from the lining of the cervical stump, which is the part of the cervix left after removal of the uterus.

Coding Tips

This code is used for the dilation and curettage of the cervical stump, and should not be confused with 58120. When 57558 is performed with another separately identifiable procedure, the highest dollar value code is listed as the primary procedure and subsequent procedures are appended with modifier 51. However, this code is often misused when larger invasive procedures are performed, in which case it is not separately reported. Local anesthesia is included in this service. However, this procedure may be performed under general anesthesia, depending on the age and/or condition of the patient. Surgical trays, A4550, are not separately reimbursed by Medicare; however, other third-party payers may cover them. Check with the specific payer to determine coverage.

ICD-9-CM Procedural

69.09 Other dilation and curettage of uterus

Anesthesia

57558 00940

ICD-9-CM Diagnostic

180.0	Malignant neoplasm of endocervix
180.8	Malignant neoplasm of other specified sites of cervix
233.1	Carcinoma in situ of cervix uteri
236.0	Neoplasm of uncertain behavior of uterus
239.5	Neoplasm of unspecified nature of other genitourinary organs
616.0	Cervicitis and endocervicitis — (Use additional code to identify organism: 041.00-041.09, 041.10-041.19)
617.0	Endometriosis of uterus
622.0	Erosion and ectropion of cervix
622.10	Dysplasia of cervix, unspecified
622.11	Mild dysplasia of cervix
622.12	Moderate dysplasia of cervix
622.2	Leukoplakia of cervix (uteri)
622.4	Stricture and stenosis of cervix
622.7	Mucous polyp of cervix
622.8	Other specified noninflammatory disorder of cervix
627.1	Postmenopausal bleeding

Terms To Know

cervical ectropion. Eversion or turning outward of the cervical canal with epithelium extending further out of the external os of the cervix.

curettage. Removal of tissue by scraping.

dilation. Artificial increase in the diameter of an opening or lumen made by medication or by instrumentation.

dysplasia. Abnormality or alteration in the size, shape, and organization of cells from their normal pattern of development.

endometriosis. Aberrant uterine mucosal tissue appearing in areas of the pelvic cavity outside of its normal location, lining the uterus and inflaming surrounding tissues, and can result in infertility and spontaneous abortion.

leukoplakia. Thickened white patches or lesions appearing on a mucous membrane.

malignant. Any condition tending to progress toward death, specifically an invasive tumor with a loss of cellular differentiation that has the ability to spread or metastasize to other areas in the body.

mucous polyp. Outgrowth or projection of the mucous membrane tissue lining a body cavity.

polyp. Small growth on a stalk-like attachment projecting from a mucous membrane.

stenosis. Narrowing or constriction of a passage.

stricture. Narrowing of an anatomical structure.

CCI Version 18.3

0213T, 0216T, 0228T, 0230T, 12001-12007, 12011-12057, 13100-13153, 36000, 36400-36410, 36420-36430, 36440, 36600, 36640, 37202, 43752, 51701-51703, 57100, 57180, 57400-57410, 57420, 57452, 57500, 57530, 57800, 58100, 62310-62319, 64400-64435, 64445-64450, 64479, 64483, 64490, 64493, 64505-64530, 69990, 93000-93010, 93040-93042, 93318, 94002, 94200, 94250, 94680-94690, 94770, 95812-95816, 95819, 95822, 95829, 95955, 96360, 96365, 96372, 96374-96376, 99148-99149, 99150, J2001

Note: These CCI edits are used for Medicare. Other payers may reimburse on codes listed above.

Medicare Edits

	Fac RVU	Non-Fac RVU	FUD	Status
57558	3.4	3.73	10	A

	MUE		Modifiers		
57558	1	51	N/A	N/A	N/A

* with documentation

Medicare References: None

Cervix Uteri

57700

57700 Cerclage of uterine cervix, nonobstetrical

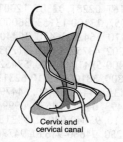

Suture material inserted around cervix

Cervix and cervical canal

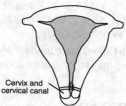

Cervix and cervical canal

Explanation

The physician inserts a speculum into the vagina to view the cervix of a nonpregnant patient. Suture or wire is threaded around the cervix and pulled in pursestring fashion to make the opening smaller.

Coding Tips

Depending on the patient's anatomy, there may be additional complications. When 57700 is performed with another separately identifiable procedure, the highest dollar value code is listed as the primary procedure and subsequent procedures are appended with modifier 51. If the patient is pregnant, see 59320 or 59325. Surgical trays, A4550, are not separately reimbursed by Medicare; however, other third-party payers may cover them. Check with the specific payer to determine coverage.

ICD-9-CM Procedural

67.59   Other repair of cervical os

Anesthesia

57700   00948

ICD-9-CM Diagnostic

622.5   Incompetence of cervix

654.54   Cervical incompetence, postpartum condition or complication — (Code first any associated obstructed labor, 660.2)

867.4   Uterus injury without mention of open wound into cavity

Terms To Know

cerclage. Looping or encircling an organ or tissue with wire or ligature for positional support.

endocervix. Region of the cervix uteri that opens into the uterus or the mucous membrane lining the cervical canal.

external os. Uterine opening through the cervix and into the vagina.

internal os. Opening through the cervix into the uterus.

postpartum. Period of time following childbirth.

speculum. Tool used to enlarge the opening of any canal or cavity.

suture. Numerous stitching techniques employed in wound closure: 1) Buried suture: Continuous or interrupted suture placed under the skin for a layered closure. 2) Continuous suture: Running stitch with tension evenly distributed across a single strand to provide a leakproof closure line. 3) Interrupted suture: Series of single stitches with tension isolated at each stitch, in which all stitches are not affected if one becomes loose, and the isolated sutures cannot act as a wick to transport an infection. 4) Purse-string suture: Continuous suture placed around a tubular structure and tightened, to reduce or close the lumen. 5) Retention suture: Secondary stitching that bridges the primary suture, providing support for the primary repair; a plastic or rubber bolster may be placed over the primary repair and under the retention sutures.

CCI Version 18.3

0213T, 0216T, 0228T, 0230T, 12001-12007, 12011-12057, 13100-13153, 36000, 36400-36410, 36420-36430, 36440, 36600, 36640, 37202, 43752, 51701-51703, 57100, 57180, 57400-57410, 57420, 57452, 57500, 57530, 57800, 58100, 62310-62319, 64400-64435, 64445-64450, 64479, 64483, 64490, 64493, 64505-64530, 69990, 93000-93010, 93040-93042, 93318, 94002, 94200, 94250, 94680-94690, 94770, 95812-95816, 95819, 95822, 95829, 95955, 96360, 96365, 96372, 96374-96376, 99148-99149, 99150, P9612

Note: These CCI edits are used for Medicare. Other payers may reimburse on codes listed above.

Medicare Edits

	Fac RVU	Non-Fac RVU	FUD	Status
57700	9.29	9.29	90	A

	MUE		Modifiers		
57700	1	51	N/A	N/A	80*

* with documentation

Medicare References: None

57720

57720 Trachelorrhaphy, plastic repair of uterine cervix, vaginal approach

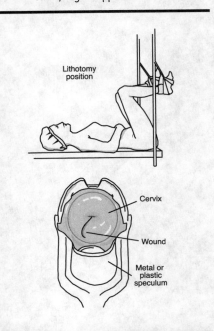

Lithotomy position

Cervix

Wound

Metal or plastic speculum

Explanation

The physician inserts a speculum into the vagina to view the cervix. The physician performs a plastic suture repair of a laceration or wound on the cervix. A plastic repair also can encompass excising scar tissue or tightening an incompetent cervix.

Coding Tips

A more complex plastic repair may also encompass an excision of scar tissue or tightening of the cervix. Any manipulation or dilation of the vagina is not reported separately. Electrocautery may be used to stop small bleeding points. When 57720 is performed with another separately identifiable procedure, the highest dollar value code is listed as the primary procedure and subsequent procedures are appended with modifier 51. For repairs of the vagina, see 57200–57270.

ICD-9-CM Procedural

67.69   Other repair of cervix

Anesthesia

57720   00940, 00942

ICD-9-CM Diagnostic

622.3   Old laceration of cervix

622.5   Incompetence of cervix

665.31   Laceration of cervix, with delivery

665.34   Laceration of cervix, postpartum condition or complication

867.4   Uterus injury without mention of open wound into cavity

Terms To Know

approach. Method or anatomical location used to gain access to a body organ or specific area for procedures. The approach is not coded separately although it may be a specified component of the procedure, such as laparoscopic vs. incisional, or spinal procedures in which the amount of dissection required to expose the spine significantly alters with the site of approach.

endocervical canal. Opening between the uterus and the vagina, through the cervix, lined with mucous membrane.

external os. Uterine opening through the cervix and into the vagina.

incompetent cervix. Narrow end of the uterus opening into the birth canal that abnormally dilates during the second trimester of the pregnancy and can lead to a miscarriage or premature delivery.

internal os. Opening through the cervix into the uterus.

laceration. Tearing injury; a torn, ragged-edged wound.

scar tissue. Fibrous connective tissue that forms around a wounded area or injury, composed mainly of fibroblasts or collagenous fibers.

speculum. Tool used to enlarge the opening of any canal or cavity.

CCI Version 18.3

0213T, 0216T, 0228T, 0230T, 12001-12007, 12011-12057, 13100-13153, 36000, 36400-36410, 36420-36430, 36440, 36600, 36640, 37202, 43752, 51701-51703, 57100, 57180, 57400-57410, 57420, 57452, 57500, 57530, 57800, 58100, 62310-62319, 64400-64435, 64445-64450, 64479, 64483, 64490, 64493, 64505-64530, 69990, 93000-93010, 93040-93042, 93318, 94002, 94200, 94250, 94680-94690, 94770, 95812-95816, 95819, 95822, 95829, 95955, 96360, 96365, 96372, 96374-96376, 99148-99149, 99150, J2001, P9612

Note: These CCI edits are used for Medicare. Other payers may reimburse on codes listed above.

Medicare Edits

	Fac RVU	Non-Fac RVU	FUD	Status
57720	9.18	9.18	90	A

	MUE		Modifiers		
57720	1	51	N/A	N/A	80

* with documentation

Medicare References: None

57800

57800 Dilation of cervical canal, instrumental (separate procedure)

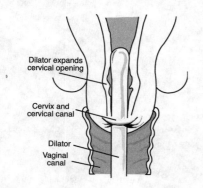

Dilator expands cervical opening

Cervix and cervical canal

Dilator

Vaginal canal

Explanation

The physician inserts a speculum into the vagina to view the cervix. A tool is used to grasp the cervix and pull it down. A dilator or series of dilators is inserted into the endocervix and passed through the cervical canal.

Coding Tips

This separate procedure by definition is usually a component of a more complex service and is not identified separately. When performed alone or with other unrelated procedures/services it may be reported. If performed alone, list the code; if performed with other procedures/services, list the code and append modifier 59. For dilation and curettage of cervical stump, see 57558. For endometrial and/or endocervical sampling (biopsy), without cervical dilation, any method, see 58100. For dilation and curettage, diagnostic and/or therapeutic (nonobstetrical), see 58120. For treatment of a missed abortion, see 59820–59821. Surgical trays, A4550, are not separately reimbursed by Medicare; however, other third-party payers may cover them. Check with the specific payer to determine coverage.

ICD-9-CM Procedural

67.0 Dilation of cervical canal

Anesthesia

57800 00940

ICD-9-CM Diagnostic

622.4 Stricture and stenosis of cervix

622.8 Other specified noninflammatory disorder of cervix

626.8 Other disorder of menstruation and other abnormal bleeding from female genital tract

628.4 Female infertility of cervical or vaginal origin

789.00 Abdominal pain, unspecified site

Terms To Know

dilation. Artificial increase in the diameter of an opening or lumen made by medication or by instrumentation.

endocervix. Region of the cervix uteri that opens into the uterus or the mucous membrane lining the cervical canal.

speculum. Tool used to enlarge the opening of any canal or cavity.

stenosis. Narrowing or constriction of a passage.

stricture. Narrowing of an anatomical structure.

CCI Version 18.3

0213T, 0216T, 0228T, 0230T, 12001-12007, 12011-12057, 13100-13153, 36000, 36400-36410, 36420-36430, 36440, 36600, 36640, 37202, 43752, 51701-51703, 57100, 57420, 57452, 57500, 57530, 62310-62319, 64400-64435, 64445-64450, 64479, 64483, 64490, 64493, 64505-64530, 69990, 93000-93010, 93040-93042, 93318, 94002, 94200, 94250, 94680-94690, 94770, 95812-95816, 95819, 95822, 95829, 95955, 96360, 96365, 96372, 96374-96376, 99148-99149, 99150, J2001

Note: These CCI edits are used for Medicare. Other payers may reimburse on codes listed above.

Medicare Edits

	Fac RVU	Non-Fac RVU	FUD	Status
57800	1.44	1.79	0	A

	MUE		Modifiers		
57800	1	51	N/A	N/A	N/A

* with documentation

Medicare References: None

Cervix Uteri

58100

58100 Endometrial sampling (biopsy) with or without endocervical sampling (biopsy), without cervical dilation, any method (separate procedure)

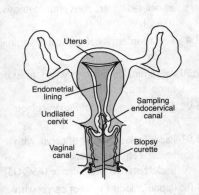

Labels: Uterus; Endometrial lining; Undilated cervix; Vaginal canal; Sampling endocervical canal; Biopsy curette

Explanation
The physician inserts a speculum into the vagina to view the cervix. A tool is used to grasp the cervix and pull it down. The physician places a curette in the endocervical canal and passes it into the uterus. The endometrial lining of the uterus is scraped on all sides to obtain tissue for diagnosis. Biopsy(ies) may also be taken from the endocervix. Cervical dilation is not required.

Coding Tips
This separate procedure by definition is usually a component of a more complex service and is not identified separately. When performed alone or with other unrelated procedures/services it may be reported. If performed alone, list the code; if performed with other procedures/services, list the code and append modifier 59. If a specimen is transported to an outside laboratory, report 99000 for handling or conveyance. For endocervical curettage (not done as part of a dilation and curettage), see 57505. For dilation and curettage, diagnostic and/or therapeutic (nonobstetrical), see 58120. For curettage for postpartum hemorrhage, see 59160.

ICD-9-CM Procedural
67.11   Endocervical biopsy
67.12   Other cervical biopsy
68.16   Closed biopsy of uterus

Anesthesia
58100 00940

ICD-9-CM Diagnostic
179   Malignant neoplasm of uterus, part unspecified
180.0   Malignant neoplasm of endocervix
180.1   Malignant neoplasm of exocervix
180.8   Malignant neoplasm of other specified sites of cervix
182.0   Malignant neoplasm of corpus uteri, except isthmus
182.8   Malignant neoplasm of other specified sites of body of uterus
218.0   Submucous leiomyoma of uterus
218.1   Intramural leiomyoma of uterus
219.8   Benign neoplasm of other specified parts of uterus
233.1   Carcinoma in situ of cervix uteri
256.31 Premature menopause — (Use additional code for states associated with natural menopause: 627.2)
256.39 Other ovarian failure — (Use additional code for states associated with natural menopause: 627.2)
256.4   Polycystic ovaries
615.0   Acute inflammatory disease of uterus, except cervix — (Use additional code to identify organism: 041.00-041.09, 041.10-041.19)
615.1   Chronic inflammatory disease of uterus, except cervix — (Use additional code to identify organism: 041.00-041.09, 041.10-041.19)
616.0   Cervicitis and endocervicitis — (Use additional code to identify organism: 041.00-041.09, 041.10-041.19)
617.0   Endometriosis of uterus
621.0   Polyp of corpus uteri
621.2   Hypertrophy of uterus
621.31 Simple endometrial hyperplasia without atypia
621.32 Complex endometrial hyperplasia without atypia
621.33 Endometrial hyperplasia with atypia
621.4   Hematometra
621.5   Intrauterine synechiae
622.10 Dysplasia of cervix, unspecified
622.4   Stricture and stenosis of cervix
622.7   Mucous polyp of cervix
623.5   Leukorrhea, not specified as infective
625.3   Dysmenorrhea
626.0   Absence of menstruation
626.1   Scanty or infrequent menstruation
626.2   Excessive or frequent menstruation
626.3   Puberty bleeding
626.4   Irregular menstrual cycle
626.5   Ovulation bleeding
626.6   Metrorrhagia
626.8   Other disorder of menstruation and other abnormal bleeding from female genital tract
627.1   Postmenopausal bleeding
627.2   Symptomatic menopausal or female climacteric states
628.3   Female infertility of uterine origin — (Use additional code for any associated tuberculous endometriosis: 016.7)
628.4   Female infertility of cervical or vaginal origin
629.0   Hematocele, female, not elsewhere classified
646.30 Pregnancy complication, recurrent pregnancy loss, unspecified as to episode of care — (Use additional code to further specify complication)
795.02 Papanicolaou smear of cervix with atypical squamous cells cannot exclude high grade squamous intraepithelial lesion (ASC-H)
795.04 Papanicolaou smear of cervix with high grade squamous intraepithelial lesion (HGSIL)
795.05 Cervical high risk human papillomavirus (HPV) DNA test positive

CCI Version 18.3
0213T, 0216T, 0228T, 0230T, 10021-10022, 12001-12007, 12011-12057, 13100-13153, 36000, 36400-36410, 36420-36430, 36440, 36600, 36640, 37202, 43752, 51701-51703, 57100, 57180, 57452, 57500, 57800, 62310-62319, 64400-64435, 64445-64450, 64479, 64483, 64490, 64493, 64505-64530, 69990, 93000-93010, 93040-93042, 93318, 94002, 94200, 94250, 94680-94690, 94770, 95812-95816, 95819, 95822, 95829, 95955, 96360, 96365, 96372, 96374-96376, 99148-99149, 99150

Note: These CCI edits are used for Medicare. Other payers may reimburse on codes listed above.

Medicare Edits

	Fac RVU	Non-Fac RVU	FUD	Status
58100	2.62	3.27	0	A

	MUE		Modifiers		
58100	1	51	N/A	N/A	N/A

* with documentation

Medicare References: 100-3,230.6

58110

58110 Endometrial sampling (biopsy) performed in conjunction with colposcopy (List separately in addition to code for primary procedure)

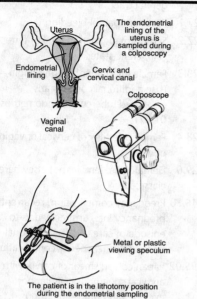

The endometrial lining of the uterus is sampled during a colposcopy

Uterus

Endometrial lining

Cervix and cervical canal

Colposcope

Vaginal canal

Metal or plastic viewing speculum

The patient is in the lithotomy position during the endometrial sampling

Explanation

A tool is used to grasp the cervix and pull it down. The physician places a curette in the endocervical canal and passes it into the uterus. The endometrial lining of the uterus is scraped in several places to obtain tissue for a biopsy sample. The endometrial sampling is performed in conjunction with direct visualization of the vagina and cervix and is reported in addition to the separately reportable primary colposcopy.

Coding Tips

As an "add-on" code, 58110 is not subject to multiple procedure rules. No reimbursement reduction or modifier 51 is applied. "Add-on" codes describe additional intra-service work associated with the primary procedure. They are performed by the same physician on the same date of service as the primary service/procedure, and must never be reported as a stand-alone code. Report 58110 in conjunction with 57420, 57421, and 57452–57461.

ICD-9-CM Procedural

68.16   Closed biopsy of uterus

Anesthesia

58110   N/A

ICD-9-CM Diagnostic

179	Malignant neoplasm of uterus, part unspecified
180.0	Malignant neoplasm of endocervix
180.1	Malignant neoplasm of exocervix
180.8	Malignant neoplasm of other specified sites of cervix
182.0	Malignant neoplasm of corpus uteri, except isthmus
182.8	Malignant neoplasm of other specified sites of body of uterus
218.0	Submucous leiomyoma of uterus
218.1	Intramural leiomyoma of uterus
219.0	Benign neoplasm of cervix uteri
219.1	Benign neoplasm of corpus uteri
233.1	Carcinoma in situ of cervix uteri
233.2	Carcinoma in situ of other and unspecified parts of uterus
256.31	Premature menopause — (Use additional code for states associated with natural menopause: 627.2)
615.0	Acute inflammatory disease of uterus, except cervix — (Use additional code to identify organism: 041.00-041.09, 041.10-041.19)
615.1	Chronic inflammatory disease of uterus, except cervix — (Use additional code to identify organism: 041.00-041.09, 041.10-041.19)
616.0	Cervicitis and endocervicitis — (Use additional code to identify organism: 041.00-041.09, 041.10-041.19)
617.0	Endometriosis of uterus
621.0	Polyp of corpus uteri
621.2	Hypertrophy of uterus
621.30	Endometrial hyperplasia, unspecified
621.31	Simple endometrial hyperplasia without atypia
621.32	Complex endometrial hyperplasia without atypia
621.33	Endometrial hyperplasia with atypia
621.4	Hematometra
621.5	Intrauterine synechiae
622.10	Dysplasia of cervix, unspecified
622.11	Mild dysplasia of cervix
622.12	Moderate dysplasia of cervix
622.7	Mucous polyp of cervix
623.5	Leukorrhea, not specified as infective
623.7	Polyp of vagina
625.3	Dysmenorrhea
626.0	Absence of menstruation
626.1	Scanty or infrequent menstruation
626.2	Excessive or frequent menstruation
626.3	Puberty bleeding
626.4	Irregular menstrual cycle
626.5	Ovulation bleeding
626.6	Metrorrhagia
626.8	Other disorder of menstruation and other abnormal bleeding from female genital tract
627.1	Postmenopausal bleeding
628.3	Female infertility of uterine origin — (Use additional code for any associated tuberculous endometriosis: 016.7)
628.4	Female infertility of cervical or vaginal origin
789.30	Abdominal or pelvic swelling, mass or lump, unspecified site
795.00	Abnormal glandular Papanicolaou smear of cervix
795.01	Papanicolaou smear of cervix with atypical squamous cells of undetermined significance (ASC-US)
795.02	Papanicolaou smear of cervix with atypical squamous cells cannot exclude high grade squamous intraepithelial lesion (ASC-H)
795.03	Papanicolaou smear of cervix with low grade squamous intraepithelial lesion (LGSIL)
795.04	Papanicolaou smear of cervix with high grade squamous intraepithelial lesion (HGSIL)
795.05	Cervical high risk human papillomavirus (HPV) DNA test positive

CCI Version 18.3

0213T, 0216T, 36000, 36410, 37202, 43752, 62318-62319, 64415-64417, 64450, 64490, 64493, 69990, 96360, 96365, 96372, 96374-96376

Note: These CCI edits are used for Medicare. Other payers may reimburse on codes listed above.

Medicare Edits

	Fac RVU	Non-Fac RVU	FUD	Status
58110	1.22	1.43	N/A	A

	MUE		Modifiers		
58110	1	N/A	N/A	N/A	80*

* with documentation

Medicare References: None

Corpus Uteri

58120

58120 Dilation and curettage, diagnostic and/or therapeutic (nonobstetrical)

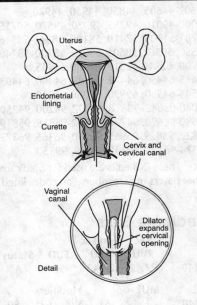

Labels on figure: Uterus; Endometrial lining; Curette; Cervix and cervical canal; Vaginal canal; Detail; Dilator expands cervical opening

Explanation

The physician inserts a speculum into the vagina to view the cervix. A tool is used to grasp the cervix and pull it down. A dilator is inserted into the endocervix and through the cervical canal to enlarge the opening. The physician places a curette in the endocervical canal and passes it into the uterus. The endometrial lining of the uterus is scraped on all sides for diagnostic or therapeutic purposes.

Coding Tips

This code includes a biopsy, single or multiple, whether being performed with a curette or another method. This procedure should not be separately identified when being used in conjunction with the hysterectomy procedures. When 58120 is performed with another separately identifiable procedure, the highest dollar value code is listed as the primary procedure and subsequent procedures are appended with modifier 51. Local anesthesia is included in this service. However, this procedure may be performed under general anesthesia, depending on the age and/or condition of the patient. For curettage due to postpartum hemorrhage, see 59160.

ICD-9-CM Procedural

69.09   Other dilation and curettage of uterus

Anesthesia

58120   00940, 01962

ICD-9-CM Diagnostic

180.0	Malignant neoplasm of endocervix
180.1	Malignant neoplasm of exocervix
180.8	Malignant neoplasm of other specified sites of cervix
180.9	Malignant neoplasm of cervix uteri, unspecified site
182.0	Malignant neoplasm of corpus uteri, except isthmus
182.1	Malignant neoplasm of isthmus
182.8	Malignant neoplasm of other specified sites of body of uterus
184.0	Malignant neoplasm of vagina
198.82	Secondary malignant neoplasm of genital organs
218.0	Submucous leiomyoma of uterus
218.1	Intramural leiomyoma of uterus
233.1	Carcinoma in situ of cervix uteri
233.2	Carcinoma in situ of other and unspecified parts of uterus
233.30	Carcinoma in situ, unspecified female genital organ
233.31	Carcinoma in situ, vagina
233.32	Carcinoma in situ, vulva
233.39	Carcinoma in situ, other female genital organ
236.0	Neoplasm of uncertain behavior of uterus
239.5	Neoplasm of unspecified nature of other genitourinary organs
615.1	Chronic inflammatory disease of uterus, except cervix — (Use additional code to identify organism: 041.00-041.09, 041.10-041.19)
616.0	Cervicitis and endocervicitis — (Use additional code to identify organism: 041.00-041.09, 041.10-041.19)
616.10	Unspecified vaginitis and vulvovaginitis — (Use additional code to identify organism, such as: 041.00-041.09, 041.10-041.19, 041.41-041.49)
617.0	Endometriosis of uterus
617.9	Endometriosis, site unspecified
621.0	Polyp of corpus uteri
621.2	Hypertrophy of uterus
621.31	Simple endometrial hyperplasia without atypia
621.32	Complex endometrial hyperplasia without atypia
621.33	Endometrial hyperplasia with atypia
621.34	Benign endometrial hyperplasia
621.35	Endometrial intraepithelial neoplasia [EIN]
621.8	Other specified disorders of uterus, not elsewhere classified
622.10	Dysplasia of cervix, unspecified
622.11	Mild dysplasia of cervix
622.12	Moderate dysplasia of cervix
622.4	Stricture and stenosis of cervix
622.7	Mucous polyp of cervix
623.8	Other specified noninflammatory disorder of vagina
625.0	Dyspareunia
625.3	Dysmenorrhea
625.8	Other specified symptom associated with female genital organs
626.0	Absence of menstruation
626.1	Scanty or infrequent menstruation
626.2	Excessive or frequent menstruation
626.3	Puberty bleeding
626.4	Irregular menstrual cycle
626.6	Metrorrhagia
626.8	Other disorder of menstruation and other abnormal bleeding from female genital tract
627.0	Premenopausal menorrhagia
627.1	Postmenopausal bleeding
628.9	Female infertility of unspecified origin
677	Late effect of complication of pregnancy, childbirth, and the puerperium — (Code first any sequelae)

CCI Version 18.3

0213T, 0216T, 0228T, 0230T, 12001-12007, 12011-12057, 13100-13153, 36000, 36400-36410, 36420-36430, 36440, 36600, 36640, 37202, 43752, 51701-51703, 57100, 57180, 57400-57410, 57452, 57500, 57530, 57800, 58100, 62310-62319, 64400-64435, 64445-64450, 64479, 64483, 64490, 64493, 64505-64530, 69990, 93000-93010, 93040-93042, 93318, 94002, 94200, 94250, 94680-94690, 94770, 95812-95816, 95819, 95822, 95829, 95955, 96360, 96365, 96372, 96374-96376, 99148-99149, 99150, J0670, J2001, P9612

Note: These CCI edits are used for Medicare. Other payers may reimburse on codes listed above.

Medicare Edits

	Fac RVU	Non-Fac RVU	FUD	Status
58120	6.5	7.63	10	A

	MUE		Modifiers		
58120	1	51	N/A	N/A	N/A

* with documentation

Medicare References: None

Coding Companion for Ob/Gyn

58140

58140 Myomectomy, excision of fibroid tumor(s) of uterus, 1 to 4 intramural myoma(s) with total weight of 250 g or less and/or removal of surface myomas; abdominal approach

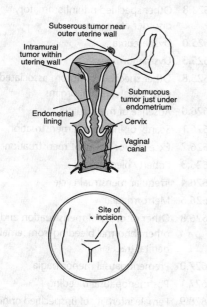

Subserous tumor near outer uterine wall
Intramural tumor within uterine wall
Submucous tumor just under endometrium
Endometrial lining
Cervix
Vaginal canal

Site of incision

Explanation

The physician removes one to four fibroid tumors from the wall of the uterus (intramural myomas) with a total weight of 250 gm or less and/or removes surface myomas by abdominal approach. A transverse incision is made in the abdomen, the anterior sheath of the rectus abdominis muscle is dissected, and muscles are retracted. Vasoconstrictors are injected and a tourniquet is applied to encompass the uterine mass and the adnexa to limit blood flow. A scalpel, electrocautery, and/or laser may be used to remove small surface myomas. The physician incises the uterus through the myometrium to expose the myoma, which is grasped with a clamp and dissected free from the surrounding myometrium with sharp and blunt dissection. The pedicle is isolated, clamped, and ligated and the myoma is dissected down to the pedicular blood supply. Other myomas are identified by palpating the uterine wall through the defect created by the already excised myoma. Adjacent myomas are reached and removed by tunneling further through the initial incision to avoid additional uterine trauma. The uterine wall defects are repaired by approximating the tissues to restore previous anatomy. The serosa is closed so as to minimize adhesion formation. Antiadhesion prophylaxis may be instilled in the abdominal cavity and the wound is closed.

Coding Tips

This code is often misused when the fibroid tumor is excised through laparoscopy or hysteroscopy. For removal of 5 or more intramural myomas with a total weight greater than 250 grams, see 58146. For the laparoscopic removal of intramural myomas, see 58545–58546. If removal of leiomyomata is performed through hysteroscopy, report 58561. If myomectomy is performed through a vaginal approach, see 58145.

ICD-9-CM Procedural

68.29   Other excision or destruction of lesion of uterus

Anesthesia

58140   00840

ICD-9-CM Diagnostic

218.0   Submucous leiomyoma of uterus
218.1   Intramural leiomyoma of uterus
218.2   Subserous leiomyoma of uterus
218.9   Leiomyoma of uterus, unspecified
V64.41 Laparoscopic surgical procedure converted to open procedure

Terms To Know

adhesion. Abnormal fibrous connection between two structures, soft tissue or bony structures, that may occur as the result of surgery, infection, or trauma.

approach. Method or anatomical location used to gain access to a body organ or specific area for procedures. The approach is not coded separately although it may be a specified component of the procedure, such as laparoscopic vs. incisional, or spinal procedures in which the amount of dissection required to expose the spine significantly alters with the site of approach.

defect. Imperfection, flaw, or absence.

intramural uterine leiomyoma. Benign, smooth muscle tumor within the wall of the uterus.

myometrium. Muscular middle layer of the uterine wall responsible for contractions associated with childbirth.

prophylaxis. Intervention or protective therapy intended to prevent a disease.

submucous uterine leiomyoma. Benign, smooth muscle tumor beneath the inner lining of the uterus.

subserous uterine leiomyoma. Benign, smooth muscle tumor beneath the serous membrane lining of the uterus.

CCI Version 18.3

0071T-0072T, 0213T, 0216T, 0228T, 0230T, 12001-12007, 12011-12057, 13100-13153, 36000, 36400-36410, 36420-36430, 36440, 36600, 36640, 37202, 43752, 44005, 44180, 44602-44605, 44850, 44950, 44970, 49000-49010, 49255, 49320, 49570, 50715, 51701-51703, 57410, 58100, 58545-58546, 58550, 58561, 58605, 58662, 58700, 58740, 58900, 62310-62319, 64400-64435, 64445-64450, 64479, 64483, 64490, 64493, 64505-64530, 69990, 93000-93010, 93040-93042, 93318, 94002, 94200, 94250, 94680-94690, 94770, 95812-95816, 95819, 95822, 95829, 95955, 96360, 96365, 96372, 96374-96376, 99148-99149, 99150

Note: These CCI edits are used for Medicare. Other payers may reimburse on codes listed above.

Medicare Edits

	Fac RVU	Non-Fac RVU	FUD	Status
58140	27.42	27.42	90	A

	MUE		Modifiers		
58140	1	51	N/A	62*	80

* with documentation

Medicare References: None

Corpus Uteri

58145

58145 Myomectomy, excision of fibroid tumor(s) of uterus, 1 to 4 intramural myoma(s) with total weight of 250 g or less and/or removal of surface myomas; vaginal approach

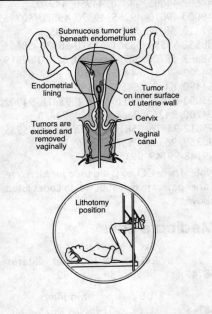

Submucous tumor just beneath endometrium

Endometrial lining

Tumor on inner surface of uterine wall

Tumors are excised and removed vaginally

Cervix

Vaginal canal

Lithotomy position

Explanation

The physician removes one to four fibroid tumors from the wall of the uterus (intramural myomas) with a total weight of 250 gm or less and/or removes surface myomas by vaginal approach. This approach is used for pedunculated myomas protruding through the cervix and prolapsed myomas. The cervix is dilated with laminaria to facilitate exposure and a tonsil snare or other appropriate device is passed through to reach the myoma. Prolapsed myomas are usually attached to the cervical or endometrial cavity by a stalk. The tumor is removed by ligating or twisting the stalk or a tonsil snare is employed to encircle the tumor, cut it from its stalk, and remove it. The instruments are then removed.

Coding Tips

Any manipulation or dilation of the vagina is not reported separately. This code is often misused when the fibroid tumor is excised through laparoscopy or hysteroscopy. For the laparoscopic removal of leiomyomata, see 58545 and 58546. If performed through hysteroscopy, report 58561. If myomectomy is performed through an abdominal approach, see 58140 and 58146.

ICD-9-CM Procedural

68.29 Other excision or destruction of lesion of uterus

Anesthesia

58145 00860, 00940

ICD-9-CM Diagnostic

218.0 Submucous leiomyoma of uterus
218.1 Intramural leiomyoma of uterus
218.2 Subserous leiomyoma of uterus
218.9 Leiomyoma of uterus, unspecified
V64.41 Laparoscopic surgical procedure converted to open procedure

Terms To Know

approach. Method or anatomical location used to gain access to a body organ or specific area for procedures. The approach is not coded separately although it may be a specified component of the procedure, such as laparoscopic vs. incisional, or spinal procedures in which the amount of dissection required to expose the spine significantly alters with the site of approach.

corpus uteri. Main body of the uterus, which is located above the isthmus and below the openings of the fallopian tubes.

dilation. Artificial increase in the diameter of an opening or lumen made by medication or by instrumentation.

endometrium. Lining of the uterus, which thickens in preparation for fertilization. A fertilized ovum embeds into the thickened endometrium. When no fertilization takes place, the endometrial lining sheds during the process of menstruation.

intramural uterine leiomyoma. Benign, smooth muscle tumor within the wall of the uterus.

ligate. To tie off a blood vessel or duct with a suture or a soft, thin wire (ligature wire).

myometrium. Muscular middle layer of the uterine wall responsible for contractions associated with childbirth.

parametrium. Connective tissue between the uterus and the broad ligament.

snare. Wire used as a loop to excise a polyp or lesion.

submucous uterine leiomyoma. Benign, smooth muscle tumor beneath the inner lining of the uterus.

CCI Version 18.3

0071T-0072T, 0213T, 0216T, 0228T, 0230T, 12001-12007, 12011-12057, 13100-13153, 36000, 36400-36410, 36420-36430, 36440, 36600, 36640, 37202, 43752, 50715, 51701-51703, 57410, 57420, 57452, 57500, 57800, 58100, 58120-58140, 58545-58546, 58561❖, 58605, 58662, 58700, 58900,

62310-62319, 64400-64435, 64445-64450, 64479, 64483, 64490, 64493, 64505-64530, 69990, 93000-93010, 93040-93042, 93318, 94002, 94200, 94250, 94680-94690, 94770, 95812-95816, 95819, 95822, 95829, 95955, 96360, 96365, 96372, 96374-96376, 99148-99149, 99150, P9612

Note: These CCI edits are used for Medicare. Other payers may reimburse on codes listed above.

Medicare Edits

	Fac RVU	Non-Fac RVU	FUD	Status
58145	16.24	16.24	90	A

	MUE		Modifiers		
58145	1	51	N/A	62*	80

* with documentation

Medicare References: None

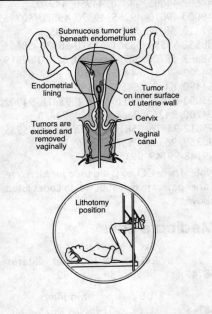

Coding Companion for Ob/Gyn

Corpus Uteri

58146

58146 Myomectomy, excision of fibroid tumor(s) of uterus, 5 or more intramural myomas and/or intramural myomas with total weight greater than 250 g, abdominal approach

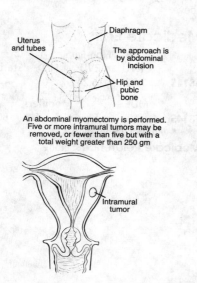

Uterus and tubes

Diaphragm

The approach is by abdominal incision

Hip and pubic bone

An abdominal myomectomy is performed. Five or more intramural tumors may be removed, or fewer than five but with a total weight greater than 250 gm

Intramural tumor

Explanation

The physician removes five or more fibroid tumors from the wall of the uterus and/or intramural myomas with a total weight greater than 250 gm by abdominal approach. A transverse incision is made in the abdomen (a midline incision is made for large myomas) and the anterior sheath of the rectus abdominis muscle is dissected and muscles are retracted. Vasoconstrictors are injected and a tourniquet is applied to encompass the uterine mass and the adnexa to limit blood flow. The physician incises the uterus down through the myometrium to expose the myoma, which is grasped with a clamp and dissected free from the surrounding myometrium with sharp and blunt dissection. For deep intramural myomas, the endometrial cavity may be exposed. The pedicle is isolated, clamped, and ligated and the myoma is dissected down to the pedicular blood supply. Other myomas are identified by palpating the uterine wall through the defect created by the already excised myoma. Adjacent myomas are reached and removed by tunneling further through the initial incision to avoid additional uterine trauma. The uterine wall defects are repaired by approximating the tissues to restore previous anatomy. The serosa is closed so as to minimize adhesion formation. Antiadhesion prophylaxis may be instilled in the abdominal cavity and the wound is closed.

Coding Tips

This code is often misused when fibroid tumors are excised through laparoscopy or hysteroscopy. For the laparoscopic removal of intramural myomas, see 58545–58546. If removal of leiomyomata is performed through a hysteroscope, see 58561. If myomectomy if performed through a vaginal approach, see 58145.

ICD-9-CM Procedural

68.29 Other excision or destruction of lesion of uterus

Anesthesia

58146 00840

ICD-9-CM Diagnostic

218.0 Submucous leiomyoma of uterus
218.1 Intramural leiomyoma of uterus
218.2 Subserous leiomyoma of uterus
218.9 Leiomyoma of uterus, unspecified
V64.41 Laparoscopic surgical procedure converted to open procedure

Terms To Know

approach. Method or anatomical location used to gain access to a body organ or specific area for procedures. The approach is not coded separately although it may be a specified component of the procedure, such as laparoscopic vs. incisional, or spinal procedures in which the amount of dissection required to expose the spine significantly alters with the site of approach.

defect. Imperfection, flaw, or absence.

dissect. Cut apart or separate tissue for surgical purposes or for visual or microscopic study.

intramural uterine leiomyoma. Benign, smooth muscle tumor within the wall of the uterus.

ligate. To tie off a blood vessel or duct with a suture or a soft, thin wire (ligature wire).

myometrium. Muscular middle layer of the uterine wall responsible for contractions associated with childbirth.

prophylaxis. Intervention or protective therapy intended to prevent a disease.

submucous uterine leiomyoma. Benign, smooth muscle tumor beneath the inner lining of the uterus.

subserous uterine leiomyoma. Benign, smooth muscle tumor beneath the serous membrane lining of the uterus.

transverse. Crosswise at right angles to the long axis of a structure or part.

CCI Version 18.3

0071T-0072T, 0213T, 0216T, 0228T, 0230T, 12001-12007, 12011-12057, 13100-13153, 36000, 36400-36410, 36420-36430, 36440, 36600, 36640, 37202, 43752, 44005, 44180, 44602-44605, 44850, 44950, 44970, 49000-49010, 49255, 49320, 49570, 50715, 57410, 58100, 58140-58145, 58550, 58552-58553, 58561, 58570-58572, 58605, 58662, 58700, 58740, 58900, 62310-62319, 64400-64435, 64445-64450, 64479, 64483, 64490, 64493, 64505-64530, 69990, 93000-93010, 93040-93042, 93318, 94002, 94200, 94250, 94680-94690, 94770, 95812-95816, 95819, 95822, 95829, 95955, 96360, 96365, 96372, 96374-96376, 99148-99149, 99150

Note: These CCI edits are used for Medicare. Other payers may reimburse on codes listed above.

Medicare Edits

	Fac RVU	Non-Fac RVU	FUD	Status
58146	34.5	34.5	90	A

	MUE		Modifiers		
58146	1	51	N/A	62*	80

* with documentation

Medicare References: None

Corpus Uteri

58150

58150 Total abdominal hysterectomy (corpus and cervix), with or without removal of tube(s), with or without removal of ovary(s);

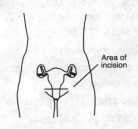

Area of incision

Surgeon may elect to leave any combination of tubes and ovaries

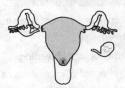

Explanation

Through a horizontal incision just within the pubic hairline, the physician removes the uterus including the cervix and may elect to remove one or both of the ovaries and one or both of the fallopian tubes (salpingo-oophorectomy). The supporting pedicles containing the tubes, ligaments, and arteries are clamped and cut free. The uterus and cervix are removed along with a narrow rim or cuff of vaginal lining. The vaginal defect may be left open for drainage. The abdominal incision is closed by suturing.

Coding Tips

If a colpo-urethrocystopexy (Marshall-Marchetti-Krantz type) is performed in conjunction with the total abdominal hysterectomy, report 58152.

ICD-9-CM Procedural

59.5	Retropubic urethral suspension
65.39	Other unilateral oophorectomy
65.49	Other unilateral salpingo-oophorectomy
65.51	Other removal of both ovaries at same operative episode
65.52	Other removal of remaining ovary
65.61	Other removal of both ovaries and tubes at same operative episode
65.62	Other removal of remaining ovary and tube

68.49	Other and unspecified total abdominal hysterectomy

Anesthesia
58150 00840

ICD-9-CM Diagnostic

180.0	Malignant neoplasm of endocervix
182.0	Malignant neoplasm of corpus uteri, except isthmus
182.1	Malignant neoplasm of isthmus
183.0	Malignant neoplasm of ovary — (Use additional code to identify any functional activity)
183.2	Malignant neoplasm of fallopian tube
198.6	Secondary malignant neoplasm of ovary
198.82	Secondary malignant neoplasm of genital organs
218.0	Submucous leiomyoma of uterus
218.1	Intramural leiomyoma of uterus
218.2	Subserous leiomyoma of uterus
233.1	Carcinoma in situ of cervix uteri
233.31	Carcinoma in situ, vagina
614.1	Chronic salpingitis and oophoritis — (Use additional code to identify organism: 041.00-041.09, 041.10-041.19)
614.2	Salpingitis and oophoritis not specified as acute, subacute, or chronic — (Use additional code to identify organism: 041.00-041.09, 041.10-041.19)
614.4	Chronic or unspecified parametritis and pelvic cellulitis — (Use additional code to identify organism: 041.00-041.09, 041.10-041.19)
614.5	Acute or unspecified pelvic peritonitis, female — (Use additional code to identify organism: 041.00-041.09, 041.10-041.19)
614.6	Pelvic peritoneal adhesions, female (postoperative) (postinfection) — (Use additional code to identify organism: 041.00-041.09, 041.10-041.19) (Use additional code to identify any associated infertility: 628.2)
617.0	Endometriosis of uterus
617.1	Endometriosis of ovary
617.2	Endometriosis of fallopian tube
617.3	Endometriosis of pelvic peritoneum
618.1	Uterine prolapse without mention of vaginal wall prolapse — (Use additional code to identify urinary incontinence: 625.6, 788.31, 788.33-788.39)

618.2	Uterovaginal prolapse, incomplete — (Use additional code to identify urinary incontinence: 625.6, 788.31, 788.33-788.39)
618.3	Uterovaginal prolapse, complete — (Use additional code to identify urinary incontinence: 625.6, 788.31, 788.33-788.39)
621.2	Hypertrophy of uterus
621.32	Complex endometrial hyperplasia without atypia
621.33	Endometrial hyperplasia with atypia
622.11	Mild dysplasia of cervix
622.12	Moderate dysplasia of cervix
625.3	Dysmenorrhea
625.5	Pelvic congestion syndrome
625.6	Female stress incontinence
626.2	Excessive or frequent menstruation
626.6	Metrorrhagia
627.1	Postmenopausal bleeding
677	Late effect of complication of pregnancy, childbirth, and the puerperium — (Code first any sequelae)
752.2	Congenital doubling of uterus

CCI Version 18.3

0071T-0072T, 01962-01963, 01969, 0213T, 0216T, 0228T, 0230T, 12001-12007, 12011-12057, 13100-13153, 36000, 36400-36410, 36420-36430, 36440, 36600, 36640, 37202, 43752, 44005, 44180, 44602-44605, 44850, 44950, 44970, 49000-49010, 49082-49084, 49180, 49255, 49320, 49322, 49560-49566, 49570, 50715, 51701-51703, 51840, 57410, 57522, 57540-57545, 58100, 58120-58146, 58180, 58353-58356, 58541-58543, 58545-58546, 58550, 58552-58554, 58558, 58570, 58660-58673, 58700-58740, 58805, 58822, 58900-58940, 62310-62319, 64400-64435, 64445-64450, 64479, 64483, 64490, 64493, 64505-64530, 69990, 93000-93010, 93040-93042, 93318, 94002, 94200, 94250, 94680-94690, 94770, 95812-95816, 95819, 95822, 95829, 95955, 96360, 96365, 96372, 96374-96376, 99148-99149, 99150, P9612

Note: These CCI edits are used for Medicare. Other payers may reimburse on codes listed above.

Medicare Edits

	Fac RVU	Non-Fac RVU	FUD	Status
58150	29.73	29.73	90	A

	MUE		Modifiers		
58150	1	51	N/A	62*	80

* with documentation

Medicare References: 100-3,230.3

Coding Companion for Ob/Gyn

Corpus Uteri

58152

58152 Total abdominal hysterectomy (corpus and cervix), with or without removal of tube(s), with or without removal of ovary(s); with colpo-urethrocystopexy (eg, Marshall-Marchetti-Krantz, Burch)

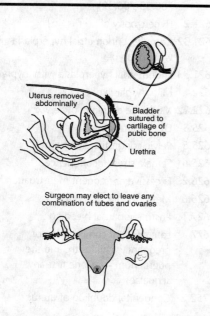

Uterus removed abdominally

Bladder sutured to cartilage of pubic bone

Urethra

Surgeon may elect to leave any combination of tubes and ovaries

Explanation

Through a horizontal incision just within the pubic hairline, the physician removes the uterus including the cervix and may elect to remove one or both of the ovaries and one or both of the fallopian tubes (salpingo-oophorectomy). The supporting pedicles containing the tubes, ligaments, and arteries are clamped and cut free. The uterus and cervix are removed. The bladder neck is suspended by placing sutures through the tissue surrounding the urethra and into the back of the symphysis pubis, which is the midline junction of the pubic bones in the front (Marshall-Marchetti-Krantz). The sutures are pulled tight so that the tissues are tacked to the symphysis pubis and the urethra is moved forward. The abdominal incision is closed by suturing.

Coding Tips

For a urethrocystopexy without hysterectomy, see 51840 and 51841.

ICD-9-CM Procedural

59.5	Retropubic urethral suspension
65.39	Other unilateral oophorectomy
65.49	Other unilateral salpingo-oophorectomy
65.51	Other removal of both ovaries at same operative episode
65.52	Other removal of remaining ovary
65.61	Other removal of both ovaries and tubes at same operative episode
65.62	Other removal of remaining ovary and tube
68.49	Other and unspecified total abdominal hysterectomy

Anesthesia

58152 00840

ICD-9-CM Diagnostic

180.0	Malignant neoplasm of endocervix
182.0	Malignant neoplasm of corpus uteri, except isthmus
182.1	Malignant neoplasm of isthmus
183.0	Malignant neoplasm of ovary — (Use additional code to identify any functional activity)
183.2	Malignant neoplasm of fallopian tube
198.6	Secondary malignant neoplasm of ovary
218.0	Submucous leiomyoma of uterus
218.1	Intramural leiomyoma of uterus
218.2	Subserous leiomyoma of uterus
233.1	Carcinoma in situ of cervix uteri
233.2	Carcinoma in situ of other and unspecified parts of uterus
233.30	Carcinoma in situ, unspecified female genital organ
614.1	Chronic salpingitis and oophoritis — (Use additional code to identify organism: 041.00-041.09, 041.10-041.19)
614.4	Chronic or unspecified parametritis and pelvic cellulitis — (Use additional code to identify organism: 041.00-041.09, 041.10-041.19)
614.5	Acute or unspecified pelvic peritonitis, female — (Use additional code to identify organism: 041.00-041.09, 041.10-041.19)
614.6	Pelvic peritoneal adhesions, female (postoperative) (postinfection) — (Use additional code to identify organism: 041.00-041.09, 041.10-041.19) (Use additional code to identify any associated infertility: 628.2)
617.0	Endometriosis of uterus
617.1	Endometriosis of ovary
617.2	Endometriosis of fallopian tube
617.3	Endometriosis of pelvic peritoneum
618.1	Uterine prolapse without mention of vaginal wall prolapse — (Use additional code to identify urinary incontinence: 625.6, 788.31, 788.33-788.39)
618.2	Uterovaginal prolapse, incomplete — (Use additional code to identify urinary incontinence: 625.6, 788.31, 788.33-788.39)
618.3	Uterovaginal prolapse, complete — (Use additional code to identify urinary incontinence: 625.6, 788.31, 788.33-788.39)
621.2	Hypertrophy of uterus
621.32	Complex endometrial hyperplasia without atypia
621.33	Endometrial hyperplasia with atypia
622.11	Mild dysplasia of cervix
622.12	Moderate dysplasia of cervix
625.6	Female stress incontinence
626.2	Excessive or frequent menstruation
626.6	Metrorrhagia
627.1	Postmenopausal bleeding
677	Late effect of complication of pregnancy, childbirth, and the puerperium — (Code first any sequelae)
752.2	Congenital doubling of uterus

CCI Version 18.3

0071T-0072T, 01962-01963, 01969, 0213T, 0216T, 0228T, 0230T, 12001-12007, 12011-12057, 13100-13153, 36000, 36400-36410, 36420-36430, 36440, 36600, 36640, 37202, 43752, 44005, 44180, 44602-44605, 44850, 44950, 44970, 49000-49010, 49082-49084, 49255, 49320, 49322, 49560-49566, 49570, 50715, 51701-51703, 51840-51841, 57284, 57410, 57423, 57500, 57522-57530, 57540-57545, 58100, 58120-58150, 58180, 58353-58356, 58541-58546, 58550, 58552-58554, 58558, 58570-58572❖, 58660, 58662, 58700-58740, 58805, 58900, 58925-58940, 62310-62319, 64400-64435, 64445-64450, 64479, 64483, 64490, 64493, 64505-64530, 69990, 93000-93010, 93040-93042, 93318, 94002, 94200, 94250, 94680-94690, 94770, 95812-95816, 95819, 95822, 95829, 95955, 96360, 96365, 96372, 96374-96376, 99148-99149, 99150, P9612

Note: These CCI edits are used for Medicare. Other payers may reimburse on codes listed above.

Medicare Edits

	Fac RVU	Non-Fac RVU	FUD	Status
58152	37.23	37.23	90	A

	MUE			Modifiers	
58152	1	51	N/A	62*	80

* with documentation

Medicare References: 100-3,230.3

Corpus Uteri

58180

58180 Supracervical abdominal hysterectomy (subtotal hysterectomy), with or without removal of tube(s), with or without removal of ovary(s)

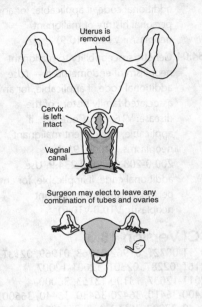

Uterus is removed

Cervix is left intact

Vaginal canal

Surgeon may elect to leave any combination of tubes and ovaries

Explanation

Through a horizontal incision just within the pubic hairline, the physician removes the uterus above the cervix and may elect to remove one or both of the ovaries and one or both of the fallopian tubes (salpingo-oophorectomy). The supporting pedicles containing the tubes, ligaments, and arteries are clamped and cut free. The uterus is cut free from the cervix leaving the cervix still attached to the vagina. The abdominal incision is closed by suturing.

Coding Tips

When 58180 is performed with another separately identifiable procedure, the highest dollar value code is listed as the primary procedure and subsequent procedures are appended with modifier 51. For excision of a remaining cervical stump, see 57540–57556.

ICD-9-CM Procedural

65.39 Other unilateral oophorectomy

65.49 Other unilateral salpingo-oophorectomy

65.51 Other removal of both ovaries at same operative episode

65.52 Other removal of remaining ovary

65.61 Other removal of both ovaries and tubes at same operative episode

65.62 Other removal of remaining ovary and tube

68.39 Other and unspecified subtotal abdominal hysterectomy

Anesthesia

58180 00840, 01962

ICD-9-CM Diagnostic

182.0 Malignant neoplasm of corpus uteri, except isthmus

182.1 Malignant neoplasm of isthmus

182.8 Malignant neoplasm of other specified sites of body of uterus

183.8 Malignant neoplasm of other specified sites of uterine adnexa

183.9 Malignant neoplasm of uterine adnexa, unspecified site

184.8 Malignant neoplasm of other specified sites of female genital organs

218.0 Submucous leiomyoma of uterus

218.1 Intramural leiomyoma of uterus

218.2 Subserous leiomyoma of uterus

219.1 Benign neoplasm of corpus uteri

219.9 Benign neoplasm of uterus, part unspecified

236.0 Neoplasm of uncertain behavior of uterus

236.3 Neoplasm of uncertain behavior of other and unspecified female genital organs

239.5 Neoplasm of unspecified nature of other genitourinary organs

617.0 Endometriosis of uterus

617.1 Endometriosis of ovary

617.2 Endometriosis of fallopian tube

618.1 Uterine prolapse without mention of vaginal wall prolapse — (Use additional code to identify urinary incontinence: 625.6, 788.31, 788.33-788.39)

625.3 Dysmenorrhea

626.8 Other disorder of menstruation and other abnormal bleeding from female genital tract

677 Late effect of complication of pregnancy, childbirth, and the puerperium — (Code first any sequelae)

V84.02 Genetic susceptibility to malignant neoplasm of ovary — (Use additional code, if applicable, for any associated family history of the disease: V16-V19. Code first, if applicable, any current malignant neoplasms: 140.0-195.8, 200.0-208.9, 230.0-234.9. Use additional code, if applicable, for any personal history of malignant neoplasm: V10.0-V10.9)

V84.04 Genetic susceptibility to malignant neoplasm of endometrium — (Use additional code, if applicable, for any associated family history of the disease: V16-V19. Code first, if applicable, any current malignant neoplasms: 140.0-195.8, 200.0-208.9, 230.0-234.9. Use additional code, if applicable, for any personal history of malignant neoplasm: V10.0-V10.9)

Terms To Know

submucous uterine leiomyoma. Benign, smooth muscle tumor beneath the inner lining of the uterus.

subserous uterine leiomyoma. Benign, smooth muscle tumor beneath the serous membrane lining of the uterus.

CCI Version 18.3

0071T-0072T, 01962-01963, 01969, 0213T, 0216T, 0228T, 0230T, 12001-12007, 12011-12057, 13100-13153, 36000, 36400-36410, 36420-36430, 36440, 36600, 36640, 37202, 43752, 44005, 44180, 44602-44605, 44850, 44950, 44970, 49000-49010, 49082-49084, 49255, 49320, 49322, 49560-49566, 49570, 50715, 51701-51703, 57410, 57522-57530, 57540-57545, 58100, 58120-58146, 58353-58356, 58541❖, 58545-58546, 58550, 58552-58554, 58558, 58570❖, 58660-58673, 58700-58740, 58805, 58900-58940, 62310-62319, 64400-64435, 64445-64450, 64479, 64483, 64490, 64493, 64505-64530, 69990, 93000-93010, 93040-93042, 93318, 94002, 94200, 94250, 94680-94690, 94770, 95812-95816, 95819, 95822, 95829, 95955, 96360, 96365, 96372, 96374-96376, 99148-99149, 99150, P9612

Note: These CCI edits are used for Medicare. Other payers may reimburse on codes listed above.

Medicare Edits

	Fac RVU	Non-Fac RVU	FUD	Status
58180	28.55	28.55	90	A

	MUE			Modifiers		
58180	1	51	N/A	62*	80

* with documentation

Medicare References: 100-3,230.3

Corpus Uteri

58200

58200 Total abdominal hysterectomy, including partial vaginectomy, with para-aortic and pelvic lymph node sampling, with or without removal of tube(s), with or without removal of ovary(s)

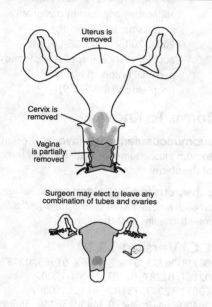

Uterus is removed

Cervix is removed

Vagina is partially removed

Surgeon may elect to leave any combination of tubes and ovaries

Explanation

Through a horizontal incision just within the pubic hairline, the physician removes the uterus, including the cervix and part of the vagina. The supporting pedicles containing the tubes, ligaments and arteries are clamped and cut free and the uterus, cervix, and part of the vagina are removed. A biopsy is taken of the para-aortic and pelvic lymph nodes. The physician may elect to remove one or both of the ovaries and one or both of the fallopian tubes (salpingo-oophorectomy). The abdominal incision is closed by suturing.

Coding Tips

Removal of the tubes and ovaries is included in this procedure and should not be reported separately. For a hysterectomy with pelvic lymphadenectomy, report 58210. Several hysterectomy codes exist, see 58150–58285 for open procedures and 58550–58554 for a laparoscopic vaginal hysterectomy.

ICD-9-CM Procedural

40.11 Biopsy of lymphatic structure
65.39 Other unilateral oophorectomy
65.49 Other unilateral salpingo-oophorectomy
65.51 Other removal of both ovaries at same operative episode
65.52 Other removal of remaining ovary

65.61 Other removal of both ovaries and tubes at same operative episode
65.62 Other removal of remaining ovary and tube
68.49 Other and unspecified total abdominal hysterectomy
70.8 Obliteration of vaginal vault

Anesthesia
58200 00840, 00846

ICD-9-CM Diagnostic

179 Malignant neoplasm of uterus, part unspecified
180.0 Malignant neoplasm of endocervix
180.1 Malignant neoplasm of exocervix
180.8 Malignant neoplasm of other specified sites of cervix
182.0 Malignant neoplasm of corpus uteri, except isthmus
182.1 Malignant neoplasm of isthmus
182.8 Malignant neoplasm of other specified sites of body of uterus
183.0 Malignant neoplasm of ovary — (Use additional code to identify any functional activity)
183.2 Malignant neoplasm of fallopian tube
183.3 Malignant neoplasm of broad ligament of uterus
183.4 Malignant neoplasm of parametrium of uterus
183.5 Malignant neoplasm of round ligament of uterus
183.8 Malignant neoplasm of other specified sites of uterine adnexa
184.0 Malignant neoplasm of vagina
184.8 Malignant neoplasm of other specified sites of female genital organs
196.2 Secondary and unspecified malignant neoplasm of intra-abdominal lymph nodes
196.6 Secondary and unspecified malignant neoplasm of intrapelvic lymph nodes
196.8 Secondary and unspecified malignant neoplasm of lymph nodes of multiple sites
198.82 Secondary malignant neoplasm of genital organs
209.74 Secondary neuroendocrine tumor of peritoneum
233.1 Carcinoma in situ of cervix uteri
236.0 Neoplasm of uncertain behavior of uterus
236.2 Neoplasm of uncertain behavior of ovary — (Use additional code to identify any functional activity)

V84.02 Genetic susceptibility to malignant neoplasm of ovary — (Use additional code, if applicable, for any associated family history of the disease: V16-V19. Code first, if applicable, any current malignant neoplasms: 140.0-195.8, 200.0-208.9, 230.0-234.9. Use additional code, if applicable, for any personal history of malignant neoplasm: V10.0-V10.9)
V84.04 Genetic susceptibility to malignant neoplasm of endometrium — (Use additional code, if applicable, for any associated family history of the disease: V16-V19. Code first, if applicable, any current malignant neoplasms: 140.0-195.8, 200.0-208.9, 230.0-234.9. Use additional code, if applicable, for any personal history of malignant neoplasm: V10.0-V10.9)

CCI Version 18.3

0071T-0072T, 01962-01963, 01969, 0213T, 0216T, 0228T, 0230T, 12001-12007, 12011-12057, 13100-13153, 36000, 36400-36410, 36420-36430, 36440, 36600, 36640, 37202, 38562, 43752, 44005, 44180, 44602-44605, 44820-44850, 44950, 44970, 49000-49010, 49082-49084, 49203, 49255, 49320, 49322, 49560-49566, 49570, 50715, 51701-51703, 51840, 57105-57107, 57109-57112, 57410, 57522-57530, 57540-57545, 58100, 58120-58180, 58260-58263, 58267-58280, 58290-58294, 58353-58356, 58541-58546, 58550, 58552-58554, 58558, 58570-58573❖, 58660-58673, 58700-58740, 58805, 58822, 58900-58940, 58943, 62310-62319, 64400-64435, 64445-64450, 64479, 64483, 64490, 64493, 64505-64530, 69990, 93000-93010, 93040-93042, 93318, 94002, 94200, 94250, 94680-94690, 94770, 95812-95816, 95819, 95822, 95829, 95955, 96360, 96365, 96372, 96374-96376, 99148-99149, 99150, P9612

Note: These CCI edits are used for Medicare. Other payers may reimburse on codes listed above.

Medicare Edits

	Fac RVU	Non-Fac RVU	FUD	Status
58200	39.23	39.23	90	A

	MUE		Modifiers	
58200	1	51	N/A 62*	80

* with documentation
Medicare References: 100-3,230.3

Corpus Uteri

58210

58210 Radical abdominal hysterectomy, with bilateral total pelvic lymphadenectomy and para-aortic lymph node sampling (biopsy), with or without removal of tube(s), with or without removal of ovary(s)

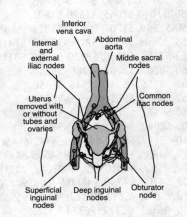

Inferior vena cava
Internal and external iliac nodes
Abdominal aorta
Middle sacral nodes
Uterus removed with or without tubes and ovaries
Common iliac nodes
Superficial inguinal nodes
Deep inguinal nodes
Obturator node

Explanation

Through a horizontal incision just within the pubic hairline, the physician removes the uterus, including the cervix and the pelvic lymph nodes on both sides and takes a biopsy of the para-aortic lymph nodes. The supporting pedicles containing the tubes, ligaments, and arteries are clamped and cut free and the uterus, cervix, all or part of the vagina, and all pelvic lymph nodes are removed. The physician may elect to remove one or both of the ovaries and one or both of the fallopian tubes (salpingo-oophorectomy). The abdominal incision is closed by suturing.

Coding Tips

For total abdominal hysterectomy with or without removal of a tube(s) and/or ovary(s), see 58150. For ovarian transposition, report 58825. Several hysterectomy codes exist; see 58150–58240 for abdominal procedures, 58260–58294 for vaginal procedures, and 58550–58554 for a laparoscopic vaginal hysterectomy.

ICD-9-CM Procedural

- 40.11 Biopsy of lymphatic structure
- 40.3 Regional lymph node excision
- 40.59 Radical excision of other lymph nodes
- 65.39 Other unilateral oophorectomy
- 65.49 Other unilateral salpingo-oophorectomy
- 65.51 Other removal of both ovaries at same operative episode
- 65.52 Other removal of remaining ovary
- 65.61 Other removal of both ovaries and tubes at same operative episode
- 65.62 Other removal of remaining ovary and tube
- 68.69 Other and unspecified radical abdominal hysterectomy

Anesthesia

58210 00846

ICD-9-CM Diagnostic

- 179 Malignant neoplasm of uterus, part unspecified
- 180.0 Malignant neoplasm of endocervix
- 180.1 Malignant neoplasm of exocervix
- 180.8 Malignant neoplasm of other specified sites of cervix
- 182.0 Malignant neoplasm of corpus uteri, except isthmus
- 182.1 Malignant neoplasm of isthmus
- 182.8 Malignant neoplasm of other specified sites of body of uterus
- 183.0 Malignant neoplasm of ovary — (Use additional code to identify any functional activity)
- 183.2 Malignant neoplasm of fallopian tube
- 183.3 Malignant neoplasm of broad ligament of uterus
- 183.4 Malignant neoplasm of parametrium of uterus
- 183.5 Malignant neoplasm of round ligament of uterus
- 183.8 Malignant neoplasm of other specified sites of uterine adnexa
- 183.9 Malignant neoplasm of uterine adnexa, unspecified site
- 184.0 Malignant neoplasm of vagina
- 184.8 Malignant neoplasm of other specified sites of female genital organs
- 196.2 Secondary and unspecified malignant neoplasm of intra-abdominal lymph nodes
- 196.6 Secondary and unspecified malignant neoplasm of intrapelvic lymph nodes
- 196.8 Secondary and unspecified malignant neoplasm of lymph nodes of multiple sites
- 198.82 Secondary malignant neoplasm of genital organs
- 209.74 Secondary neuroendocrine tumor of peritoneum
- 233.1 Carcinoma in situ of cervix uteri
- 236.0 Neoplasm of uncertain behavior of uterus
- 236.2 Neoplasm of uncertain behavior of ovary — (Use additional code to identify any functional activity)
- 238.8 Neoplasm of uncertain behavior of other specified sites
- 239.5 Neoplasm of unspecified nature of other genitourinary organs
- 239.89 Neoplasms of unspecified nature, other specified sites
- V84.09 Genetic susceptibility to other malignant neoplasm — (Use additional code, if applicable, for any associated family history of the disease: V16-V19. Code first, if applicable, any current malignant neoplasms: 140.0-195.8, 200.0-208.9, 230.0-234.9. Use additional code, if applicable, for any personal history of malignant neoplasm: V10.0-V10.9)

CCI Version 18.3

0071T-0072T, 01962-01963, 01969, 0213T, 0216T, 0228T, 0230T, 12001-12007, 12011-12057, 13100-13153, 36000, 36400-36410, 36420-36430, 36440, 36600, 36640, 37202, 38562, 38570-38572, 38770, 38780, 43752, 44005, 44180, 44602-44605, 44820-44850, 44950, 44970, 49000-49010, 49082-49084, 49180, 49203-49205, 49255, 49320, 49322, 49560-49566, 49570, 50715, 51040, 51701-51703, 57106-57107, 57109-57112, 57410, 57522-57545, 58100, 58120-58150, 58353-58356, 58541-58550, 58552-58554, 58558, 58570-58573❖, 58660-58673, 58700-58740, 58805, 58822, 58900-58940, 58943, 62310-62319, 64400-64435, 64445-64450, 64479, 64483, 64490, 64493, 64505-64530, 69990, 93000-93010, 93040-93042, 93318, 94002, 94200, 94250, 94680-94690, 94770, 95812-95816, 95819, 95822, 95829, 95955, 96360, 96365, 96372, 96374-96376, 99148-99149, 99150, P9612

Note: These CCI edits are used for Medicare. Other payers may reimburse on codes listed above.

Medicare Edits

	Fac RVU	Non-Fac RVU	FUD	Status
58210	52.55	52.55	90	A

	MUE		Modifiers		
58210	1	51	N/A	62*	80

* with documentation

Medicare References: 100-3,230.3

Corpus Uteri

58240

58240 Pelvic exenteration for gynecologic malignancy, with total abdominal hysterectomy or cervicectomy, with or without removal of tube(s), with or without removal of ovary(s), with removal of bladder and ureteral transplantations, and/or abdominoperineal resection of rectum and colon and colostomy, or any combination thereof

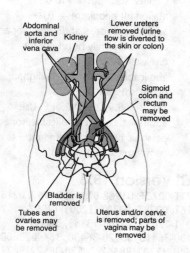

Abdominal aorta and inferior vena cava
Kidney
Lower ureters removed (urine flow is diverted to the skin or colon)
Sigmoid colon and rectum may be removed
Bladder is removed
Tubes and ovaries may be removed
Uterus and/or cervix is removed; parts of vagina may be removed

Explanation

Through a horizontal incision just within the pubic hairline, the physician removes all of the organs and adjacent structures of the pelvis including the cervix, uterus, and all or part of the vagina. The supporting pedicles containing the tubes, ligaments, and arteries are clamped and cut free and the uterus, cervix, and all or part of the vagina are removed. The physician may remove one or both of the ovaries and one or both of the fallopian tubes (salpingo-oophorectomy). The physician removes the bladder and diverts urine flow by transplanting the ureters to the skin or colon. The rectum and part of the colon may be removed and an artificial abdominal opening in the skin surface created for waste (colostomy). The abdominal incision is closed by suturing.

Coding Tips

Report 51597 for a pelvic exenteration for malignancy of the lower urinary tract. Check diagnoses carefully to ensure metastases are reported correctly.

ICD-9-CM Procedural

40.3	Regional lymph node excision
40.59	Radical excision of other lymph nodes
46.13	Permanent colostomy
56.61	Formation of other cutaneous ureterostomy
68.8	Pelvic evisceration

Anesthesia

58240 00848

ICD-9-CM Diagnostic

179	Malignant neoplasm of uterus, part unspecified
180.0	Malignant neoplasm of endocervix
180.1	Malignant neoplasm of exocervix
180.8	Malignant neoplasm of other specified sites of cervix
182.0	Malignant neoplasm of corpus uteri, except isthmus
182.1	Malignant neoplasm of isthmus
182.8	Malignant neoplasm of other specified sites of body of uterus
183.0	Malignant neoplasm of ovary — (Use additional code to identify any functional activity)
183.2	Malignant neoplasm of fallopian tube
183.3	Malignant neoplasm of broad ligament of uterus
183.4	Malignant neoplasm of parametrium of uterus
183.5	Malignant neoplasm of round ligament of uterus
183.8	Malignant neoplasm of other specified sites of uterine adnexa
183.9	Malignant neoplasm of uterine adnexa, unspecified site
184.0	Malignant neoplasm of vagina
184.8	Malignant neoplasm of other specified sites of female genital organs
184.9	Malignant neoplasm of female genital organ, site unspecified
197.5	Secondary malignant neoplasm of large intestine and rectum
198.1	Secondary malignant neoplasm of other urinary organs
198.6	Secondary malignant neoplasm of ovary
198.82	Secondary malignant neoplasm of genital organs
199.0	Disseminated malignant neoplasm

CCI Version 18.3

0071T-0072T, 0213T, 0216T, 0226T, 0228T, 0230T, 0249T, 0288T, 12001-12007, 12011-12057, 13100-13153, 36000, 36400-36410, 36420-36430, 36440, 36600, 36640, 37202, 38562-38564, 38571-38572, 38770, 38780, 43752, 44005, 44140-44151, 44155-44158, 44180, 44188, 44320-44346, 44602-44605, 44620-44625, 44820-44850, 44950-44970, 45110-45123, 45130-45135, 45160, 45171-45172, 45190, 45395-45397, 45505, 45540, 46080-46200, 46220-46280, 46285, 46600, 46940-46942, 46947, 49000-49020, 49040, 49082-49084, 49203-49205, 49255, 49320, 49322, 49560-49566, 49570, 49580, 49582-49587, 50650, 50715, 50800, 50810-50815, 50820, 50860, 51040-51045, 51520-51525, 51550-51596, 51701-51703, 55821-55845, 55866, 57106-57107, 57109-57112, 57410, 57522-57556, 58100, 58120-58200, 58210, 58260-58263, 58267-58280, 58290-58294, 58353-58356, 58541-58546, 58550, 58552-58554, 58558, 58570-58573❖, 58660-58673, 58700-58740, 58805, 58822, 58900-58940, 58943, 58950-58958, 62310-62319, 64400-64435, 64445-64450, 64479, 64483, 64490, 64493, 64505-64530, 69990, 93000-93010, 93040-93042, 93318, 94002, 94200, 94250, 94680-94690, 94770, 95812-95816, 95819, 95822, 95829, 95955, 96360, 96365, 96372, 96374-96376, 99148-99149, 99150, P9612

Note: These CCI edits are used for Medicare. Other payers may reimburse on codes listed above.

Medicare Edits

	Fac RVU	Non-Fac RVU	FUD	Status
58240	83.37	83.37	90	A

	MUE		Modifiers		
58240	1	51	N/A	62*	80

* with documentation

Medicare References: 100-3,230.3

58260

58260 Vaginal hysterectomy, for uterus 250 g or less;

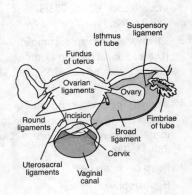

Explanation

The physician performs a vaginal hysterectomy for a uterus 250 gm or less. An incision is made around the cervix through the full thickness of the vaginal membrane. The cut vaginal edge is pulled toward the lower cervix and vaginal dissection is continued with countertraction. The posterior peritoneum is opened to admit a finger examination of the pelvis. The uterosacral ligaments are clamped and possibly shortened, cut from the uterus, and secured to the vagina. The vesicovaginal space is entered. The connective tissue fusing the bladder and vagina is dissected and the bladder is separated from the cervix. The bladder pillars are clamped, cut, and ligated near their cervical attachments, as well as the cardinal ligament tissue on each side of the cervix and the left and right uterine vessels. The physician clamps, cuts, and ligates the upper cardinal and lower broad ligament complex. Traction applied to the cervix moves the uterus down until the fundus is low in the pelvis. Hemostats are applied to the angle of the uterus on each side and the uterus is removed. The peritoneum is closed with purse-string sutures that incorporate the proximal part of the uterosacral ligaments.

Coding Tips

This code includes a hysterectomy for a uterus of 250 grams or less only. See 58262–58263 when the tubes and ovaries are also removed. For other vaginal hysterectomy codes, see 58262–58285. For vaginal hysterectomy for a uterus greater than 250 grams, see

58290–58294. For laparoscopy with vaginal hysterectomy for a uterus 250 grams or less, see 58550.

ICD-9-CM Procedural

68.59   Other and unspecified vaginal hysterectomy

Anesthesia

58260   00944

ICD-9-CM Diagnostic

180.0   Malignant neoplasm of endocervix
180.1   Malignant neoplasm of exocervix
180.8   Malignant neoplasm of other specified sites of cervix
181   Malignant neoplasm of placenta
182.0   Malignant neoplasm of corpus uteri, except isthmus
182.1   Malignant neoplasm of isthmus
182.8   Malignant neoplasm of other specified sites of body of uterus
183.0   Malignant neoplasm of ovary — (Use additional code to identify any functional activity)
198.6   Secondary malignant neoplasm of ovary
218.0   Submucous leiomyoma of uterus
218.1   Intramural leiomyoma of uterus
218.2   Subserous leiomyoma of uterus
218.9   Leiomyoma of uterus, unspecified
233.1   Carcinoma in situ of cervix uteri
233.31   Carcinoma in situ, vagina
614.4   Chronic or unspecified parametritis and pelvic cellulitis — (Use additional code to identify organism: 041.00-041.09, 041.10-041.19)
617.0   Endometriosis of uterus
618.00   Unspecified prolapse of vaginal walls without mention of uterine prolapse — (Use additional code to identify urinary incontinence: 625.6, 788.31, 788.33-788.39)
618.1   Uterine prolapse without mention of vaginal wall prolapse — (Use additional code to identify urinary incontinence: 625.6, 788.31, 788.33-788.39)
618.3   Uterovaginal prolapse, complete — (Use additional code to identify urinary incontinence: 625.6, 788.31, 788.33-788.39)
618.6   Vaginal enterocele, congenital or acquired — (Use additional code to identify urinary incontinence: 625.6, 788.31, 788.33-788.39)
621.2   Hypertrophy of uterus

621.30   Endometrial hyperplasia, unspecified
621.6   Malposition of uterus
622.10   Dysplasia of cervix, unspecified
625.3   Dysmenorrhea
625.6   Female stress incontinence
626.2   Excessive or frequent menstruation
626.6   Metrorrhagia
627.1   Postmenopausal bleeding
677   Late effect of complication of pregnancy, childbirth, and the puerperium — (Code first any sequelae)
788.33   Mixed incontinence urge and stress (male)(female) — (Code, if applicable, any causal condition first: 600.0-600.9, with fifth digit 1; 618.00-618.9; 753.23)

CCI Version 18.3

0071T-0072T, 01962-01963, 01969, 0213T, 0216T, 0228T, 0230T, 12001-12007, 12011-12057, 13100-13153, 36000, 36400-36410, 36420-36430, 36440, 36600, 36640, 37202, 43752, 50715, 51040, 51701-51703, 57106, 57180, 57268, 57410, 57420, 57452, 57500, 57522-57530, 57550, 57800, 58100, 58120-58146, 58280❖, 58353-58356, 58545-58546, 58550, 58552, 58554, 58558, 58660, 58662, 58720, 62310-62319, 64400-64435, 64445-64450, 64479, 64483, 64490, 64493, 64505-64530, 69990, 93000-93010, 93040-93042, 93318, 94002, 94200, 94250, 94680-94690, 94770, 95812-95816, 95819, 95822, 95829, 95955, 96360, 96365, 96372, 96374-96376, 99148-99149, 99150, P9612

Note: These CCI edits are used for Medicare. Other payers may reimburse on codes listed above.

Medicare Edits

	Fac RVU	Non-Fac RVU	FUD	Status
58260	24.69	24.69	90	A

	MUE			Modifiers	
58260	1	51	N/A	62*	80

* with documentation

Medicare References: 100-3, 230.3

Coding Companion for Ob/Gyn

58262

58262 Vaginal hysterectomy, for uterus 250 g or less; with removal of tube(s), and/or ovary(s)

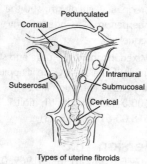
Types of uterine fibroids

Explanation

The physician performs a vaginal hysterectomy for a uterus 250 gm or less and removes the tubes and/or ovaries. An incision is made around the cervix through the full thickness of the vaginal membrane. The cut vaginal edge is pulled toward the lower cervix and vaginal dissection is continued with countertraction. The posterior peritoneum is opened to admit a finger examination of the pelvis. The uterosacral ligaments are clamped and possibly shortened, cut from the uterus, and secured to the vagina. The vesicovaginal space is entered. The connective tissue fusing the bladder and vagina is dissected and the bladder is separated from the cervix. The bladder pillars are clamped, cut, and ligated near their cervical attachments, as well as the cardinal ligament tissue on each side of the cervix and the left and right uterine vessels. The physician clamps, cuts, and ligates the upper cardinal and lower broad ligament complex. Traction applied to the cervix moves the uterus down until the fundus is low in the pelvis. Hemostats are applied to the angle of the uterus on each side and the uterus is removed. After the uterus is exteriorized, care is taken to ensure ligation of the ovarian vessels. The ovary is excised under direct vision. For removal of both tubes and ovaries, the round ligament on one side at a time is clamped and divided. A tunnel is made through the layers of the uterine broad ligament that enclose the tube and the tube and ovary are clamped together. The structure

is pulled forward, the two sheets of the broad ligament are each cut, and the broad ligament is opened completely. The whole specimen is separated from its attaching ligament, which is clamped, and the tube and ovary on that side are removed. The peritoneal and vaginal wall incisions of the hysterectomy procedure are closed.

Coding Tips

This code includes removal of the tubes and ovaries and should not be reported separately. For hysterectomy only, see 58260. For other vaginal hysterectomy codes, see 58263–58294. For laparoscopic vaginal hysterectomy of a uterus 250 gm or less, with removal of tube(s) and/or ovary(ies), report 58552.

ICD-9-CM Procedural

65.39	Other unilateral oophorectomy
65.49	Other unilateral salpingo-oophorectomy
65.51	Other removal of both ovaries at same operative episode
65.52	Other removal of remaining ovary
65.61	Other removal of both ovaries and tubes at same operative episode
65.62	Other removal of remaining ovary and tube
68.59	Other and unspecified vaginal hysterectomy

Anesthesia

58262 00944

ICD-9-CM Diagnostic

180.0	Malignant neoplasm of endocervix
180.1	Malignant neoplasm of exocervix
181	Malignant neoplasm of placenta
182.0	Malignant neoplasm of corpus uteri, except isthmus
182.1	Malignant neoplasm of isthmus
183.0	Malignant neoplasm of ovary — (Use additional code to identify any functional activity)
183.8	Malignant neoplasm of other specified sites of uterine adnexa
218.0	Submucous leiomyoma of uterus
218.1	Intramural leiomyoma of uterus
218.2	Subserous leiomyoma of uterus
233.1	Carcinoma in situ of cervix uteri
614.4	Chronic or unspecified parametritis and pelvic cellulitis — (Use additional code to identify organism: 041.00-041.09, 041.10-041.19)
617.0	Endometriosis of uterus

618.00	Unspecified prolapse of vaginal walls without mention of uterine prolapse — (Use additional code to identify urinary incontinence: 625.6, 788.31, 788.33-788.39)
618.1	Uterine prolapse without mention of vaginal wall prolapse — (Use additional code to identify urinary incontinence: 625.6, 788.31, 788.33-788.39)
618.3	Uterovaginal prolapse, complete — (Use additional code to identify urinary incontinence: 625.6, 788.31, 788.33-788.39)
618.6	Vaginal enterocele, congenital or acquired — (Use additional code to identify urinary incontinence: 625.6, 788.31, 788.33-788.39)
621.0	Polyp of corpus uteri
621.2	Hypertrophy of uterus
621.30	Endometrial hyperplasia, unspecified
621.6	Malposition of uterus
622.10	Dysplasia of cervix, unspecified
625.3	Dysmenorrhea
625.6	Female stress incontinence
626.2	Excessive or frequent menstruation
627.1	Postmenopausal bleeding

CCI Version 18.3

0071T-0072T, 01962-01963, 01969, 0213T, 0216T, 0228T, 0230T, 12001-12007, 12011-12057, 13100-13153, 36000, 36400-36410, 36420-36430, 36440, 36600, 36640, 37202, 43752, 49322, 50715, 51040, 51701-51703, 57180, 57410, 57420, 57452, 57500, 57522-57530, 57550, 57800, 58100, 58120-58146, 58260, 58290, 58353-58356, 58541❖, 58545-58546, 58550, 58552-58554, 58558, 58570❖, 58660-58673, 58700-58740, 58800, 58820, 58900, 58925-58940, 62310-62319, 64400-64435, 64445-64450, 64479, 64483, 64490, 64493, 64505-64530, 69990, 93000-93010, 93040-93042, 93318, 94002, 94200, 94250, 94680-94690, 94770, 95812-95816, 95819, 95822, 95829, 95955, 96360, 96365, 96372, 96374-96376, 99148-99149, 99150, P9612

Note: These CCI edits are used for Medicare. Other payers may reimburse on codes listed above.

Medicare Edits

	Fac RVU	Non-Fac RVU	FUD	Status
58262	27.54	27.54	90	A

	MUE		Modifiers		
58262	1	51	N/A	62	80

* with documentation

Medicare References: 100-3,230.3

Coding Companion for Ob/Gyn

Corpus Uteri

58263

58263 Vaginal hysterectomy, for uterus 250 g or less; with removal of tube(s), and/or ovary(s), with repair of enterocele

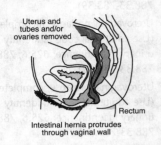

Uterus and tubes and/or ovaries removed

Rectum

Intestinal hernia protrudes through vaginal wall

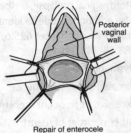

Posterior vaginal wall

Repair of enterocele

Explanation

The physician performs a vaginal hysterectomy for a uterus 250 gm or less and removes the tubes and/or ovaries. An incision is made around the cervix through the full thickness of the vaginal membrane. The cut vaginal edge is pulled toward the lower cervix and vaginal dissection is continued with countertraction. The posterior peritoneum is opened to admit a finger examination of the pelvis. The uterosacral ligaments are clamped and possibly shortened, cut from the uterus, and secured to the vagina. The vesicovaginal space is entered. The connective tissue fusing the bladder and vagina is dissected and the bladder is separated from the cervix. The bladder pillars are clamped, cut, and ligated near their cervical attachments, as well as the cardinal ligament tissue on each side of the cervix and the left and right uterine vessels. The physician clamps, cuts, and ligates the upper cardinal and lower broad ligament complex. Traction applied to the cervix moves the uterus down until the fundus is low in the pelvis. Hemostats are applied to the angle of the uterus on each side and the uterus is removed. After the uterus is exteriorized, care is taken to ensure ligation of the ovarian vessels. The ovary is excised under direct vision. For removal of both tubes and ovaries, the round ligament on one side at a time is clamped and divided. A tunnel is made through the layers of the uterine broad ligament that enclose the tube and the tube and ovary are clamped together. The structure is pulled forward, the two sheets of the broad ligament are each cut, and the broad ligament is opened completely. The whole specimen is separated from its attaching ligament, which is clamped, and the tube and ovary on that side are removed. An enterocele is repaired in addition to removing the tube and/or ovary. An enterocele is a hernia of the intestine protruding against the vaginal wall. The hernia sac is bluntly and sharply dissected from the surrounding connective tissue, excised and ligated, and the surrounding tissues are strengthened and sutured. The peritoneal and vaginal wall incisions of the hysterectomy procedure are closed.

Coding Tips

Removal of the tubes and ovaries and the enterocele repair are included in this procedure and should not be reported separately. Do not report this code in addition to 57283 as it is considered an inclusive component of 57283 when performed. For a vaginal hysterectomy with enterocele repair without removal of the tubes and ovaries, see 58270, 58280, and 58294. For other vaginal hysterectomy codes, see 58260–58262, and 58267–58294.

ICD-9-CM Procedural

65.39 Other unilateral oophorectomy

65.49 Other unilateral salpingo-oophorectomy

65.51 Other removal of both ovaries at same operative episode

65.52 Other removal of remaining ovary

65.61 Other removal of both ovaries and tubes at same operative episode

65.62 Other removal of remaining ovary and tube

68.59 Other and unspecified vaginal hysterectomy

70.92 Other operations on cul-de-sac

Anesthesia

58263 00944

ICD-9-CM Diagnostic

180.0 Malignant neoplasm of endocervix

180.1 Malignant neoplasm of exocervix

181 Malignant neoplasm of placenta

182.0 Malignant neoplasm of corpus uteri, except isthmus

182.1 Malignant neoplasm of isthmus

183.0 Malignant neoplasm of ovary — (Use additional code to identify any functional activity)

218.0 Submucous leiomyoma of uterus

218.1 Intramural leiomyoma of uterus

218.2 Subserous leiomyoma of uterus

233.1 Carcinoma in situ of cervix uteri

617.0 Endometriosis of uterus

618.1 Uterine prolapse without mention of vaginal wall prolapse — (Use additional code to identify urinary incontinence: 625.6, 788.31, 788.33-788.39)

618.3 Uterovaginal prolapse, complete — (Use additional code to identify urinary incontinence: 625.6, 788.31, 788.33-788.39)

618.6 Vaginal enterocele, congenital or acquired — (Use additional code to identify urinary incontinence: 625.6, 788.31, 788.33-788.39)

621.0 Polyp of corpus uteri

621.2 Hypertrophy of uterus

621.6 Malposition of uterus

622.10 Dysplasia of cervix, unspecified

626.2 Excessive or frequent menstruation

627.1 Postmenopausal bleeding

CCI Version 18.3

0071T-0072T, 01962-01963, 01969, 0213T, 0216T, 0228T, 0230T, 12001-12007, 12011-12057, 13100-13153, 36000, 36400-36410, 36420-36430, 36440, 36600, 36640, 37202, 43752, 45560, 49322, 50715, 51040, 51701-51703, 57180, 57268, 57283, 57410, 57420, 57452, 57500, 57522-57530, 57550-57555, 57800, 58100, 58120-58146, 58260-58262, 58270, 58290-58291, 58353-58356, 58541-58543❖, 58545-58546, 58550, 58552, 58554, 58558, 58570❖, 58660-58673, 58700-58740, 58800, 58820, 58900, 58925-58940, 62310-62319, 64400-64435, 64445-64450, 64479, 64483, 64490, 64493, 64505-64530, 69990, 93000-93010, 93040-93042, 93318, 94002, 94200, 94250, 94680-94690, 94770, 95812-95816, 95819, 95822, 95829, 95955, 96360, 96365, 96372, 96374-96376, 99148-99149, 99150, P9612

Note: These CCI edits are used for Medicare. Other payers may reimburse on codes listed above.

Medicare Edits

	Fac RVU	Non-Fac RVU	FUD	Status
58263	29.61	29.61	90	A

	MUE		Modifiers		
58263	1	51	N/A	62	80

* with documentation

Medicare References: 100-3,230.3

Corpus Uteri

58267

58267 Vaginal hysterectomy, for uterus 250 g or less; with colpo-urethrocystopexy (Marshall-Marchetti-Krantz type, Pereyra type) with or without endoscopic control

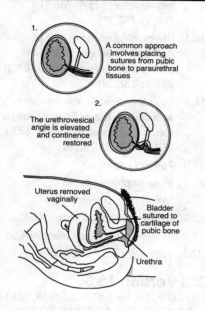

1. A common approach involves placing sutures from pubic bone to paraurethral tissues

2. The urethrovesical angle is elevated and continence restored

Uterus removed vaginally

Bladder sutured to cartilage of pubic bone

Urethra

Explanation

The physician performs a vaginal hysterectomy, for a uterus 250 gm or less with colpo-urethrocystopexy, with or without endoscopic control. An incision is made around the cervix through the full thickness of the vaginal membrane. The cut vaginal edge is pulled toward the lower cervix and vaginal dissection is continued with countertraction. The posterior peritoneum is opened to admit a finger examination of the pelvis. The uterosacral ligaments are clamped and possibly shortened, cut from the uterus, and secured to the vagina. The vesicovaginal space is entered. The connective tissue fusing the bladder and vagina is dissected and the bladder is separated from the cervix. The bladder pillars are clamped, cut, and ligated near their cervical attachments, as well as the cardinal ligament tissue on each side of the cervix and the left and right uterine vessels. The physician clamps, cuts, and ligates the upper cardinal and lower broad ligament complex. Traction applied to the cervix moves the uterus down until the fundus is low in the pelvis. Hemostats are applied to the angle of the uterus on each side and the uterus is removed. Colpo-urethrocystopexy is done in cases of urinary incontinence to elevate the lower part of the bladder that connects to the urethra (bladder neck) and the urethra to a new position higher in the pelvis so the muscles of the pelvic floor can help control urination. After the uterus has been exteriorized and the bladder and urethra separated from surrounding structures, the physician lifts the vagina upward, suspends the bladder neck and urethra by placing sutures through the fibromuscular wall of the vagina lateral to the tissue surrounding the urethra, and sutures the tissue to the symphysis pubis—the midline junction of the pubic bones at the front. An endoscope may be placed to ensure no sutures pass through the lining of the bladder and to evaluate ureteral patency. The sutures are pulled tight to tack the structures to the pubic bone and provide support.

Coding Tips

This code does not include removal of tubes or ovaries. Colpourethrocystopexy is included and should not be identified separately. For colpourethrocystopexy without hysterectomy, see 51840 and 51841. For other vaginal hysterectomy codes, see 58260–58263 and 58270–58294.

ICD-9-CM Procedural

59.5 Retropubic urethral suspension
68.59 Other and unspecified vaginal hysterectomy

Anesthesia

58267 00944

ICD-9-CM Diagnostic

180.0	Malignant neoplasm of endocervix
180.1	Malignant neoplasm of exocervix
180.8	Malignant neoplasm of other specified sites of cervix
182.0	Malignant neoplasm of corpus uteri, except isthmus
182.1	Malignant neoplasm of isthmus
182.8	Malignant neoplasm of other specified sites of body of uterus
218.0	Submucous leiomyoma of uterus
218.1	Intramural leiomyoma of uterus
218.2	Subserous leiomyoma of uterus
617.0	Endometriosis of uterus
618.00	Unspecified prolapse of vaginal walls without mention of uterine prolapse — (Use additional code to identify urinary incontinence: 625.6, 788.31, 788.33-788.39)
618.05	Perineocele without mention of uterine prolapse — (Use additional code to identify urinary incontinence: 625.6, 788.31, 788.33-788.39)
618.09	Other prolapse of vaginal walls without mention of uterine prolapse — (Use additional code to identify

	urinary incontinence: 625.6, 788.31, 788.33-788.39)
618.1	Uterine prolapse without mention of vaginal wall prolapse — (Use additional code to identify urinary incontinence: 625.6, 788.31, 788.33-788.39)
618.2	Uterovaginal prolapse, incomplete — (Use additional code to identify urinary incontinence: 625.6, 788.31, 788.33-788.39)
618.3	Uterovaginal prolapse, complete — (Use additional code to identify urinary incontinence: 625.6, 788.31, 788.33-788.39)
618.4	Uterovaginal prolapse, unspecified — (Use additional code to identify urinary incontinence: 625.6, 788.31, 788.33-788.39)
625.3	Dysmenorrhea
625.6	Female stress incontinence
626.2	Excessive or frequent menstruation
626.8	Other disorder of menstruation and other abnormal bleeding from female genital tract

CCI Version 18.3

0071T-0072T, 01962-01963, 01969, 0213T, 0216T, 0228T, 0230T, 12001-12007, 12011-12057, 13100-13153, 36000, 36400-36410, 36420-36430, 36440, 36600, 36640, 37202, 43752, 50715, 51040, 51701-51703, 51840-51845, 52000, 52204, 57180, 57220, 57284, 57289, 57410, 57420, 57423, 57452, 57500, 57522-57530, 57550-57555, 57800, 58100, 58120-58146, 58260-58263, 58270, 58290, 58353-58356, 58541-58546, 58550, 58552, 58554, 58558, 58570-58571❖, 58660, 58662, 58720, 62310-62319, 64400-64435, 64445-64450, 64479, 64483, 64490, 64493, 64505-64530, 69990, 93000-93010, 93040-93042, 93318, 94002, 94200, 94250, 94680-94690, 94770, 95812-95816, 95819, 95822, 95829, 95955, 96360, 96365, 96372, 96374-96376, 99148-99149, 99150, P9612

Note: These CCI edits are used for Medicare. Other payers may reimburse on codes listed above.

Medicare Edits

	Fac RVU	Non-Fac RVU	FUD	Status
58267	31.55	31.55	90	A

	MUE		Modifiers		
58267	1	51	N/A	62*	80

* with documentation

Medicare References: 100-3,230.3

Coding Companion for Ob/Gyn

Corpus Uteri

58270

58270 Vaginal hysterectomy, for uterus 250 g or less; with repair of enterocele

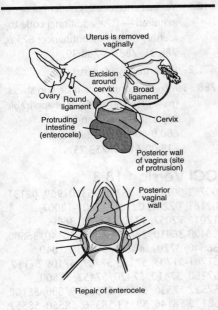

Repair of enterocele

Explanation

The physician performs a vaginal hysterectomy, for a uterus 250 gm or less, with repair of an enterocele. An incision is made around the cervix through the full thickness of the vaginal membrane. The cut vaginal edge is pulled toward the lower cervix and vaginal dissection is continued with countertraction. The posterior peritoneum is opened to admit a finger examination of the pelvis. The uterosacral ligaments are clamped and possibly shortened, cut from the uterus, and secured to the vagina. The vesicovaginal space is entered. The connective tissue fusing the bladder and vagina is dissected and the bladder is separated from the cervix. The bladder pillars are clamped, cut, and ligated near their cervical attachments as well as the cardinal ligament tissue on each side of the cervix and the left and right uterine vessels. The anterior peritoneum is opened under direct vision to avoid damaging the bladder and admit finger exploration. The physician clamps, cuts, and ligates the upper cardinal and lower broad ligament complex now that the peritoneum is open both anterior and posterior to the uterine fundus. Hemostats are applied to the angle of the uterus on each side and the uterus is removed, usually posteriorly. The physician also repairs an enterocele, a herniation of intestine that protrudes against the vaginal wall, discovered during finger exploration. The hernia sac is bluntly and sharply dissected from the surrounding connective tissue, excised and ligated, and the surrounding tissues are strengthened and

sutured. The peritoneum is closed with purse-string sutures that incorporate the proximal part of the uterosacral ligaments.

Coding Tips

Removal of the tubes and ovaries is not included in this procedure. However, the enterocele repair is included and should not be identified separately. For repair of an enterocele with removal of tubes and ovaries, report 58263. For other vaginal hysterectomy codes, see 58262–58267 and 58275–58294.

ICD-9-CM Procedural

- 68.59 Other and unspecified vaginal hysterectomy
- 70.92 Other operations on cul-de-sac

Anesthesia

58270 00944

ICD-9-CM Diagnostic

- 180.0 Malignant neoplasm of endocervix
- 180.1 Malignant neoplasm of exocervix
- 182.0 Malignant neoplasm of corpus uteri, except isthmus
- 182.1 Malignant neoplasm of isthmus
- 182.8 Malignant neoplasm of other specified sites of body of uterus
- 218.0 Submucous leiomyoma of uterus
- 218.1 Intramural leiomyoma of uterus
- 218.2 Subserous leiomyoma of uterus
- 233.1 Carcinoma in situ of cervix uteri
- 618.04 Rectocele without mention of uterine prolapse — (Use additional code to identify urinary incontinence: 625.6, 788.31, 788.33-788.39) (Use additional code for any associated fecal incontinence: 787.60-787.63)
- 618.1 Uterine prolapse without mention of vaginal wall prolapse — (Use additional code to identify urinary incontinence: 625.6, 788.31, 788.33-788.39)
- 618.2 Uterovaginal prolapse, incomplete — (Use additional code to identify urinary incontinence: 625.6, 788.31, 788.33-788.39)
- 618.3 Uterovaginal prolapse, complete — (Use additional code to identify urinary incontinence: 625.6, 788.31, 788.33-788.39)
- 618.4 Uterovaginal prolapse, unspecified — (Use additional code to identify urinary incontinence: 625.6, 788.31, 788.33-788.39)
- 618.6 Vaginal enterocele, congenital or acquired — (Use additional code to

identify urinary incontinence: 625.6, 788.31, 788.33-788.39)
- 618.83 Pelvic muscle wasting — (Use additional code to identify urinary incontinence: 625.6, 788.31, 788.33-788.39)
- 618.9 Unspecified genital prolapse — (Use additional code to identify urinary incontinence: 625.6, 788.31, 788.33-788.39)
- 621.30 Endometrial hyperplasia, unspecified
- 621.31 Simple endometrial hyperplasia without atypia
- 621.32 Complex endometrial hyperplasia without atypia
- 621.33 Endometrial hyperplasia with atypia
- 621.34 Benign endometrial hyperplasia
- 621.35 Endometrial intraepithelial neoplasia [EIN]
- 622.10 Dysplasia of cervix, unspecified
- 622.11 Mild dysplasia of cervix
- 622.12 Moderate dysplasia of cervix
- 627.1 Postmenopausal bleeding

CCI Version 18.3

0071T-0072T, 01962-01963, 01969, 0213T, 0216T, 0228T, 0230T, 12001-12007, 12011-12057, 13100-13153, 36000, 36400-36410, 36420-36430, 36440, 36600, 36640, 37202, 43752, 45560, 50715, 51040, 51701-51703, 57180, 57268-57270, 57283, 57410, 57420, 57452, 57500, 57522-57530, 57550-57555, 57800, 58100, 58120-58150❖, 58260-58262, 58290, 58353-58356, 58541❖, 58545-58546, 58550, 58552, 58554, 58558, 58660, 58662, 58720, 62310-62319, 64400-64435, 64445-64450, 64479, 64483, 64490, 64493, 64505-64530, 69990, 93000-93010, 93040-93042, 93318, 94002, 94200, 94250, 94680-94690, 94770, 95812-95816, 95819, 95822, 95829, 95955, 96360, 96365, 96372, 96374-96376, 99148-99149, 99150, P9612

Note: These CCI edits are used for Medicare. Other payers may reimburse on codes listed above.

Medicare Edits

	Fac RVU	Non-Fac RVU	FUD	Status
58270	26.32	26.32	90	A

	MUE		Modifiers		
58270	1	51	N/A	62*	80

* with documentation

Medicare References: 100-3,230.3

58275-58280

58275 Vaginal hysterectomy, with total or partial vaginectomy;

58280 with repair of enterocele

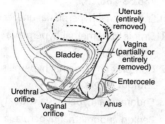

The uterus is removed by a vaginal approach. The vagina is partially or entirely removed as well. Report code 58280 when an enterocele is repaired during the same surgical session

Explanation

The physician performs a vaginal hysterectomy with total or partial vaginectomy in 58275-58280 and with enterocele repair in 58280. An incision is made around the cervix through the full thickness of the vaginal membrane. The cut vaginal edge is pulled toward the lower cervix and vaginal dissection is continued with countertraction. The posterior peritoneum is opened to admit a finger examination of the pelvis. The uterosacral ligaments are clamped and possibly shortened, cut from the uterus, and secured to the vagina. The vesicovaginal space is entered. The connective tissue fusing the bladder and vagina is dissected and the bladder is separated from the cervix. The bladder pillars are clamped, cut, and ligated near their cervical attachments, as well as the cardinal ligament tissue on each side of the cervix and the left and right uterine vessels. The anterior peritoneum is opened under direct vision to avoid damaging the bladder and admit finger exploration. The physician clamps, cuts, and ligates the upper cardinal and lower broad ligament complex now that the peritoneum is open both anterior and posterior to the uterine fundus. Traction applied to the cervix moves the uterus down until the fundus is low in the pelvis. Hemostats are applied to the angle of the uterus on each side and the uterus is removed, usually posteriorly. The vagina is everted out through its opening and totally or partially removed in sections by blunt and sharp dissection. Any

remaining vaginal tissue and the supporting tissues are inverted back into the resulting defect and are sutured in place with total vaginectomy obliterating the space. Report 58280 if the physician also repairs an enterocele, a herniation of intestine protruding through the vaginal wall. The hernia sac is bluntly and sharply dissected from the surrounding connective tissue, excised and ligated, and the surrounding tissues are strengthened and sutured. The peritoneum is closed with purse-string sutures that incorporate the proximal part of the uterosacral ligaments.

Coding Tips

Removing a narrow rim of vagina surrounding the cervix is standard with a vaginal hysterectomy; however, these codes include removing a significant amount of the vagina. For other vaginal hysterectomy codes, see 58262–58285 and 58550.

ICD-9-CM Procedural

68.59   Other and unspecified vaginal hysterectomy

70.4   Obliteration and total excision of vagina

70.8   Obliteration of vaginal vault

70.92   Other operations on cul-de-sac

Anesthesia

00944

ICD-9-CM Diagnostic

180.0   Malignant neoplasm of endocervix

180.1   Malignant neoplasm of exocervix

182.0   Malignant neoplasm of corpus uteri, except isthmus

182.1   Malignant neoplasm of isthmus

184.0   Malignant neoplasm of vagina

218.0   Submucous leiomyoma of uterus

218.1   Intramural leiomyoma of uterus

218.2   Subserous leiomyoma of uterus

618.00 Unspecified prolapse of vaginal walls without mention of uterine prolapse — (Use additional code to identify urinary incontinence: 625.6, 788.31, 788.33-788.39)

618.1   Uterine prolapse without mention of vaginal wall prolapse — (Use additional code to identify urinary incontinence: 625.6, 788.31, 788.33-788.39)

618.2   Uterovaginal prolapse, incomplete — (Use additional code to identify urinary incontinence: 625.6, 788.31, 788.33-788.39)

618.3   Uterovaginal prolapse, complete — (Use additional code to identify urinary incontinence: 625.6, 788.31, 788.33-788.39)

618.6   Vaginal enterocele, congenital or acquired — (Use additional code to identify urinary incontinence: 625.6, 788.31, 788.33-788.39)

621.2   Hypertrophy of uterus

788.33 Mixed incontinence urge and stress (male)(female) — (Code, if applicable, any causal condition first: 600.0-600.9, with fifth digit 1; 618.00-618.9; 753.23)

CCI Version 18.3

0071T-0072T, 01962-01963, 01969, 0213T, 0216T, 0228T, 0230T, 12001-12007, 12011-12057, 13100-13153, 36000, 36400-36410, 36420-36430, 36440, 36600, 36640, 37202, 43752, 50715, 51040, 51701-51703, 57106-57107, 57109-57112, 57180, 57410, 57420, 57452, 57500, 57522-57530, 57550-57555, 57800, 58100, 58120-58146, 58353-58356, 58550, 58552, 58554, 58558, 58660, 58662, 58700-58720, 58800, 58900-58940, 62310-62319, 64400-64435, 64445-64450, 64479, 64483, 64490, 64493, 64505-64530, 69990, 93000-93010, 93040-93042, 93318, 94002, 94200, 94250, 94680-94690, 94770, 95812-95816, 95819, 95822, 95829, 95955, 96360, 96365, 96372, 96374-96376, 99148-99149, 99150, P9612

Also not with 58275: 58541-58543❖, 58545-58546, 58570❖, 58820

Also not with 58280: 45560, 57260-57265, 57268-57270, 57283, 58263❖, 58270-58275, 58541-58546, 58570-58571❖

Note: These CCI edits are used for Medicare. Other payers may reimburse on codes listed above.

Medicare Edits

	Fac RVU	Non-Fac RVU	FUD	Status
58275	29.4	29.4	90	A
58280	31.45	31.45	90	A

	MUE			Modifiers	
58275	1	51	N/A	62*	80
58280	1	51	N/A	62*	80

* with documentation

Medicare References: 100-3,230.3

58285

58285 Vaginal hysterectomy, radical (Schauta type operation)

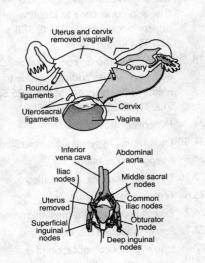

Uterus and cervix removed vaginally
Ovary
Round ligaments
Cervix
Uterosacral ligaments
Vagina

Inferior vena cava
Abdominal aorta
Iliac nodes
Middle sacral nodes
Uterus removed
Common iliac nodes
Superficial inguinal nodes
Obturator node
Deep inguinal nodes

Explanation

The physician performs a radical vaginal hysterectomy. This includes the uterus, its surrounding tissues, and the pelvic lymph nodes. An incision is made around the cervix through the full thickness of the vaginal membrane. The cut vaginal edge is pulled toward the lower cervix and vaginal dissection is continued with countertraction. The posterior peritoneum is opened to admit a finger examination of the pelvis. The uterosacral ligaments are clamped and possibly shortened, cut from the uterus, and secured to the vagina. The vesicovaginal space is entered. The connective tissue fusing the bladder and vagina is dissected and the bladder is separated from the cervix. The bladder pillars are clamped, cut, and ligated near their cervical attachments, as well as the cardinal ligament tissue on each side of the cervix and the left and right uterine vessels. The anterior peritoneum is opened under direct vision to avoid damaging the bladder and admit finger exploration. The physician clamps, cuts, and ligates the upper cardinal and lower broad ligament complex now that the peritoneum is open both anterior and posterior to the uterine fundus. Traction applied to the cervix moves the uterus down until the fundus is low in the pelvis. Hemostats are applied to the angle of the uterus on each side and the uterus is removed, usually posteriorly. The physician also removes the surrounding tissues, including part or all of the vagina and the pelvic lymph nodes. Any incisions are closed by suturing.

Coding Tips

Removal of tubes and ovaries is not included in this code. Note that 58285 includes removal of more uterine adnexal tissue than 58275 or 58280. Several vaginal hysterectomy codes exist that include many different components and amounts of uterine and adnexal tissue dissection, see 58260–58280 and 58290–58294.

ICD-9-CM Procedural

68.79 Other and unspecified radical vaginal hysterectomy

Anesthesia

58285 00944

ICD-9-CM Diagnostic

180.0 Malignant neoplasm of endocervix

180.1 Malignant neoplasm of exocervix

180.8 Malignant neoplasm of other specified sites of cervix

182.0 Malignant neoplasm of corpus uteri, except isthmus

182.1 Malignant neoplasm of isthmus

182.8 Malignant neoplasm of other specified sites of body of uterus

183.2 Malignant neoplasm of fallopian tube

183.3 Malignant neoplasm of broad ligament of uterus

183.4 Malignant neoplasm of parametrium of uterus

183.5 Malignant neoplasm of round ligament of uterus

183.8 Malignant neoplasm of other specified sites of uterine adnexa

198.82 Secondary malignant neoplasm of genital organs

236.0 Neoplasm of uncertain behavior of uterus

239.5 Neoplasm of unspecified nature of other genitourinary organs

618.1 Uterine prolapse without mention of vaginal wall prolapse — (Use additional code to identify urinary incontinence: 625.6, 788.31, 788.33-788.39)

618.2 Uterovaginal prolapse, incomplete — (Use additional code to identify urinary incontinence: 625.6, 788.31, 788.33-788.39)

618.3 Uterovaginal prolapse, complete — (Use additional code to identify urinary incontinence: 625.6, 788.31, 788.33-788.39)

618.4 Uterovaginal prolapse, unspecified — (Use additional code to identify

urinary incontinence: 625.6, 788.31, 788.33-788.39)

618.83 Pelvic muscle wasting — (Use additional code to identify urinary incontinence: 625.6, 788.31, 788.33-788.39)

618.89 Other specified genital prolapse — (Use additional code to identify urinary incontinence: 625.6, 788.31, 788.33-788.39)

625.6 Female stress incontinence

V84.02 Genetic susceptibility to malignant neoplasm of ovary — (Use additional code, if applicable, for any associated family history of the disease: V16-V19. Code first, if applicable, any current malignant neoplasms: 140.0-195.8, 200.0-208.9, 230.0-234.9. Use additional code, if applicable, for any personal history of malignant neoplasm: V10.0-V10.9)

CCI Version 18.3

0071T-0072T, 01962-01963, 01969, 0213T, 0216T, 0228T, 0230T, 12001-12007, 12011-12057, 13100-13153, 36000, 36400-36410, 36420-36430, 36440, 36600, 36640, 37202, 43752, 45560, 50715, 51040, 51701-51703, 57106-57107, 57109-57112, 57180, 57410, 57420, 57452, 57500, 57522-57530, 57550-57555, 57800, 58100, 58120-58146, 58353-58356, 58541-58546, 58550, 58552, 58554, 58558, 58570-58573❖, 58660, 58662, 58700-58720, 58800, 58900-58925, 62310-62319, 64400-64435, 64445-64450, 64479, 64483, 64490, 64493, 64505-64530, 69990, 93000-93010, 93040-93042, 93318, 94002, 94200, 94250, 94680-94690, 94770, 95812-95816, 95819, 95822, 95829, 95955, 96360, 96365, 96372, 96374-96376, 99148-99149, 99150, P9612

Note: These CCI edits are used for Medicare. Other payers may reimburse on codes listed above.

Medicare Edits

	Fac RVU	Non-Fac RVU	FUD	Status
58285	39.17	39.17	90	A

	MUE		Modifiers		
58285	1	51	N/A	62*	80

* with documentation

Medicare References: 100-3,230.3

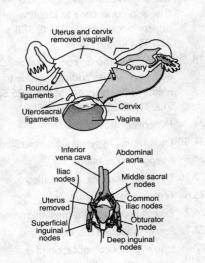

Corpus Uteri

58290

58290 Vaginal hysterectomy, for uterus greater than 250 g;

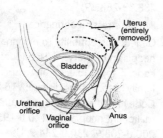

Report 58290 when the uterus is greater than 250 gm

Explanation

The physician performs a vaginal hysterectomy, for a uterus greater than 250 gm. An incision is made around the cervix through the full thickness of the vaginal membrane. The cut vaginal edge is pulled toward the lower cervix and vaginal dissection is continued with countertraction. The posterior peritoneum is opened to admit a finger examination of the pelvis. The uterosacral ligaments are clamped and possibly shortened, cut from the uterus, and secured to the vagina. The vesicovaginal space is entered. The connective tissue fusing the bladder and vagina is dissected and the bladder is separated from the cervix. The bladder pillars are clamped, cut, and ligated near their cervical attachments as well as the cardinal ligament tissue on each side of the cervix and the left and right uterine vessels. The anterior peritoneum is opened under direct vision to avoid damaging the bladder and admit finger exploration. The physician clamps, cuts, and ligates the upper cardinal and lower broad ligament complex now that the peritoneum is open both anterior and posterior to the uterine fundus. Traction applied to the cervix moves the uterus down until the fundus is low in the pelvis. Hemostats are applied to the angle of the uterus on each side and the uterus is removed, usually posteriorly. When the uterus is too large to permit delivery through the anterior or posterior peritoneal opening, the myometrium may be incised circumferentially parallel to the uterine cavity axis and removed or the uterus can be dissected and removed one half at a time. The peritoneum is closed with purse-string sutures that incorporate the proximal part of the uterosacral ligaments. Colporrhaphy may be performed before the vaginal wall is closed by running or interrupted sutures placed side to side longitudinally.

Coding Tips

This code reports a hysterectomy for a uterus greater than 250 gm only. When tubes and ovaries are also removed, see 58291–58292. For other vaginal hysterectomy codes, see 58260–58285 and 58293–58294. For laparoscopy with a vaginal hysterectomy only for a uterus greater than 250 gm, see 58553.

ICD-9-CM Procedural

68.59 Other and unspecified vaginal hysterectomy

Anesthesia

58290 00944

ICD-9-CM Diagnostic

180.0 Malignant neoplasm of endocervix
180.1 Malignant neoplasm of exocervix
180.8 Malignant neoplasm of other specified sites of cervix
181 Malignant neoplasm of placenta
182.0 Malignant neoplasm of corpus uteri, except isthmus
182.1 Malignant neoplasm of isthmus
182.8 Malignant neoplasm of other specified sites of body of uterus
183.0 Malignant neoplasm of ovary — (Use additional code to identify any functional activity)
183.8 Malignant neoplasm of other specified sites of uterine adnexa
198.6 Secondary malignant neoplasm of ovary
218.0 Submucous leiomyoma of uterus
218.1 Intramural leiomyoma of uterus
218.2 Subserous leiomyoma of uterus
218.9 Leiomyoma of uterus, unspecified
233.1 Carcinoma in situ of cervix uteri
233.31 Carcinoma in situ, vagina
614.4 Chronic or unspecified parametritis and pelvic cellulitis — (Use additional code to identify organism: 041.00-041.09, 041.10-041.19)
614.9 Unspecified inflammatory disease of female pelvic organs and tissues — (Use additional code to identify organism: 041.00-041.09, 041.10-041.19)
617.0 Endometriosis of uterus

618.1 Uterine prolapse without mention of vaginal wall prolapse — (Use additional code to identify urinary incontinence: 625.6, 788.31, 788.33-788.39)
618.3 Uterovaginal prolapse, complete — (Use additional code to identify urinary incontinence: 625.6, 788.31, 788.33-788.39)
618.6 Vaginal enterocele, congenital or acquired — (Use additional code to identify urinary incontinence: 625.6, 788.31, 788.33-788.39)
621.2 Hypertrophy of uterus
621.30 Endometrial hyperplasia, unspecified
621.6 Malposition of uterus
622.10 Dysplasia of cervix, unspecified
625.6 Female stress incontinence
626.2 Excessive or frequent menstruation
627.1 Postmenopausal bleeding
677 Late effect of complication of pregnancy, childbirth, and the puerperium — (Code first any sequelae)

CCI Version 18.3

0071T-0072T, 01962-01963, 01969, 0213T, 0216T, 0228T, 0230T, 12001-12007, 12011-12057, 13100-13153, 36000, 36400-36410, 36420-36430, 36440, 36600, 36640, 37202, 43752, 50715, 51040, 51701-51703, 57106, 57180, 57268, 57410, 57420, 57452, 57500, 57522-57530, 57550, 57800, 58100, 58120-58145, 58260, 58280❖, 58353-58356, 58541-58544❖, 58550, 58552-58554, 58558, 58570-58572❖, 58660, 58662, 58720, 62310-62319, 64400-64435, 64445-64450, 64479, 64483, 64490, 64493, 64505-64530, 69990, 93000-93010, 93040-93042, 93318, 94002, 94200, 94250, 94680-94690, 94770, 95812-95816, 95819, 95822, 95829, 95955, 96360, 96365, 96372, 96374-96376, 99148-99149, 99150, P9612

Note: These CCI edits are used for Medicare. Other payers may reimburse on codes listed above.

Medicare Edits

	Fac RVU	Non-Fac RVU	FUD	Status
58290	34.36	34.36	90	A

	MUE		Modifiers		
58290	1	51	N/A	62*	80

* with documentation

Medicare References: None

Coding Companion for Ob/Gyn

58291-58292

58291 Vaginal hysterectomy, for uterus greater than 250 g; with removal of tube(s) and/or ovary(s)

58292 with removal of tube(s) and/or ovary(s), with repair of enterocele

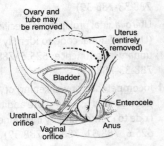

The uterus, tubes, and ovaries are removed vaginally in an open surgical session

Report 58291 for a uterus that weighs more than 250 gm and tubes and/or ovaries are removed. Report 58292 when the uterus is greater than 250 gm, tubes and/or ovaries are removed, and an enterocele is repaired

Explanation

The physician performs a vaginal hysterectomy, for a uterus greater than 250 gm and removes the tubes and/or ovaries. An incision is made around the cervix through the full thickness of the vaginal membrane. The cut vaginal edge is pulled toward the lower cervix and vaginal dissection is continued with countertraction. The posterior peritoneum is opened to admit a finger examination of the pelvis. The uterosacral ligaments are clamped and possibly shortened, cut from the uterus, and secured to the vagina. The vesicovaginal space is entered. The connective tissue fusing the bladder and vagina is dissected and the bladder is separated from the cervix. The bladder pillars are clamped, cut, and ligated near their cervical attachments, as well as the cardinal ligament tissue on each side of the cervix and the left and right uterine vessels. The anterior peritoneum is opened under direct vision to avoid damaging the bladder and admit finger exploration. The physician clamps, cuts, and ligates the upper cardinal and lower broad ligament complex now that the peritoneum is open both anterior and posterior to the uterine fundus. Traction applied to the cervix moves the uterus down until the fundus is low in the pelvis. Hemostats are applied to the angle of the uterus on each side and the uterus is removed, usually posteriorly. After the uterus is exteriorized, care is taken to ensure ligation of the ovarian vessels. The ovary is excised under direct vision. For removal of both tubes and ovaries, the round ligament on one side at a time is clamped and divided. A tunnel is made through the layers of the uterine broad ligament that enclose the tube and the tube and ovary are clamped together. The structure is pulled forward, the two sheets of the broad ligament are each cut, and the broad ligament is opened completely. The whole specimen is separated from its attaching ligament, which is clamped, and the tube and ovary on that side are removed. Report 58292 if an enterocele is repaired in addition to removing the tube and/or ovary. An enterocele is a hernia of the intestine protruding against the vaginal wall. The hernia sac is bluntly and sharply dissected from the surrounding connective tissue, excised and ligated, and the surrounding tissues are strengthened and sutured. The peritoneal and vaginal wall incisions of the hysterectomy procedure are closed.

Coding Tips

For a vaginal hysterectomy only for a uterus greater than 250 gm, see 58290. For a vaginal hysterectomy for a uterus greater than 250 gm with colpo-urethrocystopexy, see 58293. For a vaginal hysterectomy for a uterus greater than 250 gm with repair of an enterocele without removal of tubes or ovaries, see 58294. For other vaginal hysterectomy codes, see 58260–58285. For laparoscopic vaginal hysterectomy with removal of the tubes and/or ovaries for a uterus greater than 250 gm, see 58554.

ICD-9-CM Procedural

65.39 Other unilateral oophorectomy

65.49 Other unilateral salpingo-oophorectomy

65.51 Other removal of both ovaries at same operative episode

65.52 Other removal of remaining ovary

65.61 Other removal of both ovaries and tubes at same operative episode

65.62 Other removal of remaining ovary and tube

68.59 Other and unspecified vaginal hysterectomy

70.92 Other operations on cul-de-sac

Anesthesia

00944

ICD-9-CM Diagnostic

180.0 Malignant neoplasm of endocervix

180.1 Malignant neoplasm of exocervix

181 Malignant neoplasm of placenta

182.0 Malignant neoplasm of corpus uteri, except isthmus

182.1 Malignant neoplasm of isthmus

183.0 Malignant neoplasm of ovary — (Use additional code to identify any functional activity)

183.8 Malignant neoplasm of other specified sites of uterine adnexa

198.6 Secondary malignant neoplasm of ovary

218.0 Submucous leiomyoma of uterus

218.1 Intramural leiomyoma of uterus

218.2 Subserous leiomyoma of uterus

233.1 Carcinoma in situ of cervix uteri

617.0 Endometriosis of uterus

621.30 Endometrial hyperplasia, unspecified

622.10 Dysplasia of cervix, unspecified

CCI Version 18.3

0071T-0072T, 01962-01963, 01969, 0213T, 0216T, 0228T, 0230T, 12001-12007, 12011-12057, 13100-13153, 36000, 36400-36410, 36420-36430, 36440, 36600, 36640, 37202, 43752, 49322, 50715, 51040, 51701-51703, 57180, 57410, 57420, 57452, 57500, 57522-57530, 57800, 58100, 58120-58145, 58267-58270, 58353-58356, 58541-58544❖, 58550, 58552-58554, 58558, 58660-58673, 58700-58740, 58800, 58820, 58900, 58925-58940, 62310-62319, 64400-64435, 64445-64450, 64479, 64483, 64490, 64493, 64505-64530, 69990, 93000-93010, 93040-93042, 93318, 94002, 94200, 94250, 94680-94690, 94770, 95812-95816, 95819, 95822, 95829, 95955, 96360, 96365, 96372, 96374-96376, 99148-99149, 99150, P9612

Also not with 58291: 57550, 58260-58262, 58570-58572❖

Also not with 58292: 45560, 57268-57270, 57283, 57550-57555, 58260-58263, 58280❖, 58291, 58294, 58570-58573❖

Note: These CCI edits are used for Medicare. Other payers may reimburse on codes listed above.

Medicare Edits

	Fac RVU	Non-Fac RVU	FUD	Status
58291	37.23	37.23	90	A
58292	39.29	39.29	90	A

	MUE		Modifiers		
58291	1	51	N/A	62	80
58292	1	51	N/A	62	80

* with documentation

Medicare References: None

Coding Companion for Ob/Gyn

58293

58293 Vaginal hysterectomy, for uterus greater than 250 g; with colpo-urethrocystopexy (Marshall-Marchetti-Krantz type, Pereyra type) with or without endoscopic control

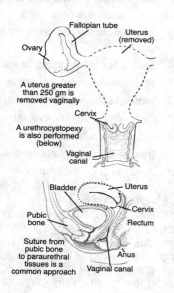

A uterus greater than 250 gm is removed vaginally

A urethrocystopexy is also performed (below)

Suture from pubic bone to paraurethral tissues is a common approach

Explanation

The physician performs a vaginal hysterectomy, for a uterus greater than 250 gm with colpo-urethrocystopexy, with or without endoscopic control. Colpo-urethrocystopexy is done after vaginal hysterectomy in cases of urinary incontinence to elevate the lower part of the bladder that connects to the urethra (bladder neck) and the urethra to a new position higher in the pelvis so the muscles of the pelvic floor can help control urination. An incision is made around the cervix through the full thickness of the vaginal membrane. The cut vaginal edge is pulled toward the lower cervix and vaginal dissection is continued with countertraction. The posterior peritoneum is opened to admit a finger examination of the pelvis. The uterosacral ligaments are clamped and possibly shortened, cut from the uterus, and secured to the vagina. The vesicovaginal space is entered. The connective tissue fusing the bladder and vagina is dissected and the bladder is separated from the cervix. The bladder pillars are clamped, cut, and ligated near their cervical attachments, as well as the cardinal ligament tissue on each side of the cervix and the left and right uterine vessels. The anterior peritoneum is opened under direct vision to avoid damaging the bladder and admit finger exploration. The physician clamps, cuts, and ligates the upper cardinal and lower broad ligament complex now that the peritoneum is open both anterior and

posterior to the uterine fundus. Traction applied to the cervix moves the uterus down until the fundus is low in the pelvis. Hemostats are applied to the angle of the uterus on each side and the uterus is removed, usually posteriorly. When the uterus is too large to permit delivery through the anterior or posterior peritoneal opening, the myometrium may be incised circumferentially parallel to the uterine cavity axis and removed or the uterus can be dissected and removed one half at a time. After the uterus has been exteriorized and the bladder and urethra separated from surrounding structures, the physician lifts the vagina upward, suspends the bladder neck and urethra by placing sutures through the fibromuscular wall of the vagina lateral to the tissue surrounding the urethra, and sutures the tissue to the symphysis pubis—the midline junction of the pubic bones at the front. An endoscope may be placed to ensure no sutures pass through the lining of the bladder and to evaluate ureteral patency. The sutures are pulled tight to tack the structures to the pubic bone and provide support. Packing may be placed in the vagina to be removed later and urine is drained by a catheter placed intraoperatively.

Coding Tips

This code does not include removal of tubes or ovaries. Colpourethrocystopexy is included and should not be identified separately. For colpourethrocystopexy without a hysterectomy, see 51840 and 51841. For other vaginal hysterectomy codes, see 58260–58292 and 58294.

ICD-9-CM Procedural

59.5   Retropubic urethral suspension

68.59   Other and unspecified vaginal hysterectomy

Anesthesia

58293   00944

ICD-9-CM Diagnostic

180.0   Malignant neoplasm of endocervix

180.1   Malignant neoplasm of exocervix

182.0   Malignant neoplasm of corpus uteri, except isthmus

182.1   Malignant neoplasm of isthmus

218.0   Submucous leiomyoma of uterus

218.1   Intramural leiomyoma of uterus

218.2   Subserous leiomyoma of uterus

614.4   Chronic or unspecified parametritis and pelvic cellulitis — (Use additional code to identify organism: 041.00-041.09, 041.10-041.19)

617.0   Endometriosis of uterus

618.1   Uterine prolapse without mention of vaginal wall prolapse — (Use additional code to identify urinary incontinence: 625.6, 788.31, 788.33-788.39)

618.2   Uterovaginal prolapse, incomplete — (Use additional code to identify urinary incontinence: 625.6, 788.31, 788.33-788.39)

618.3   Uterovaginal prolapse, complete — (Use additional code to identify urinary incontinence: 625.6, 788.31, 788.33-788.39)

618.4   Uterovaginal prolapse, unspecified — (Use additional code to identify urinary incontinence: 625.6, 788.31, 788.33-788.39)

618.81   Incompetence or weakening of pubocervical tissue — (Use additional code to identify urinary incontinence: 625.6, 788.31, 788.33-788.39)

618.82   Incompetence or weakening of rectovaginal tissue — (Use additional code to identify urinary incontinence: 625.6, 788.31, 788.33-788.39)

625.6   Female stress incontinence

626.2   Excessive or frequent menstruation

CCI Version 18.3

0071T-0072T, 01962-01963, 01969, 0213T, 0216T, 0228T, 0230T, 12001-12007, 12011-12057, 13100-13153, 36000, 36400-36410, 36420-36430, 36440, 36600, 36640, 37202, 43752, 50715, 51040, 51701-51703, 51840-51845, 52000, 52204, 57180, 57220, 57289, 57410, 57420, 57452, 57500, 57522-57530, 57550-57555, 57800, 58100, 58120-58145, 58260-58263, 58267-58270, 58291-58292, 58353-58356, 58541-58544❖, 58550, 58552-58554, 58558, 58570-58573❖, 58660, 58662, 58720, 62310-62319, 64400-64435, 64445-64450, 64479, 64483, 64490, 64493, 64505-64530, 69990, 93000-93010, 93040-93042, 93318, 94002, 94200, 94250, 94680-94690, 94770, 95812-95816, 95819, 95822, 95829, 95955, 96360, 96365, 96372, 96374-96376, 99148-99149, 99150, P9612

Note: These CCI edits are used for Medicare. Other payers may reimburse on codes listed above.

Medicare Edits

	Fac RVU	Non-Fac RVU	FUD	Status
58293	40.85	40.85	90	A

	MUE			Modifiers	
58293	1	51	N/A	62*	80

* with documentation

Medicare References: None

Corpus Uteri

58294

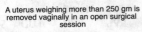

58294 Vaginal hysterectomy, for uterus greater than 250 g; with repair of enterocele

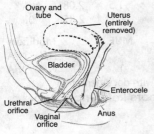

A uterus weighing more than 250 gm is removed vaginally in an open surgical session

A repair of an enterocele is performed during the same surgical session

Explanation

The physician performs a vaginal hysterectomy, for a uterus greater than 250 gm, with repair of an enterocele. An incision is made around the cervix through the full thickness of the vaginal membrane. The cut vaginal edge is pulled toward the lower cervix and vaginal dissection is continued with countertraction. The posterior peritoneum is opened to admit a finger examination of the pelvis. The uterosacral ligaments are clamped and possibly shortened, cut from the uterus, and secured to the vagina. The vesicovaginal space is entered. The connective tissue fusing the bladder and vagina is dissected and the bladder is separated from the cervix. The bladder pillars are clamped, cut, and ligated near their cervical attachments, as well as the cardinal ligament tissue on each side of the cervix and the left and right uterine vessels. The anterior peritoneum is opened under direct vision. The physician clamps, cuts, and ligates the upper cardinal and lower broad ligament complex now that the peritoneum is open both anterior and posterior to the uterine fundus. Traction applied to the cervix moves the uterus down until the fundus is low in the pelvis. Hemostats are applied to the angle of the uterus on each side and the uterus is removed, usually posteriorly. The physician also repairs an enterocele, a herniation of intestine that protrudes against the vaginal wall, discovered during finger exploration. The hernia sac is bluntly and sharply dissected from the surrounding connective tissue, excised and ligated, and the surrounding tissues are strengthened and sutured. The peritoneum is closed with purse-string sutures that incorporate the proximal part of the uterosacral ligaments.

Coding Tips

This code does not include removal of tubes or ovaries. The enterocele repair is included and should not be identified separately. For repair of an enterocele with removal of tubes and ovaries, see 58292. For other vaginal hysterectomy codes, see 58260–58293.

ICD-9-CM Procedural

68.59 Other and unspecified vaginal hysterectomy

70.92 Other operations on cul-de-sac

Anesthesia

58294 00944

ICD-9-CM Diagnostic

180.0 Malignant neoplasm of endocervix

180.1 Malignant neoplasm of exocervix

182.0 Malignant neoplasm of corpus uteri, except isthmus

182.1 Malignant neoplasm of isthmus

182.8 Malignant neoplasm of other specified sites of body of uterus

218.0 Submucous leiomyoma of uterus

218.1 Intramural leiomyoma of uterus

218.2 Subserous leiomyoma of uterus

233.1 Carcinoma in situ of cervix uteri

618.00 Unspecified prolapse of vaginal walls without mention of uterine prolapse — (Use additional code to identify urinary incontinence: 625.6, 788.31, 788.33-788.39)

618.1 Uterine prolapse without mention of vaginal wall prolapse — (Use additional code to identify urinary incontinence: 625.6, 788.31, 788.33-788.39)

618.2 Uterovaginal prolapse, incomplete — (Use additional code to identify urinary incontinence: 625.6, 788.31, 788.33-788.39)

618.3 Uterovaginal prolapse, complete — (Use additional code to identify urinary incontinence: 625.6, 788.31, 788.33-788.39)

618.4 Uterovaginal prolapse, unspecified — (Use additional code to identify urinary incontinence: 625.6, 788.31, 788.33-788.39)

618.6 Vaginal enterocele, congenital or acquired — (Use additional code to identify urinary incontinence: 625.6, 788.31, 788.33-788.39)

618.82 Incompetence or weakening of rectovaginal tissue — (Use additional code to identify urinary incontinence: 625.6, 788.31, 788.33-788.39)

621.30 Endometrial hyperplasia, unspecified

621.31 Simple endometrial hyperplasia without atypia

621.32 Complex endometrial hyperplasia without atypia

621.33 Endometrial hyperplasia with atypia

621.34 Benign endometrial hyperplasia

621.35 Endometrial intraepithelial neoplasia [EIN]

622.10 Dysplasia of cervix, unspecified

625.6 Female stress incontinence

626.8 Other disorder of menstruation and other abnormal bleeding from female genital tract

627.1 Postmenopausal bleeding

CCI Version 18.3

0071T-0072T, 01962-01963, 01969, 0213T, 0216T, 0228T, 0230T, 12001-12007, 12011-12057, 13100-13153, 36000, 36400-36410, 36420-36430, 36440, 36600, 36640, 37202, 43752, 45560, 50715, 51040, 51701-51703, 57180, 57268-57270, 57283, 57410, 57420, 57452, 57500, 57522-57530, 57550-57555, 57800, 58100, 58120-58145, 58150❖, 58260-58263, 58267-58270, 58280❖, 58291, 58293, 58353-58356, 58541-58544❖, 58550, 58552-58554, 58558, 58570-58572❖, 58660, 58662, 58720, 62310-62319, 64400-64435, 64445-64450, 64479, 64483, 64490, 64493, 64505-64530, 69990, 93000-93010, 93040-93042, 93318, 94002, 94200, 94250, 94680-94690, 94770, 95812-95816, 95819, 95822, 95829, 95955, 96360, 96365, 96372, 96374-96376, 99148-99149, 99150, P9612

Note: These CCI edits are used for Medicare. Other payers may reimburse on codes listed above.

Medicare Edits

	Fac RVU	Non-Fac RVU	FUD	Status
58294	36.42	36.42	90	A

	MUE		Modifiers		
58294	1	51	N/A	62*	80

* with documentation

Medicare References: None

58300-58301

58300 Insertion of intrauterine device (IUD)
58301 Removal of intrauterine device (IUD)

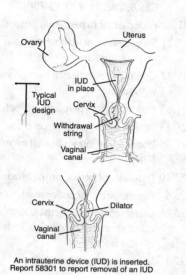

An intrauterine device (IUD) is inserted. Report 58301 to report removal of an IUD

Explanation

The physician inserts a speculum into the vagina to visualize the cervix. A tool is used to gently pull down the cervix; it is dilated. In 58300, an intrauterine device (IUD), any of a variety of shapes (coil, loop, T, 7), is guided into the uterus through an insertion tube placed in the cervical os. In 58301, to remove a previously placed IUD from the uterus, a device is inserted through the cervical os and used to grasp and remove the IUD.

Coding Tips

These procedures may be performed by a registered nurse, physician assistant, nurse practitioner, or other trained paramedical person under a physician's supervision. For IUD removal and insertion of a new device during the same visit, report both the IUD removal (58301) and insertion (58300) codes separately. The cost of the IUD is not included in these codes and should be reported separately using the appropriate HCPCS Level II code (J7300 or J7302). These procedures are usually not done out of medical necessity; therefore, the patient may be responsible for charges. Verify with the insurance carrier for coverage. Local anesthesia is included in these services. Surgical trays, A4550, are not separately reimbursed by Medicare; however, other third-party payers may cover them. Check with the specific payer to determine coverage.

ICD-9-CM Procedural

69.7 Insertion of intrauterine contraceptive device
97.71 Removal of intrauterine contraceptive device

Anesthesia
00940

ICD-9-CM Diagnostic

996.32 Mechanical complication due to intrauterine contraceptive device
996.65 Infection and inflammatory reaction due to other genitourinary device, implant, and graft — (Use additional code to identify specified infections)
996.76 Other complications due to genitourinary device, implant, and graft — (Use additional code to identify complication: 338.18-338.19, 338.28-338.29)
V25.11 Encounter for insertion of intrauterine contraceptive device
V25.12 Encounter for removal of intrauterine contraceptive device
V25.13 Encounter for removal and reinsertion of intrauterine contraceptive device
V25.42 Surveillance of previously prescribed intrauterine contraceptive device

Terms To Know

dilation. Artificial increase in the diameter of an opening or lumen made by medication or by instrumentation.

insertion. Placement or implantation into a body part.

IUD. Intrauterine device.

medical necessity. Medically appropriate and necessary to meet basic health needs; consistent with the diagnosis or condition and national medical practice guidelines regarding type, frequency, and duration of treatment; rendered in a cost-effective manner.

removal. Process of moving out of or away from, or the fact of being removed.

speculum. Tool used to enlarge the opening of any canal or cavity.

CCI Version 18.3

Also not with 58301: 0213T, 0216T, 0228T, 0230T, 12001-12007, 12011-12057, 13100-13153, 36000, 36400-36410, 36420-36430, 36440, 36600, 36640, 37202, 43752, 51701-51703, 57410, 57500, 62310-62319, 64400-64435, 64445-64450, 64479, 64483, 64490, 64493, 64505-64530, 69990, 93000-93010, 93040-93042, 93318, 94002, 94200, 94250, 94680-94690, 94770, 95812-95816, 95819, 95822, 95829, 95955, 96360, 96365, 96372, 96374-96376, 99148-99149, 99150, J0670, J2001

Note: These CCI edits are used for Medicare. Other payers may reimburse on codes listed above.

Medicare Edits

	Fac RVU	Non-Fac RVU	FUD	Status
58300	1.5	2.08	N/A	N
58301	2.03	2.85	0	A

	MUE		Modifiers		
58300	-	N/A	N/A	N/A	N/A
58301	1	51	N/A	N/A	80*

* with documentation

Medicare References: None

Corpus Uteri

58321-58322

58321 Artificial insemination; intra-cervical
58322 intra-uterine

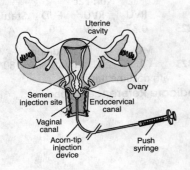

The physician injects semen into the endocervical canal in 58321

The physician injects semen into the uterine cavity in 58322

Explanation

In 58321, the physician performs artificial insemination by injecting semen into the endocervical canal by applying the blunt tip of a plastic syringe to the external os (opening) of the cervix. Sometimes a cervical cap is used to keep the semen in and around the cervix for eight to 16 hours. In 58322, the physician dilates the cervix and inserts a long flexible tube into the cavity of the uterus. Semen is injected into the uterus by a syringe connected to the tube.

Coding Tips

These procedures include only the semen injection and not the sperm preparation. For sperm preparation, see 58323. Because this procedure is usually not done out of medical necessity, the patient may be responsible for charges. Verify with the insurance carrier for coverage. For in vitro fertilization, see 58970–58976. Diagnostic coding should include male infertility in addition to the codes for female infertility. Surgical trays, A4550, are not separately reimbursed by Medicare; however, other third-party payers may cover them. Check with the specific payer to determine coverage.

ICD-9-CM Procedural

69.92   Artificial insemination

Anesthesia

N/A

ICD-9-CM Diagnostic

606.0   Azoospermia
606.1   Oligospermia
606.8   Infertility due to extratesticular causes
606.9   Unspecified male infertility
617.0   Endometriosis of uterus
622.4   Stricture and stenosis of cervix
628.0   Female infertility associated with anovulation — (Use additional code for any associated Stein-Leventhal syndrome: 256.4)
628.1   Female infertility of pituitary-hypothalamic origin — (Code first underlying cause: 253.0-253.4, 253.8)
628.3   Female infertility of uterine origin — (Use additional code for any associated tuberculous endometriosis: 016.7)
628.4   Female infertility of cervical or vaginal origin
628.8   Female infertility of other specified origin
628.9   Female infertility of unspecified origin
V26.1   Artificial insemination

Terms To Know

anovulation. Abnormal condition in which an ovum is not released each month. Anovulation is a prime factor in female infertility.

azoospermia. Failure of the development of sperm or the absence of sperm in semen; one of the most common factors in male infertility.

external os. Uterine opening through the cervix and into the vagina.

medical necessity. Medically appropriate and necessary to meet basic health needs; consistent with the diagnosis or condition and national medical practice guidelines regarding type, frequency, and duration of treatment; rendered in a cost-effective manner.

oligospermia. Insufficient production of sperm in semen, a common factor in male infertility.

stenosis. Narrowing or constriction of a passage.

stricture. Narrowing of an anatomical structure.

CCI Version 18.3

0213T, 0216T, 0228T, 0230T, 12001-12007, 12011-12057, 13100-13153, 36000, 36400-36410, 36420-36430, 36440, 36600, 36640, 37202, 43752, 51701-51703, 57410, 62310-62319, 64400-64435, 64445-64450, 64479, 64483, 64490, 64493, 64505-64530, 69990, 93000-93010, 93040-93042, 93318, 94002, 94200, 94250, 94680-94690, 94770, 95812-95816, 95819, 95822, 95829, 95955, 96360, 96365, 96372, 96374-96376, 99148-99149, 99150, J0670, J2001

Note: These CCI edits are used for Medicare. Other payers may reimburse on codes listed above.

Medicare Edits

	Fac RVU	Non-Fac RVU	FUD	Status
58321	1.37	2.2	0	A
58322	1.75	2.57	0	A

	MUE			Modifiers	
58321	1	51	N/A	N/A	80*
58322	1	51	N/A	N/A	80*

* with documentation

Medicare References: None

Coding Companion for Ob/Gyn

© 2012 OptumInsight, Inc.

Corpus Uteri

58323

58323 Sperm washing for artificial insemination

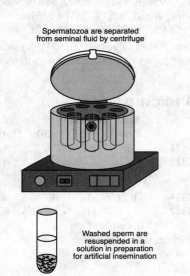

Spermatozoa are separated from seminal fluid by centrifuge

Washed sperm are resuspended in a solution in preparation for artificial insemination

Explanation

Sperm are spun in a centrifuge that removes the superficial antibodies on the sperm in order to facilitate fertilization. The sperm are first washed in a medium three times the volume of the collected semen. This mixture is spun in a centrifuge and the layer of liquid is discarded. The sperm are resuspended in a fresh medium. This method removes debris, bacteria, antibodies, and abnormal spermatozoa.

Coding Tips

Sperm washing is not routinely done with all sperm samples. Diagnostic coding should include codes for male infertility in addition to the codes for female infertility when applicable. Because this procedure is usually performed for the treatment of infertility, the patient may be responsible for charges. Verify with the insurance carrier for coverage. For artificial insemination, see 58321 and 58322. Surgical trays, A4550, are not separately reimbursed by Medicare; however, other third-party payers may cover them. Check with the specific payer to determine coverage.

ICD-9-CM Procedural

99.99   Other miscellaneous procedures

Anesthesia

58323 N/A

ICD-9-CM Diagnostic

606.0   Azoospermia

606.1   Oligospermia

606.8   Infertility due to extratesticular causes

606.9   Unspecified male infertility

622.4   Stricture and stenosis of cervix

628.0   Female infertility associated with anovulation — (Use additional code for any associated Stein-Leventhal syndrome: 256.4)

628.1   Female infertility of pituitary-hypothalamic origin — (Code first underlying cause: 253.0-253.4, 253.8)

628.4   Female infertility of cervical or vaginal origin

628.8   Female infertility of other specified origin

628.9   Female infertility of unspecified origin

V26.1   Artificial insemination

Terms To Know

anovulation. Abnormal condition in which an ovum is not released each month. Anovulation is a prime factor in female infertility.

antibody. Protein that B cells of the immune system produce in response to the presence of a foreign antigen.

azoospermia. Failure of the development of sperm or the absence of sperm in semen; one of the most common factors in male infertility.

centrifuge. Machine used to simulate gravitational effects or centrifugal force to separate substances of different densities.

medical necessity. Medically appropriate and necessary to meet basic health needs; consistent with the diagnosis or condition and national medical practice guidelines regarding type, frequency, and duration of treatment; rendered in a cost-effective manner.

oligospermia. Insufficient production of sperm in semen, a common factor in male infertility.

stenosis. Narrowing or constriction of a passage.

stricture. Narrowing of an anatomical structure.

CCI Version 18.3

0213T, 0216T, 0228T, 0230T, 12001-12007, 12011-12057, 13100-13153, 36000, 36400-36410, 36420-36430, 36440, 36600, 36640, 37202, 43752, 51701-51703, 57410, 62310-62319, 64400-64435, 64445-64450, 64479, 64483, 64490, 64493, 64505-64530, 69990, 93000-93010, 93040-93042, 93318, 94002, 94200, 94250, 94680-94690, 94770, 95812-95816, 95819, 95822, 95829, 95955, 96360, 96365, 96372, 96374-96376, 99148-99149, 99150

Note: These CCI edits are used for Medicare. Other payers may reimburse on codes listed above.

Medicare Edits

	Fac RVU	Non-Fac RVU	FUD	Status
58323	0.37	0.49	0	A

	MUE		Modifiers		
58323	1	51	N/A	N/A	80*

* with documentation

Medicare References: None

Corpus Uteri

58340

58340 Catheterization and introduction of saline or contrast material for saline infusion sonohysterography (SIS) or hysterosalpingography

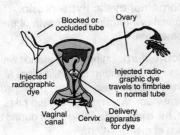

Explanation

A small catheter is introduced into the cervical opening and a saline solution (for saline infusion sonohysterography [SIS]) or liquid radiographic contrast material (for hysterosalpingography) is injected into the endometrial cavity with mild pressure to force the material into the fallopian tubes. The shadow of the contrast material appears on separately reported x-ray films, permitting examination of the uterus and fallopian tubes for any abnormalities or blockages. When sonohysterography is performed, a thin catheter is inserted into the uterus and one to two teaspoons of saline solution is injected into the uterine cavity. Separately reported, fluid enhanced endovaginal ultrasound is performed with the saline solution acting as a contrast medium to view any abnormal anatomic findings in the uterus.

Coding Tips

Report radiology services for this procedure separately. For hysterosonography, see 76831; hysterosalpingography, see 74740. For chromotubation of oviduct, see 58350. For transcervical introduction of fallopian tube or catheter, see 58345.

ICD-9-CM Procedural

68.19	Other diagnostic procedures on uterus and supporting structures
87.82	Gas contrast hysterosalpingogram
87.83	Opaque dye contrast hysterosalpingogram
87.84	Percutaneous hysterogram

Anesthesia

58340 00952

ICD-9-CM Diagnostic

218.0	Submucous leiomyoma of uterus
218.1	Intramural leiomyoma of uterus
218.2	Subserous leiomyoma of uterus
218.9	Leiomyoma of uterus, unspecified
256.31	Premature menopause — (Use additional code for states associated with natural menopause: 627.2)
256.39	Other ovarian failure — (Use additional code for states associated with natural menopause: 627.2)
256.4	Polycystic ovaries
256.8	Other ovarian dysfunction
614.1	Chronic salpingitis and oophoritis — (Use additional code to identify organism: 041.00-041.09, 041.10-041.19)
614.2	Salpingitis and oophoritis not specified as acute, subacute, or chronic — (Use additional code to identify organism: 041.00-041.09, 041.10-041.19)
614.6	Pelvic peritoneal adhesions, female (postoperative) (postinfection) — (Use additional code to identify organism: 041.00-041.09, 041.10-041.19) (Use additional code to identify any associated infertility: 628.2)
614.9	Unspecified inflammatory disease of female pelvic organs and tissues — (Use additional code to identify organism: 041.00-041.09, 041.10-041.19)
617.0	Endometriosis of uterus
617.1	Endometriosis of ovary
617.2	Endometriosis of fallopian tube
617.3	Endometriosis of pelvic peritoneum
617.9	Endometriosis, site unspecified
620.5	Torsion of ovary, ovarian pedicle, or fallopian tube
620.8	Other noninflammatory disorder of ovary, fallopian tube, and broad ligament
621.1	Chronic subinvolution of uterus
621.2	Hypertrophy of uterus
625.3	Dysmenorrhea
625.5	Pelvic congestion syndrome
626.0	Absence of menstruation
626.1	Scanty or infrequent menstruation
626.2	Excessive or frequent menstruation
626.4	Irregular menstrual cycle
626.6	Metrorrhagia
628.0	Female infertility associated with anovulation — (Use additional code for any associated Stein-Leventhal syndrome: 256.4)
628.2	Female infertility of tubal origin — (Use additional code for any associated peritubal adhesions: 614.6)
628.3	Female infertility of uterine origin — (Use additional code for any associated tuberculous endometriosis: 016.7)
628.8	Female infertility of other specified origin
629.0	Hematocele, female, not elsewhere classified
752.2	Congenital doubling of uterus
752.32	Hypoplasia of uterus
752.33	Unicornuate uterus
752.34	Bicornuate uterus
752.35	Septate uterus
752.36	Arcuate uterus
752.39	Other anomalies of uterus
793.5	Nonspecific (abnormal) findings on radiological and other examination of genitourinary organs

CCI Version 18.3

00952, 0213T, 0216T, 0228T, 0230T, 12001-12007, 12011-12057, 13100-13153, 36000, 36400-36410, 36420-36430, 36440, 36600, 36640, 37202, 43752, 51701-51703, 57410, 62310-62319, 64400-64435, 64445-64450, 64479, 64483, 64490, 64493, 64505-64530, 69990, 76000-76001, 76942, 77001-77002, 93000-93010, 93040-93042, 93318, 94002, 94200, 94250, 94680-94690, 94770, 95812-95816, 95819, 95822, 95829, 95955, 96360, 96365, 96372, 96374-96376, 99148-99149, 99150, J0670, J1644, J2001

Note: These CCI edits are used for Medicare. Other payers may reimburse on codes listed above.

Medicare Edits

	Fac RVU	Non-Fac RVU	FUD	Status
58340	1.72	3.58	0	A

	MUE		Modifiers		
58340	1	51	N/A	N/A	N/A

* with documentation

Medicare References: None

Corpus Uteri

58345

58345 Transcervical introduction of fallopian tube catheter for diagnosis and/or re-establishing patency (any method), with or without hysterosalpingography

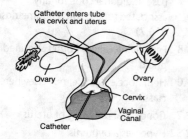

Catheter enters tube via cervix and uterus

Ovary — Ovary

Cervix

Vaginal Canal

Catheter

Explanation

The physician introduces a catheter into the cervix, and takes it into the uterus and through the fallopian tube. The catheter must be made of a material that will show on x-ray film so that any blockages or abnormalities in the tube can be seen. The physician may inject radiographic contrast material into the endometrial cavity with mild pressure to force the material into the tubes. The shadow of this material on separately reported x-ray film permits examination of the uterus and tubes for any abnormalities or blockages.

Coding Tips

This procedure can be accomplished in a physician's office when radiology equipment is present or in a radiology facility. This code includes any method of re-establishing patency of the tube and a hysterosalpingography performed by the physician. For radiological supervision and interpretation of transcervical catheterization of a fallopian tube, see 74742. Because this procedure is usually performed for the treatment of infertility, the patient may be responsible for charges. Verify with the insurance carrier for coverage. For surgical treatment of an ectopic pregnancy, see 59120–59140. For laparoscopic treatment of an ectopic pregnancy, see 59150–59151.

ICD-9-CM Procedural

66.79	Other repair of fallopian tube
66.8	Insufflation of fallopian tube
66.95	Insufflation of therapeutic agent into fallopian tubes
66.96	Dilation of fallopian tube
87.85	Other x-ray of fallopian tubes and uterus

Anesthesia

58345 00952

ICD-9-CM Diagnostic

256.4	Polycystic ovaries
256.8	Other ovarian dysfunction
614.1	Chronic salpingitis and oophoritis — (Use additional code to identify organism: 041.00-041.09, 041.10-041.19)
614.2	Salpingitis and oophoritis not specified as acute, subacute, or chronic — (Use additional code to identify organism: 041.00-041.09, 041.10-041.19)
614.6	Pelvic peritoneal adhesions, female (postoperative) (postinfection) — (Use additional code to identify organism: 041.00-041.09, 041.10-041.19) (Use additional code to identify any associated infertility: 628.2)
617.2	Endometriosis of fallopian tube
620.8	Other noninflammatory disorder of ovary, fallopian tube, and broad ligament
621.1	Chronic subinvolution of uterus
621.2	Hypertrophy of uterus
621.30	Endometrial hyperplasia, unspecified
621.31	Simple endometrial hyperplasia without atypia
621.32	Complex endometrial hyperplasia without atypia
621.33	Endometrial hyperplasia with atypia
621.34	Benign endometrial hyperplasia
621.35	Endometrial intraepithelial neoplasia [EIN]
621.7	Chronic inversion of uterus
622.4	Stricture and stenosis of cervix
622.8	Other specified noninflammatory disorder of cervix
628.2	Female infertility of tubal origin — (Use additional code for any associated peritubal adhesions: 614.6)
628.8	Female infertility of other specified origin
628.9	Female infertility of unspecified origin
752.19	Other congenital anomaly of fallopian tubes and broad ligaments
V26.21	Fertility testing
V26.22	Aftercare following sterilization reversal
V26.29	Other investigation and testing

Terms To Know

chronic inversion of uterus. Persistent abnormality in which the uterus turns inside out.

endometrial cystic hyperplasia. Abnormal cyst-forming overgrowth of the endometrium.

endometrium. Lining of the uterus, which thickens in preparation for fertilization. A fertilized ovum embeds into the thickened endometrium. When no fertilization takes place, the endometrial lining sheds during the process of menstruation.

hysterosalpingography. Radiographic pictures taken of the uterus and the fallopian tubes after the injection of a radiopaque dye.

oophoritis. Inflammation or infection of one or both ovaries that can cause chronic pelvic pain, ectopic pregnancy, or sterilization.

salpingitis. Inflammation of the fallopian tubes, usually caused by a bacterial infection and occurring in conjunction with inflammation of the ovaries (oophoritis).

stenosis. Narrowing or constriction of a passage.

CCI Version 18.3

00952, 0213T, 0216T, 0228T, 0230T, 12001-12007, 12011-12057, 13100-13153, 36000, 36400-36410, 36420-36430, 36440, 36600, 36640, 37202, 43752, 51701-51703, 57410, 58340, 62310-62319, 64400-64435, 64445-64450, 64479, 64483, 64490, 64493, 64505-64530, 69990, 76000-76001, 76942, 77001-77002, 93000-93010, 93040-93042, 93318, 94002, 94200, 94250, 94680-94690, 94770, 95812-95816, 95819, 95822, 95829, 95955, 96360, 96365, 96372, 96374-96376, 99148-99149, 99150

Note: These CCI edits are used for Medicare. Other payers may reimburse on codes listed above.

Medicare Edits

	Fac RVU	Non-Fac RVU	FUD	Status
58345	8.35	8.35	10	A

	MUE		Modifiers		
58345	1	51	50	62	80

* with documentation

Medicare References: None

Corpus Uteri

58346

58346 Insertion of Heyman capsules for clinical brachytherapy

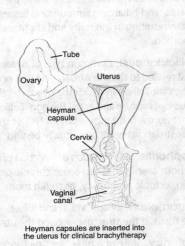

Heyman capsules are inserted into the uterus for clinical brachytherapy

Explanation

The physician inserts radioactive Heyman capsules into the uterus to treat endometrial cancer. Radiotherapy is often the prescribed treatment for patients who are medically inoperable for endometrial carcinoma. Brachytherapy is administered via low dose radiation (LDR) or high dose radiation (HDR) technique, with the goal of achieving coverage of all uterine tissue. This is achieved with the placement of multiple Heyman capsules, inserted through the cervical os and placed in the uterus with consideration of appropriate radiation field. For low-dose treatment, Heyman capsules are used for patients with a large uterus to help expand the uterine cavity and cover the uterus. Heyman capsules also may be prescribed for patients with early-stage disease and low-grade histology, when radiation alone is the preferred therapy. Use this code once to report multiple capsules inserted during the same session.

Coding Tips

For insertion of intracavitary radioelement sources, see 77761–77763. For interstitial application of radioelement sources or ribbons, see 77776–77778. For high intensity brachytherapy remote afterloading, see 77781–77784.

ICD-9-CM Procedural

68.0   Hysterotomy
92.27   Implantation or insertion of radioactive elements

Anesthesia

58346   00940

ICD-9-CM Diagnostic

179   Malignant neoplasm of uterus, part unspecified
180.0   Malignant neoplasm of endocervix
180.1   Malignant neoplasm of exocervix
180.8   Malignant neoplasm of other specified sites of cervix
180.9   Malignant neoplasm of cervix uteri, unspecified site
182.0   Malignant neoplasm of corpus uteri, except isthmus
182.1   Malignant neoplasm of isthmus
182.8   Malignant neoplasm of other specified sites of body of uterus
198.82   Secondary malignant neoplasm of genital organs
233.1   Carcinoma in situ of cervix uteri
233.2   Carcinoma in situ of other and unspecified parts of uterus
233.30   Carcinoma in situ, unspecified female genital organ
233.31   Carcinoma in situ, vagina
233.32   Carcinoma in situ, vulva
233.39   Carcinoma in situ, other female genital organ
236.0   Neoplasm of uncertain behavior of uterus
236.3   Neoplasm of uncertain behavior of other and unspecified female genital organs

Terms To Know

brachytherapy. Form of radiation therapy in which radioactive pellets or seeds are implanted directly into the tissue being treated to deliver their dose of radiation in a more directed fashion. Brachytherapy provides radiation to the prescribed body area while minimizing exposure to normal tissue.

carcinoma in situ. Malignancy that arises from the cells of the vessel, gland, or organ of origin that remains confined to that site or has not invaded neighboring tissue. Carcinoma in situ codes are found in their own subchapter of neoplasms according to site.

endometrial carcinoma. Cancer of the inner lining of the uterine wall.

malignant. Any condition tending to progress toward death, specifically an invasive tumor with a loss of cellular differentiation that has the ability to spread or metastasize to other areas in the body.

secondary. Second in order of occurrence or importance, or appearing during the course of another disease or condition.

CCI Version 18.3

0213T, 0216T, 0228T, 0230T, 12001-12007, 12011-12057, 13100-13153, 36000, 36400-36410, 36420-36430, 36440, 36600, 36640, 37202, 43752, 51701-51703, 57400-57410, 57558, 57800, 58100, 62310-62319, 64400-64435, 64445-64450, 64479, 64483, 64490, 64493, 64505-64530, 69990, 93000-93010, 93040-93042, 93318, 94002, 94200, 94250, 94680-94690, 94770, 95812-95816, 95819, 95822, 95829, 95955, 96360, 96365, 96372, 96374-96376, 99148-99149, 99150

Note: These CCI edits are used for Medicare. Other payers may reimburse on codes listed above.

Medicare Edits

	Fac RVU	Non-Fac RVU	FUD	Status
58346	13.21	13.21	90	A

	MUE		Modifiers		
58346	1	51	N/A	N/A	N/A

* with documentation

Medicare References: None

58350

58350 Chromotubation of oviduct, including materials

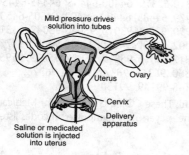

Mild pressure drives solution into tubes

Uterus

Ovary

Cervix

Delivery apparatus

Saline or medicated solution is injected into uterus

Explanation

The physician injects a liquid dye or solution into the uterine cavity or directly into the fallopian tubes. This procedure is frequently performed during a separately reported surgery, open or laparoscopic, to verify patency of tubes.

Coding Tips

When 58350 is performed with another separately identifiable procedure, the highest dollar value code is listed as the primary procedure and subsequent procedures are appended with modifier 51. Supply of materials should be reported separately with code 99070.

ICD-9-CM Procedural

66.8   Insufflation of fallopian tube
66.95   Insufflation of therapeutic agent into fallopian tubes

Anesthesia

58350   00952

ICD-9-CM Diagnostic

614.1   Chronic salpingitis and oophoritis — (Use additional code to identify organism: 041.00-041.09, 041.10-041.19)

614.2   Salpingitis and oophoritis not specified as acute, subacute, or chronic — (Use additional code to identify organism: 041.00-041.09, 041.10-041.19)

614.3   Acute parametritis and pelvic cellulitis — (Use additional code to identify organism: 041.00-041.09, 041.10-041.19)

614.4   Chronic or unspecified parametritis and pelvic cellulitis — (Use additional code to identify organism: 041.00-041.09, 041.10-041.19)

614.5   Acute or unspecified pelvic peritonitis, female — (Use additional code to identify organism: 041.00-041.09, 041.10-041.19)

614.6   Pelvic peritoneal adhesions, female (postoperative) (postinfection) — (Use additional code to identify organism: 041.00-041.09, 041.10-041.19) (Use additional code to identify any associated infertility: 628.2)

617.0   Endometriosis of uterus
617.2   Endometriosis of fallopian tube
617.3   Endometriosis of pelvic peritoneum
617.8   Endometriosis of other specified sites
620.0   Follicular cyst of ovary
620.2   Other and unspecified ovarian cyst
620.3   Acquired atrophy of ovary and fallopian tube
620.8   Other noninflammatory disorder of ovary, fallopian tube, and broad ligament
625.3   Dysmenorrhea
628.2   Female infertility of tubal origin — (Use additional code for any associated peritubal adhesions: 614.6)
628.8   Female infertility of other specified origin
628.9   Female infertility of unspecified origin
752.19 Other congenital anomaly of fallopian tubes and broad ligaments
V26.21 Fertility testing
V26.22 Aftercare following sterilization reversal
V26.29 Other investigation and testing

Terms To Know

adhesion. Abnormal fibrous connection between two structures, soft tissue or bony structures, that may occur as the result of surgery, infection, or trauma.

cellulitis. Sudden, severe, suppurative inflammation and edema in subcutaneous tissue or muscle, most often caused by bacterial infection secondary to a cutaneous lesion.

chromotubation. Injection of a medication or saline solution into the uterine cavity and fallopian tubes to verify patency of the tubes.

endometriosis. Aberrant uterine mucosal tissue appearing in areas of the pelvic cavity outside of its normal location, lining the uterus, and inflaming surrounding tissues often resulting in infertility and spontaneous abortion.

follicular cyst. Common type of ovarian cyst related to the menstrual cycle that occurs when the follicle in which the ovum develops does not rupture and expel the egg. Follicular cysts normally disappear within two or three menstrual cycles and are usually benign.

oophoritis. Inflammation or infection of one or both ovaries that can cause chronic pelvic pain, ectopic pregnancy, or sterilization.

parametritis. Inflammation and infection of the tissue in the structures around the uterus.

patency. State of a tube-like structure or conduit being open and unobstructed.

peritonitis. Inflammation and infection within the peritoneal cavity, the space between the membrane lining the abdominopelvic walls and covering the internal organs.

salpingitis. Inflammation of the fallopian tubes, usually caused by a bacterial infection and occurring in conjunction with inflammation of the ovaries (oophoritis).

CCI Version 18.3

0213T, 0216T, 0228T, 0230T, 12001-12007, 12011-12057, 13100-13153, 36000, 36400-36410, 36420-36430, 36440, 36600, 36640, 37202, 43752, 51701-51703, 57410, 62310-62319, 64400-64435, 64445-64450, 64479, 64483, 64490, 64493, 64505-64530, 69990, 93000-93010, 93040-93042, 93318, 94002, 94200, 94250, 94680-94690, 94770, 95812-95816, 95819, 95822, 95829, 95955, 96360, 96365, 96372, 96374-96376, 99148-99149, 99150, J0670, J2001

Note: These CCI edits are used for Medicare. Other payers may reimburse on codes listed above.

Medicare Edits

	Fac RVU	Non-Fac RVU	FUD	Status
58350	2.36	2.89	10	A

	MUE		Modifiers		
58350	2	51	N/A	N/A	N/A

* with documentation

Medicare References: None

58353

58353 Endometrial ablation, thermal, without hysteroscopic guidance

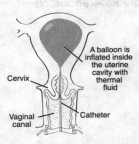

A balloon is inflated inside the uterine cavity with thermal fluid

Cervix

Vaginal canal

Catheter

Fluid in the balloon is heated to a scalding temperature, causing the lining to slough away

The endometrial lining of the uterus is ablated using a thermal method, without hysteroscopic guidance

Explanation

The physician performs an endometrial ablation, using heat without hysteroscopic guidance. The physician inserts a soft, flexible balloon attached to a thin catheter into the vagina through the cervix and into the uterus. The balloon is inflated with fluid, which expands to fit the size and shape of the patient's uterus. The fluid in the balloon is heated to 87°C or 188°F and maintained for eight to nine minutes while the uterine lining is treated. When the treatment cycle is complete, all the fluid is withdrawn from the balloon and the balloon and catheter are removed.

Coding Tips

When 58353 is performed with another separately identifiable procedure, the highest dollar value code is listed as the primary procedure and subsequent procedures are appended with modifier 51. Local anesthesia is included in this service; however, this procedure may be performed under general anesthesia depending on the age and/or condition of the patient. For endometrial ablation with hysteroscopy, see 58563. Surgical trays, A4550, are not separately reimbursed by Medicare; however, other third-party payers may cover them. Check with the specific payer to determine coverage.

ICD-9-CM Procedural

68.23 Endometrial ablation

69.09 Other dilation and curettage of uterus

69.59 Other aspiration curettage of uterus

88.79 Other diagnostic ultrasound

Anesthesia

58353 00940

ICD-9-CM Diagnostic

617.0 Endometriosis of uterus

617.9 Endometriosis, site unspecified

626.2 Excessive or frequent menstruation

626.6 Metrorrhagia

626.8 Other disorder of menstruation and other abnormal bleeding from female genital tract

627.1 Postmenopausal bleeding

Terms To Know

ablation. Removal or destruction of a body part or tissue or its function. Ablation may be performed by surgical means, hormones, drugs, radiofrequency, heat, chemical application, or other methods.

catheter. Flexible tube inserted into an area of the body for introducing or withdrawing fluid.

endometriosis. Aberrant uterine mucosal tissue appearing in areas of the pelvic cavity outside of its normal location, lining the uterus and inflaming surrounding tissues, and can result in infertility and spontaneous abortion.

metrorrhagia. Prolonged, irregular uterine bleeding of an inconsistent amount occurring in frequent bouts.

CCI Version 18.3

0213T, 0216T, 0228T, 0230T, 12001-12007, 12011-12057, 13100-13153, 36000, 36400-36410, 36420-36430, 36440, 36600, 36640, 37202, 43752, 51701-51703, 57100, 57400-57410, 57800, 58100, 58120, 58555-58560, 58562-58563, 62310-62319, 64400-64435, 64445-64450, 64479, 64483, 64490, 64493, 64505-64530, 69990, 93000-93010, 93040-93042, 93318, 94002, 94200, 94250, 94680-94690, 94770, 95812-95816, 95819, 95822, 95829, 95955, 96360, 96365, 96372, 96374-96376, 99148-99149, 99150, J0670, J2001

Note: These CCI edits are used for Medicare. Other payers may reimburse on codes listed above.

Medicare Edits

	Fac RVU	Non-Fac RVU	FUD	Status
58353	6.56	31.13	10	A

	MUE		Modifiers		
58353	1	51	N/A	62	N/A

* with documentation

Medicare References: 100-3,230.6

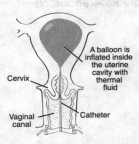

Coding Companion for Ob/Gyn

Corpus Uteri

58356

58356 Endometrial cryoablation with ultrasonic guidance, including endometrial curettage, when performed

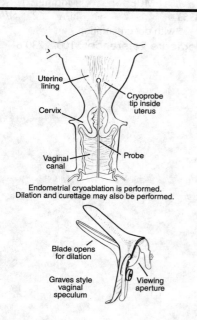

Endometrial cryoablation is performed. Dilation and curettage may also be performed.

Blade opens for dilation

Graves style vaginal speculum

Viewing aperture

Explanation

The physician performs endometrial cryoablation with any required endometrial curettage using ultrasound guidance. The physician inserts a speculum for visualization of the cervix. A numbing block is placed in the cervix. A thin cryoablation device is inserted through the cervix into the uterus. The cryoablation device freezes targeted uterine endometrial tissue. The instrument is withdrawn following completion of the procedure. Ultrasound provides visualization of probe placement and real-time monitoring of the ice ball growth. If endometrial curettage is required, the physician passes a curette into the uterus through the endocervical canal. The lining of the uterus is scraped.

Coding Tips

Biopsy of the endometrium, dilation and curettage, catheterization and contrast medium or saline infusion, and pelvic or abdominal ultrasound are included in 58356 and should not be reported separately. Surgical trays, A4550, are not separately reimbursed by Medicare; however, other third-party payers may cover them. Check with the specific payer to determine coverage.

ICD-9-CM Procedural

68.23 Endometrial ablation
69.09 Other dilation and curettage of uterus
69.59 Other aspiration curettage of uterus

88.79 Other diagnostic ultrasound

Anesthesia

58356 00840, 00940, 00944

ICD-9-CM Diagnostic

617.0 Endometriosis of uterus
617.9 Endometriosis, site unspecified
626.2 Excessive or frequent menstruation
626.6 Metrorrhagia
626.8 Other disorder of menstruation and other abnormal bleeding from female genital tract
627.1 Postmenopausal bleeding

Terms To Know

ablation. Removal or destruction of a body part or tissue or its function. Ablation may be performed by surgical means, hormones, drugs, radiofrequency, heat, chemical application, or other methods.

cryotherapy. Any surgical procedure that uses intense cold for treatment.

curettage. Removal of tissue by scraping.

curette. Spoon-shaped instrument used to scrape out abnormal tissue from a cavity or bone.

endometrium. Lining of the uterus, which thickens in preparation for fertilization. A fertilized ovum embeds into the thickened endometrium. When no fertilization takes place, the endometrial lining sheds during the process of menstruation.

speculum. Tool used to enlarge the opening of any canal or cavity.

ultrasound. Imaging using ultra-high sound frequency bounced off body structures.

CCI Version 18.3

00940, 0213T, 0216T, 0228T, 0230T, 12001-12007, 12011-12057, 13100-13153, 36000, 36400-36410, 36420-36430, 36440, 36600, 36640, 37202, 43752, 51701-51703, 57180, 57400-57410, 57452, 57500, 57800, 58100, 58120, 58340, 58353❖, 58558, 58563❖, 62310-62319, 64400-64435, 64445-64450, 64479, 64483, 64490, 64493, 64505-64530, 69990, 76700, 76830, 76856-76857, 76940, 76942, 76998, 77013, 77022, 93000-93010, 93040-93042, 93318, 94002, 94200, 94250, 94680-94690, 94770, 95812-95816, 95819, 95822, 95829, 95955, 96360, 96365, 96372, 96374-96376, 99148-99149, 99150, J0670, J2001

Note: These CCI edits are used for Medicare. Other payers may reimburse on codes listed above.

58400

58400   Uterine suspension, with or without shortening of round ligaments, with or without shortening of sacrouterine ligaments; (separate procedure)

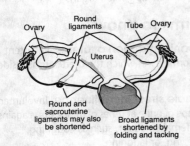

Ovary   Round ligaments   Tube   Ovary

Uterus

Round and sacrouterine ligaments may also be shortened

Broad ligaments shortened by folding and tacking

Explanation

The physician plicates stretched uterine broad ligaments, bringing the uterus back into place. Plication shortens the ligament by folding and tacking it. The physician may elect to plicate the round and sacrouterine ligaments as well. This procedure may be done through a small abdominal incision or through an incision in the vagina.

Coding Tips

This separate procedure by definition is usually a component of a more complex service and is not identified separately. When performed alone or with other unrelated procedures/services it may be reported. If performed alone, list the code; if performed with other procedures/services, list the code and append modifier 59. When 58400 is performed with another separately identifiable procedure, the highest dollar value code is listed as the primary procedure and subsequent procedures are appended with modifier 51. For uterine suspension, with or without shortening of round ligaments, with or without shortening of sacrouterine ligaments, with presacral sympathectomy, report 58410.

ICD-9-CM Procedural

69.21   Interposition operation of uterine supporting structures

69.22   Other uterine suspension

69.29   Other repair of uterus and supporting structures

69.98   Other operations on supporting structures of uterus

Anesthesia

58400   00840

ICD-9-CM Diagnostic

618.00   Unspecified prolapse of vaginal walls without mention of uterine prolapse — (Use additional code to identify urinary incontinence: 625.6, 788.31, 788.33-788.39)

618.01   Cystocele without mention of uterine prolapse, midline — (Use additional code to identify urinary incontinence: 625.6, 788.31, 788.33-788.39)

618.02   Cystocele without mention of uterine prolapse, lateral — (Use additional code to identify urinary incontinence: 625.6, 788.31, 788.33-788.39)

618.03   Urethrocele without mention of uterine prolapse — (Use additional code to identify urinary incontinence: 625.6, 788.31, 788.33-788.39)

618.04   Rectocele without mention of uterine prolapse — (Use additional code to identify urinary incontinence: 625.6, 788.31, 788.33-788.39) (Use additional code for any associated fecal incontinence: 787.60-787.63)

618.05   Perineocele without mention of uterine prolapse — (Use additional code to identify urinary incontinence: 625.6, 788.31, 788.33-788.39)

618.1   Uterine prolapse without mention of vaginal wall prolapse — (Use additional code to identify urinary incontinence: 625.6, 788.31, 788.33-788.39)

618.2   Uterovaginal prolapse, incomplete — (Use additional code to identify urinary incontinence: 625.6, 788.31, 788.33-788.39)

618.3   Uterovaginal prolapse, complete — (Use additional code to identify urinary incontinence: 625.6, 788.31, 788.33-788.39)

618.81   Incompetence or weakening of pubocervical tissue — (Use additional code to identify urinary incontinence: 625.6, 788.31, 788.33-788.39)

618.82   Incompetence or weakening of rectovaginal tissue — (Use additional code to identify urinary incontinence: 625.6, 788.31, 788.33-788.39)

618.83   Pelvic muscle wasting — (Use additional code to identify urinary incontinence: 625.6, 788.31, 788.33-788.39)

618.89   Other specified genital prolapse — (Use additional code to identify urinary incontinence: 625.6, 788.31, 788.33-788.39)

621.6   Malposition of uterus

621.7   Chronic inversion of uterus

625.0   Dyspareunia

625.3   Dysmenorrhea

625.6   Female stress incontinence

625.8   Other specified symptom associated with female genital organs

625.9   Unspecified symptom associated with female genital organs

Terms To Know

broad ligament. Fold of peritoneum extending from the side of the uterus to the wall of the pelvis.

chronic inversion of uterus. Persistent abnormality in which the uterus turns inside out.

round ligament. Ligament between the uterus and the pelvic wall.

suspension. Fixation of an organ for support; temporary state of cessation of an activity, process, or experience.

CCI Version 18.3

0213T, 0216T, 0228T, 0230T, 12001-12007, 12011-12057, 13100-13153, 36000, 36400-36410, 36420-36430, 36440, 36600, 36640, 37202, 43752, 44005, 44180, 44602-44605, 44820-44850, 44950, 44970, 49000-49010, 49255, 49320, 49570, 50715, 51701-51703, 57410, 62310-62319, 64400-64435, 64445-64450, 64479, 64483, 64490, 64493, 64505-64530, 69990, 93000-93010, 93040-93042, 93318, 94002, 94200, 94250, 94680-94690, 94770, 95812-95816, 95819, 95822, 95829, 95955, 96360, 96365, 96372, 96374-96376, 99148-99149, 99150

Note: These CCI edits are used for Medicare. Other payers may reimburse on codes listed above.

Medicare Edits

	Fac RVU	Non-Fac RVU	FUD	Status
58400	13.09	13.09	90	A

	MUE		Modifiers		
58400	1	51	N/A	62*	80

* with documentation

Medicare References: None

Coding Companion for Ob/Gyn

Corpus Uteri

58410

58410 Uterine suspension, with or without shortening of round ligaments, with or without shortening of sacrouterine ligaments; with presacral sympathectomy

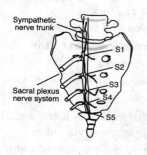

Sympathetic nerve trunk
S1
S2
S3
Sacral plexus nerve system
S4
S5

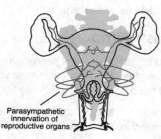

Parasympathetic innervation of reproductive organs

Explanation

The physician plicates stretched uterine broad ligaments, bringing the uterus back into place. Plication shortens the ligament by folding and tacking it. The physician may elect to plicate the round and sacrouterine ligaments as well. A portion of the presacral sympathetic nerve is removed or destroyed to alleviate pelvic pain. The procedure may be done through a small abdominal incision or through an incision in the vagina.

Coding Tips

When 58410 is performed with another separately identifiable procedure, the highest dollar value code is listed as the primary procedure and subsequent procedures are appended with modifier 51. For uterine suspension, with or without shortening of round ligaments, with or without shortening of sacrouterine ligaments, without presacral sympathectomy, report 58400.

ICD-9-CM Procedural

05.24	Presacral sympathectomy
69.21	Interposition operation of uterine supporting structures
69.22	Other uterine suspension
69.29	Other repair of uterus and supporting structures
69.98	Other operations on supporting structures of uterus

Anesthesia

58410 00840

ICD-9-CM Diagnostic

618.00	Unspecified prolapse of vaginal walls without mention of uterine prolapse — (Use additional code to identify urinary incontinence: 625.6, 788.31, 788.33-788.39)
618.01	Cystocele without mention of uterine prolapse, midline — (Use additional code to identify urinary incontinence: 625.6, 788.31, 788.33-788.39)
618.02	Cystocele without mention of uterine prolapse, lateral — (Use additional code to identify urinary incontinence: 625.6, 788.31, 788.33-788.39)
618.03	Urethrocele without mention of uterine prolapse — (Use additional code to identify urinary incontinence: 625.6, 788.31, 788.33-788.39)
618.04	Rectocele without mention of uterine prolapse — (Use additional code to identify urinary incontinence: 625.6, 788.31, 788.33-788.39) (Use additional code for any associated fecal incontinence: 787.60-787.63)
618.05	Perineocele without mention of uterine prolapse — (Use additional code to identify urinary incontinence: 625.6, 788.31, 788.33-788.39)
618.1	Uterine prolapse without mention of vaginal wall prolapse — (Use additional code to identify urinary incontinence: 625.6, 788.31, 788.33-788.39)
618.2	Uterovaginal prolapse, incomplete — (Use additional code to identify urinary incontinence: 625.6, 788.31, 788.33-788.39)
618.3	Uterovaginal prolapse, complete — (Use additional code to identify urinary incontinence: 625.6, 788.31, 788.33-788.39)
618.81	Incompetence or weakening of pubocervical tissue — (Use additional code to identify urinary incontinence: 625.6, 788.31, 788.33-788.39)
618.82	Incompetence or weakening of rectovaginal tissue — (Use additional code to identify urinary incontinence: 625.6, 788.31, 788.33-788.39)
618.83	Pelvic muscle wasting — (Use additional code to identify urinary incontinence: 625.6, 788.31, 788.33-788.39)
618.89	Other specified genital prolapse — (Use additional code to identify urinary incontinence: 625.6, 788.31, 788.33-788.39)
621.6	Malposition of uterus
621.7	Chronic inversion of uterus
625.0	Dyspareunia
625.3	Dysmenorrhea
625.6	Female stress incontinence
625.8	Other specified symptom associated with female genital organs
625.9	Unspecified symptom associated with female genital organs

Terms To Know

chronic inversion of uterus. Persistent abnormality in which the uterus turns inside out.

female stress incontinence. Involuntary escape of urine at times of minor stress against the female bladder, such as coughing, sneezing, or laughing.

round ligament. Ligament between the uterus and the pelvic wall.

suspension. Fixation of an organ for support; temporary state of cessation of an activity, process, or experience.

uterovaginal prolapse. Uterus displaces downward and is exposed in the external genitalia.

CCI Version 18.3

0213T, 0216T, 0228T, 0230T, 12001-12007, 12011-12057, 13100-13153, 36000, 36400-36410, 36420-36430, 36440, 36600, 36640, 37202, 43752, 44005, 44180, 44602-44605, 44820-44850, 44950, 44970, 49000-49010, 49255, 49320, 49570, 50715, 51701-51703, 57410, 58400, 62310-62319, 64400-64435, 64445-64450, 64479, 64483, 64490, 64493, 64505-64530, 69990, 93000-93010, 93040-93042, 93318, 94002, 94200, 94250, 94680-94690, 94770, 95812-95816, 95819, 95822, 95829, 95955, 96360, 96365, 96372, 96374-96376, 99148-99149, 99150

Note: These CCI edits are used for Medicare. Other payers may reimburse on codes listed above.

Medicare Edits

	Fac RVU	Non-Fac RVU	FUD	Status
58410	24.0	24.0	90	A

	MUE			Modifiers	
58410	1	51	N/A	62*	80

* with documentation

Medicare References: None

Corpus Uteri

58520

58520 Hysterorrhaphy, repair of ruptured uterus (nonobstetrical)

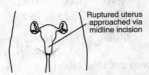

Ruptured uterus approached via midline incision

The injury may require additional procedures

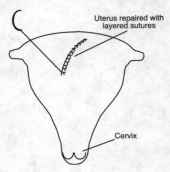

Uterus repaired with layered sutures

Cervix

Explanation

The physician repairs a uterus that became lacerated or ruptured by nonobstetrical means. A large incision is made in the abdomen and the uterus is repaired with layered suturing of torn, crushed, or deeply lacerated tissue. The physician debrides the wound by removing foreign material or damaged tissue. Irrigation of the wound is performed and antimicrobial solutions are used to decontaminate and cleanse the wound. The physician may trim skin margins with a scalpel or scissors to allow for proper closure. The abdominal incision is closed.

Coding Tips

This code applies only to ruptures caused by injury or trauma, not by pregnancy. When 58520 is performed with another separately identifiable procedure, the highest dollar value code is listed as the primary procedure and subsequent procedures are appended with modifier 51. For repair of a ruptured uterus in an obstetrical setting, report 59350. When hysteroplasty is done to correct an anomaly present from birth, not an acquired condition due to trauma, age, or disease, see 58540.

ICD-9-CM Procedural

69.29 Other repair of uterus and supporting structures

69.49 Other repair of uterus

Anesthesia

58520 00840

ICD-9-CM Diagnostic

621.8 Other specified disorders of uterus, not elsewhere classified

867.4 Uterus injury without mention of open wound into cavity

867.5 Uterus injury with open wound into cavity

Terms To Know

debride. To remove all foreign objects and devitalized or infected tissue from a burn or wound to prevent infection and promote healing.

irrigation. To wash out or cleanse a body cavity, wound, or tissue with water or other fluid.

repair. Surgical closure of a wound. The wound may be a result of injury/trauma or it may be a surgically created defect. Repairs are divided into three categories: simple, intermediate, and complex.

rupture. Tearing or breaking open of tissue.

suture. Numerous stitching techniques employed in wound closure.

buried suture. Continuous or interrupted suture placed under the skin for a layered closure.

continuous suture. Running stitch with tension evenly distributed across a single strand to provide a leakproof closure line.

interrupted suture. Series of single stitches with tension isolated at each stitch, in which all stitches are not affected if one becomes loose, and the isolated sutures cannot act as a wick to transport an infection.

purse-string suture. Continuous suture placed around a tubular structure and tightened, to reduce or close the lumen.

retention suture. Secondary stitching that bridges the primary suture, providing support for the primary repair; a plastic or rubber bolster may be placed over the primary repair and under the retention sutures.

wound. Injury to living tissue often involving a cut or break in the skin.

CCI Version 18.3

0213T, 0216T, 0228T, 0230T, 12001-12007, 12011-12057, 13100-13153, 36000, 36400-36410, 36420-36430, 36440, 36600, 36640, 37202, 43752, 44005, 44180, 44602-44605, 44820-44850, 44950, 44970, 49000-49010, 49255, 49320, 49570, 50715, 51701-51703, 57410, 58140-58146, 62310-62319, 64400-64435, 64445-64450, 64479, 64483, 64490, 64493, 64505-64530, 69990, 93000-93010, 93040-93042, 93318, 94002, 94200, 94250, 94680-94690, 94770,

95812-95816, 95819, 95822, 95829, 95955, 96360, 96365, 96372, 96374-96376, 99148-99149, 99150

Note: These CCI edits are used for Medicare. Other payers may reimburse on codes listed above.

Medicare Edits

	Fac RVU	Non-Fac RVU	FUD	Status
58520	24.11	24.11	90	A

	MUE		Modifiers	
58520	1	51	N/A 62*	80

* with documentation

Medicare References: None

58540

58540 Hysteroplasty, repair of uterine anomaly (Strassman type)

Some types of uterine anomalies

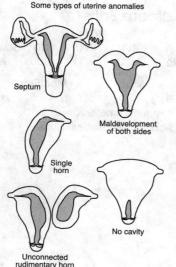

Septum

Maldevelopment of both sides

Single horn

No cavity

Unconnected rudimentary horn

Explanation

Through a small incision in the lower abdomen, the physician performs a plastic repair of a malformed uterus. This often is an extensive procedure that involves removing abnormal tissues, rearranging the uterine walls, and suturing.

Coding Tips

This code should be used when the hysteroplasty is done to correct an anomaly present from birth, not an acquired condition due to trauma, age, or disease. Use 58520 to report the repair of an acquired ruptured uterus. When 58540 is performed with another separately identifiable procedure, the highest dollar value code is listed as the primary procedure and subsequent procedures are appended with modifier 51. For repair of a ruptured uterus in an obstetrical setting, report 59350.

ICD-9-CM Procedural

68.22 Incision or excision of congenital septum of uterus

69.23 Vaginal repair of chronic inversion of uterus

69.49 Other repair of uterus

Anesthesia

58540 00840

ICD-9-CM Diagnostic

621.5 Intrauterine synechiae

621.8 Other specified disorders of uterus, not elsewhere classified

752.2 Congenital doubling of uterus

752.31 Agenesis of uterus

752.32 Hypoplasia of uterus

752.33 Unicornuate uterus

752.34 Bicornuate uterus

752.35 Septate uterus

752.36 Arcuate uterus

752.39 Other anomalies of uterus

Terms To Know

anomaly. Irregularity in the structure or position of an organ or tissue.

congenital. Present at birth, occurring through heredity or an influence during gestation up to the moment of birth.

incision. Act of cutting into tissue or an organ.

intrauterine synechiae. Abnormal joining of tissues within the uterus.

suture. Numerous stitching techniques employed in wound closure.

buried suture. Continuous or interrupted suture placed under the skin for a layered closure.

continuous suture. Running stitch with tension evenly distributed across a single strand to provide a leakproof closure line.

interrupted suture. Series of single stitches with tension isolated at each stitch, in which all stitches are not affected if one becomes loose, and the isolated sutures cannot act as a wick to transport an infection.

purse-string suture. Continuous suture placed around a tubular structure and tightened, to reduce or close the lumen.

retention suture. Secondary stitching that bridges the primary suture, providing support for the primary repair; a plastic or rubber bolster may be placed over the primary repair and under the retention sutures.

CCI Version 18.3

0213T, 0216T, 0228T, 0230T, 12001-12007, 12011-12057, 13100-13153, 36000, 36400-36410, 36420-36430, 36440, 36600, 36640, 37202, 43752, 44005, 44180, 44602-44605, 44820-44850, 44950, 44970, 49000-49010, 49255, 49320, 49570, 50715, 51701-51703, 57410, 58140-58146, 58520, 62310-62319, 64400-64435, 64445-64450, 64479, 64483, 64490, 64493, 64505-64530, 69990, 93000-93010, 93040-93042, 93318, 94002, 94200, 94250, 94680-94690, 94770, 95812-95816, 95819, 95822, 95829, 95955, 96360, 96365, 96372, 96374-96376, 99148-99149, 99150

Note: These CCI edits are used for Medicare. Other payers may reimburse on codes listed above.

Medicare Edits

	Fac RVU	Non-Fac RVU	FUD	Status
58540	27.13	27.13	90	A

	MUE		Modifiers		
58540	1	51	N/A	N/A	80

* with documentation

Medicare References: None

© 2012 OptumInsight, Inc.

218 — Corpus Uteri

CPT only © 2012 American Medical Association. All Rights Reserved.

Coding Companion for Ob/Gyn

Corpus Uteri

58541-58542

58541 Laparoscopy, surgical, supracervical hysterectomy, for uterus 250 g or less;

58542 with removal of tube(s) and/or ovary(s)

Laparoscope

Trocars deliver surgical instruments

Ovary

Instruments may be also be inserted via vaginal canal

A hysterectomy is performed via laparoscopy and the cervix is preserved. The uterus weighs 250 g or less

Tubes and ovaries

In 58542, tube(s) and ovary(ies) are removed as well

Uterus

Cervix

Vagina

Explanation

The physician performs a laparoscopic hysterectomy, removing a uterus with a total weight of 250 gm or less while preserving the cervix. The patient is placed in the dorsal lithotomy position. After the insertion of a speculum in the vagina, the physician grasps the cervix with an instrument to manipulate the uterus during the surgery. A trocar is inserted periumbilically and the abdomen is insufflated with gas. Additional trocars are placed in the right and left lower quadrants. The uterus is dissected free from the bladder and surrounding tissue and its body is separated from the cervix. Coagulation is achieved with the aid of electrocautery instruments. Alternatively, some vessels may be ligated. The uterus is morcellized and removed using endoscopic tools. In 58542, one or both ovaries and/or one or both fallopian tubes are removed in similar fashion. Once the excisions are complete, the abdominal cavity is deflated and instruments and trocars removed. The fascia and skin are closed with sutures.

Coding Tips

Surgical laparoscopy always includes diagnostic laparoscopy. For diagnostic laparoscopy, see 49350. For laparoscopic supracervical hysterectomy, for a uterus greater than 250 gm, see 58543; with removal of tubes and/or ovaries, see 58544. Do not report these codes with 49320, 57000, 57180,

57410, 58140–58146, 58545–58546, 58561, 58661, or 58670-58671.

ICD-9-CM Procedural

65.31	Laparoscopic unilateral oophorectomy
65.41	Laparoscopic unilateral salpingo-oophorectomy
65.53	Laparoscopic removal of both ovaries at same operative episode
65.54	Laparoscopic removal of remaining ovary
65.63	Laparoscopic removal of both ovaries and tubes at same operative episode
65.64	Laparoscopic removal of remaining ovary and tube
68.31	Laparoscopic supracervical hysterectomy [LSH]

Anesthesia

00840

ICD-9-CM Diagnostic

180.8	Malignant neoplasm of other specified sites of cervix
181	Malignant neoplasm of placenta
182.0	Malignant neoplasm of corpus uteri, except isthmus
183.0	Malignant neoplasm of ovary — (Use additional code to identify any functional activity)
218.0	Submucous leiomyoma of uterus
218.1	Intramural leiomyoma of uterus
218.2	Subserous leiomyoma of uterus
233.1	Carcinoma in situ of cervix uteri
233.2	Carcinoma in situ of other and unspecified parts of uterus
614.4	Chronic or unspecified parametritis and pelvic cellulitis — (Use additional code to identify organism: 041.00-041.09, 041.10-041.19)
617.0	Endometriosis of uterus
617.9	Endometriosis, site unspecified
618.1	Uterine prolapse without mention of vaginal wall prolapse — (Use additional code to identify urinary incontinence: 625.6, 788.31, 788.33-788.39)
618.2	Uterovaginal prolapse, incomplete — (Use additional code to identify urinary incontinence: 625.6, 788.31, 788.33-788.39)
618.3	Uterovaginal prolapse, complete — (Use additional code to identify urinary incontinence: 625.6, 788.31, 788.33-788.39)
618.89	Other specified genital prolapse — (Use additional code to identify

urinary incontinence: 625.6, 788.31, 788.33-788.39)

621.0	Polyp of corpus uteri
621.2	Hypertrophy of uterus
621.30	Endometrial hyperplasia, unspecified
621.31	Simple endometrial hyperplasia without atypia
621.32	Complex endometrial hyperplasia without atypia
621.33	Endometrial hyperplasia with atypia
621.6	Malposition of uterus
621.8	Other specified disorders of uterus, not elsewhere classified
625.3	Dysmenorrhea
626.2	Excessive or frequent menstruation
626.6	Metrorrhagia
627.1	Postmenopausal bleeding
677	Late effect of complication of pregnancy, childbirth, and the puerperium — (Code first any sequelae)

CCI Version 18.3

0213T, 0216T, 0228T, 0230T, 12001-12007, 12011-12057, 13100-13153, 36000, 36400-36410, 36420-36430, 36440, 36600, 36640, 37202, 43752, 44005, 44180, 44602-44605, 44950, 44970, 49320, 50715, 51701-51703, 57000, 57020, 57100, 57180, 57400-57420, 57452, 57500, 57530, 57800, 58100, 58140-58146, 58545-58546, 58558, 58561, 58660-58661, 58670-58673, 58700-58720, 58940, 62310-62319, 64400-64435, 64445-64450, 64479, 64483, 64490, 64493, 64505-64530, 69990, 76000-76001, 77001-77002, 93000-93010, 93040-93042, 93318, 94002, 94200, 94250, 94680-94690, 94770, 95812-95816, 95819, 95822, 95829, 95955, 96360, 96365, 96372, 96374-96376, 99148-99149, 99150, P9612

Also not with 58541: 58260❖

Also not with 58542: 58180❖, 58260-58262❖, 58270❖, 58541, 58550❖, 58570❖

Note: These CCI edits are used for Medicare. Other payers may reimburse on codes listed above.

Medicare Edits

	Fac RVU	Non-Fac RVU	FUD	Status
58541	25.74	25.74	90	A
58542	28.75	28.75	90	A

	MUE		Modifiers		
58541	1	51	N/A	62	80
58542	1	51	N/A	62	80

* with documentation

Medicare References: None

Corpus Uteri

58543-58544

58543 Laparoscopy, surgical, supracervical hysterectomy, for uterus greater than 250 g;

58544 with removal of tube(s) and/or ovary(s)

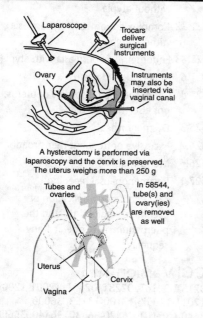

Laparoscope

Trocars deliver surgical instruments

Ovary

Instruments may also be inserted via vaginal canal

A hysterectomy is performed via laparoscopy and the cervix is preserved. The uterus weighs more than 250 g

Tubes and ovaries

In 58544, tube(s) and ovary(ies) are removed as well

Uterus

Cervix

Vagina

Explanation

The physician performs a laparoscopic hysterectomy, removing a uterus with a total weight of more than 250 gm while preserving the cervix. The patient is placed in the dorsal lithotomy position. After the insertion of a speculum in the vagina, the physician grasps the cervix with an instrument to manipulate the uterus during the surgery. A trocar is inserted periumbilically and the abdomen is insufflated with gas. Additional trocars are placed in the right and left lower quadrants. The uterus is dissected free from the bladder and surrounding tissue and its body is separated from the cervix. Coagulation is achieved with the aid of electrocautery instruments. Alternatively, some vessels may be ligated. The uterus is morcellized and removed using endoscopic tools. In 58544, one or both ovaries and/or one or both fallopian tubes are removed in similar fashion. Once the excisions are complete, the abdominal cavity is deflated and instruments and trocars removed. The fascia and skin are closed with sutures.

Coding Tips

Surgical laparoscopy always includes diagnostic laparoscopy. For diagnostic laparoscopy, see 49320. For laparoscopic supracervical hysterectomy, for a uterus 250 gm or less, see 58541; with removal of tubes and/or ovaries, see 58542. Do not report these codes with 49320, 57000, 57180, 57410,

58140–58146, 58545–58546, 58561, 58661, or 58670-58671.

ICD-9-CM Procedural

65.31 Laparoscopic unilateral oophorectomy
65.41 Laparoscopic unilateral salpingo-oophorectomy
65.53 Laparoscopic removal of both ovaries at same operative episode
65.54 Laparoscopic removal of remaining ovary
65.63 Laparoscopic removal of both ovaries and tubes at same operative episode
65.64 Laparoscopic removal of remaining ovary and tube
68.31 Laparoscopic supracervical hysterectomy [LSH]

Anesthesia
00840

ICD-9-CM Diagnostic

180.0 Malignant neoplasm of endocervix
180.1 Malignant neoplasm of exocervix
181 Malignant neoplasm of placenta
182.0 Malignant neoplasm of corpus uteri, except isthmus
182.1 Malignant neoplasm of isthmus
182.8 Malignant neoplasm of other specified sites of body of uterus
183.0 Malignant neoplasm of ovary — (Use additional code to identify any functional activity)
183.8 Malignant neoplasm of other specified sites of uterine adnexa
183.9 Malignant neoplasm of uterine adnexa, unspecified site
218.0 Submucous leiomyoma of uterus
218.1 Intramural leiomyoma of uterus
218.2 Subserous leiomyoma of uterus
218.9 Leiomyoma of uterus, unspecified
233.1 Carcinoma in situ of cervix uteri
233.2 Carcinoma in situ of other and unspecified parts of uterus
614.4 Chronic or unspecified parametritis and pelvic cellulitis — (Use additional code to identify organism: 041.00-041.09, 041.10-041.19)
614.9 Unspecified inflammatory disease of female pelvic organs and tissues — (Use additional code to identify organism: 041.00-041.09, 041.10-041.19)
617.0 Endometriosis of uterus
618.1 Uterine prolapse without mention of vaginal wall prolapse — (Use

additional code to identify urinary incontinence: 625.6, 788.31, 788.33-788.39)
618.2 Uterovaginal prolapse, incomplete — (Use additional code to identify urinary incontinence: 625.6, 788.31, 788.33-788.39)
618.3 Uterovaginal prolapse, complete — (Use additional code to identify urinary incontinence: 625.6, 788.31, 788.33-788.39)
618.4 Uterovaginal prolapse, unspecified — (Use additional code to identify urinary incontinence: 625.6, 788.31, 788.33-788.39)
621.31 Simple endometrial hyperplasia without atypia
621.32 Complex endometrial hyperplasia without atypia
621.33 Endometrial hyperplasia with atypia

CCI Version 18.3

0213T, 0216T, 0228T, 0230T, 12001-12007, 12011-12057, 13100-13153, 36000, 36400-36410, 36420-36430, 36440, 36600, 36640, 37202, 43752, 44005, 44180, 44602-44605, 44950, 44970, 49320, 50715, 51701-51703, 57000, 57020, 57100, 57180, 57400-57420, 57452, 57500, 57530, 57800, 58100, 58180❖, 58545-58546, 58550❖, 58552❖, 58558, 58561, 58660-58661, 58670-58673, 58700-58720, 58940, 62310-62319, 64400-64435, 64445-64450, 64479, 64483, 64490, 64493, 64505-64530, 69990, 76000-76001, 77001-77002, 93000-93010, 93040-93042, 93318, 94002, 94200, 94250, 94680-94690, 94770, 95812-95816, 95819, 95822, 95829, 95955, 96360, 96365, 96372, 96374-96376, 99148-99149, 99150, P9612

Also not with 58543: 58140-58146, 58260-58262❖, 58270❖, 58541-58542❖, 58570❖

Also not with 58544: 58140-58150, 58260-58263❖, 58270-58275❖, 58541-58543, 58570-58571❖

Note: These CCI edits are used for Medicare. Other payers may reimburse on codes listed above.

Medicare Edits

	Fac RVU	Non-Fac RVU	FUD	Status
58543	29.23	29.23	90	A
58544	31.64	31.64	90	A

	MUE			Modifiers	
58543	1	51	N/A	62	80
58544	1	51	N/A	62	80

* with documentation

Medicare References: None

Corpus Uteri

58545

58545 Laparoscopy, surgical, myomectomy, excision; 1 to 4 intramural myomas with total weight of 250 g or less and/or removal of surface myomas

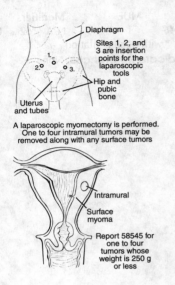

Diaphragm

Sites 1, 2, and 3 are insertion points for the laparoscopic tools

Hip and pubic bone

Uterus and tubes

A laparoscopic myomectomy is performed. One to four intramural tumors may be removed along with any surface tumors

Intramural

Surface myoma

Report 58545 for one to four tumors whose weight is 250 g or less

Explanation

The physician performs a laparoscopic myomectomy, removing one to four fibroid tumors from the wall of the uterus (intramural myomas) with a total weight of 250 gm or less and/or removes surface myomas. The patient is placed in the dorsal lithotomy position. A trocar is inserted periumbilically and the abdomen is insufflated with gas. Additional trocars are placed in the right and left lower quadrants. Electrocautery instruments and/or laser may be used to remove small surface myomas. Pedunculated myomas are removed by ligating, twisting, or snaring the stalk. The physician incises the uterus through the myometrium to expose the myoma, which is dissected free from the surrounding myometrium. The pedicle is isolated, clamped, and ligated and the myoma is dissected down to the pedicular blood supply. The adjacent myomas may be reached and removed by tunneling further through the initial incision. The uterine wall defects are sutured laparoscopically, the trocars are removed, and the wounds are closed.

Coding Tips

Surgical laparoscopy always includes diagnostic laparoscopy. For diagnostic laparoscopy, see 49320. Myomectomy performed via an abdominal (open) approach is reported with 58140 or 58146; vaginal approach, see 58145. Hysteroscopy with removal of leiomyomata should be reported with 58561.

ICD-9-CM Procedural

68.29   Other excision or destruction of lesion of uterus

Anesthesia

58545   00840

ICD-9-CM Diagnostic

218.0   Submucous leiomyoma of uterus

218.1   Intramural leiomyoma of uterus

218.2   Subserous leiomyoma of uterus

218.9   Leiomyoma of uterus, unspecified

Terms To Know

dissect. Cut apart or separate tissue for surgical purposes or for visual or microscopic study.

electrocautery. Division or cutting of tissue using high-frequency electrical current to produce heat, which destroys cells.

insufflation. Blowing air or gas into a body cavity.

intramural uterine leiomyoma. Benign, smooth muscle tumor within the wall of the uterus.

laparoscopy. Direct visualization of the peritoneal cavity, outer fallopian tubes, uterus, and ovaries utilizing a laparoscope, a thin, flexible fiberoptic tube.

ligate. To tie off a blood vessel or duct with a suture or a soft, thin wire (ligature wire).

myometrium. Muscular middle layer of the uterine wall responsible for contractions associated with childbirth.

submucous uterine leiomyoma. Benign, smooth muscle tumor beneath the inner lining of the uterus.

subserous uterine leiomyoma. Benign, smooth muscle tumor beneath the serous membrane lining of the uterus.

trocar. Cannula or a sharp pointed instrument used to puncture and aspirate fluid from cavities.

CCI Version 18.3

0213T, 0216T, 0228T, 0230T, 12001-12007, 12011-12057, 13100-13153, 36000, 36400-36410, 36420-36430, 36440, 36600, 36640, 37202, 43653, 43752, 44005, 44180, 44602-44605, 44950, 44970, 49320, 50715, 51701-51703, 57410, 58550, 58660, 62310-62319, 64400-64435, 64445-64450, 64479, 64483, 64490, 64493, 64505-64530, 69990, 76000-76001, 77001-77002,

93000-93010, 93040-93042, 93318, 94002, 94200, 94250, 94680-94690, 94770, 95812-95816, 95819, 95822, 95829, 95955, 96360, 96365, 96372, 96374-96376, 99148-99149, 99150

Note: These CCI edits are used for Medicare. Other payers may reimburse on codes listed above.

Medicare Edits

	Fac RVU	Non-Fac RVU	FUD	Status
58545	26.71	26.71	90	A

	MUE		Modifiers		
58545	1	51	N/A	62	80

* with documentation

Medicare References: None

Coding Companion for Ob/Gyn

Corpus Uteri

58546

58546 Laparoscopy, surgical, myomectomy, excision; 5 or more intramural myomas and/or intramural myomas with total weight greater than 250 g

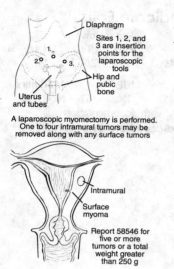

A laparoscopic myomectomy is performed. One to four intramural tumors may be removed along with any surface tumors

Report 58546 for five or more tumors or a total weight greater than 250 g

Explanation

The physician performs a laparoscopic myomectomy, removing five or more fibroid tumors from the wall of the uterus (intramural myomas) and/or intramural myomas with a total weight greater than 250 gm. The patient is placed in the dorsal lithotomy position. A trocar is inserted periumbilically and the abdomen is insufflated with gas. Additional trocars are placed in the right and left lower quadrants. The physician incises the uterus through the myometrium to expose the myoma, which is dissected free from the surrounding myometrium. The pedicle is isolated, clamped, and ligated and the myoma is dissected to the pedicular blood supply. The adjacent myomas may be reached and removed by tunneling further through the initial incision. After resecting large intramural myomas, removing them from the abdominal cavity may require making a culdotomy incision or using morcellation techniques. A minilaparotomy may be done with laparoscopic myomectomy as myomas are brought to the abdominal wall for removal and the uterus may be closed with some layered suturing. The laparoscopic instruments are removed and the wounds are closed.

Coding Tips

Surgical laparoscopy always includes diagnostic laparoscopy; the diagnostic laparoscopy should not be reported separately.

For diagnostic laparoscopy, see 49320. For myomectomy performed via an abdominal approach, see 58140 and 58146; vaginal approach, see 58145. Hysteroscopy with removal of leiomyomata is reported with 58561.

ICD-9-CM Procedural

68.29   Other excision or destruction of lesion of uterus

Anesthesia

58546   00840

ICD-9-CM Diagnostic

218.0   Submucous leiomyoma of uterus
218.1   Intramural leiomyoma of uterus
218.2   Subserous leiomyoma of uterus
218.9   Leiomyoma of uterus, unspecified

Terms To Know

blunt dissection. Surgical technique used to expose an underlying area by separating along natural cleavage lines of tissue, without cutting.

culdotomy/colpotomy. Incision through the vaginal wall into the cul-de-sac of Douglas (retro uterine pouch).

intramural uterine leiomyoma. Benign, smooth muscle tumor within the wall of the uterus.

laparoscopy. Direct visualization of the peritoneal cavity, outer fallopian tubes, uterus, and ovaries utilizing a laparoscope, a thin, flexible fiberoptic tube.

leiomyoma. Benign tumor consisting of smooth muscle in the uterus.

myometrium. Muscular middle layer of the uterine wall responsible for contractions associated with childbirth.

trocar. Cannula or a sharp pointed instrument used to puncture and aspirate fluid from cavities.

CCI Version 18.3

0213T, 0216T, 0228T, 0230T, 12001-12007, 12011-12057, 13100-13153, 36000, 36400-36410, 36420-36430, 36440, 36600, 36640, 37202, 43653, 43752, 44005, 44180, 44602-44605, 44950, 44970, 49320, 50715, 51701-51703, 57410, 58545, 58550, 58552, 58570-58571, 58660, 62310-62319, 64400-64435, 64445-64450, 64479, 64483, 64490, 64493, 64505-64530, 69990, 76000-76001, 77001-77002, 93000-93010, 93040-93042, 93318, 94002, 94200, 94250, 94680-94690, 94770, 95812-95816, 95819, 95822, 95829, 95955, 96360, 96365, 96372, 96374-96376, 99148-99149, 99150

Note: These CCI edits are used for Medicare. Other payers may reimburse on codes listed above.

Medicare Edits

	Fac RVU	Non-Fac RVU	FUD	Status
58546	33.67	33.67	90	A

	MUE		Modifiers		
58546	1	51	N/A	62	80

* with documentation

Medicare References: None

Coding Companion for Ob/Gyn

Corpus Uteri

58548

58548 Laparoscopy, surgical, with radical hysterectomy, with bilateral total pelvic lymphadenectomy and para-aortic lymph node sampling (biopsy), with removal of tube(s) and ovary(s), if performed

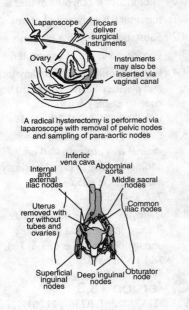

Laparoscope / Trocars deliver surgical instruments
Ovary / Instruments may also be inserted via vaginal canal

A radical hysterectomy is performed via laparoscope with removal of pelvic nodes and sampling of para-aortic nodes

Inferior vena cava / Abdominal aorta
Internal and external iliac nodes / Middle sacral nodes
Uterus removed with or without tubes and ovaries / Common iliac nodes
Superficial inguinal nodes / Deep inguinal nodes / Obturator node

Explanation

The physician performs a laparoscopic hysterectomy, bilateral total pelvic lymphadenectomy, and para-aortic lymph node sampling, and may remove all or portions of the fallopian tubes and ovaries. The patient is placed in the dorsal lithotomy position. After the insertion of a speculum in the vagina, the physician grasps the cervix with an instrument to manipulate the uterus during the surgery. A trocar is inserted periumbilically and the abdomen is insufflated with gas. Additional trocars are placed in the right and left lower quadrants. The uterus is dissected free from the bladder and surrounding tissue and its body with the cervix is dissected from the vagina. Alternately, the vagina may also be excised. Coagulation is achieved with the aid of electrocautery instruments. Some vessels may be ligated. The uterus is morcellized and removed using endoscopic tools. One or both ovaries and/or one or both fallopian tubes are removed in similar fashion. The physician removes the pelvic lymph nodes on both sides and takes samples or biopsies of the para-aortic lymph nodes. Once the excisions are complete, the abdominal cavity is deflated and instruments and trocars removed. The fascia and skin of the abdomen and vagina are closed with sutures.

Coding Tips

A surgical laparoscopy always includes a diagnostic laparoscopy; the diagnostic laparoscopy should not be reported separately. This code should not be reported with 38570–38572, 58210, 58285, 58550–58554.

ICD-9-CM Procedural

40.11	Biopsy of lymphatic structure
40.3	Regional lymph node excision
40.59	Radical excision of other lymph nodes
65.31	Laparoscopic unilateral oophorectomy
65.41	Laparoscopic unilateral salpingo-oophorectomy
65.53	Laparoscopic removal of both ovaries at same operative episode
65.54	Laparoscopic removal of remaining ovary
65.63	Laparoscopic removal of both ovaries and tubes at same operative episode
65.64	Laparoscopic removal of remaining ovary and tube
68.61	Laparoscopic radical abdominal hysterectomy
68.71	Laparoscopic radical vaginal hysterectomy [LRVH]

Anesthesia

58548 00846

ICD-9-CM Diagnostic

179	Malignant neoplasm of uterus, part unspecified
180.0	Malignant neoplasm of endocervix
180.1	Malignant neoplasm of exocervix
180.8	Malignant neoplasm of other specified sites of cervix
182.0	Malignant neoplasm of corpus uteri, except isthmus
182.1	Malignant neoplasm of isthmus
182.8	Malignant neoplasm of other specified sites of body of uterus
183.0	Malignant neoplasm of ovary — (Use additional code to identify any functional activity)
183.2	Malignant neoplasm of fallopian tube
183.3	Malignant neoplasm of broad ligament of uterus
183.4	Malignant neoplasm of parametrium of uterus
183.5	Malignant neoplasm of round ligament of uterus
184.0	Malignant neoplasm of vagina
196.6	Secondary and unspecified malignant neoplasm of intrapelvic lymph nodes
198.82	Secondary malignant neoplasm of genital organs
233.1	Carcinoma in situ of cervix uteri
236.0	Neoplasm of uncertain behavior of uterus
236.2	Neoplasm of uncertain behavior of ovary — (Use additional code to identify any functional activity)
V84.02	Genetic susceptibility to malignant neoplasm of ovary — (Use additional code, if applicable, for any associated family history of the disease: V16-V19. Code first, if applicable, any current malignant neoplasms: 140.0-195.8, 200.0-208.9, 230.0-234.9. Use additional code, if applicable, for any personal history of malignant neoplasm: V10.0-V10.9)

CCI Version 18.3

0213T, 0216T, 0228T, 0230T, 12001-12007, 12011-12057, 13100-13153, 36000, 36400-36410, 36420-36430, 36440, 36600, 36640, 37202, 38562-38572, 38770, 38780, 43653, 43752, 44005, 44180, 44602-44605, 44950, 44970, 49320, 50715, 51701-51703, 57020, 57100, 57180, 57400-57420, 57452, 57500, 57530, 57800, 58100, 58140-58200❖, 58260-58263❖, 58267-58294❖, 58541-58546, 58550, 58552-58554, 58570-58573, 58660-58673, 58700-58720, 58940, 62310-62319, 64400-64435, 64445-64450, 64479, 64483, 64490, 64493, 64505-64530, 69990, 76000-76001, 77001-77002, 93000-93010, 93040-93042, 93318, 94002, 94200, 94250, 94680-94690, 94770, 95812-95816, 95819, 95822, 95829, 95955, 96360, 96365, 96372, 96374-96376, 99148-99149, 99150, P9612

Note: These CCI edits are used for Medicare. Other payers may reimburse on codes listed above.

Medicare Edits

	Fac RVU	Non-Fac RVU	FUD	Status
58548	53.8	53.8	90	A

	MUE			Modifiers	
58548	1	51	N/A	62	80

* with documentation

Medicare References: None

Coding Companion for Ob/Gyn

58550-58552

58550 Laparoscopy, surgical, with vaginal hysterectomy, for uterus 250 g or less;

58552 with removal of tube(s) and/or ovary(s)

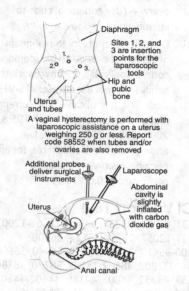

A vaginal hysterectomy is performed with laparoscopic assistance on a uterus weighing 250 g or less. Report code 58552 when tubes and/or ovaries are also removed

Explanation

The physician performs surgical laparoscopy with vaginal hysterectomy for a uterus with a total weight of 250 gm or less. The laparoscope is used to perform the initial operative portion of the hysterectomy. The patient is placed in the dorsal lithotomy position for the endoscopic portion. For the vaginal portion, the patient is positioned in stirrups. A trocar is inserted periumbilically and the abdomen is insufflated with gas. Additional trocars are placed in the right and left lower quadrants. An intra-abdominal and pelvic survey is done and any adhesions are lysed. The round ligaments are ligated and incised. Starting on the left round ligament, the vesicouterine peritoneal fold is incised and the peritoneal vessels are dissected and desiccated. The physician continues the incision across the lower uterine segment to the round ligament on the other side and dissects the bladder off the uterus and cervix. Staples are inserted through one port on the side to be stapled or a bipolar coagulation unit is inserted for electrocautery. At this point, if tubes and/or ovaries are to be removed, the infundibulopelvic ligament is now ligated lateral to the ovary. If not, the ligation is done medial to the ovary. Staple ligation or electrodesiccation of the uterine vasculature is accomplished on both sides, followed by ligation or electrodesiccation of the cardinal ligaments. An anterior colpotomy incision is made to enter the vagina and the vaginal portion of the procedure is begun. The remaining supporting structures attached to the cervix and uterus are detached and the hysterectomy proceeds through a posterior cul-de-sac incision. The uterus is removed, the vaginal incision is closed, and hemostasis is confirmed before the trocars are removed and the skin incisions are closed. Report 58550 for removal of uterus or 58552 if uterus, tubes, and/or ovaries are removed.

Coding Tips

A surgical laparoscopy always includes a diagnostic laparoscopy; the diagnostic laparoscopy should not be reported separately. For a vaginal hysterectomy for a uterus 250 gm or less without laparoscopy, see 58260; with removal of the tubes and/or ovaries, see 58262–58263. For a vaginal hysterectomy for a uterus greater than 250 gm without laparoscopy, see 58290; with removal of the tubes and/or ovaries, see 58291–58292. For surgical laparoscopy with a vaginal hysterectomy for a uterus greater than 250 gm, see 58553–58554.

ICD-9-CM Procedural

65.31	Laparoscopic unilateral oophorectomy
65.41	Laparoscopic unilateral salpingo-oophorectomy
65.53	Laparoscopic removal of both ovaries at same operative episode
65.54	Laparoscopic removal of remaining ovary
65.63	Laparoscopic removal of both ovaries and tubes at same operative episode
65.64	Laparoscopic removal of remaining ovary and tube
68.51	Laparoscopically assisted vaginal hysterectomy (LAVH)
68.71	Laparoscopic radical vaginal hysterectomy [LRVH]

Anesthesia

58550 00840
58552 00840, 00944

ICD-9-CM Diagnostic

180.0	Malignant neoplasm of endocervix
180.1	Malignant neoplasm of exocervix
180.8	Malignant neoplasm of other specified sites of cervix
181	Malignant neoplasm of placenta
182.0	Malignant neoplasm of corpus uteri, except isthmus
182.1	Malignant neoplasm of isthmus
182.8	Malignant neoplasm of other specified sites of body of uterus
183.0	Malignant neoplasm of ovary — (Use additional code to identify any functional activity)
183.8	Malignant neoplasm of other specified sites of uterine adnexa
198.6	Secondary malignant neoplasm of ovary
218.0	Submucous leiomyoma of uterus
218.1	Intramural leiomyoma of uterus
218.2	Subserous leiomyoma of uterus
233.1	Carcinoma in situ of cervix uteri
614.4	Chronic or unspecified parametritis and pelvic cellulitis — (Use additional code to identify organism: 041.00-041.09, 041.10-041.19)
618.1	Uterine prolapse without mention of vaginal wall prolapse — (Use additional code to identify urinary incontinence: 625.6, 788.31, 788.33-788.39)
618.3	Uterovaginal prolapse, complete — (Use additional code to identify urinary incontinence: 625.6, 788.31, 788.33-788.39)

CCI Version 18.3

0213T, 0216T, 0228T, 0230T, 12001-12007, 12011-12057, 13100-13153, 36000, 36400-36410, 36420-36430, 36440, 36600, 36640, 37202, 43653, 43752, 44005, 44180, 44602-44605, 44950, 44970, 49320, 49322, 50715, 51701-51703, 57000, 57020, 57100, 57180, 57400-57420, 57452, 57500, 57530, 57800, 58100, 58558, 58561, 58660-58661, 58670-58673, 58700-58720, 58940, 62310-62319, 64400-64435, 64445-64450, 64479, 64483, 64490, 64493, 64505-64530, 69990, 76000-76001, 77001-77002, 93000-93010, 93040-93042, 93318, 94002, 94200, 94250, 94680-94690, 94770, 95812-95816, 95819, 95822, 95829, 95955, 96360, 96365, 96372, 96374-96376, 99148-99149, 99150, P9612

Also not with 58550: 58145, 58541❖

Also not with 58552: 58140-58145, 58541-58542❖, 58545, 58550, 58570❖

Note: These CCI edits are used for Medicare. Other payers may reimburse on codes listed above.

Medicare Edits

	Fac RVU	Non-Fac RVU	FUD	Status
58550	26.36	26.36	90	A
58552	29.28	29.28	90	A

	MUE			Modifiers	
58550	1	51	N/A	62	80
58552	1	51	N/A	62	80

* with documentation

Medicare References: 100-3,230.3

Corpus Uteri

58553-58554

58553 Laparoscopy, surgical, with vaginal hysterectomy, for uterus greater than 250 g;

58554 with removal of tube(s) and/or ovary(s)

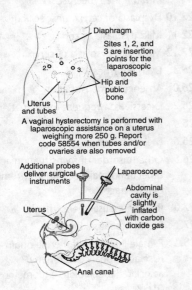

Diaphragm

Sites 1, 2, and 3 are insertion points for the laparoscopic tools

Hip and pubic bone

Uterus and tubes

A vaginal hysterectomy is performed with laparoscopic assistance on a uterus weighing more 250 g. Report code 58554 when tubes and/or ovaries are also removed

Additional probes deliver surgical instruments

Laparoscope

Abdominal cavity is slightly inflated with carbon dioxide gas

Uterus

Anal canal

Explanation

The physician performs surgical laparoscopy with vaginal hysterectomy for a uterus with a total weight of more than 250 gm. The laparoscope is used to perform the initial operative portion of the hysterectomy. The patient is placed in the dorsal lithotomy position for the endoscopic portion. For the vaginal portion, the patient is positioned in stirrups. A trocar is inserted periumbilically and the abdomen is insufflated with gas. Additional trocars are placed in the right and left lower quadrants. An intra-abdominal and pelvic survey is done and any adhesions are lysed. The round ligaments are ligated and incised. Starting on the left round ligament, the vesicouterine peritoneal fold is incised and the peritoneal vessels are dissected and desiccated. The physician continues the incision across the lower uterine segment to the round ligament on the other side and dissects the bladder off the uterus and cervix. Staples are inserted through one port on the side to be stapled or a bipolar coagulation unit is inserted for electrocautery. At this point, if tubes and/or ovaries are to be removed, the infundibulopelvic ligament is now ligated lateral to the ovary. If not, the ligation is done medial to the ovary. Staple-ligation or electrodesiccation of the uterine vasculature is accomplished on both sides, followed by ligation or electrodesiccation of the cardinal ligaments. An anterior colpotomy incision is made to enter the vagina and the vaginal

portion of the procedure is begun. The remaining supporting structures attached to the cervix and uterus are detached and the hysterectomy proceeds through a posterior cul-de-sac incision. The uterus is removed, the vaginal incision is closed, and hemostasis is confirmed before the trocars are removed and the skin incisions are closed. Report 58553 for removal of uterus or 58554 if uterus, tubes, and/or ovaries are removed.

Coding Tips

For surgical laparoscopy with a vaginal hysterectomy for a uterus weighing less than 250 gm, see 58550–58552. For a vaginal hysterectomy for a uterus 250 gm or less without laparoscopy, see 58260; with removal of the tubes and/or ovaries, see 58262–58263. For a vaginal hysterectomy for a uterus greater than 250 gm without laparoscopy, see 58290; with removal of the tubes and/or ovaries, see 58291–58292.

ICD-9-CM Procedural

65.31 Laparoscopic unilateral oophorectomy

65.41 Laparoscopic unilateral salpingo-oophorectomy

65.53 Laparoscopic removal of both ovaries at same operative episode

65.54 Laparoscopic removal of remaining ovary

65.63 Laparoscopic removal of both ovaries and tubes at same operative episode

65.64 Laparoscopic removal of remaining ovary and tube

68.51 Laparoscopically assisted vaginal hysterectomy (LAVH)

68.71 Laparoscopic radical vaginal hysterectomy [LRVH]

Anesthesia

00840, 00944

ICD-9-CM Diagnostic

180.0 Malignant neoplasm of endocervix

180.1 Malignant neoplasm of exocervix

180.8 Malignant neoplasm of other specified sites of cervix

181 Malignant neoplasm of placenta

182.0 Malignant neoplasm of corpus uteri, except isthmus

182.1 Malignant neoplasm of isthmus

183.0 Malignant neoplasm of ovary — (Use additional code to identify any functional activity)

198.6 Secondary malignant neoplasm of ovary

218.0 Submucous leiomyoma of uterus

218.1 Intramural leiomyoma of uterus

218.2 Subserous leiomyoma of uterus

233.1 Carcinoma in situ of cervix uteri

614.4 Chronic or unspecified parametritis and pelvic cellulitis — (Use additional code to identify organism: 041.00-041.09, 041.10-041.19)

618.00 Unspecified prolapse of vaginal walls without mention of uterine prolapse — (Use additional code to identify urinary incontinence: 625.6, 788.31, 788.33-788.39)

618.1 Uterine prolapse without mention of vaginal wall prolapse — (Use additional code to identify urinary incontinence: 625.6, 788.31, 788.33-788.39)

618.3 Uterovaginal prolapse, complete — (Use additional code to identify urinary incontinence: 625.6, 788.31, 788.33-788.39)

621.30 Endometrial hyperplasia, unspecified

CCI Version 18.3

0213T, 0216T, 0228T, 0230T, 12001-12007, 12011-12057, 13100-13153, 36000, 36400-36410, 36420-36430, 36440, 36600, 36640, 37202, 43653, 43752, 44005, 44180, 44602-44605, 44950, 44970, 49320, 50715, 51701-51703, 57000, 57020, 57100, 57180, 57400-57420, 57452, 57500, 57530, 57800, 58100, 58541-58546, 58550, 58561, 58670-58673, 58700-58720, 62310-62319, 64400-64435, 64445-64450, 64479, 64483, 64490, 64493, 64505-64530, 69990, 76000-76001, 77001-77002, 93000-93010, 93040-93042, 93318, 94002, 94200, 94250, 94680-94690, 94770, 95812-95816, 95819, 95822, 95829, 95955, 96360, 96365, 96372, 96374-96376, 99148-99149, 99150, P9612

Also not with 58553: 58140-58145, 58552, 58570-58571❖, 58661

Also not with 58554: 49322, 58140-58146, 58552-58553, 58558, 58570-58572❖, 58660-58661, 58940

Note: These CCI edits are used for Medicare. Other payers may reimburse on codes listed above.

Medicare Edits

	Fac RVU	Non-Fac RVU	FUD	Status
58553	33.9	33.9	90	A
58554	39.21	39.21	90	A

	MUE			Modifiers	
58553	1	51	N/A	62	80
58554	1	51	N/A	62	80

* with documentation

Medicare References: None

Corpus Uteri

58555

58555 Hysteroscopy, diagnostic (separate procedure)

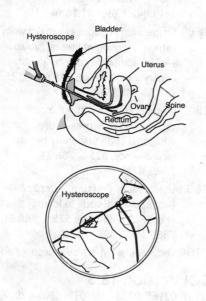

Explanation

The physician performs a diagnostic inspection of the uterus using a hysteroscope. The physician advances the hysteroscope through the vagina and into the cervical os to gain entry into the uterine cavity. The physician inspects the uterine cavity with the fiberoptic scope for diagnostic purposes.

Coding Tips

This separate procedure by definition is usually a component of a more complex service and is not identified separately. When performed alone or with other unrelated procedures/services it may be reported. If performed alone, list the code; if performed with other procedures/services, list the code and append modifier 59. If biopsies or samplings are taken from the endometrial surface, report 58558. If hysteroscopy is performed with lysis of intrauterine adhesions, report 58559. If a laparoscopy is performed in conjunction with this procedure, report the appropriate laparoscopy code in addition to the hysteroscopy code. Local anesthesia is included in this service; however, this procedure may be performed under general anesthesia depending on the age and/or condition of the patient.

ICD-9-CM Procedural

68.12   Hysteroscopy

Anesthesia

58555   00952

ICD-9-CM Diagnostic

180.0	Malignant neoplasm of endocervix
180.1	Malignant neoplasm of exocervix
182.0	Malignant neoplasm of corpus uteri, except isthmus
182.1	Malignant neoplasm of isthmus
183.2	Malignant neoplasm of fallopian tube
183.3	Malignant neoplasm of broad ligament of uterus
183.4	Malignant neoplasm of parametrium of uterus
183.5	Malignant neoplasm of round ligament of uterus
198.82	Secondary malignant neoplasm of genital organs
218.0	Submucous leiomyoma of uterus
218.1	Intramural leiomyoma of uterus
218.2	Subserous leiomyoma of uterus
219.0	Benign neoplasm of cervix uteri
219.1	Benign neoplasm of corpus uteri
221.0	Benign neoplasm of fallopian tube and uterine ligaments
233.1	Carcinoma in situ of cervix uteri
233.2	Carcinoma in situ of other and unspecified parts of uterus
233.30	Carcinoma in situ, unspecified female genital organ
233.31	Carcinoma in situ, vagina
233.32	Carcinoma in situ, vulva
233.39	Carcinoma in situ, other female genital organ
614.4	Chronic or unspecified parametritis and pelvic cellulitis — (Use additional code to identify organism: 041.00-041.09, 041.10-041.19)
615.0	Acute inflammatory disease of uterus, except cervix — (Use additional code to identify organism: 041.00-041.09, 041.10-041.19)
615.1	Chronic inflammatory disease of uterus, except cervix — (Use additional code to identify organism: 041.00-041.09, 041.10-041.19)
616.0	Cervicitis and endocervicitis — (Use additional code to identify organism: 041.00-041.09, 041.10-041.19)
617.0	Endometriosis of uterus
618.1	Uterine prolapse without mention of vaginal wall prolapse — (Use additional code to identify urinary incontinence: 625.6, 788.31, 788.33-788.39)
621.0	Polyp of corpus uteri
621.2	Hypertrophy of uterus
621.30	Endometrial hyperplasia, unspecified
621.31	Simple endometrial hyperplasia without atypia
621.32	Complex endometrial hyperplasia without atypia
621.33	Endometrial hyperplasia with atypia
621.4	Hematometra
621.5	Intrauterine synechiae
622.10	Dysplasia of cervix, unspecified
622.11	Mild dysplasia of cervix
622.12	Moderate dysplasia of cervix
625.3	Dysmenorrhea
626.0	Absence of menstruation
626.2	Excessive or frequent menstruation
626.4	Irregular menstrual cycle
626.6	Metrorrhagia
626.8	Other disorder of menstruation and other abnormal bleeding from female genital tract
627.0	Premenopausal menorrhagia
627.1	Postmenopausal bleeding
628.3	Female infertility of uterine origin — (Use additional code for any associated tuberculous endometriosis: 016.7)
629.0	Hematocele, female, not elsewhere classified
629.1	Hydrocele, canal of Nuck
789.03	Abdominal pain, right lower quadrant
789.04	Abdominal pain, left lower quadrant

CCI Version 18.3

00952, 0213T, 0216T, 0228T, 0230T, 12001-12007, 12011-12057, 13100-13153, 36000, 36400-36410, 36420-36430, 36440, 36600, 36640, 37202, 43752, 50715, 51701-51703, 57100, 57410, 57800, 58100, 62310-62319, 64400-64435, 64445-64450, 64479, 64483, 64490, 64493, 64505-64530, 69990, 76000-76001, 77001-77002, 93000-93010, 93040-93042, 93318, 94002, 94200, 94250, 94680-94690, 94770, 95812-95816, 95819, 95822, 95829, 95955, 96360, 96365, 96372, 96374-96376, 99148-99149, 99150, J0670, J2001

Note: These CCI edits are used for Medicare. Other payers may reimburse on codes listed above.

Medicare Edits

	Fac RVU	Non-Fac RVU	FUD	Status
58555	5.67	8.56	0	A

	MUE		Modifiers	
58555	1	51	N/A	62	80*

* with documentation

Medicare References: None

Corpus Uteri

58558

58558 Hysteroscopy, surgical; with sampling (biopsy) of endometrium and/or polypectomy, with or without D & C

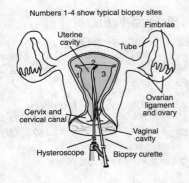

Numbers 1-4 show typical biopsy sites

Explanation

The physician performs a diagnostic inspection of the uterus using a hysteroscope and removes a uterine polyp, removes uterine tissue for biopsy, and may perform cervical dilation and uterine curettage (D&C). The physician advances the hysteroscope through the vagina and into the cervical os to gain entry into the uterine cavity. The physician inspects the uterine cavity with the fiberoptic scope and removes a sample of the uterine lining and/or removes a growth (polypectomy) within the uterus and may perform a cervical dilation and uterine curettage, scraping (D&C) to take a complete sampling of the uterine lining.

Coding Tips

An excisional biopsy is not separately reported if a therapeutic excision is performed during the same surgical session. Surgical hysteroscopy always includes diagnostic hysteroscopy. For diagnostic hysteroscopy only, see 58555. When 58558 is performed with another separately identifiable procedure, the highest dollar value code is listed as the primary procedure and subsequent procedures are appended with modifier 51. If a hysteroscopy is performed with lysis of intrauterine adhesions, report 58559.

ICD-9-CM Procedural

68.16   Closed biopsy of uterus

68.29   Other excision or destruction of lesion of uterus

69.09   Other dilation and curettage of uterus

Anesthesia

58558   00952

ICD-9-CM Diagnostic

179   Malignant neoplasm of uterus, part unspecified

180.0   Malignant neoplasm of endocervix

180.1   Malignant neoplasm of exocervix

182.0   Malignant neoplasm of corpus uteri, except isthmus

182.1   Malignant neoplasm of isthmus

218.0   Submucous leiomyoma of uterus

218.1   Intramural leiomyoma of uterus

218.2   Subserous leiomyoma of uterus

219.0   Benign neoplasm of cervix uteri

219.1   Benign neoplasm of corpus uteri

233.1   Carcinoma in situ of cervix uteri

233.2   Carcinoma in situ of other and unspecified parts of uterus

233.30   Carcinoma in situ, unspecified female genital organ

233.31   Carcinoma in situ, vagina

233.32   Carcinoma in situ, vulva

236.0   Neoplasm of uncertain behavior of uterus

236.3   Neoplasm of uncertain behavior of other and unspecified female genital organs

614.6   Pelvic peritoneal adhesions, female (postoperative) (postinfection) — (Use additional code to identify organism: 041.00-041.09, 041.10-041.19) (Use additional code to identify any associated infertility: 628.2)

617.0   Endometriosis of uterus

617.1   Endometriosis of ovary

617.3   Endometriosis of pelvic peritoneum

618.1   Uterine prolapse without mention of vaginal wall prolapse — (Use additional code to identify urinary incontinence: 625.6, 788.31, 788.33-788.39)

621.0   Polyp of corpus uteri

621.2   Hypertrophy of uterus

621.30   Endometrial hyperplasia, unspecified

622.10   Dysplasia of cervix, unspecified

622.4   Stricture and stenosis of cervix

622.7   Mucous polyp of cervix

625.3   Dysmenorrhea

625.6   Female stress incontinence

626.0   Absence of menstruation

626.2   Excessive or frequent menstruation

626.4   Irregular menstrual cycle

626.6   Metrorrhagia

626.8   Other disorder of menstruation and other abnormal bleeding from female genital tract

627.0   Premenopausal menorrhagia

627.1   Postmenopausal bleeding

628.2   Female infertility of tubal origin — (Use additional code for any associated peritubal adhesions: 614.6)

628.3   Female infertility of uterine origin — (Use additional code for any associated tuberculous endometriosis: 016.7)

628.4   Female infertility of cervical or vaginal origin

789.33   Abdominal or pelvic swelling, mass, or lump, right lower quadrant

789.34   Abdominal or pelvic swelling, mass, or lump, left lower quadrant

795.01   Papanicolaou smear of cervix with atypical squamous cells of undetermined significance (ASC-US)

795.02   Papanicolaou smear of cervix with atypical squamous cells cannot exclude high grade squamous intraepithelial lesion (ASC-H)

CCI Version 18.3

00952, 0213T, 0216T, 0228T, 0230T, 12001-12007, 12011-12057, 13100-13153, 36000, 36400-36410, 36420-36430, 36440, 36600, 36640, 37202, 43752, 50715, 51701-51703, 57100, 57410, 57800, 58100, 58120, 58555, 62310-62319, 64400-64435, 64445-64450, 64479, 64483, 64490, 64493, 64505-64530, 69990, 76000-76001, 77001-77002, 93000-93010, 93040-93042, 93318, 94002, 94200, 94250, 94680-94690, 94770, 95812-95816, 95819, 95822, 95829, 95955, 96360, 96365, 96372, 96374-96376, 99148-99149, 99150, J0670, J2001

Note: These CCI edits are used for Medicare. Other payers may reimburse on codes listed above.

Medicare Edits

	Fac RVU	Non-Fac RVU	FUD	Status
58558	7.97	11.27	0	A

	MUE		Modifiers		
58558	1	51	N/A	62	N/A

* with documentation

Medicare References: None

58559-58560

58559 Hysteroscopy, surgical; with lysis of intrauterine adhesions (any method)

58560 with division or resection of intrauterine septum (any method)

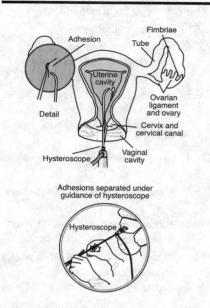

Adhesions separated under guidance of hysteroscope

Explanation

The physician removes scar tissue (adhesions) from within the uterus using a fiberoptic hysteroscope. The physician advances the hysteroscope through the vagina and into the cervical os to gain entry into the uterine cavity. The physician inspects the uterine cavity with the fiberoptic scope and removes or divides adhesions (fibrous scar tissue) that are artificially connecting the walls of the uterus. In 58560, the physician divides or resects an intrauterine septum (tissue creating an abnormal partition in the uterus).

Coding Tips

An excisional biopsy is not separately reported if a therapeutic excision is performed during the same surgical session. Surgical hysteroscopy always includes diagnostic hysteroscopy. For diagnostic hysteroscopy only, see 58555. When either procedure is performed with another separately identifiable procedure, the highest dollar value code is listed as the primary procedure and subsequent procedures are appended with modifier 51. For excision of a vaginal septum, see 57130.

ICD-9-CM Procedural

68.21 Division of endometrial synechiae

68.22 Incision or excision of congenital septum of uterus

Anesthesia
00952

ICD-9-CM Diagnostic

621.5 Intrauterine synechiae

626.2 Excessive or frequent menstruation

752.2 Congenital doubling of uterus

752.31 Agenesis of uterus

752.32 Hypoplasia of uterus

752.33 Unicornuate uterus

752.34 Bicornuate uterus

752.35 Septate uterus

752.36 Arcuate uterus

752.39 Other anomalies of uterus

908.1 Late effect of internal injury to intra-abdominal organs

908.2 Late effect of internal injury to other internal organs

908.6 Late effect of certain complications of trauma

909.3 Late effect of complications of surgical and medical care

Terms To Know

adhesion. Abnormal fibrous connection between two structures, soft tissue or bony structures, that may occur as the result of surgery, infection, or trauma.

complication. Condition arising after the beginning of observation and treatment that modifies the course of the patient's illness or the medical care required, or an undesired result or misadventure in medical care.

congenital. Present at birth, occurring through heredity or an influence during gestation up to the moment of birth.

intrauterine synechiae. Abnormal joining of tissues within the uterus.

lysis. Destruction, breakdown, dissolution, or decomposition of cells or substances by a specific catalyzing agent.

resection. Surgical removal of a part or all of an organ or body part.

scar tissue. Fibrous connective tissue that forms around a wounded area or injury, composed mainly of fibroblasts or collagenous fibers.

septum. Anatomical partition or dividing wall.

CCI Version 18.3

00952, 0213T, 0216T, 0228T, 0230T, 12001-12007, 12011-12057, 13100-13153, 36000, 36400-36410, 36420-36430, 36440, 36600, 36640, 37202, 43752, 50715, 51701-51703, 57100, 57410, 57800, 58100, 58555, 62310-62319, 64400-64435, 64445-64450, 64479, 64483, 64490, 64493, 64505-64530, 69990, 76000-76001, 77001-77002, 93000-93010, 93040-93042, 93318, 94002, 94200, 94250, 94680-94690, 94770, 95812-95816, 95819, 95822, 95829, 95955, 96360, 96365, 96372, 96374-96376, 99148-99149, 99150

Note: These CCI edits are used for Medicare. Other payers may reimburse on codes listed above.

Medicare Edits

	Fac RVU	Non-Fac RVU	FUD	Status
58559	10.26	10.26	0	A
58560	11.57	11.57	0	A

	MUE		Modifiers		
58559	1	51	N/A	62	N/A
58560	1	51	N/A	62	80

* with documentation

Medicare References: None

Corpus Uteri

58561

58561 Hysteroscopy, surgical; with removal of leiomyomata

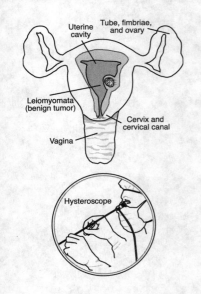

Explanation

The physician surgically removes a leiomyomata (uterine fibroid tumor) with the assistance of a fiberoptic hysteroscope. The physician advances the hysteroscope through the vagina and into the cervical os to gain entry into the uterine cavity. The physician inspects the uterine cavity with the fiberoptic scope and removes uterine leiomyomata with the assistance of the fiberoptic scope.

Coding Tips

An excisional biopsy is not separately reported if a therapeutic excision is performed during the same surgical session. Surgical hysteroscopy always includes diagnostic hysteroscopy. For diagnostic hysteroscopy only, see 58555. When 58561 is performed with another separately identifiable procedure, the highest dollar value code is listed as the primary procedure and subsequent procedures are appended with modifier 51. If hysteroscopy is performed with lysis of intrauterine adhesions, report 58559.

ICD-9-CM Procedural

68.29 Other excision or destruction of lesion of uterus

Anesthesia

58561 00952

ICD-9-CM Diagnostic

218.0 Submucous leiomyoma of uterus

218.1 Intramural leiomyoma of uterus
218.2 Subserous leiomyoma of uterus
218.9 Leiomyoma of uterus, unspecified
626.2 Excessive or frequent menstruation
626.6 Metrorrhagia

Terms To Know

intramural uterine leiomyoma. Benign, smooth muscle tumor within the wall of the uterus.

leiomyoma. Benign tumor consisting of smooth muscle in the uterus.

metrorrhagia. Prolonged, irregular uterine bleeding of an inconsistent amount occurring in frequent bouts.

submucous uterine leiomyoma. Benign, smooth muscle tumor beneath the inner lining of the uterus.

subserous uterine leiomyoma. Benign, smooth muscle tumor beneath the serous membrane lining of the uterus.

CCI Version 18.3

00952, 0213T, 0216T, 0228T, 0230T, 12001-12007, 12011-12057, 13100-13153, 36000, 36400-36410, 36420-36430, 36440, 36600, 36640, 37202, 43752, 50715, 51701-51703, 57100, 57410, 57800, 58100, 58353, 58555, 62310-62319, 64400-64435, 64445-64450, 64479, 64483, 64490, 64493, 64505-64530, 69990, 76000-76001, 77001-77002, 93000-93010, 93040-93042, 93318, 94002, 94200, 94250, 94680-94690, 94770, 95812-95816, 95819, 95822, 95829, 95955, 96360, 96365, 96372, 96374-96376, 99148-99149, 99150

Note: These CCI edits are used for Medicare. Other payers may reimburse on codes listed above.

Medicare Edits

	Fac RVU	Non-Fac RVU	FUD	Status
58561	16.36	16.36	0	A

	MUE			Modifiers	
58561	1	51	N/A	62	80*

* with documentation

Medicare References: None

Coding Companion for Ob/Gyn

58562

58562 Hysteroscopy, surgical; with removal of impacted foreign body

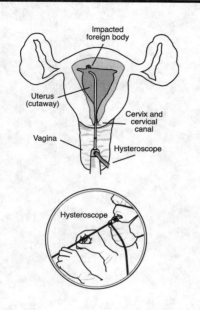

Impacted foreign body

Uterus (cutaway)

Cervix and cervical canal

Vagina

Hysteroscope

Hysteroscope

Explanation

The physician surgically removes an impacted foreign body with the assistance of a fiberoptic hysteroscope. The physician advances the hysteroscope through the vagina and into the cervical os to gain entry into the uterine cavity. The physician inspects the uterine cavity with the fiberoptic scope and removes an impacted foreign body from the uterine wall with the assistance of the hysteroscope.

Coding Tips

Surgical hysteroscopy always includes diagnostic hysteroscopy. For diagnostic hysteroscopy only, see 58555. When 58562 is performed with another separately identifiable procedure, the highest dollar value code is listed as the primary procedure and subsequent procedures are appended with modifier 51. For removal of an impacted vaginal foreign body under anesthesia, report 57415. If a laparoscopy is performed in conjunction with this procedure, report the appropriate laparoscopy code in addition to the hysteroscopy code.

ICD-9-CM Procedural

97.71   Removal of intrauterine contraceptive device
98.16   Removal of intraluminal foreign body from uterus without incision

Anesthesia

58562   00952

ICD-9-CM Diagnostic

939.1   Foreign body in uterus, any part
996.32   Mechanical complication due to intrauterine contraceptive device
996.65   Infection and inflammatory reaction due to other genitourinary device, implant, and graft — (Use additional code to identify specified infections)

Terms To Know

foreign body. Any object or substance found in an organ and tissue that does not belong under normal circumstances.

CCI Version 18.3

00952, 0213T, 0216T, 0228T, 0230T, 12001-12007, 12011-12057, 13100-13153, 36000, 36400-36410, 36420-36430, 36440, 36600, 36640, 37202, 43752, 50715, 51701-51703, 57100, 57410, 57800, 58100, 58301, 58555, 62310-62319, 64400-64435, 64445-64450, 64479, 64483, 64490, 64493, 64505-64530, 69990, 76000-76001, 77001-77002, 93000-93010, 93040-93042, 93318, 94002, 94200, 94250, 94680-94690, 94770, 95812-95816, 95819, 95822, 95829, 95955, 96360, 96365, 96372, 96374-96376, 99148-99149, 99150, J0670, J2001

Note: These CCI edits are used for Medicare. Other payers may reimburse on codes listed above.

Medicare Edits

	Fac RVU	Non-Fac RVU	FUD	Status
58562	8.66	11.72	0	A

	MUE		Modifiers		
58562	1	51	N/A	62	N/A

* with documentation

Medicare References: None

Corpus Uteri

58563

58563 Hysteroscopy, surgical; with endometrial ablation (eg, endometrial resection, electrosurgical ablation, thermoablation)

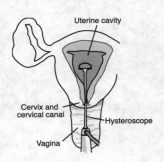

Uterine cavity

Cervix and cervical canal

Hysteroscope

Vagina

Explanation

The physician surgically removes (ablates) the inner lining of the uterus with the assistance of a fiberoptic hysteroscope. The physician advances the hysteroscope through the vagina and into the cervical os to gain entry into the uterine cavity. The physician inspects the uterine cavity with the fiberoptic scope and ablates the endometrium by various methods, such as resection, electrosurgical ablation, or thermoablation.

Coding Tips

Surgical hysteroscopy always includes diagnostic hysteroscopy. For diagnostic hysteroscopy only, see 58555. When 58563 is performed with another separately identifiable procedure, the highest dollar value code is listed as the primary procedure and subsequent procedures are appended with modifier 51. If a laparoscopy is performed in conjunction with this procedure, report the appropriate laparoscopy code in addition to the hysteroscopy code. For endometrial ablation without hysteroscopy, see 58353. Local anesthesia is included in this service; however, this procedure may be performed under general anesthesia depending on the age and/or condition of the patient.

ICD-9-CM Procedural

68.23   Endometrial ablation

Anesthesia

58563   00952

ICD-9-CM Diagnostic

617.0   Endometriosis of uterus

617.9   Endometriosis, site unspecified

626.2   Excessive or frequent menstruation

626.6   Metrorrhagia

626.8   Other disorder of menstruation and other abnormal bleeding from female genital tract

627.1   Postmenopausal bleeding

Terms To Know

ablation. Removal or destruction of a body part or tissue or its function. Ablation may be performed by surgical means, hormones, drugs, radiofrequency, heat, chemical application, or other methods.

endometriosis. Aberrant uterine mucosal tissue appearing in areas of the pelvic cavity outside of its normal location, lining the uterus and inflaming surrounding tissues, and can result in infertility and spontaneous abortion.

metrorrhagia. Prolonged, irregular uterine bleeding of an inconsistent amount occurring in frequent bouts.

CCI Version 18.3

00952, 0213T, 0216T, 0228T, 0230T, 12001-12007, 12011-12057, 13100-13153, 36000, 36400-36410, 36420-36430, 36440, 36600, 36640, 37202, 43752, 50715, 51701-51703, 57100, 57410, 57800, 58100, 58120, 58555-58558, 62310-62319, 64400-64435, 64445-64450, 64479, 64483, 64490, 64493, 64505-64530, 69990, 76000-76001, 77001-77002, 93000-93010, 93040-93042, 93318, 94002, 94200, 94250, 94680-94690, 94770, 95812-95816, 95819, 95822, 95829, 95955, 96360, 96365, 96372, 96374-96376, 99148-99149, 99150, J0670, J2001

Note: These CCI edits are used for Medicare. Other payers may reimburse on codes listed above.

Medicare Edits

	Fac RVU	Non-Fac RVU	FUD	Status
58563	10.25	51.18	0	A

	MUE		Modifiers		
58563	1	51	N/A	62	80*

* with documentation

Medicare References: 100-3,230.6

58565

58565 Hysteroscopy, surgical; with bilateral fallopian tube cannulation to induce occlusion by placement of permanent implants

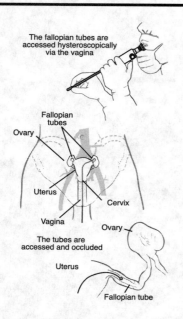

The fallopian tubes are accessed hysteroscopically via the vagina

Fallopian tubes
Ovary
Uterus
Cervix
Vagina
Ovary

The tubes are accessed and occluded

Uterus
Fallopian tube

Explanation

The physician performs a hysteroscopy with bilateral fallopian tube cannulation and placement of permanent implants to occlude the fallopian tubes. The physician advances the hysteroscope through the vagina and into the cervical os to gain entry into the uterine cavity. The physician inserts a catheter into each fallopian tube. The catheter delivers a small metallic implant into each fallopian tube. The presence of the obstructive implant causes scar tissue to form, completely blocking the fallopian tube as a means of birth control.

Coding Tips

This is a bilateral procedure and as such is reported once even if the procedure is performed on both sides. If performed only on one side, append modifier 52. This procedure includes hysteroscopy and cervical dilation and should not be reported with 58555 or 57800.

ICD-9-CM Procedural

66.29 Other bilateral endoscopic destruction or occlusion of fallopian tubes

Anesthesia

58565 00952

ICD-9-CM Diagnostic

659.41 Grand multiparity, delivered, with or without mention of antepartum condition
V25.2 Sterilization
V61.5 Multiparity

Terms To Know

cannulation. Insertion of a flexible length of hollow tubing into a blood vessel, duct, or body cavity, usually for extracorporeal circulation or chemotherapy infusion to a particular region of the body.

grand multiparity. Condition of having had five or more pregnancies that resulted in viable fetuses.

implant. Material or device inserted or placed within the body for therapeutic, reconstructive, or diagnostic purposes.

multiparity. Condition of having had two or more pregnancies that resulted in viable fetuses; producing more than one fetus or offspring in the same gestation.

sterile. Unable to reproduce; aseptic condition free of microorganisms.

CCI Version 18.3

00952, 0213T, 0216T, 0228T, 0230T, 12001-12007, 12011-12057, 13100-13153, 36000, 36400-36410, 36420-36430, 36440, 36600, 36640, 37202, 43752, 51701-51703, 57400-57410, 57800, 58100, 58555, 58615❖, 58671❖, 62310-62319, 64400-64435, 64445-64450, 64479, 64483, 64490, 64493, 64505-64530, 69990, 76000-76001, 77001-77002, 93000-93010, 93040-93042, 93318, 94002, 94200, 94250, 94680-94690, 94770, 95812-95816, 95819, 95822, 95829, 95955, 96360, 96365, 96372, 96374-96376, 99148-99149, 99150, J0670, J2001

Note: These CCI edits are used for Medicare. Other payers may reimburse on codes listed above.

Medicare Edits

	Fac RVU	Non-Fac RVU	FUD	Status
58565	12.96	56.82	90	A

	MUE		Modifiers		
58565	1	51	N/A	62	N/A

* with documentation

Medicare References: None

Coding Companion for Ob/Gyn

Corpus Uteri

58570-58571

58570 Laparoscopy, surgical, with total hysterectomy, for uterus 250 g or less;

58571 with removal of tube(s) and/or ovary(s)

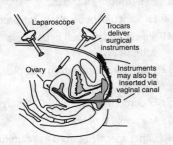

Report 58570 for a uterus up to 250 g and 58571 if also removing tubes and ovaries

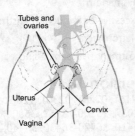

Explanation

The physician performs a total laparoscopic hysterectomy (TLH), removing a uterus with a total weight of 250 gm or less. Following appropriate anesthesia, the patient is placed in the dorsal lithotomy position. A Foley catheter ensures that the bladder is emptied during the procedure. A trocar is inserted periumbilically and the abdomen is insufflated with gas. Ancillary trocars are also placed suprapubically. Following abdominal pelvic inspection and lysis of any adhesions present, the uterus is mobilized. The uterine ligaments are sectioned, and the uterus and cervix are dissected free from the bladder and surrounding tissues. Coagulation is achieved with the aid of electrocautery instruments. Alternately, some vessels may be ligated. The uterus and cervix are morcellized using endoscopic tools and removed through the abdominal incisions or the vagina. In 58571, one or both ovaries and/or one or both fallopian tubes are removed in similar fashion. Once the excisions are complete, the abdominal cavity is deflated and instruments and trocars are removed. The fascia and skin are closed with sutures.

Coding Tips

Surgical laparoscopy always includes a diagnostic laparoscopy; the diagnostic laparoscopy should not be reported separately. For a diagnostic laparoscopy, see 49320. For a laparoscopic supracervical hysterectomy, for a uterus 250 gm or less, see 58541 and

58542; greater than 250 gm, see 58543 and 58544.

ICD-9-CM Procedural

65.31	Laparoscopic unilateral oophorectomy
65.41	Laparoscopic unilateral salpingo-oophorectomy
65.53	Laparoscopic removal of both ovaries at same operative episode
65.54	Laparoscopic removal of remaining ovary
65.63	Laparoscopic removal of both ovaries and tubes at same operative episode
65.64	Laparoscopic removal of remaining ovary and tube
68.41	Laparoscopic total abdominal hysterectomy
68.51	Laparoscopically assisted vaginal hysterectomy (LAVH)
68.61	Laparoscopic radical abdominal hysterectomy
68.71	Laparoscopic radical vaginal hysterectomy [LRVH]

Anesthesia

00840

ICD-9-CM Diagnostic

180.8	Malignant neoplasm of other specified sites of cervix
181	Malignant neoplasm of placenta
182.0	Malignant neoplasm of corpus uteri, except isthmus
183.0	Malignant neoplasm of ovary — (Use additional code to identify any functional activity)
218.0	Submucous leiomyoma of uterus
218.1	Intramural leiomyoma of uterus
218.2	Subserous leiomyoma of uterus
233.1	Carcinoma in situ of cervix uteri
233.2	Carcinoma in situ of other and unspecified parts of uterus
233.30	Carcinoma in situ, unspecified female genital organ
233.31	Carcinoma in situ, vagina
233.32	Carcinoma in situ, vulva
617.0	Endometriosis of uterus
618.1	Uterine prolapse without mention of vaginal wall prolapse — (Use additional code to identify urinary incontinence: 625.6, 788.31, 788.33-788.39)
618.2	Uterovaginal prolapse, incomplete — (Use additional code to identify urinary incontinence: 625.6, 788.31, 788.33-788.39)
618.3	Uterovaginal prolapse, complete — (Use additional code to identify urinary incontinence: 625.6, 788.31, 788.33-788.39)
621.0	Polyp of corpus uteri
621.2	Hypertrophy of uterus
621.30	Endometrial hyperplasia, unspecified
621.31	Simple endometrial hyperplasia without atypia
621.32	Complex endometrial hyperplasia without atypia
621.33	Endometrial hyperplasia with atypia
621.6	Malposition of uterus
621.8	Other specified disorders of uterus, not elsewhere classified
625.3	Dysmenorrhea
626.2	Excessive or frequent menstruation
626.6	Metrorrhagia
627.1	Postmenopausal bleeding

CCI Version 18.3

0213T, 0216T, 0228T, 0230T, 12001-12007, 12011-12057, 13100-13153, 36000, 36400-36410, 36420-36430, 36440, 36600, 36640, 37202, 43752, 44180, 44602-44605, 44950, 44970, 49320, 51701-51703, 57000, 57020, 57100, 57180, 57400-57420, 57452, 57500, 57530, 57800, 58100, 58140-58145, 58545, 58550❖, 58558, 58561, 58660-58661, 58670-58673, 58700-58720, 58940, 62310-62319, 64400-64435, 64445-64450, 64479, 64483, 64490, 64493, 64505-64530, 69990, 76000-76001, 77001-77002, 93000-93010, 93040-93042, 93318, 94002, 94200, 94250, 94680-94690, 94770, 95812-95816, 95819, 95822, 95829, 95955, 96360, 96365, 96372, 96374-96376, 99148-99149, 99150, P9612

Also not with 58570: 58260❖, 58270❖, 58541❖

Also not with 58571: 58150, 58180❖, 58260-58263❖, 58270-58275❖, 58541-58543❖, 58552❖, 58570

Note: These CCI edits are used for Medicare. Other payers may reimburse on codes listed above.

Medicare Edits

	Fac RVU	Non-Fac RVU	FUD	Status
58570	27.68	27.68	90	A
58571	30.77	30.77	90	A

	MUE		Modifiers		
58570	1	51	N/A	62	80
58571	1	51	N/A	62	80

* with documentation

Medicare References: None

Corpus Uteri

58572-58573

58572 Laparoscopy, surgical, with total hysterectomy, for uterus greater than 250 g;

58573   with removal of tube(s) and/or ovary(s)

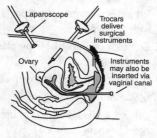

Report 58572 for a uterus over 250 g and 58573 if also removing tubes and ovaries.

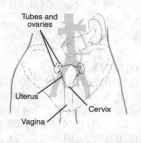

Explanation

The physician performs a total laparoscopic hysterectomy (TLH), removing a uterus with a total weight greater than 250 gm. Following appropriate anesthesia, the patient is placed in the dorsal lithotomy position. A Foley catheter ensures that the bladder is emptied during the procedure. A trocar is inserted periumbilically and the abdomen is insufflated with gas. Ancillary trocars are also placed suprapubically. Following abdominal pelvic inspection and lysis of any adhesions present, the uterus is mobilized. The uterine ligaments are sectioned, and the uterus and cervix are dissected free from the bladder and surrounding tissues. Coagulation is achieved with the aid of electrocautery instruments. Alternately, some vessels may be ligated. The uterus and cervix are morcellized using endoscopic tools and removed through the abdominal incisions or the vagina. In 58573, one or both ovaries and/or one or both fallopian tubes are removed in similar fashion. Once the excisions are complete, the abdominal cavity is deflated and instruments and trocars are removed. The fascia and skin are closed with sutures.

Coding Tips

A surgical laparoscopy always includes a diagnostic laparoscopy; the diagnostic laparoscopy should not be reported separately. For a diagnostic laparoscopy, see 49320. For a surgical laparoscopy, supracervical

hysterectomy, for a uterus 250 gm or less, see 58541 and 58542; for a uterus greater than 250 gm, see 58543 and 58544.

ICD-9-CM Procedural

65.31	Laparoscopic unilateral oophorectomy
65.41	Laparoscopic unilateral salpingo-oophorectomy
65.53	Laparoscopic removal of both ovaries at same operative episode
65.54	Laparoscopic removal of remaining ovary
65.63	Laparoscopic removal of both ovaries and tubes at same operative episode
65.64	Laparoscopic removal of remaining ovary and tube
68.41	Laparoscopic total abdominal hysterectomy
68.51	Laparoscopically assisted vaginal hysterectomy (LAVH)
68.61	Laparoscopic radical abdominal hysterectomy
68.71	Laparoscopic radical vaginal hysterectomy [LRVH]

Anesthesia
00840

ICD-9-CM Diagnostic

180.8	Malignant neoplasm of other specified sites of cervix
181	Malignant neoplasm of placenta
182.0	Malignant neoplasm of corpus uteri, except isthmus
183.0	Malignant neoplasm of ovary — (Use additional code to identify any functional activity)
218.0	Submucous leiomyoma of uterus
218.1	Intramural leiomyoma of uterus
218.2	Subserous leiomyoma of uterus
233.1	Carcinoma in situ of cervix uteri
233.2	Carcinoma in situ of other and unspecified parts of uterus
233.31	Carcinoma in situ, vagina
233.32	Carcinoma in situ, vulva
617.0	Endometriosis of uterus
618.1	Uterine prolapse without mention of vaginal wall prolapse — (Use additional code to identify urinary incontinence: 625.6, 788.31, 788.33-788.39)
618.2	Uterovaginal prolapse, incomplete — (Use additional code to identify urinary incontinence: 625.6, 788.31, 788.33-788.39)
618.3	Uterovaginal prolapse, complete — (Use additional code to identify urinary incontinence: 625.6, 788.31, 788.33-788.39)
621.0	Polyp of corpus uteri
621.2	Hypertrophy of uterus
621.30	Endometrial hyperplasia, unspecified
621.31	Simple endometrial hyperplasia without atypia
621.32	Complex endometrial hyperplasia without atypia
621.33	Endometrial hyperplasia with atypia
621.6	Malposition of uterus
621.8	Other specified disorders of uterus, not elsewhere classified
625.3	Dysmenorrhea
626.2	Excessive or frequent menstruation
626.6	Metrorrhagia
627.1	Postmenopausal bleeding

CCI Version 18.3

0213T, 0216T, 0228T, 0230T, 12001-12007, 12011-12057, 13100-13153, 36000, 36400-36410, 36420-36430, 36440, 36600, 36640, 37202, 43752, 44005, 44180, 44602-44605, 44950, 44970, 49320, 50715, 51701-51703, 57000, 57020, 57100, 57180, 57400-57420, 57452, 57500, 57530, 57800, 58100, 58260-58263❖, 58267-58280❖, 58541-58546, 58550❖, 58558, 58561, 58660-58661, 58670-58673, 58700-58720, 58940, 58943, 58950, 62310-62319, 64400-64435, 64445-64450, 64479, 64483, 64490, 64493, 64505-64530, 69990, 76000-76001, 77001-77002, 93000-93010, 93040-93042, 93318, 94002, 94200, 94250, 94680-94690, 94770, 95812-95816, 95819, 95822, 95829, 95955, 96360, 96365, 96372, 96374-96376, 99148-99149, 99150, P9612

Also not with 58572: 58140-58145, 58150, 58180❖, 58552-58553❖, 58570-58571❖

Also not with 58573: 58140-58180❖, 58290-58291❖, 58294❖, 58552-58554❖, 58570-58572, 58956

Note: These CCI edits are used for Medicare. Other payers may reimburse on codes listed above.

Medicare Edits

	Fac RVU	Non-Fac RVU	FUD	Status
58572	34.46	34.46	90	A
58573	39.4	39.4	90	A

	MUE		Modifiers		
58572	1	51	N/A	62	80
58573	1	51	N/A	62	80

* with documentation

Medicare References: None

Corpus Uteri

58600-58605

58600 Ligation or transection of fallopian tube(s), abdominal or vaginal approach, unilateral or bilateral

58605 Ligation or transection of fallopian tube(s), abdominal or vaginal approach, postpartum, unilateral or bilateral, during same hospitalization (separate procedure)

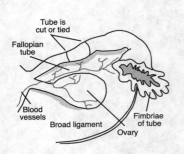

Tube is cut or tied
Fallopian tube
Blood vessels
Broad ligament
Ovary
Fimbriae of tube

Explanation

The physician ties off the fallopian tube or removes a portion of it on one side or both. The procedure may be done through the vagina or through a small incision just above the pubic hairline. In 58605, the procedure is done during the same hospital stay as the delivery of a baby.

Coding Tips

Report 58605 only when a tubal ligation is completed while the patient is hospitalized following a delivery. Note that 58605, a separate procedure by definition, is usually a component of a more complex service and is not identified separately. When performed alone or with other unrelated procedures/services it may be reported. If performed alone, list the code; if performed with other procedures/services, list the code and append modifier 59. When 58600 is performed with another separately identifiable procedure, the highest dollar value code is listed as the primary procedure and subsequent procedures are appended with modifier 51. For tubal ligation performed with a laparoscope, see 58670 and 58671.

ICD-9-CM Procedural

66.32 Other bilateral ligation and division of fallopian tubes

Anesthesia
00851

ICD-9-CM Diagnostic

659.41 Grand multiparity, delivered, with or without mention of antepartum condition

V25.2 Sterilization

V61.5 Multiparity

Terms To Know

approach. Method or anatomical location used to gain access to a body organ or specific area for procedures. The approach is not coded separately although it may be a specified component of the procedure, such as laparoscopic vs. incisional, or spinal procedures in which the amount of dissection required to expose the spine significantly alters with the site of approach.

incision. Act of cutting into tissue or an organ.

ligation. Tying off a blood vessel or duct with a suture or a soft, thin wire.

multiparity. Condition of having had two or more pregnancies that resulted in viable fetuses; producing more than one fetus or offspring in the same gestation.

transection. Transverse dissection; to cut across a long axis; cross section.

CCI Version 18.3

00851, 0213T, 0216T, 0228T, 0230T, 12001-12007, 12011-12057, 13100-13153, 36000, 36400-36410, 36420-36430, 36440, 36600, 36640, 37202, 43752, 44005, 44180, 44602-44605, 44820-44850, 44950, 44970, 49000-49010, 49255, 49320, 49570, 50715, 51701-51703, 57410, 58350, 58670-58671, 58805, 58900, 62310-62319, 64400-64435, 64445-64450, 64479, 64483, 64490, 64493, 64505-64530, 69990, 93000-93010, 93040-93042, 93318, 94002, 94200, 94250, 94680-94690, 94770, 95812-95816, 95819, 95822, 95829, 95955, 96360, 96365, 96372, 96374-96376, 99148-99149, 99150

Also not with 58600: 58605, 58700

Note: These CCI edits are used for Medicare. Other payers may reimburse on codes listed above.

Medicare Edits

	Fac RVU	Non-Fac RVU	FUD	Status
58600	10.89	10.89	90	A
58605	9.83	9.83	90	A

	MUE		Modifiers		
58600	1	51	N/A	62*	80
58605	1	51	N/A	N/A	80

* with documentation

Medicare References: 100-3,230.3

Oviduct

Coding Companion for Ob/Gyn

58611

58611 Ligation or transection of fallopian tube(s) when done at the time of cesarean delivery or intra-abdominal surgery (not a separate procedure) (List separately in addition to code for primary procedure)

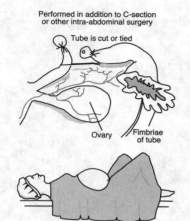

Performed in addition to C-section or other intra-abdominal surgery

Tube is cut or tied

Ovary

Fimbriae of tube

Explanation

The physician ties off the fallopian tube or removes a portion of it on one side or both. This procedure is done at the time of a cesarean section or during intra-abdominal surgery.

Coding Tips

This code should only be used for a tubal ligation completed during a cesarean section or during intra-abdominal surgery. Unlike other minor procedures, 58611 is reported along with the primary procedure. As an "add-on" code, 58611 is not subject to multiple procedure rules. No reimbursement reduction or modifier 51 is applied. "Add-on" codes describe additional intra-service work associated with the primary procedure. They are performed by the same physician on the same date of service as the primary service/procedure, and must never be reported as a stand-alone code. To report a tubal ligation performed with a laparoscope, see 58670 and 58671.

ICD-9-CM Procedural

66.32 Other bilateral ligation and division of fallopian tubes

Anesthesia

58611 N/A

ICD-9-CM Diagnostic

V25.2 Sterilization
V61.5 Multiparity

Terms To Know

cesarean section. Delivery of fetus by incision made in the upper part of the uterus, or corpus uteri, via an abdominal peritoneal approach when a vaginal delivery is not possible or advisable; often referred to as a classic c-section. Low cervical approach is a type of c-section by an incision in the lower segment of the uterus, either through a transperitoneal incision or extraperitoneally with the peritoneal fold being displaced upwards.

ligation. Tying off a blood vessel or duct with a suture or a soft, thin wire.

multiparity. Condition of having had two or more pregnancies that resulted in viable fetuses; producing more than one fetus or offspring in the same gestation.

transection. Transverse dissection; to cut across a long axis; cross section.

CCI Version 18.3

00851, 44180, 50715, 57410, 58350, 58670-58671

Note: These CCI edits are used for Medicare. Other payers may reimburse on codes listed above.

Medicare Edits

	Fac RVU	Non-Fac RVU	FUD	Status
58611	2.31	2.31	N/A	A

	MUE		Modifiers		
58611	1	N/A	N/A	N/A	80

* with documentation

Medicare References: 100-3,230.3

58615

58615 Occlusion of fallopian tube(s) by device (eg, band, clip, Falope ring) vaginal or suprapubic approach

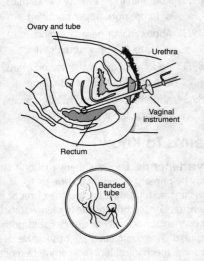

Ovary and tube
Urethra
Vaginal instrument
Rectum

Banded tube

Explanation

The physician blocks one or both of the fallopian tubes with a band, clip, or Falope ring. The physician may elect to do the procedure through the vagina or through a small incision just above the pubic hairline.

Coding Tips

This procedure is a reversible sterilization procedure. This code is appropriate when performed with any combination of techniques (e.g., band, clip, Falope ring). When 58615 is performed with another separately identifiable procedure, the highest dollar value code is listed as the primary procedure and subsequent procedures are appended with modifier 51. To report a tubal occlusion performed with a laparoscope, see 58671.

ICD-9-CM Procedural

66.31 Other bilateral ligation and crushing of fallopian tubes

66.39 Other bilateral destruction or occlusion of fallopian tubes

66.92 Unilateral destruction or occlusion of fallopian tube

Anesthesia

58615 00851

ICD-9-CM Diagnostic

V25.2 Sterilization

V61.5 Multiparity

Terms To Know

approach. Method or anatomical location used to gain access to a body organ or specific area for procedures. The approach is not coded separately although it may be a specified component of the procedure, such as laparoscopic vs. incisional, or spinal procedures in which the amount of dissection required to expose the spine significantly alters with the site of approach.

incision. Act of cutting into tissue or an organ.

multiparity. Condition of having had two or more pregnancies that resulted in viable fetuses; producing more than one fetus or offspring in the same gestation.

occlusion. Constriction, closure, or blockage of a passage.

CCI Version 18.3

00851, 0213T, 0216T, 0228T, 0230T, 12001-12007, 12011-12057, 13100-13153, 36000, 36400-36410, 36420-36430, 36440, 36600, 36640, 37202, 43752, 44005, 44180, 44602-44605, 44820-44850, 44950, 44970, 49000-49010, 49255, 49570, 50715, 51701-51703, 57410, 58350, 58605, 58700-58720, 58805, 58900, 62310-62319, 64400-64435, 64445-64450, 64479, 64483, 64490, 64493, 64505-64530, 69990, 93000-93010, 93040-93042, 93318, 94002, 94200, 94250, 94680-94690, 94770, 95812-95816, 95819, 95822, 95829, 95955, 96360, 96365, 96372, 96374-96376, 99148-99149, 99150

Note: These CCI edits are used for Medicare. Other payers may reimburse on codes listed above.

Medicare Edits

	Fac RVU	Non-Fac RVU	FUD	Status
58615	7.33	7.33	10	A

	MUE		Modifiers		
58615	1	51	N/A	N/A	80

* with documentation

Medicare References: 100-3,230.3

Coding Companion for Ob/Gyn

© 2012 OptumInsight, Inc.

58660

58660 Laparoscopy, surgical; with lysis of adhesions (salpingolysis, ovariolysis) (separate procedure)

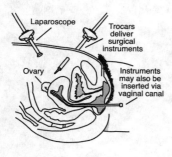

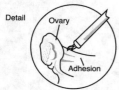

Explanation

The physician performs a laparoscopic surgical cutting/releasing (lysis) of scar tissue (adhesions) surrounding the ovaries and/or fallopian tubes with the assistance of a fiberoptic laparoscope. The physician may first insert an instrument through the vagina to grasp the cervix and manipulate the uterus during surgery. Next, the physician makes a small incision just below the umbilicus through which a fiberoptic laparoscope is inserted. A second incision is made in the abdomen with additional instruments being placed through these incisions into the abdomen or pelvis. The physician manipulates the tools so that the pelvic organs can be observed, manipulated and lysis of adhesions can be performed. The abdomen is deflated, the trocars removed, and the incisions are closed with sutures.

Coding Tips

Surgical laparoscopy always includes diagnostic laparoscopy. For diagnostic laparoscopy only, see 49230. This separate procedure by definition is usually a component of a more complex service and is not identified separately. When performed alone or with other unrelated procedures/services it may be reported. If performed alone, list the code; if performed with other procedures/services, list the code and append modifier 59. For hysteroscopic lysis of adhesions, see 58559. For open lysis of adhesions (salpingolysis, ovariolysis), see 58740.

ICD-9-CM Procedural

65.81 Laparoscopic lysis of adhesions of ovary and fallopian tube

Anesthesia

58660 00840

ICD-9-CM Diagnostic

568.0 Peritoneal adhesions (postoperative) (postinfection)

568.89 Other specified disorder of peritoneum

614.1 Chronic salpingitis and oophoritis — (Use additional code to identify organism: 041.00-041.09, 041.10-041.19)

614.2 Salpingitis and oophoritis not specified as acute, subacute, or chronic — (Use additional code to identify organism: 041.00-041.09, 041.10-041.19)

614.5 Acute or unspecified pelvic peritonitis, female — (Use additional code to identify organism: 041.00-041.09, 041.10-041.19)

614.6 Pelvic peritoneal adhesions, female (postoperative) (postinfection) — (Use additional code to identify organism: 041.00-041.09, 041.10-041.19) (Use additional code to identify any associated infertility: 628.2)

614.9 Unspecified inflammatory disease of female pelvic organs and tissues — (Use additional code to identify organism: 041.00-041.09, 041.10-041.19)

617.0 Endometriosis of uterus

617.1 Endometriosis of ovary

617.2 Endometriosis of fallopian tube

617.3 Endometriosis of pelvic peritoneum

617.8 Endometriosis of other specified sites

625.3 Dysmenorrhea

625.8 Other specified symptom associated with female genital organs

628.2 Female infertility of tubal origin — (Use additional code for any associated peritubal adhesions: 614.6)

628.3 Female infertility of uterine origin — (Use additional code for any associated tuberculous endometriosis: 016.7)

628.8 Female infertility of other specified origin

628.9 Female infertility of unspecified origin

789.00 Abdominal pain, unspecified site

789.01 Abdominal pain, right upper quadrant

789.02 Abdominal pain, left upper quadrant

789.03 Abdominal pain, right lower quadrant

789.04 Abdominal pain, left lower quadrant

789.05 Abdominal pain, periumbilic

789.30 Abdominal or pelvic swelling, mass or lump, unspecified site

789.31 Abdominal or pelvic swelling, mass, or lump, right upper quadrant

789.32 Abdominal or pelvic swelling, mass, or lump, left upper quadrant

789.33 Abdominal or pelvic swelling, mass, or lump, right lower quadrant

789.34 Abdominal or pelvic swelling, mass, or lump, left lower quadrant

Terms To Know

dysmenorrhea. Painful menstruation that may be primary, or essential, due to prostaglandin production and the onset of menstruation; secondary due to uterine, tubal, or ovarian abnormality or disease; spasmodic arising uterine contractions; or obstructive due to some mechanical blockage or interference with the menstrual flow.

oophoritis. Inflammation or infection of one or both ovaries that can cause chronic pelvic pain, ectopic pregnancy, or sterilization.

salpingitis. Inflammation of the fallopian tubes, usually caused by a bacterial infection and occurring in conjunction with inflammation of the ovaries (oophoritis).

CCI Version 18.3

0213T, 0216T, 0228T, 0230T, 12001-12007, 12011-12057, 13100-13153, 36000, 36400-36410, 36420-36430, 36440, 36600, 36640, 37202, 43653, 43752, 44005, 44180, 44602-44605, 49320, 50715, 51701-51703, 57410, 58350, 58740, 62310-62319, 64400-64435, 64445-64450, 64479, 64483, 64490, 64493, 64505-64530, 69990, 76000-76001, 77001-77002, 93000-93010, 93040-93042, 93318, 94002, 94200, 94250, 94680-94690, 94770, 95812-95816, 95819, 95822, 95829, 95955, 96360, 96365, 96372, 96374-96376, 99148-99149, 99150

Note: These CCI edits are used for Medicare. Other payers may reimburse on codes listed above.

Medicare Edits

	Fac RVU	Non-Fac RVU	FUD	Status
58660	20.06	20.06	90	A

	MUE		Modifiers		
58660	1	51	N/A	62	80

* with documentation

Medicare References: 100-3,230.3

Coding Companion for Ob/Gyn

58661

58661 Laparoscopy, surgical; with removal of adnexal structures (partial or total oophorectomy and/or salpingectomy)

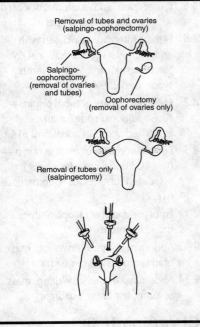

Removal of tubes and ovaries (salpingo-oophorectomy)

Salpingo-oophorectomy (removal of ovaries and tubes)

Oophorectomy (removal of ovaries only)

Removal of tubes only (salpingectomy)

Explanation

The physician performs a laparoscopic surgical removal of one or both ovaries and their accompanying fallopian tubes with the assistance of a fiberoptic laparoscope. The physician may first insert an instrument through the vagina to grasp the cervix and manipulate the uterus during surgery. Next, the physician makes a small incision just below the umbilicus through which a fiberoptic laparoscope is inserted. A second incision is made on the left or right side of the abdomen with additional instruments being placed through these incisions into the abdomen or pelvis. The physician manipulates the tools so that the pelvic organs can be observed, manipulated and removal of one or both ovaries and fallopian tubes can be performed with the laparoscope. The abdomen is deflated, the trocars removed and the incisions are closed with sutures.

Coding Tips

This is a bilateral code and is reported once even if the procedure is performed on both sides. Surgical laparoscopy always includes diagnostic laparoscopy. For diagnostic laparoscopy only, see 49230. If the procedure is performed to treat an ectopic pregnancy, see 59151. When 58661 is performed with another separately identifiable procedure, the highest dollar value code is listed as the primary procedure and subsequent procedures are appended with modifier 51. To report open salpingectomy, see 58700; for open salpingo-oophorectomy, see 58720. If a hysteroscopy is performed in conjunction with this procedure, report the appropriate hysteroscopy code.

ICD-9-CM Procedural

65.24	Laparoscopic wedge resection of ovary
65.31	Laparoscopic unilateral oophorectomy
65.41	Laparoscopic unilateral salpingo-oophorectomy
65.53	Laparoscopic removal of both ovaries at same operative episode
65.54	Laparoscopic removal of remaining ovary
65.63	Laparoscopic removal of both ovaries and tubes at same operative episode
65.64	Laparoscopic removal of remaining ovary and tube
66.4	Total unilateral salpingectomy
66.51	Removal of both fallopian tubes at same operative episode
66.52	Removal of remaining fallopian tube
66.62	Salpingectomy with removal of tubal pregnancy
66.63	Bilateral partial salpingectomy, not otherwise specified
66.69	Other partial salpingectomy

Anesthesia

58661 00840

ICD-9-CM Diagnostic

183.2	Malignant neoplasm of fallopian tube
183.8	Malignant neoplasm of other specified sites of uterine adnexa
198.6	Secondary malignant neoplasm of ovary
220	Benign neoplasm of ovary — (Use additional code to identify any functional activity: 256.0-256.1)
221.0	Benign neoplasm of fallopian tube and uterine ligaments
221.8	Benign neoplasm of other specified sites of female genital organs
233.30	Carcinoma in situ, unspecified female genital organ
233.31	Carcinoma in situ, vagina
233.32	Carcinoma in situ, vulva
233.39	Carcinoma in situ, other female genital organ
256.0	Hyperestrogenism
614.1	Chronic salpingitis and oophoritis — (Use additional code to identify organism: 041.00-041.09, 041.10-041.19)
614.2	Salpingitis and oophoritis not specified as acute, subacute, or chronic — (Use additional code to identify organism: 041.00-041.09, 041.10-041.19)
614.6	Pelvic peritoneal adhesions, female (postoperative) (postinfection) — (Use additional code to identify organism: 041.00-041.09, 041.10-041.19) (Use additional code to identify any associated infertility: 628.2)
617.1	Endometriosis of ovary
617.2	Endometriosis of fallopian tube
617.3	Endometriosis of pelvic peritoneum
617.9	Endometriosis, site unspecified
620.0	Follicular cyst of ovary
620.1	Corpus luteum cyst or hematoma
620.2	Other and unspecified ovarian cyst
620.5	Torsion of ovary, ovarian pedicle, or fallopian tube
628.2	Female infertility of tubal origin — (Use additional code for any associated peritubal adhesions: 614.6)

CCI Version 18.3

0213T, 0216T, 0228T, 0230T, 12001-12007, 12011-12057, 13100-13153, 36000, 36400-36410, 36420-36430, 36440, 36600, 36640, 37202, 43653, 43752, 44005, 44180, 44602-44605, 44950, 44970, 49320, 49322, 50715, 51701-51703, 57410, 58660, 58670, 58672-58673, 58740, 62310-62319, 64400-64435, 64445-64450, 64479, 64483, 64490, 64493, 64505-64530, 69990, 76000-76001, 77001-77002, 93000-93010, 93040-93042, 93318, 94002, 94200, 94250, 94680-94690, 94770, 95812-95816, 95819, 95822, 95829, 95955, 96360, 96365, 96372, 96374-96376, 99148-99149, 99150

Note: These CCI edits are used for Medicare. Other payers may reimburse on codes listed above.

Medicare Edits

	Fac RVU	Non-Fac RVU	FUD	Status
58661	19.2	19.2	10	A

	MUE		Modifiers		
58661	1	51	50	62	80

* with documentation

Medicare References: 100-3,230.3

58662

58662 Laparoscopy, surgical; with fulguration or excision of lesions of the ovary, pelvic viscera, or peritoneal surface by any method

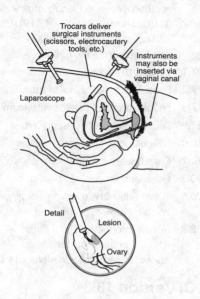

Trocars deliver surgical instruments (scissors, electrocautery tools, etc.)

Instruments may also be inserted via vaginal canal

Laparoscope

Detail

Lesion

Ovary

Explanation

The physician performs a laparoscopic electrical cautery destruction of an ovarian, pelvic or peritoneal lesion with the assistance of a fiberoptic laparoscope. The physician may first insert an instrument through the vagina to grasp the cervix and manipulate the uterus during surgery. Next, the physician makes a small incision just below the umbilicus through which a fiberoptic laparoscope is inserted. A second incision is made on the left or right side of the abdomen with additional instruments being placed through these incisions into the abdomen or pelvis. The physician manipulates the tools so that the pelvic organs can be observed, manipulated and operated upon with the laparoscope. Once lesions are identified with the laparoscope, a third incision is typically made adjacent to the lesion through which an electric cautery tool, knife, or laser is inserted for lesion fulguration. The abdomen is deflated, the trocars removed and the incisions are closed with sutures.

Coding Tips

Surgical laparoscopy always includes diagnostic laparoscopy. For diagnostic laparoscopy only, see 49230. When 58662 is performed with another separately identifiable procedure, the highest dollar value code is listed as the primary procedure and subsequent procedures are appended with modifier 51. If a hysteroscopy is performed in conjunction with this procedure, report the appropriate hysteroscopy code. For laparotomy with excision or destruction of intra-abdominal or retroperitoneal tumors, cysts, or endometriomas, see 49203–49205.

ICD-9-CM Procedural

54.4 Excision or destruction of peritoneal tissue
65.25 Other laparoscopic local excision or destruction of ovary
69.19 Other excision or destruction of uterus and supporting structures

Anesthesia

58662 00840

ICD-9-CM Diagnostic

158.8 Malignant neoplasm of specified parts of peritoneum
158.9 Malignant neoplasm of peritoneum, unspecified
159.8 Malignant neoplasm of other sites of digestive system and intra-abdominal organs
197.6 Secondary malignant neoplasm of retroperitoneum and peritoneum
211.8 Benign neoplasm of retroperitoneum and peritoneum
219.1 Benign neoplasm of corpus uteri
220 Benign neoplasm of ovary — (Use additional code to identify any functional activity: 256.0-256.1)
221.0 Benign neoplasm of fallopian tube and uterine ligaments
235.4 Neoplasm of uncertain behavior of retroperitoneum and peritoneum
256.4 Polycystic ovaries
614.6 Pelvic peritoneal adhesions, female (postoperative) (postinfection) — (Use additional code to identify organism: 041.00-041.09, 041.10-041.19) (Use additional code to identify any associated infertility: 628.2)
617.0 Endometriosis of uterus
617.1 Endometriosis of ovary
617.2 Endometriosis of fallopian tube
617.3 Endometriosis of pelvic peritoneum
620.0 Follicular cyst of ovary
620.1 Corpus luteum cyst or hematoma
620.2 Other and unspecified ovarian cyst
620.8 Other noninflammatory disorder of ovary, fallopian tube, and broad ligament
621.0 Polyp of corpus uteri
621.30 Endometrial hyperplasia, unspecified
621.31 Simple endometrial hyperplasia without atypia
621.32 Complex endometrial hyperplasia without atypia
625.3 Dysmenorrhea
625.8 Other specified symptom associated with female genital organs
628.0 Female infertility associated with anovulation — (Use additional code for any associated Stein-Leventhal syndrome: 256.4)
628.2 Female infertility of tubal origin — (Use additional code for any associated peritubal adhesions: 614.6)
628.3 Female infertility of uterine origin — (Use additional code for any associated tuberculous endometriosis: 016.7)
752.11 Embryonic cyst of fallopian tubes and broad ligaments
789.33 Abdominal or pelvic swelling, mass, or lump, right lower quadrant
789.34 Abdominal or pelvic swelling, mass, or lump, left lower quadrant

CCI Version 18.3

0213T, 0216T, 0228T, 0230T, 12001-12007, 12011-12057, 13100-13153, 36000, 36400-36410, 36420-36430, 36440, 36600, 36640, 37202, 43653, 43752, 44005, 44180, 44602-44605, 44950, 44970, 49320, 50715, 51701-51703, 57410, 58350, 58660, 62310-62319, 64400-64435, 64445-64450, 64479, 64483, 64490, 64493, 64505-64530, 69990, 76000-76001, 77001-77002, 93000-93010, 93040-93042, 93318, 94002, 94200, 94250, 94680-94690, 94770, 95812-95816, 95819, 95822, 95829, 95955, 96360, 96365, 96372, 96374-96376, 99148-99149, 99150

Note: These CCI edits are used for Medicare. Other payers may reimburse on codes listed above.

Medicare Edits

	Fac RVU	Non-Fac RVU	FUD	Status
58662	21.04	21.04	90	A

	MUE			Modifiers	
58662	1	51	N/A	62	80

* with documentation

Medicare References: 100-3,230.3

58670-58671

58670 Laparoscopy, surgical; with fulguration of oviducts (with or without transection)

58671 with occlusion of oviducts by device (eg, band, clip, or Falope ring)

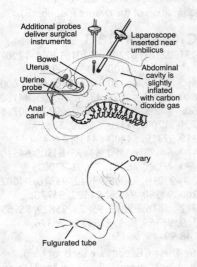

Additional probes deliver surgical instruments

Laparoscope inserted near umbilicus

Bowel
Uterus

Abdominal cavity is slightly inflated with carbon dioxide gas

Uterine probe

Anal canal

Ovary

Fulgurated tube

Explanation

The physician performs a laparoscopic electrical cautery destruction of an oviduct (the uterine tube) with or without complete cutting through the fallopian tubes (transection) with the assistance of a fiberoptic laparoscope. The physician may first insert an instrument through the vagina to grasp the cervix and manipulate the uterus during surgery. Next, the physician makes a small incision just below the umbilicus through which a fiberoptic laparoscope is inserted. A second incision is made on the left or right side of the abdomen with additional instruments being placed through these incisions into the abdomen or pelvis. The physician manipulates the tools so that the pelvic organs can be observed, manipulated and operated upon with the laparoscope. A third incision is typically made adjacent to the fallopian tubes. To fulgurate the fallopian tube the physician inserts an electric cautery tool or a laser. The physician may cut the tubes and fulgurate or burn the ends. Additionally, the physician may transect (cut through) the fallopian tubes. The abdomen is deflated, the trocars removed and the incisions are closed with sutures.

Coding Tips

Surgical laparoscopy always includes diagnostic laparoscopy. For diagnostic laparoscopy only, see 49230. When either

procedure is performed with another separately identifiable procedure, the highest dollar value code is listed as the primary procedure and subsequent procedures are appended with modifier 51. If a hysteroscopy is performed in conjunction with this procedure, report the appropriate hysteroscopy code. For occlusion of oviducts by vaginal or suprapubic approach, see 58615.

ICD-9-CM Procedural

66.21 Bilateral endoscopic ligation and crushing of fallopian tubes

66.22 Bilateral endoscopic ligation and division of fallopian tubes

66.29 Other bilateral endoscopic destruction or occlusion of fallopian tubes

Anesthesia

00851

ICD-9-CM Diagnostic

V25.2 Sterilization

V61.5 Multiparity

Terms To Know

electrocautery. Division or cutting of tissue using high-frequency electrical current to produce heat, which destroys cells.

fulguration. Destruction of living tissue by using sparks from a high-frequency electric current.

laparoscopy. Direct visualization of the peritoneal cavity, outer fallopian tubes, uterus, and ovaries utilizing a laparoscope, a thin, flexible fiberoptic tube.

multiparity. Condition of having had two or more pregnancies that resulted in viable fetuses; producing more than one fetus or offspring in the same gestation.

occlusion. Constriction, closure, or blockage of a passage.

transection. Transverse dissection; to cut across a long axis; cross section.

trocar. Cannula or a sharp pointed instrument used to puncture and aspirate fluid from cavities.

CCI Version 18.3

00851, 0213T, 0216T, 0228T, 0230T, 12001-12007, 12011-12057, 13100-13153, 36000, 36400-36410, 36420-36430, 36440, 36600, 36640, 37202, 43653, 43752, 44005, 44180, 44602-44605, 44950, 44970, 49320, 50715, 51701-51703, 57410, 58350, 58660, 62310-62319, 64400-64435, 64445-64450, 64479, 64483, 64490, 64493, 64505-64530, 69990, 76000-76001, 77001-77002, 93000-93010, 93040-93042, 93318, 94002,

94200, 94250, 94680-94690, 94770, 95812-95816, 95819, 95822, 95829, 95955, 96360, 96365, 96372, 96374-96376, 99148-99149, 99150

Also not with 58670: 58671❖

Note: These CCI edits are used for Medicare. Other payers may reimburse on codes listed above.

Medicare Edits

	Fac RVU	Non-Fac RVU	FUD	Status
58670	10.92	10.92	90	A
58671	10.91	10.91	90	A

	MUE		Modifiers		
58670	1	51	N/A	62	N/A
58671	1	51	N/A	62	N/A

* with documentation

Medicare References: 100-3, 230.3

© 2012 OptumInsight, Inc.

58672

58672 Laparoscopy, surgical; with fimbrioplasty

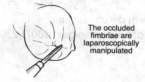

Fallopian tube
Ovary
Uterus
Fimbriae
Cervix
Vaginal canal

The occluded fimbriae are laparoscopically manipulated

Explanation

The physician performs a laparoscopic surgical repair of the ovarian fimbria (fingerlike processes on the distal part of the infundibulum of the uterine tube) with the assistance of a fiberoptic laparoscope. The physician may first insert an instrument through the vagina to grasp the cervix and manipulate the uterus during surgery. Next, the physician makes a small incision just below the umbilicus through which a fiberoptic laparoscope is inserted. A second incision is made on the left or right side of the abdomen with additional instruments being placed through these incisions into the abdomen or pelvis. The physician manipulates the tools so that the pelvic organs can be observed, manipulated and operated upon with the laparoscope. A third incision is typically made adjacent to the fallopian tubes. The physician performs surgical repair of the ovarian fimbria using instruments placed through the abdomen and pelvic trocars. The abdomen is deflated, the trocars removed and the incisions are closed with sutures.

Coding Tips

Report this code when the documentation specifies reconstruction of the fimbriae (hair-like projections) at the end of the tube. This code should not be used to report other tubal reconstruction. Surgical laparoscopy always includes diagnostic laparoscopy. For diagnostic laparoscopy only, see 49230. This is a unilateral procedure. If performed bilaterally, some payers require that the service be reported twice with modifier 50 appended to the second code while others require identification of the service only once with modifier 50 appended. Check with individual payers. Modifier 50 identifies a procedure performed identically on the opposite side of the body (mirror image). For open fimbrioplasty, see 58760. For tubotubal anastomosis, see 58750. For tubouterine implantation, see 58752. Because this procedure is usually not done out of medical necessity, the patient may be responsible for charges. Verify with the insurance carrier for coverage.

ICD-9-CM Procedural

66.79   Other repair of fallopian tube

Anesthesia

58672   00840

ICD-9-CM Diagnostic

614.1   Chronic salpingitis and oophoritis — (Use additional code to identify organism: 041.00-041.09, 041.10-041.19)

614.2   Salpingitis and oophoritis not specified as acute, subacute, or chronic — (Use additional code to identify organism: 041.00-041.09, 041.10-041.19)

614.4   Chronic or unspecified parametritis and pelvic cellulitis — (Use additional code to identify organism: 041.00-041.09, 041.10-041.19)

614.6   Pelvic peritoneal adhesions, female (postoperative) (postinfection) — (Use additional code to identify organism: 041.00-041.09, 041.10-041.19) (Use additional code to identify any associated infertility: 628.2)

614.8   Other specified inflammatory disease of female pelvic organs and tissues — (Use additional code to identify organism: 041.00-041.09, 041.10-041.19)

617.2   Endometriosis of fallopian tube

628.2   Female infertility of tubal origin — (Use additional code for any associated peritubal adhesions: 614.6)

752.19   Other congenital anomaly of fallopian tubes and broad ligaments

Terms To Know

endometriosis. Aberrant uterine mucosal tissue appearing in areas of the pelvic cavity outside of its normal location, lining the uterus and inflaming surrounding tissues, and can result in infertility and spontaneous abortion.

oophoritis. Inflammation or infection of one or both ovaries that can cause chronic pelvic pain, ectopic pregnancy, or sterilization.

parametritis. Inflammation and infection of the tissue in the structures around the uterus.

salpingitis. Inflammation of the fallopian tubes, usually caused by a bacterial infection and occurring in conjunction with inflammation of the ovaries (oophoritis).

CCI Version 18.3

0213T, 0216T, 0228T, 0230T, 12001-12007, 12011-12057, 13100-13153, 36000, 36400-36410, 36420-36430, 36440, 36600, 36640, 37202, 43653, 43752, 44005, 44180, 44602-44605, 44950, 44970, 49320, 50715, 51701-51703, 57410, 58350, 58660, 62310-62319, 64400-64435, 64445-64450, 64479, 64483, 64490, 64493, 64505-64530, 69990, 76000-76001, 77001-77002, 93000-93010, 93040-93042, 93318, 94002, 94200, 94250, 94680-94690, 94770, 95812-95816, 95819, 95822, 95829, 95955, 96360, 96365, 96372, 96374-96376, 99148-99149, 99150

Note: These CCI edits are used for Medicare. Other payers may reimburse on codes listed above.

Medicare Edits

	Fac RVU	Non-Fac RVU	FUD	Status
58672	21.98	21.98	90	A

	MUE		Modifiers		
58672	1	51	50	N/A	80

* with documentation

Medicare References: 100-3,230.3

58673

58673 Laparoscopy, surgical; with salpingostomy (salpingoneostomy)

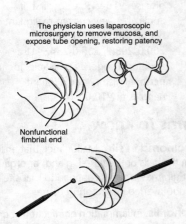

The physician uses laparoscopic microsurgery to remove mucosa, and expose tube opening, restoring patency

Nonfunctional fimbrial end

A new opening can be created in any location

Explanation

The physician performs a laparoscopic surgical restoration of the patency of the uterine tube damaged typically by infection, tumor or endometriosis. The physician may first insert an instrument through the vagina to grasp the cervix and manipulate the uterus during surgery. Next, the physician makes a small incision just below the umbilicus through which a fiberoptic laparoscope is inserted. A second incision is made on the left or right side of the abdomen with additional instruments being placed through these incisions into the abdomen or pelvis. The physician then manipulates the tools so that the pelvic organs can be observed, manipulated and operated upon with the laparoscope. A third incision is typically made adjacent to the fallopian tubes. The physician performs surgical restoration of the fallopian tube (salpingostomy) using instruments placed through the abdomen and pelvic trocars. The abdomen is then deflated, the trocars removed and the incisions are closed with sutures.

Coding Tips

Report 58673 for repair of the fimbrial end of the tube, not reconstruction of the fimbriae, which should be coded with 58672. Surgical laparoscopy always includes diagnostic laparoscopy. For diagnostic laparoscopy only, see 49230. This is a unilateral procedure. If performed bilaterally, some payers require that the service be reported twice with modifier 50 appended to the second code while others require identification of the service only once with modifier 50 appended. Check with individual payers. Modifier 50 identifies a procedure performed identically on the opposite side of the body (mirror image). For open salpingostomy, see 58770. Because this procedure is usually not done out of medical necessity, the patient may be responsible for charges. Verify with the insurance carrier for coverage.

ICD-9-CM Procedural

66.02   Salpingostomy

Anesthesia

58673   00840

ICD-9-CM Diagnostic

139.8   Late effects of other and unspecified infectious and parasitic diseases — (Note: This category is to be used to indicate conditions classifiable to categories 001-009, 020-041, 046-136 as the cause of late effects, which are themselves classified elsewhere. The "late effects" include conditions specified as such, as sequelae of diseases classifiable to the above categories if there is evidence that the disease itself is no longer present.)

614.1   Chronic salpingitis and oophoritis — (Use additional code to identify organism: 041.00-041.09, 041.10-041.19)

614.2   Salpingitis and oophoritis not specified as acute, subacute, or chronic — (Use additional code to identify organism: 041.00-041.09, 041.10-041.19)

614.4   Chronic or unspecified parametritis and pelvic cellulitis — (Use additional code to identify organism: 041.00-041.09, 041.10-041.19)

614.6   Pelvic peritoneal adhesions, female (postoperative) (postinfection) — (Use additional code to identify organism: 041.00-041.09, 041.10-041.19) (Use additional code to identify any associated infertility: 628.2)

614.8   Other specified inflammatory disease of female pelvic organs and tissues — (Use additional code to identify organism: 041.00-041.09, 041.10-041.19)

617.2   Endometriosis of fallopian tube

628.2   Female infertility of tubal origin — (Use additional code for any associated peritubal adhesions: 614.6)

908.2   Late effect of internal injury to other internal organs

V51.8   Other aftercare involving the use of plastic surgery

Terms To Know

salpingitis. Inflammation of the fallopian tubes, usually caused by a bacterial infection and occurring in conjunction with inflammation of the ovaries (oophoritis).

CCI Version 18.3

0213T, 0216T, 0228T, 0230T, 12001-12007, 12011-12057, 13100-13153, 36000, 36400-36410, 36420-36430, 36440, 36600, 36640, 37202, 43653, 43752, 44005, 44180, 44602-44605, 44950, 44970, 49320, 50715, 51701-51703, 57410, 58350, 58660, 62310-62319, 64400-64435, 64445-64450, 64479, 64483, 64490, 64493, 64505-64530, 69990, 76000-76001, 77001-77002, 93000-93010, 93040-93042, 93318, 94002, 94200, 94250, 94680-94690, 94770, 95812-95816, 95819, 95822, 95829, 95955, 96360, 96365, 96372, 96374-96376, 99148-99149, 99150

Note: These CCI edits are used for Medicare. Other payers may reimburse on codes listed above.

Medicare Edits

	Fac RVU	Non-Fac RVU	FUD	Status
58673	23.89	23.89	90	A

	MUE		Modifiers		
58673	1	51	50	N/A	80

* with documentation

Medicare References: 100-3,230.3

58700

58700 Salpingectomy, complete or partial, unilateral or bilateral (separate procedure)

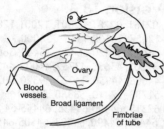

All or part of tube is removed

Ovary

Blood vessels

Broad ligament

Fimbriae of tube

Explanation

Through a small incision in the lower abdomen just above the pubic hairline, the physician removes part or all of the fallopian tube on one or both sides. The incision is closed by suturing.

Coding Tips

This separate procedure by definition is usually a component of a more complex service and is not identified separately. When performed alone or with other unrelated procedures/services it may be reported. If performed alone, list the code; if performed with other procedures/services, list the code and append modifier 59. When 58700 is performed with another separately identifiable procedure, the highest dollar value code is listed as the primary procedure and subsequent procedures are appended with modifier 51. This code should only be used when completing an open invasive procedure, not when being performed through a laparoscopy; for laparoscopic salpingectomy, see 58661. If the ovary and fallopian tube are excised in an open approach, report 58720.

ICD-9-CM Procedural

66.4	Total unilateral salpingectomy
66.51	Removal of both fallopian tubes at same operative episode
66.52	Removal of remaining fallopian tube
66.63	Bilateral partial salpingectomy, not otherwise specified
66.69	Other partial salpingectomy

Anesthesia

58700 00840

ICD-9-CM Diagnostic

183.2	Malignant neoplasm of fallopian tube
198.82	Secondary malignant neoplasm of genital organs
221.0	Benign neoplasm of fallopian tube and uterine ligaments
233.30	Carcinoma in situ, unspecified female genital organ
233.31	Carcinoma in situ, vagina
233.32	Carcinoma in situ, vulva
233.39	Carcinoma in situ, other female genital organ
236.3	Neoplasm of uncertain behavior of other and unspecified female genital organs
239.5	Neoplasm of unspecified nature of other genitourinary organs
614.1	Chronic salpingitis and oophoritis — (Use additional code to identify organism: 041.00-041.09, 041.10-041.19)
614.2	Salpingitis and oophoritis not specified as acute, subacute, or chronic — (Use additional code to identify organism: 041.00-041.09, 041.10-041.19)
617.2	Endometriosis of fallopian tube
620.4	Prolapse or hernia of ovary and fallopian tube
620.5	Torsion of ovary, ovarian pedicle, or fallopian tube
789.00	Abdominal pain, unspecified site
V50.49	Other prophylactic organ removal
V84.02	Genetic susceptibility to malignant neoplasm of ovary — (Use additional code, if applicable, for any associated family history of the disease: V16-V19. Code first, if applicable, any current malignant neoplasms: 140.0-195.8, 200.0-208.9, 230.0-234.9. Use additional code, if applicable, for any personal history of malignant neoplasm: V10.0-V10.9)
V84.04	Genetic susceptibility to malignant neoplasm of endometrium — (Use additional code, if applicable, for any associated family history of the disease: V16-V19. Code first, if applicable, any current malignant neoplasms: 140.0-195.8, 200.0-208.9, 230.0-234.9. Use additional code, if applicable, for any personal history of malignant neoplasm: V10.0-V10.9)
V84.09	Genetic susceptibility to other malignant neoplasm — (Use additional code, if applicable, for any associated family history of the disease: V16-V19. Code first, if applicable, any current malignant neoplasms: 140.0-195.8, 200.0-208.9, 230.0-234.9. Use additional code, if applicable, for any personal history of malignant neoplasm: V10.0-V10.9)

Terms To Know

carcinoma in situ. Malignancy that arises from the cells of the vessel, gland, or organ of origin that remains confined to that site or has not invaded neighboring tissue.

oophoritis. Inflammation or infection of one or both ovaries that can cause chronic pelvic pain, ectopic pregnancy, or sterilization.

prolapse. Falling, sliding, or sinking of an organ from its normal location in the body.

salpingitis. Inflammation of the fallopian tubes, usually caused by a bacterial infection and occurring in conjunction with inflammation of the ovaries (oophoritis).

torsion of ovary or fallopian tube. Twisting or rotation of the ovary or fallopian tube upon itself, so as to compromise or cut off the blood supply.

CCI Version 18.3

0213T, 0216T, 0228T, 0230T, 12001-12007, 12011-12057, 13100-13153, 36000, 36400-36410, 36420-36430, 36440, 36600, 36640, 37202, 43752, 44005, 44180, 44602-44605, 44820-44850, 44950, 44970, 49000-49010, 49255, 49320, 49570, 50715, 51701-51703, 57410, 58605, 58661-58673, 58740, 58900, 62310-62319, 64400-64435, 64445-64450, 64479, 64483, 64490, 64493, 64505-64530, 69990, 93000-93010, 93040-93042, 93318, 94002, 94200, 94250, 94680-94690, 94770, 95812-95816, 95819, 95822, 95829, 95955, 96360, 96365, 96372, 96374-96376, 99148-99149, 99150

Note: These CCI edits are used for Medicare. Other payers may reimburse on codes listed above.

Medicare Edits

	Fac RVU	Non-Fac RVU	FUD	Status
58700	23.1	23.1	90	A

	MUE			Modifiers	
58700	1	51	N/A	62*	80

* with documentation

Medicare References: None

Coding Companion for Ob/Gyn

58720

58720 Salpingo-oophorectomy, complete or partial, unilateral or bilateral (separate procedure)

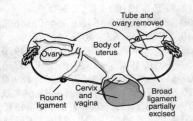

Tube and ovary removed

Body of uterus

Ovary

Round ligament

Cervix and vagina

Broad ligament partially excised

Explanation

Through a small incision in the abdomen just above the pubic hairline, the physician removes part or all of the ovary and part or all of its fallopian tube on one or both sides. The incision is closed by suturing.

Coding Tips

This code should only be used when completing an open invasive procedure, not when being performed through a laparoscopy; if performed through a laparoscopy, see 58661. This separate procedure by definition is usually a component of a more complex service and is not identified separately. When performed alone or with other unrelated procedures/services it may be reported. If performed alone, list the code; if performed with other procedures/services, list the code and append modifier 59. When 58720 is performed with another separately identifiable procedure, the highest dollar value code is listed as the primary procedure and subsequent procedures are appended with modifier 51. If only the fallopian tubes are excised, report 58700.

ICD-9-CM Procedural

65.49   Other unilateral salpingo-oophorectomy

65.61   Other removal of both ovaries and tubes at same operative episode

65.62   Other removal of remaining ovary and tube

Anesthesia

58720   00840

ICD-9-CM Diagnostic

183.0   Malignant neoplasm of ovary — (Use additional code to identify any functional activity)

183.2   Malignant neoplasm of fallopian tube

198.6   Secondary malignant neoplasm of ovary

220   Benign neoplasm of ovary — (Use additional code to identify any functional activity: 256.0-256.1)

221.0   Benign neoplasm of fallopian tube and uterine ligaments

233.30   Carcinoma in situ, unspecified female genital organ

233.31   Carcinoma in situ, vagina

233.32   Carcinoma in situ, vulva

233.39   Carcinoma in situ, other female genital organ

236.2   Neoplasm of uncertain behavior of ovary — (Use additional code to identify any functional activity)

236.3   Neoplasm of uncertain behavior of other and unspecified female genital organs

239.5   Neoplasm of unspecified nature of other genitourinary organs

256.0   Hyperestrogenism

256.4   Polycystic ovaries

614.0   Acute salpingitis and oophoritis — (Use additional code to identify organism: 041.00-041.09, 041.10-041.19)

614.1   Chronic salpingitis and oophoritis — (Use additional code to identify organism: 041.00-041.09, 041.10-041.19)

614.2   Salpingitis and oophoritis not specified as acute, subacute, or chronic — (Use additional code to identify organism: 041.00-041.09, 041.10-041.19)

614.6   Pelvic peritoneal adhesions, female (postoperative) (postinfection) — (Use additional code to identify organism: 041.00-041.09, 041.10-041.19) (Use additional code to identify any associated infertility: 628.2)

617.1   Endometriosis of ovary

617.2   Endometriosis of fallopian tube

620.0   Follicular cyst of ovary

620.1   Corpus luteum cyst or hematoma

620.2   Other and unspecified ovarian cyst

620.4   Prolapse or hernia of ovary and fallopian tube

620.5   Torsion of ovary, ovarian pedicle, or fallopian tube

620.8   Other noninflammatory disorder of ovary, fallopian tube, and broad ligament

625.3   Dysmenorrhea

625.8   Other specified symptom associated with female genital organs

626.2   Excessive or frequent menstruation

626.8   Other disorder of menstruation and other abnormal bleeding from female genital tract

628.2   Female infertility of tubal origin — (Use additional code for any associated peritubal adhesions: 614.6)

752.0   Congenital anomalies of ovaries

752.10   Unspecified congenital anomaly of fallopian tubes and broad ligaments

752.11   Embryonic cyst of fallopian tubes and broad ligaments

CCI Version 18.3

0213T, 0216T, 0228T, 0230T, 12001-12007, 12011-12057, 13100-13153, 36000, 36400-36410, 36420-36430, 36440, 36600, 36640, 37202, 43752, 44005, 44180, 44602-44605, 44820-44850, 44950, 44970, 49000-49010, 49255, 49320, 49570, 50715, 51701-51703, 57410, 58605, 58661-58673, 58700, 58740, 58805, 58900, 62310-62319, 64400-64435, 64445-64450, 64479, 64483, 64490, 64493, 64505-64530, 69990, 93000-93010, 93040-93042, 93318, 94002, 94200, 94250, 94680-94690, 94770, 95812-95816, 95819, 95822, 95829, 95955, 96360, 96365, 96372, 96374-96376, 99148-99149, 99150

Note: These CCI edits are used for Medicare. Other payers may reimburse on codes listed above.

Medicare Edits

	Fac RVU	Non-Fac RVU	FUD	Status
58720	21.53	21.53	90	A

	MUE		Modifiers		
58720	1	51	N/A	62*	80

* with documentation

Medicare References: None

58740

58740 Lysis of adhesions (salpingolysis, ovariolysis)

Oviduct

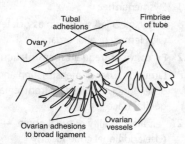

Labels on illustration:
Tubal adhesions
Fimbriae of tube
Ovary
Ovarian adhesions to broad ligament
Ovarian vessels

Explanation

The physician cuts free any fibrous tissue adhering to the ovaries or tubes through a small incision just above the pubic hairline.

Coding Tips

This is a procedure to restore fertility and should not be coded for minor freeing of the tube and ovary as part of another procedure. For laparoscopic lysis of adhesions (salpingostomy, ovariolysis), see 58660. For laparoscopic fulguration or excision of lesions of the ovary, pelvic viscera, or peritoneal surface, see 58662.

ICD-9-CM Procedural

65.89 Other lysis of adhesions of ovary and fallopian tube

Anesthesia

58740 00840

ICD-9-CM Diagnostic

614.1 Chronic salpingitis and oophoritis — (Use additional code to identify organism: 041.00-041.09, 041.10-041.19)

614.2 Salpingitis and oophoritis not specified as acute, subacute, or chronic — (Use additional code to identify organism: 041.00-041.09, 041.10-041.19)

614.5 Acute or unspecified pelvic peritonitis, female — (Use additional code to identify organism: 041.00-041.09, 041.10-041.19)

614.6 Pelvic peritoneal adhesions, female (postoperative) (postinfection) — (Use additional code to identify organism: 041.00-041.09, 041.10-041.19) (Use additional code to identify any associated infertility: 628.2)

617.0 Endometriosis of uterus

617.1 Endometriosis of ovary

617.2 Endometriosis of fallopian tube

617.3 Endometriosis of pelvic peritoneum

625.3 Dysmenorrhea

625.8 Other specified symptom associated with female genital organs

626.2 Excessive or frequent menstruation

628.2 Female infertility of tubal origin — (Use additional code for any associated peritubal adhesions: 614.6)

628.8 Female infertility of other specified origin

752.19 Other congenital anomaly of fallopian tubes and broad ligaments

789.01 Abdominal pain, right upper quadrant

789.02 Abdominal pain, left upper quadrant

789.03 Abdominal pain, right lower quadrant

789.04 Abdominal pain, left lower quadrant

789.31 Abdominal or pelvic swelling, mass, or lump, right upper quadrant

789.32 Abdominal or pelvic swelling, mass, or lump, left upper quadrant

789.33 Abdominal or pelvic swelling, mass, or lump, right lower quadrant

789.34 Abdominal or pelvic swelling, mass, or lump, left lower quadrant

V64.41 Laparoscopic surgical procedure converted to open procedure

Terms To Know

dysmenorrhea. Painful menstruation that may be primary, or essential, due to prostaglandin production and the onset of menstruation; secondary due to uterine, tubal, or ovarian abnormality or disease; spasmodic arising uterine contractions; or obstructive due to some mechanical blockage or interference with the menstrual flow.

oophoritis. Inflammation or infection of one or both ovaries that can cause chronic pelvic pain, ectopic pregnancy, or sterilization.

peritonitis. Inflammation and infection within the peritoneal cavity, the space between the membrane lining the abdominopelvic walls and covering the internal organs.

salpingitis. Inflammation of the fallopian tubes, usually caused by a bacterial infection and occurring in conjunction with inflammation of the ovaries (oophoritis).

CCI Version 18.3

0213T, 0216T, 0228T, 0230T, 12001-12007, 12011-12057, 13100-13153, 36000, 36400-36410, 36420-36430, 36440, 36600, 36640, 37202, 43752, 44005, 44180, 44602-44605, 44820-44850, 44950, 44970, 49000-49010, 49255, 49320, 49570, 50715, 51701-51703, 57410, 58350, 58805, 58900, 62310-62319, 64400-64435, 64445-64450, 64479, 64483, 64490, 64493, 64505-64530, 69990, 93000-93010, 93040-93042, 93318, 94002, 94200, 94250, 94680-94690, 94770, 95812-95816, 95819, 95822, 95829, 95955, 96360, 96365, 96372, 96374-96376, 99148-99149, 99150

Note: These CCI edits are used for Medicare. Other payers may reimburse on codes listed above.

Medicare Edits

	Fac RVU	Non-Fac RVU	FUD	Status
58740	26.14	26.14	90	A

	MUE		Modifiers		
58740	1	51	N/A	62*	80

* with documentation

Medicare References: None

58750

58750 Tubotubal anastomosis

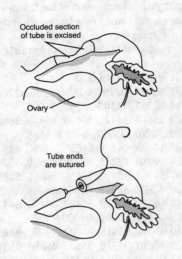

Occluded section of tube is excised

Ovary

Tube ends are sutured

Explanation

Through a small incision just above the pubic hairline, the physician excises the closed or blocked portion of the tube and sutures the clean edges together. The procedure is generally performed microsurgically in order to do an accurate repair.

Coding Tips

This is usually an elective procedure to reverse prior sterilization. If performed to restore patency after a tubal pregnancy or after excision of a tubal lesion, submit a cover letter and operative report. This is a unilateral procedure. If performed bilaterally, some payers require that the service be reported twice with modifier 50 appended to the second code while others require identification of the service only once with modifier 50 appended. Check with individual payers. Modifier 50 identifies a procedure performed identically on the opposite side of the body (mirror image). Because this procedure is usually not done out of medical necessity, the patient may be responsible for charges. Verify with the insurance carrier for coverage.

ICD-9-CM Procedural

66.73   Salpingo-salpingostomy

Anesthesia

58750   00840

ICD-9-CM Diagnostic

221.0   Benign neoplasm of fallopian tube and uterine ligaments

614.1   Chronic salpingitis and oophoritis — (Use additional code to identify organism: 041.00-041.09, 041.10-041.19)

614.2   Salpingitis and oophoritis not specified as acute, subacute, or chronic — (Use additional code to identify organism: 041.00-041.09, 041.10-041.19)

614.6   Pelvic peritoneal adhesions, female (postoperative) (postinfection) — (Use additional code to identify organism: 041.00-041.09, 041.10-041.19) (Use additional code to identify any associated infertility: 628.2)

614.7   Other chronic pelvic peritonitis, female — (Use additional code to identify organism: 041.00-041.09, 041.10-041.19)

614.8   Other specified inflammatory disease of female pelvic organs and tissues — (Use additional code to identify organism: 041.00-041.09, 041.10-041.19)

628.2   Female infertility of tubal origin — (Use additional code for any associated peritubal adhesions: 614.6)

628.8   Female infertility of other specified origin

628.9   Female infertility of unspecified origin

752.19   Other congenital anomaly of fallopian tubes and broad ligaments

V26.0   Tuboplasty or vasoplasty after previous sterilization

Terms To Know

anastomosis. Surgically created connection between ducts, blood vessels, or bowel segments to allow flow from one to the other.

chronic. Persistent, continuing, or recurring.

occlusion. Constriction, closure, or blockage of a passage.

oophoritis. Inflammation or infection of one or both ovaries that can cause chronic pelvic pain, ectopic pregnancy, or sterilization.

peritonitis. Inflammation and infection within the peritoneal cavity, the space between the membrane lining the abdominopelvic walls and covering the internal organs.

salpingitis. Inflammation of the fallopian tubes, usually caused by a bacterial infection and occurring in conjunction with inflammation of the ovaries (oophoritis).

CCI Version 18.3

0213T, 0216T, 0228T, 0230T, 12001-12007, 12011-12057, 13100-13153, 36000, 36400-36410, 36420-36430, 36440, 36600, 36640, 37202, 43752, 44005, 44180, 44602-44605, 44820-44850, 44950, 44970, 49000-49010, 49255, 49320, 49570, 50715, 51701-51703, 57410, 58350, 58660, 58805, 58900, 62310-62319, 64400-64435, 64445-64450, 64479, 64483, 64490, 64493, 64505-64530, 69990, 93000-93010, 93040-93042, 93318, 94002, 94200, 94250, 94680-94690, 94770, 95812-95816, 95819, 95822, 95829, 95955, 96360, 96365, 96372, 96374-96376, 99148-99149, 99150

Note: These CCI edits are used for Medicare. Other payers may reimburse on codes listed above.

Medicare Edits

	Fac RVU	Non-Fac RVU	FUD	Status
58750	26.94	26.94	90	A

	MUE		Modifiers		
58750	2	51	N/A	62*	80

* with documentation

Medicare References: None

Coding Companion for Ob/Gyn

© 2012 OptumInsight, Inc.

58752

58752 Tubouterine implantation

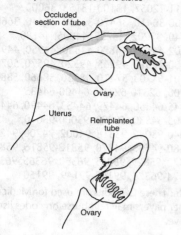

The physician excises a blocked section of fallopian tube and reattaches the remaining portion of the tube to the uterus

Occluded section of tube

Ovary

Uterus

Reimplanted tube

Ovary

Tube is reimplanted into the uterus

Explanation

Through a small incision just above the pubic hairline, the physician removes a blocked portion of the tube near its junction with the uterus and reimplants the tube into the uterus in the same place.

Coding Tips

This code should not be confused with 58750, tubotubal anastomosis, in which a portion of the tube is excised and the two ends are sutured together. Report this code when the procedure involves the tube and the uterus. This is a unilateral procedure. If performed bilaterally, some payers require that the service be reported twice with modifier 50 appended to the second code while others require identification of the service only once with modifier 50 appended. Check with individual payers. Modifier 50 identifies a procedure performed identically on the opposite side of the body (mirror image). Because this procedure is usually not done out of medical necessity, the patient may be responsible for charges. Verify with the insurance carrier for coverage.

ICD-9-CM Procedural

66.74   Salpingo-uterostomy

Anesthesia

58752   00840

ICD-9-CM Diagnostic

221.0   Benign neoplasm of fallopian tube and uterine ligaments

614.1   Chronic salpingitis and oophoritis — (Use additional code to identify organism: 041.00-041.09, 041.10-041.19)

614.2   Salpingitis and oophoritis not specified as acute, subacute, or chronic — (Use additional code to identify organism: 041.00-041.09, 041.10-041.19)

614.6   Pelvic peritoneal adhesions, female (postoperative) (postinfection) — (Use additional code to identify organism: 041.00-041.09, 041.10-041.19) (Use additional code to identify any associated infertility: 628.2)

614.7   Other chronic pelvic peritonitis, female — (Use additional code to identify organism: 041.00-041.09, 041.10-041.19)

614.8   Other specified inflammatory disease of female pelvic organs and tissues — (Use additional code to identify organism: 041.00-041.09, 041.10-041.19)

628.2   Female infertility of tubal origin — (Use additional code for any associated peritubal adhesions: 614.6)

752.19 Other congenital anomaly of fallopian tubes and broad ligaments

V26.0   Tuboplasty or vasoplasty after previous sterilization

Terms To Know

adhesion. Abnormal fibrous connection between two structures, soft tissue or bony structures, that may occur as the result of surgery, infection, or trauma.

anomaly. Irregularity in the structure or position of an organ or tissue.

benign. Mild or nonmalignant in nature.

broad ligament. Fold of peritoneum extending from the side of the uterus to the wall of the pelvis.

chronic. Persistent, continuing, or recurring.

congenital. Present at birth, occurring through heredity or an influence during gestation up to the moment of birth.

neoplasm. New abnormal growth, tumor.

oophoritis. Inflammation or infection of one or both ovaries that can cause chronic pelvic pain, ectopic pregnancy, or sterilization.

peritonitis. Inflammation and infection within the peritoneal cavity, the space between the membrane lining the abdominopelvic walls and covering the internal organs.

salpingitis. Inflammation of the fallopian tubes, usually caused by a bacterial infection and occurring in conjunction with inflammation of the ovaries (oophoritis).

CCI Version 18.3

0213T, 0216T, 0228T, 0230T, 12001-12007, 12011-12057, 13100-13153, 36000, 36400-36410, 36420-36430, 36440, 36600, 36640, 37202, 43752, 44005, 44180, 44602-44605, 44820-44850, 44950, 44970, 49000-49010, 49255, 49320, 49570, 50715, 51701-51703, 57410, 58350, 58660, 58805, 58900, 62310-62319, 64400-64435, 64445-64450, 64479, 64483, 64490, 64493, 64505-64530, 69990, 93000-93010, 93040-93042, 93318, 94002, 94200, 94250, 94680-94690, 94770, 95812-95816, 95819, 95822, 95829, 95955, 96360, 96365, 96372, 96374-96376, 99148-99149, 99150

Note: These CCI edits are used for Medicare. Other payers may reimburse on codes listed above.

Medicare Edits

	Fac RVU	Non-Fac RVU	FUD	Status
58752	25.41	25.41	90	A

	MUE		Modifiers		
58752	2	51	N/A	N/A	80

* with documentation

Medicare References: None

58760

58760 Fimbrioplasty

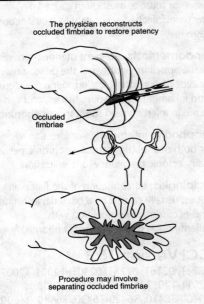

The physician reconstructs occluded fimbriae to restore patency

Occluded fimbriae

Procedure may involve separating occluded fimbriae

Explanation

Through a small incision just above the pubic hairline, the physician reconstructs the existing fimbriae in a partially or totally obstructed (occluded) or closed off oviduct. Fimbriae are the hairlike fringes at the end of the fallopian tubes. Depending on the nature of the blockage, the physician may separate the fimbriae by gentle dilation or by electrosurgical dissection. The procedure is generally performed microsurgically in order to do an accurate repair.

Coding Tips

Report this code when the documentation specifies reconstruction of the fimbriae (hair-like projections) at the end of the tube. This code should not be used to report other tubal reconstruction. This is a unilateral procedure. If performed bilaterally, some payers require that the service be reported twice with modifier 50 appended to the second code while others require identification of the service only once with modifier 50 appended. Check with individual payers. Modifier 50 identifies a procedure performed identically on the opposite side of the body (mirror image). If significant additional time and effort is documented, append modifier 22 and submit a cover letter and operative report. For laparoscopic fimbrioplasty, see 58672. For tubotubal anastomosis, see 58750. For tubouterine implantation, see 58752. Because this procedure is usually not done out of medical necessity, the patient may be responsible for charges. Verify with the insurance carrier for coverage.

ICD-9-CM Procedural

66.79 Other repair of fallopian tube

Anesthesia

58760 00840

ICD-9-CM Diagnostic

614.1 Chronic salpingitis and oophoritis — (Use additional code to identify organism: 041.00-041.09, 041.10-041.19)

614.2 Salpingitis and oophoritis not specified as acute, subacute, or chronic — (Use additional code to identify organism: 041.00-041.09, 041.10-041.19)

614.3 Acute parametritis and pelvic cellulitis — (Use additional code to identify organism: 041.00-041.09, 041.10-041.19)

614.4 Chronic or unspecified parametritis and pelvic cellulitis — (Use additional code to identify organism: 041.00-041.09, 041.10-041.19)

614.5 Acute or unspecified pelvic peritonitis, female — (Use additional code to identify organism: 041.00-041.09, 041.10-041.19)

614.6 Pelvic peritoneal adhesions, female (postoperative) (postinfection) — (Use additional code to identify organism: 041.00-041.09, 041.10-041.19) (Use additional code to identify any associated infertility: 628.2)

614.8 Other specified inflammatory disease of female pelvic organs and tissues — (Use additional code to identify organism: 041.00-041.09, 041.10-041.19)

617.2 Endometriosis of fallopian tube

628.2 Female infertility of tubal origin — (Use additional code for any associated peritubal adhesions: 614.6)

752.19 Other congenital anomaly of fallopian tubes and broad ligaments

909.3 Late effect of complications of surgical and medical care

V64.41 Laparoscopic surgical procedure converted to open procedure

Terms To Know

acute. Sudden, severe. Documentation and reporting of an acute condition is important to establishing medical necessity.

adhesion. Abnormal fibrous connection between two structures, soft tissue or bony structures, that may occur as the result of surgery, infection, or trauma.

cellulitis. Sudden, severe, suppurative inflammation and edema in subcutaneous tissue or muscle, most often caused by bacterial infection secondary to a cutaneous lesion.

endometriosis. Aberrant uterine mucosal tissue appearing in areas of the pelvic cavity outside of its normal location, lining the uterus and inflaming surrounding tissues, and can result in infertility and spontaneous abortion.

parametritis. Inflammation and infection of the tissue in the structures around the uterus.

salpingitis. Inflammation of the fallopian tubes, usually caused by a bacterial infection and occurring in conjunction with inflammation of the ovaries (oophoritis).

CCI Version 18.3

0213T, 0216T, 0228T, 0230T, 12001-12007, 12011-12057, 13100-13153, 36000, 36400-36410, 36420-36430, 36440, 36600, 36640, 37202, 43752, 44005, 44180, 44602-44605, 44820-44850, 44950, 44970, 49000-49010, 49255, 49320, 49570, 50715, 51701-51703, 57410, 58350, 58660, 58672, 58805, 58900, 62310-62319, 64400-64435, 64445-64450, 64479, 64483, 64490, 64493, 64505-64530, 69990, 93000-93010, 93040-93042, 93318, 94002, 94200, 94250, 94680-94690, 94770, 95812-95816, 95819, 95822, 95829, 95955, 96360, 96365, 96372, 96374-96376, 99148-99149, 99150

Note: These CCI edits are used for Medicare. Other payers may reimburse on codes listed above.

Medicare Edits

	Fac RVU	Non-Fac RVU	FUD	Status
58760	24.22	24.22	90	A

	MUE		Modifiers		
58760	1	51	50	62*	80

* with documentation

Medicare References: None

Coding Companion for Ob/Gyn

© 2012 OptumInsight, Inc.

58770

58770 Salpingostomy (salpingoneostomy)

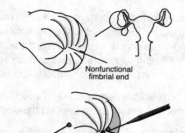

The physician uses microsurgery to remove mucosa, and expose tube opening, restoring patency

Nonfunctional fimbrial end

A new opening can be created in any location

Explanation

Through a small incision just above the pubic hairline, the physician creates a new opening in the fallopian tube where the fimbrial end has been closed by inflammation, infection, or injury. The procedure is generally performed microsurgically in order to do an accurate repair.

Coding Tips

Report 58770 for repair of the fimbrial end of the tube, not reconstruction of the fimbriae, which should be coded with 58760. This is a unilateral procedure. If performed bilaterally, some payers require that the service be reported twice with modifier 50 appended to the second code while others require identification of the service only once with modifier 50 appended. Check with individual payers. Modifier 50 identifies a procedure performed identically on the opposite side of the body (mirror image). For laparoscopic salpingostomy, see 58673. For tubotubal anastomosis, see 58750. For tubouterine implantation, see 58752. Because this procedure is usually not done out of medical necessity, the patient may be responsible for charges. Verify with the insurance carrier for coverage.

ICD-9-CM Procedural

66.02 Salpingostomy

66.72 Salpingo-oophorostomy

Anesthesia

58770 00840

ICD-9-CM Diagnostic

221.0 Benign neoplasm of fallopian tube and uterine ligaments

256.9 Unspecified ovarian dysfunction

614.1 Chronic salpingitis and oophoritis — (Use additional code to identify organism: 041.00-041.09, 041.10-041.19)

614.2 Salpingitis and oophoritis not specified as acute, subacute, or chronic — (Use additional code to identify organism: 041.00-041.09, 041.10-041.19)

614.3 Acute parametritis and pelvic cellulitis — (Use additional code to identify organism: 041.00-041.09, 041.10-041.19)

614.4 Chronic or unspecified parametritis and pelvic cellulitis — (Use additional code to identify organism: 041.00-041.09, 041.10-041.19)

614.5 Acute or unspecified pelvic peritonitis, female — (Use additional code to identify organism: 041.00-041.09, 041.10-041.19)

614.6 Pelvic peritoneal adhesions, female (postoperative) (postinfection) — (Use additional code to identify organism: 041.00-041.09, 041.10-041.19) (Use additional code to identify any associated infertility: 628.2)

614.8 Other specified inflammatory disease of female pelvic organs and tissues — (Use additional code to identify organism: 041.00-041.09, 041.10-041.19)

617.2 Endometriosis of fallopian tube

620.9 Unspecified noninflammatory disorder of ovary, fallopian tube, and broad ligament

625.9 Unspecified symptom associated with female genital organs

628.2 Female infertility of tubal origin — (Use additional code for any associated peritubal adhesions: 614.6)

908.2 Late effect of internal injury to other internal organs

909.3 Late effect of complications of surgical and medical care

V64.41 Laparoscopic surgical procedure converted to open procedure

Terms To Know

cellulitis. Sudden, severe, suppurative inflammation and edema in subcutaneous tissue or muscle, most often caused by bacterial infection secondary to a cutaneous lesion.

endometriosis. Aberrant uterine mucosal tissue appearing in areas of the pelvic cavity outside of its normal location, lining the uterus and inflaming surrounding tissues, and can result in infertility and spontaneous abortion.

oophoritis. Inflammation or infection of one or both ovaries that can cause chronic pelvic pain, ectopic pregnancy, or sterilization.

salpingitis. Inflammation of the fallopian tubes, usually caused by a bacterial infection and occurring in conjunction with inflammation of the ovaries (oophoritis).

CCI Version 18.3

0213T, 0216T, 0228T, 0230T, 12001-12007, 12011-12057, 13100-13153, 36000, 36400-36410, 36420-36430, 36440, 36600, 36640, 37202, 43752, 44005, 44180, 44602-44605, 44820-44850, 44950, 44970, 49000-49010, 49255, 49320, 49570, 50715, 51701-51703, 57410, 58350, 58660, 58673, 58805, 58900, 62310-62319, 64400-64435, 64445-64450, 64479, 64483, 64490, 64493, 64505-64530, 69990, 93000-93010, 93040-93042, 93318, 94002, 94200, 94250, 94680-94690, 94770, 95812-95816, 95819, 95822, 95829, 95955, 96360, 96365, 96372, 96374-96376, 99148-99149, 99150

Note: These CCI edits are used for Medicare. Other payers may reimburse on codes listed above.

Medicare Edits

	Fac RVU	Non-Fac RVU	FUD	Status
58770	25.35	25.35	90	A

	MUE		Modifiers		
58770	1	51	50	N/A	80

* with documentation

Medicare References: None

58800-58805

58800 Drainage of ovarian cyst(s), unilateral or bilateral (separate procedure); vaginal approach

58805 abdominal approach

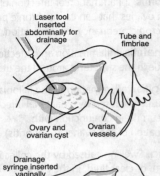

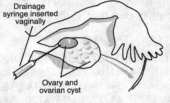

Vaginal approach 58800
Abdominal approach 58805

Explanation

The physician drains a cyst or cysts on one or both ovaries through an incision in the vagina in 58800 and through an incision in the abdominal wall just above the pubic hairline in 58805. A cyst is a sac containing fluid or semisolid material. The cyst is ruptured with a surgical instrument, electrocautery, or a laser, and the fluid is removed.

Coding Tips

These separate procedures by definition are usually a component of a more complex service and are not identified separately. When performed alone or with other unrelated procedures/services they may be reported. If performed alone, list the code; if performed with other procedures/services, list the code and append modifier 59. For drainage of an ovarian abscess vaginally, see 58820; abdominally, see 58822.

ICD-9-CM Procedural

65.09 Other oophorotomy
65.91 Aspiration of ovary
65.93 Manual rupture of ovarian cyst

Anesthesia

58800 00940
58805 00840

ICD-9-CM Diagnostic

220 Benign neoplasm of ovary — (Use additional code to identify any functional activity: 256.0-256.1)

256.4 Polycystic ovaries

620.0 Follicular cyst of ovary

620.1 Corpus luteum cyst or hematoma

620.2 Other and unspecified ovarian cyst

789.31 Abdominal or pelvic swelling, mass, or lump, right upper quadrant

789.32 Abdominal or pelvic swelling, mass, or lump, left upper quadrant

789.33 Abdominal or pelvic swelling, mass, or lump, right lower quadrant

789.34 Abdominal or pelvic swelling, mass, or lump, left lower quadrant

V84.02 Genetic susceptibility to malignant neoplasm of ovary — (Use additional code, if applicable, for any associated family history of the disease: V16-V19. Code first, if applicable, any current malignant neoplasms: 140.0-195.8, 200.0-208.9, 230.0-234.9. Use additional code, if applicable, for any personal history of malignant neoplasm: V10.0-V10.9)

V84.04 Genetic susceptibility to malignant neoplasm of endometrium — (Use additional code, if applicable, for any associated family history of the disease: V16-V19. Code first, if applicable, any current malignant neoplasms: 140.0-195.8, 200.0-208.9, 230.0-234.9. Use additional code, if applicable, for any personal history of malignant neoplasm: V10.0-V10.9)

V84.09 Genetic susceptibility to other malignant neoplasm — (Use additional code, if applicable, for any associated family history of the disease: V16-V19. Code first, if applicable, any current malignant neoplasms: 140.0-195.8, 200.0-208.9, 230.0-234.9. Use additional code, if applicable, for any personal history of malignant neoplasm: V10.0-V10.9)

Terms To Know

benign. Mild or nonmalignant in nature.

corpus luteum cyst or hematoma. Fluid-filled cyst or pocket of blood formed on the ovary at the site where a follicle has discharged its egg.

electrocautery. Division or cutting of tissue using high-frequency electrical current to produce heat, which destroys cells.

follicular cyst. Common type of ovarian cyst related to the menstrual cycle that occurs when the follicle in which the ovum develops does not rupture and expel the egg. Follicular cysts normally disappear within two or three menstrual cycles and are usually benign.

neoplasm. New abnormal growth, tumor.

polycystic. Multiple cysts.

CCI Version 18.3

0213T, 0216T, 0228T, 0230T, 12001-12007, 12011-12057, 13100-13153, 36000, 36400-36410, 36420-36430, 36440, 36600, 36640, 37202, 43752, 49322, 50715, 51701-51703, 57410, 58660, 62310-62319, 64400-64435, 64445-64450, 64479, 64483, 64490, 64493, 64505-64530, 69990, 93000-93010, 93040-93042, 93318, 94002, 94200, 94250, 94680-94690, 94770, 95812-95816, 95819, 95822, 95829, 95955, 96360, 96365, 96372, 96374-96376, 99148-99149, 99150

Also not with 58800: 58900, J0670, J2001

Also not with 58805: 44005, 44180, 44602-44605, 44820-44850, 44950, 44970, 49000-49010, 49255, 49320, 49570, 58700, 58800❖

Note: These CCI edits are used for Medicare. Other payers may reimburse on codes listed above.

Medicare Edits

	Fac RVU	Non-Fac RVU	FUD	Status
58800	8.92	9.52	90	A
58805	12.02	12.02	90	A

	MUE		Modifiers		
58800	1	51	N/A	N/A	N/A
58805	1	51	N/A	62*	80

* with documentation

Medicare References: None

Coding Companion for Ob/Gyn

© 2012 OptumInsight, Inc.

58820-58822

58820 Drainage of ovarian abscess; vaginal approach, open

58822 abdominal approach

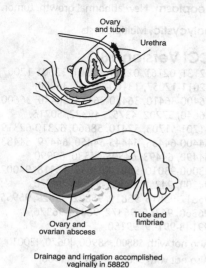

Ovary and tube

Urethra

Ovary and ovarian abscess

Tube and fimbriae

Drainage and irrigation accomplished vaginally in 58820

Drainage and irrigation accomplished abdominally in 58822

Explanation

The physician drains an abscess (infection) on the ovary through an incision in the vagina in 58820 and through a small abdominal incision just above the pubic hairline in 58822. The abscess is drained, cleaned out, and irrigated with antibiotics. Temporary catheters and tubes are often left in place to help drainage.

Coding Tips

These are unilateral procedures. If performed bilaterally, some payers require that the service be reported twice with modifier 50 appended to the second code while others require identification of the service only once with modifier 50 appended. Check with individual payers. Modifier 50 identifies a procedure performed identically on the opposite side of the body (mirror image). For drainage of an ovarian cyst, vaginal approach, see 58800; abdominal approach, see 58805.

ICD-9-CM Procedural

65.09 Other oophorotomy

65.11 Aspiration biopsy of ovary

65.91 Aspiration of ovary

Anesthesia

58820 00840, 00940

58822 00840

ICD-9-CM Diagnostic

614.0 Acute salpingitis and oophoritis — (Use additional code to identify organism: 041.00-041.09, 041.10-041.19)

614.1 Chronic salpingitis and oophoritis — (Use additional code to identify organism: 041.00-041.09, 041.10-041.19)

614.2 Salpingitis and oophoritis not specified as acute, subacute, or chronic — (Use additional code to identify organism: 041.00-041.09, 041.10-041.19)

614.3 Acute parametritis and pelvic cellulitis — (Use additional code to identify organism: 041.00-041.09, 041.10-041.19)

614.4 Chronic or unspecified parametritis and pelvic cellulitis — (Use additional code to identify organism: 041.00-041.09, 041.10-041.19)

780.60 Fever, unspecified

789.01 Abdominal pain, right upper quadrant

789.02 Abdominal pain, left upper quadrant

789.03 Abdominal pain, right lower quadrant

789.04 Abdominal pain, left lower quadrant

789.31 Abdominal or pelvic swelling, mass, or lump, right upper quadrant

789.32 Abdominal or pelvic swelling, mass, or lump, left upper quadrant

789.33 Abdominal or pelvic swelling, mass, or lump, right lower quadrant

789.34 Abdominal or pelvic swelling, mass, or lump, left lower quadrant

998.51 Infected postoperative seroma — (Use additional code to identify organism)

998.59 Other postoperative infection — (Use additional code to identify infection)

Terms To Know

abscess. Circumscribed collection of pus resulting from bacteria, frequently associated with swelling and other signs of inflammation.

acute. Sudden, severe. Documentation and reporting of an acute condition is important to establishing medical necessity.

aspiration. Drawing fluid out by suction.

cellulitis. Sudden, severe, suppurative inflammation and edema in subcutaneous tissue or muscle, most often caused by bacterial infection secondary to a cutaneous lesion.

chronic. Persistent, continuing, or recurring.

incision and drainage. Cutting open body tissue for the removal of tissue fluids or infected discharge from a wound or cavity.

irrigation. To wash out or cleanse a body cavity, wound, or tissue with water or other fluid.

oophoritis. Inflammation or infection of one or both ovaries that can cause chronic pelvic pain, ectopic pregnancy, or sterilization.

parametritis. Inflammation and infection of the tissue in the structures around the uterus.

salpingitis. Inflammation of the fallopian tubes, usually caused by a bacterial infection and occurring in conjunction with inflammation of the ovaries (oophoritis).

seroma. Swelling caused by the collection of serum, or clear fluid, in the tissues.

CCI Version 18.3

0213T, 0216T, 0228T, 0230T, 12001-12007, 12011-12057, 13100-13153, 36000, 36400-36410, 36420-36430, 36440, 36600, 36640, 37202, 43752, 50715, 51701-51703, 57410, 58660, 58900, 62310-62319, 64400-64435, 64445-64450, 64479, 64483, 64490, 64493, 64505-64530, 93000-93010, 93040-93042, 93318, 94002, 94200, 94250, 94680-94690, 94770, 95812-95816, 95819, 95822, 95829, 95955, 96360, 96365, 96372, 96374-96376, 99148-99149, 99150

Also not with 58820: 58800-58805, 58822❖, 69990

Also not with 58822: 44005, 44180, 44602-44605, 44850, 44950, 44970, 49000-49010, 49255, 49320, 49570, 58700, 58800

Note: These CCI edits are used for Medicare. Other payers may reimburse on codes listed above.

Medicare Edits

	Fac RVU	Non-Fac RVU	FUD	Status
58820	9.34	9.34	90	A
58822	22.0	22.0	90	A

	MUE			Modifiers	
58820	2	51	N/A	N/A	80
58822	2	51	N/A	62*	80

* with documentation

Medicare References: None

58823

58823 Drainage of pelvic abscess, transvaginal or transrectal approach, percutaneous (eg, ovarian, pericolic)

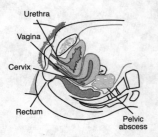

Code 58823 reports percutaneous drainage of a pelvic abscess via the vagina or rectum

Explanation

The physician drains an abscess (infection) in the pelvis percutaneously. The abscess is drained, cleaned out, and irrigated with antibiotics. Temporary catheters and tubes are often left in place to help drainage.

Coding Tips

Moderate sedation performed with 58823 is considered to be an integral part of the procedure and is not reported separately. However, anesthesia services (00100-01999) may be billed separately when performed by a physician (or other qualified provider) other than the physician performing the procedure. When 58823 is performed with another separately identifiable procedure, the highest dollar value code is listed as the primary procedure and subsequent procedures are appended with modifier 51. For drainage of an ovarian abscess, vaginal approach, open, see 58820; abdominal approach, see 58822. For drainage of an ovarian cyst, vaginal approach, see 58800; abdominal approach, see 58805. For radiological supervision and interpretation, see 75989.

ICD-9-CM Procedural

54.91 Percutaneous abdominal drainage

65.91 Aspiration of ovary

Anesthesia

58823 00940

ICD-9-CM Diagnostic

614.0 Acute salpingitis and oophoritis — (Use additional code to identify organism: 041.00-041.09, 041.10-041.19)

614.1 Chronic salpingitis and oophoritis — (Use additional code to identify organism: 041.00-041.09, 041.10-041.19)

614.2 Salpingitis and oophoritis not specified as acute, subacute, or chronic — (Use additional code to identify organism: 041.00-041.09, 041.10-041.19)

614.3 Acute parametritis and pelvic cellulitis — (Use additional code to identify organism: 041.00-041.09, 041.10-041.19)

614.4 Chronic or unspecified parametritis and pelvic cellulitis — (Use additional code to identify organism: 041.00-041.09, 041.10-041.19)

789.01 Abdominal pain, right upper quadrant

789.02 Abdominal pain, left upper quadrant

789.03 Abdominal pain, right lower quadrant

789.04 Abdominal pain, left lower quadrant

789.33 Abdominal or pelvic swelling, mass, or lump, right lower quadrant

789.34 Abdominal or pelvic swelling, mass, or lump, left lower quadrant

998.51 Infected postoperative seroma — (Use additional code to identify organism)

998.59 Other postoperative infection — (Use additional code to identify infection)

Terms To Know

abscess. Circumscribed collection of pus resulting from bacteria, frequently associated with swelling and other signs of inflammation.

chronic. Persistent, continuing, or recurring.

oophoritis. Inflammation or infection of one or both ovaries that can cause chronic pelvic pain, ectopic pregnancy, or sterilization.

parametritis. Inflammation and infection of the tissue in the structures around the uterus.

salpingitis. Inflammation of the fallopian tubes, usually caused by a bacterial infection and occurring in conjunction with inflammation of the ovaries (oophoritis).

seroma. Swelling caused by the collection of serum, or clear fluid, in the tissues.

CCI Version 18.3

0213T, 0216T, 0228T, 0230T, 12001-12007, 12011-12057, 13100-13153, 36000, 36400-36410, 36420-36430, 36440, 36600, 36640, 37202, 43752, 49021❖, 49061❖, 49423-49424, 50715, 51701-51703, 57410, 58660, 62310-62319, 64400-64435, 64445-64450, 64479, 64483, 64490, 64493, 64505-64530, 69990, 76000-76001, 76942, 77001-77002, 93000-93010, 93040-93042, 93318, 94002, 94200, 94250, 94680-94690, 94770, 95812-95816, 95819, 95822, 95829, 95955, 96360, 96365, 96372, 96374-96376, 99143-99149, 99150, J0670, J2001

Note: These CCI edits are used for Medicare. Other payers may reimburse on codes listed above.

Medicare Edits

	Fac RVU	Non-Fac RVU	FUD	Status
58823	5.02	27.24	0	A

	MUE		Modifiers		
58823	2	51	N/A	N/A	N/A

* with documentation

Medicare References: None

Ovary

58825

58825 Transposition, ovary(s)

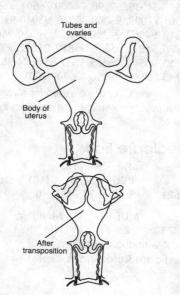

Tubes and ovaries

Body of uterus

After transposition

Explanation

The ovaries are placed behind the uterus and sutured in place prior to radiation therapy of the pelvis. The uterus acts as a shield protecting the ovaries from the radiation. The procedure is done through a small abdominal incision just above the pubic hairline.

Coding Tips

This is a bilateral code and is reported once even if the procedure is performed on both sides. When 58825 is performed with another separately identifiable procedure, the highest dollar value code is listed as the primary procedure and subsequent procedures are appended with modifier 51.

ICD-9-CM Procedural

65.99   Other operations on ovary

Anesthesia

58825   00840

ICD-9-CM Diagnostic

153.3   Malignant neoplasm of sigmoid colon

153.8   Malignant neoplasm of other specified sites of large intestine

154.0   Malignant neoplasm of rectosigmoid junction

154.1   Malignant neoplasm of rectum

154.8   Malignant neoplasm of other sites of rectum, rectosigmoid junction, and anus

158.0   Malignant neoplasm of retroperitoneum

158.8   Malignant neoplasm of specified parts of peritoneum

188.0   Malignant neoplasm of trigone of urinary bladder

188.1   Malignant neoplasm of dome of urinary bladder

188.2   Malignant neoplasm of lateral wall of urinary bladder

188.3   Malignant neoplasm of anterior wall of urinary bladder

188.4   Malignant neoplasm of posterior wall of urinary bladder

188.5   Malignant neoplasm of bladder neck

189.2   Malignant neoplasm of ureter

189.3   Malignant neoplasm of urethra

752.0   Congenital anomalies of ovaries

Terms To Know

malignant neoplasm. Any cancerous tumor or lesion exhibiting uncontrolled tissue growth that can progressively invade other parts of the body with its disease-generating cells.

CCI Version 18.3

0213T, 0216T, 0228T, 0230T, 12001-12007, 12011-12057, 13100-13153, 36000, 36400-36410, 36420-36430, 36440, 36600, 36640, 37202, 43752, 44005, 44180, 44602-44605, 44820-44850, 44950, 44970, 49000-49010, 49255, 49320, 49570, 50715, 51701-51703, 57410, 58660, 58805, 58900, 62310-62319, 64400-64435, 64445-64450, 64479, 64483, 64490, 64493, 64505-64530, 69990, 93000-93010, 93040-93042, 93318, 94002, 94200, 94250, 94680-94690, 94770, 95812-95816, 95819, 95822, 95829, 95955, 96360, 96365, 96372, 96374-96376, 99148-99149, 99150

Note: These CCI edits are used for Medicare. Other payers may reimburse on codes listed above.

Medicare Edits

	Fac RVU	Non-Fac RVU	FUD	Status
58825	21.13	21.13	90	A

	MUE		Modifiers		
58825	1	51	N/A	62*	80

* with documentation

Medicare References: None

58900

58900 Biopsy of ovary, unilateral or bilateral (separate procedure)

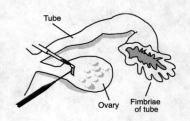

Tissue sample removed for analysis

Explanation

The physician takes a tissue sample from one or both ovaries for diagnosis. This procedure may be done through the vagina or abdominally through a small incision just above the pubic hairline.

Coding Tips

This separate procedure by definition is usually a component of a more complex service and is not identified separately. When performed alone or with other unrelated procedures/services it may be reported. If performed alone, list the code; if performed with other procedures/ services, list the code and append modifier 59. If performing a wedge resection or bisection of the ovary, see 58920. For an oophorectomy, partial or complete, see 58940.

ICD-9-CM Procedural

65.11 Aspiration biopsy of ovary
65.12 Other biopsy of ovary

Anesthesia

58900 00840

ICD-9-CM Diagnostic

183.0 Malignant neoplasm of ovary — (Use additional code to identify any functional activity)
183.8 Malignant neoplasm of other specified sites of uterine adnexa

198.82 Secondary malignant neoplasm of genital organs
220 Benign neoplasm of ovary — (Use additional code to identify any functional activity: 256.0-256.1)
236.2 Neoplasm of uncertain behavior of ovary — (Use additional code to identify any functional activity)
239.5 Neoplasm of unspecified nature of other genitourinary organs
256.0 Hyperestrogenism
617.1 Endometriosis of ovary
620.0 Follicular cyst of ovary
620.1 Corpus luteum cyst or hematoma
620.2 Other and unspecified ovarian cyst
620.8 Other noninflammatory disorder of ovary, fallopian tube, and broad ligament
789.01 Abdominal pain, right upper quadrant
789.02 Abdominal pain, left upper quadrant
789.03 Abdominal pain, right lower quadrant
789.04 Abdominal pain, left lower quadrant
789.30 Abdominal or pelvic swelling, mass or lump, unspecified site
789.31 Abdominal or pelvic swelling, mass, or lump, right upper quadrant
789.32 Abdominal or pelvic swelling, mass, or lump, left upper quadrant
789.33 Abdominal or pelvic swelling, mass, or lump, right lower quadrant
789.34 Abdominal or pelvic swelling, mass, or lump, left lower quadrant
V84.02 Genetic susceptibility to malignant neoplasm of ovary — (Use additional code, if applicable, for any associated family history of the disease: V16-V19. Code first, if applicable, any current malignant neoplasms: 140.0-195.8, 200.0-208.9, 230.0-234.9. Use additional code, if applicable, for any personal history of malignant neoplasm: V10.0-V10.9)
V84.04 Genetic susceptibility to malignant neoplasm of endometrium — (Use additional code, if applicable, for any associated family history of the disease: V16-V19. Code first, if applicable, any current malignant neoplasms: 140.0-195.8, 200.0-208.9, 230.0-234.9. Use additional code, if applicable, for any personal history of malignant neoplasm: V10.0-V10.9)
V84.09 Genetic susceptibility to other malignant neoplasm — (Use additional code, if applicable, for any associated family history of the

disease: V16-V19. Code first, if applicable, any current malignant neoplasms: 140.0-195.8, 200.0-208.9, 230.0-234.9. Use additional code, if applicable, for any personal history of malignant neoplasm: V10.0-V10.9)

Terms To Know

biopsy. Tissue or fluid removed for diagnostic purposes through analysis of the cells in the biopsy material.

tissue. Group of similar cells with a similar function that form definite structures and organs. Tissue types include epithelial tissue, muscle tissue, connective tissue, and nervous tissue.

CCI Version 18.3

0213T, 0216T, 0228T, 0230T, 10021-10022, 12001-12007, 12011-12057, 13100-13153, 36000, 36400-36410, 36420-36430, 36440, 36600, 36640, 37202, 43752, 44005, 44180, 44602-44605, 44820-44850, 44950, 44970, 49000-49010, 49255, 49320, 49570, 50715, 51701-51703, 57410, 58660, 58805, 62310-62319, 64400-64435, 64445-64450, 64479, 64483, 64490, 64493, 64505-64530, 69990, 93000-93010, 93040-93042, 93318, 94002, 94200, 94250, 94680-94690, 94770, 95812-95816, 95819, 95822, 95829, 95955, 96360, 96365, 96372, 96374-96376, 99148-99149, 99150

Note: These CCI edits are used for Medicare. Other payers may reimburse on codes listed above.

Medicare Edits

	Fac RVU	Non-Fac RVU	FUD	Status
58900	13.2	13.2	90	A

	MUE			Modifiers	
58900	1	51	N/A	62*	80

* with documentation

Medicare References: None

58920

58920 Wedge resection or bisection of ovary, unilateral or bilateral

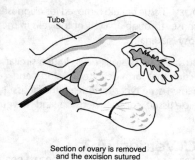

Tube

Section of ovary is removed and the excision sutured

Explanation

Through a small abdominal incision just above the pubic hairline, the physician takes a pie-shaped section or half of one or both of the ovaries to reduce the size and repairs each ovary with sutures.

Coding Tips

The documentation should reflect that a wedge or half of the ovary was removed, not simply a sample biopsy taken. This procedure can be performed unilaterally or bilaterally and is only reported once. For an open oophorectomy, partial or complete, see 58940. For laparoscopic oophorectomy, see 58661.

ICD-9-CM Procedural

65.22 Wedge resection of ovary

65.29 Other local excision or destruction of ovary

Anesthesia

58920 00840

ICD-9-CM Diagnostic

220 Benign neoplasm of ovary — (Use additional code to identify any functional activity: 256.0-256.1)

256.0 Hyperestrogenism

256.1 Other ovarian hyperfunction

256.4 Polycystic ovaries

256.8 Other ovarian dysfunction

620.0 Follicular cyst of ovary

620.1 Corpus luteum cyst or hematoma

620.2 Other and unspecified ovarian cyst

789.31 Abdominal or pelvic swelling, mass, or lump, right upper quadrant

789.32 Abdominal or pelvic swelling, mass, or lump, left upper quadrant

789.33 Abdominal or pelvic swelling, mass, or lump, right lower quadrant

789.34 Abdominal or pelvic swelling, mass, or lump, left lower quadrant

Terms To Know

bilateral. Consisting of or affecting two sides.

corpus luteum cyst or hematoma. Fluid-filled cyst or pocket of blood formed on the ovary at the site where a follicle has discharged its egg.

follicular cyst. Common type of ovarian cyst related to the menstrual cycle that occurs when the follicle in which the ovum develops does not rupture and expel the egg. Follicular cysts normally disappear within two or three menstrual cycles and are usually benign.

neoplasm. New abnormal growth, tumor.

polycystic. Multiple cysts.

resection. Surgical removal of a part or all of an organ or body part.

unilateral. Located on or affecting one side.

wedge excision. Surgical removal of a section of tissue that is thick at one edge and tapers to a thin edge.

CCI Version 18.3

0213T, 0216T, 0228T, 0230T, 12001-12007, 12011-12057, 13100-13153, 36000, 36400-36410, 36420-36430, 36440, 36600, 36640, 37202, 43752, 44005, 44180, 44602-44605, 44820-44850, 44950, 44970, 49000-49010, 49255, 49320, 49322, 49570, 50715, 51701-51703, 57410, 58660-58662, 58805, 58900, 62310-62319, 64400-64435, 64445-64450, 64479, 64483, 64490, 64493, 64505-64530, 69990, 93000-93010, 93040-93042, 93318, 94002, 94200, 94250, 94680-94690, 94770, 95812-95816, 95819, 95822, 95829, 95955, 96360, 96365, 96372, 96374-96376, 99148-99149, 99150

Note: These CCI edits are used for Medicare. Other payers may reimburse on codes listed above.

Medicare Edits

	Fac RVU	Non-Fac RVU	FUD	Status
58920	20.88	20.88	90	A

	MUE		Modifiers		
58920	1	51	N/A	62*	80

* with documentation

Medicare References: None

58925

58925 Ovarian cystectomy, unilateral or bilateral

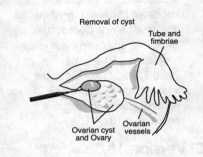

Removal of cyst

Tube and fimbriae

Ovarian cyst and Ovary

Ovarian vessels

Explanation

Through a small abdominal incision just above the pubic hairline, the physician removes a cyst or cysts on one or both of the ovaries.

Coding Tips

This can be performed unilaterally or bilaterally and is only reported once. For an open oophorectomy, partial or complete, see 58940. For laparoscopic oophorectomy, see 58661. For drainage of an ovarian cyst, see 58800–58805.

ICD-9-CM Procedural

65.21 Marsupialization of ovarian cyst

65.29 Other local excision or destruction of ovary

Anesthesia

58925 00840

ICD-9-CM Diagnostic

220 Benign neoplasm of ovary — (Use additional code to identify any functional activity: 256.0-256.1)

236.2 Neoplasm of uncertain behavior of ovary — (Use additional code to identify any functional activity)

256.0 Hyperestrogenism

256.4 Polycystic ovaries

620.0 Follicular cyst of ovary

620.1 Corpus luteum cyst or hematoma

620.2 Other and unspecified ovarian cyst

625.8 Other specified symptom associated with female genital organs

625.9 Unspecified symptom associated with female genital organs

752.11 Embryonic cyst of fallopian tubes and broad ligaments

789.01 Abdominal pain, right upper quadrant

789.02 Abdominal pain, left upper quadrant

789.03 Abdominal pain, right lower quadrant

789.04 Abdominal pain, left lower quadrant

789.31 Abdominal or pelvic swelling, mass, or lump, right upper quadrant

789.32 Abdominal or pelvic swelling, mass, or lump, left upper quadrant

789.33 Abdominal or pelvic swelling, mass, or lump, right lower quadrant

789.34 Abdominal or pelvic swelling, mass, or lump, left lower quadrant

Terms To Know

benign. Mild or nonmalignant in nature.

bilateral. Consisting of or affecting two sides.

corpus luteum cyst or hematoma. Fluid-filled cyst or pocket of blood formed on the ovary at the site where a follicle has discharged its egg.

follicular cyst. Common type of ovarian cyst related to the menstrual cycle that occurs when the follicle in which the ovum develops does not rupture and expel the egg. Follicular cysts normally disappear within two or three menstrual cycles and are usually benign.

neoplasm. New abnormal growth, tumor.

polycystic. Multiple cysts.

unilateral. Located on or affecting one side.

CCI Version 18.3

0213T, 0216T, 0228T, 0230T, 12001-12007, 12011-12057, 13100-13153, 36000, 36400-36410, 36420-36430, 36440, 36600, 36640, 37202, 43752, 44005, 44180, 44602-44605, 44820-44850, 44950, 44970, 49000-49010, 49255, 49320, 49322, 49570, 50715, 51701-51703, 57410, 58660-58662, 58740, 58805, 58900, 62310-62319, 64400-64435, 64445-64450, 64479, 64483, 64490, 64493, 64505-64530, 69990, 93000-93010, 93040-93042, 93318, 94002, 94200, 94250, 94680-94690, 94770, 95812-95816, 95819, 95822, 95829, 95955, 96360, 96365, 96372, 96374-96376, 99148-99149, 99150

Note: These CCI edits are used for Medicare. Other payers may reimburse on codes listed above.

Medicare Edits

	Fac RVU	Non-Fac RVU	FUD	Status
58925	22.05	22.05	90	A

	MUE		Modifiers		
58925	1	51	N/A	62*	80

* with documentation

Medicare References: None

Ovary

Coding Companion for Ob/Gyn

58940

58940 Oophorectomy, partial or total, unilateral or bilateral;

Ovary

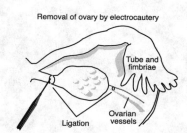

Removal of ovary by electrocautery

Tube and fimbriae

Ovarian vessels

Ligation

Explanation

Through a small abdominal incision just above the top of the pubic hairline, the physician removes part or all of one or both of the ovaries.

Coding Tips

This code should be used when completing an open invasive procedure. If performed through a laparoscope, see 58661. This can be performed unilaterally or bilaterally and is only reported once. When 58940 is performed with another separately identifiable procedure, the highest dollar value code is listed as the primary procedure and subsequent procedures are appended with modifier 51. If the ovaries and fallopian tubes are excised, report 58720. For an oophorectomy completed because of ovarian malignancy, with lymph node biopsies, report 58943.

ICD-9-CM Procedural

65.21 Marsupialization of ovarian cyst
65.29 Other local excision or destruction of ovary
65.39 Other unilateral oophorectomy
65.51 Other removal of both ovaries at same operative episode
65.52 Other removal of remaining ovary

Anesthesia

58940 00840

ICD-9-CM Diagnostic

183.0 Malignant neoplasm of ovary — (Use additional code to identify any functional activity)
198.6 Secondary malignant neoplasm of ovary
220 Benign neoplasm of ovary — (Use additional code to identify any functional activity: 256.0-256.1)
233.30 Carcinoma in situ, unspecified female genital organ
233.31 Carcinoma in situ, vagina
233.32 Carcinoma in situ, vulva
233.39 Carcinoma in situ, other female genital organ
236.2 Neoplasm of uncertain behavior of ovary — (Use additional code to identify any functional activity)
239.5 Neoplasm of unspecified nature of other genitourinary organs
256.0 Hyperestrogenism
617.1 Endometriosis of ovary
620.0 Follicular cyst of ovary
620.1 Corpus luteum cyst or hematoma
620.2 Other and unspecified ovarian cyst
620.5 Torsion of ovary, ovarian pedicle, or fallopian tube
620.8 Other noninflammatory disorder of ovary, fallopian tube, and broad ligament
625.8 Other specified symptom associated with female genital organs
625.9 Unspecified symptom associated with female genital organs
752.11 Embryonic cyst of fallopian tubes and broad ligaments
789.01 Abdominal pain, right upper quadrant
789.02 Abdominal pain, left upper quadrant
789.03 Abdominal pain, right lower quadrant
789.04 Abdominal pain, left lower quadrant
789.31 Abdominal or pelvic swelling, mass, or lump, right upper quadrant
789.32 Abdominal or pelvic swelling, mass, or lump, left upper quadrant
789.33 Abdominal or pelvic swelling, mass, or lump, right lower quadrant
789.34 Abdominal or pelvic swelling, mass, or lump, left lower quadrant
V50.42 Prophylactic ovary removal
V64.41 Laparoscopic surgical procedure converted to open procedure
V84.02 Genetic susceptibility to malignant neoplasm of ovary — (Use additional code, if applicable, for any associated family history of the disease: V16-V19)

Code first, if applicable, any current malignant neoplasms: 140.0-195.8, 200.0-208.9, 230.0-234.9. Use additional code, if applicable, for any personal history of malignant neoplasm: V10.0-V10.9)

V84.09 Genetic susceptibility to other malignant neoplasm — (Use additional code, if applicable, for any associated family history of the disease: V16-V19. Code first, if applicable, any current malignant neoplasms: 140.0-195.8, 200.0-208.9, 230.0-234.9. Use additional code, if applicable, for any personal history of malignant neoplasm: V10.0-V10.9)

CCI Version 18.3

0213T, 0216T, 0228T, 0230T, 12001-12007, 12011-12057, 13100-13153, 36000, 36400-36410, 36420-36430, 36440, 36600, 36640, 37202, 43752, 44005, 44180, 44602-44605, 44820-44850, 44950, 44970, 49000-49010, 49255, 49320, 49322, 49570, 50715, 51701-51703, 57410, 58660-58662, 58740, 58805, 62310-62319, 64400-64435, 64445-64450, 64479, 64483, 64490, 64493, 64505-64530, 69990, 93000-93010, 93040-93042, 93318, 94002, 94200, 94250, 94680-94690, 94770, 95812-95816, 95819, 95822, 95829, 95955, 96360, 96365, 96372, 96374-96376, 99148-99149, 99150

Note: These CCI edits are used for Medicare. Other payers may reimburse on codes listed above.

Medicare Edits

	Fac RVU	Non-Fac RVU	FUD	Status
58940	15.42	15.42	90	A

	MUE		Modifiers	
58940	1	51	N/A 62*	80

* with documentation

Medicare References: 100-3, 230.3

Coding Companion for Ob/Gyn

58943

58943 Oophorectomy, partial or total, unilateral or bilateral; for ovarian, tubal or primary peritoneal malignancy, with para-aortic and pelvic lymph node biopsies, peritoneal washings, peritoneal biopsies, diaphragmatic assessments, with or without salpingectomy(s), with or without omentectomy

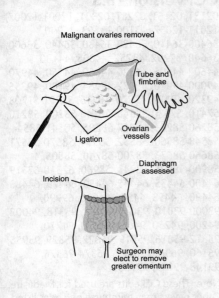

Malignant ovaries removed

Tube and fimbriae

Ligation

Ovarian vessels

Incision

Diaphragm assessed

Surgeon may elect to remove greater omentum

Explanation

Through an abdominal incision extending from the top of the pubic hairline to the rib cage, the physician removes part or all of one or both ovaries depending on the extent of the malignancy. The physician takes a sampling of the lymph nodes surrounding the lower aorta within the pelvis and flushes the peritoneum, which is the lining of the abdominal cavity, with saline. The saline solution is suctioned from the peritoneum for separately reportable examination. Multiple tissue samples are excised. The physician also examines and takes tissue samples of the diaphragm. The physician may elect to remove one or both fallopian tubes and the omentum. The abdominal incision is closed with layered sutures.

Coding Tips

For a radical resection of ovarian malignancy with bilateral salpingo-oophorectomy and omentectomy, see 58950. When 58943 is performed with another separately identifiable procedure, the highest dollar value code is listed as the primary procedure and subsequent procedures are appended with modifier 51.

ICD-9-CM Procedural

40.11	Biopsy of lymphatic structure
54.23	Biopsy of peritoneum
54.4	Excision or destruction of peritoneal tissue
65.29	Other local excision or destruction of ovary
65.39	Other unilateral oophorectomy
65.49	Other unilateral salpingo-oophorectomy
65.51	Other removal of both ovaries at same operative episode
65.52	Other removal of remaining ovary
65.61	Other removal of both ovaries and tubes at same operative episode
65.62	Other removal of remaining ovary and tube

Anesthesia

58943 00840

ICD-9-CM Diagnostic

183.0	Malignant neoplasm of ovary — (Use additional code to identify any functional activity)
183.8	Malignant neoplasm of other specified sites of uterine adnexa
196.6	Secondary and unspecified malignant neoplasm of intrapelvic lymph nodes
197.6	Secondary malignant neoplasm of retroperitoneum and peritoneum
198.6	Secondary malignant neoplasm of ovary
209.71	Secondary neuroendocrine tumor of distant lymph nodes
209.74	Secondary neuroendocrine tumor of peritoneum
236.2	Neoplasm of uncertain behavior of ovary — (Use additional code to identify any functional activity)
V84.02	Genetic susceptibility to malignant neoplasm of ovary — (Use additional code, if applicable, for any associated family history of the disease: V16-V19. Code first, if applicable, any current malignant neoplasms: 140.0-195.8, 200.0-208.9, 230.0-234.9. Use additional code, if applicable, for any personal history of malignant neoplasm: V10.0-V10.9)
V84.04	Genetic susceptibility to malignant neoplasm of endometrium — (Use additional code, if applicable, for any associated family history of the disease: V16-V19. Code first, if applicable, any current malignant neoplasms: 140.0-195.8,

200.0-208.9, 230.0-234.9. Use additional code, if applicable, for any personal history of malignant neoplasm: V10.0-V10.9)

V84.09	Genetic susceptibility to other malignant neoplasm — (Use additional code, if applicable, for any associated family history of the disease: V16-V19. Code first, if applicable, any current malignant neoplasms: 140.0-195.8, 200.0-208.9, 230.0-234.9. Use additional code, if applicable, for any personal history of malignant neoplasm: V10.0-V10.9)

Terms To Know

malignant neoplasm. Any cancerous tumor or lesion exhibiting uncontrolled tissue growth that can progressively invade other parts of the body with its disease-generating cells.

secondary. Second in order of occurrence or importance, or appearing during the course of another disease or condition.

CCI Version 18.3

0213T, 0216T, 0228T, 0230T, 12001-12007, 12011-12057, 13100-13153, 36000, 36400-36410, 36420-36430, 36440, 36600, 36640, 37202, 38562, 43752, 44005, 44180, 44602-44605, 44820-44850, 44950, 44970, 49000-49010, 49203, 49255, 49320, 49322, 49570, 50715, 51701-51703, 57410, 58541-58544, 58548-58550, 58552, 58554, 58570-58571, 58660-58673, 58740, 58805, 58900, 58940, 62310-62319, 64400-64435, 64445-64450, 64479, 64483, 64490, 64493, 64505-64530, 69990, 93000-93010, 93040-93042, 93318, 94002, 94200, 94250, 94680-94690, 94770, 95812-95816, 95819, 95822, 95829, 95955, 96360, 96365, 96372, 96374-96376, 99148-99149, 99150

Note: These CCI edits are used for Medicare. Other payers may reimburse on codes listed above.

Medicare Edits

	Fac RVU	Non-Fac RVU	FUD	Status
58943	33.75	33.75	90	A

	MUE		Modifiers		
58943	1	51	N/A	62*	80

* with documentation

Medicare References: 100-3,230.3

58950

58950 Resection (initial) of ovarian, tubal or primary peritoneal malignancy with bilateral salpingo-oophorectomy and omentectomy;

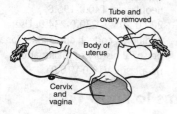

An ovarian, tubal, or primary peritoneal malignancy is removed with bilateral salpingo-oopherectomy and omentectomy

Tube and ovary removed

Body of uterus

Cervix and vagina

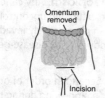

Omentum removed

Incision

This code reports the initial resection

Explanation

The physician performs the initial resection of an ovarian, tubal, or primary peritoneal malignancy. Through a full abdominal incision, the physician removes both tubes, both ovaries, and the omentum, which is a membrane of lymph nodes, blood vessels, and fat that forms a protective layer extending from the stomach to the transverse colon. The abdominal incision is closed with layered sutures.

Coding Tips

The documentation or pathology report should verify a total removal of both tubes, ovaries, and the omentum due to malignancy. This is a bilateral code and is reported once even if the procedure is performed on both sides. If performed with a total abdominal hysterectomy, see 58951. If performed with radical dissection and debulking, see 58952.

ICD-9-CM Procedural

54.4 Excision or destruction of peritoneal tissue
65.61 Other removal of both ovaries and tubes at same operative episode

Anesthesia

58950 00840

ICD-9-CM Diagnostic

158.8 Malignant neoplasm of specified parts of peritoneum
158.9 Malignant neoplasm of peritoneum, unspecified
183.0 Malignant neoplasm of ovary — (Use additional code to identify any functional activity)
183.2 Malignant neoplasm of fallopian tube
183.8 Malignant neoplasm of other specified sites of uterine adnexa
198.6 Secondary malignant neoplasm of ovary
198.82 Secondary malignant neoplasm of genital organs
209.74 Secondary neuroendocrine tumor of peritoneum
235.4 Neoplasm of uncertain behavior of retroperitoneum and peritoneum
236.2 Neoplasm of uncertain behavior of ovary — (Use additional code to identify any functional activity)
236.3 Neoplasm of uncertain behavior of other and unspecified female genital organs
V84.02 Genetic susceptibility to malignant neoplasm of ovary — (Use additional code, if applicable, for any associated family history of the disease: V16-V19. Code first, if applicable, any current malignant neoplasms: 140.0-195.8, 200.0-208.9, 230.0-234.9. Use additional code, if applicable, for any personal history of malignant neoplasm: V10.0-V10.9)
V84.04 Genetic susceptibility to malignant neoplasm of endometrium — (Use additional code, if applicable, for any associated family history of the disease: V16-V19. Code first, if applicable, any current malignant neoplasms: 140.0-195.8, 200.0-208.9, 230.0-234.9. Use additional code, if applicable, for any personal history of malignant neoplasm: V10.0-V10.9)
V84.09 Genetic susceptibility to other malignant neoplasm — (Use additional code, if applicable, for any associated family history of the disease: V16-V19. Code first, if applicable, any current malignant neoplasms: 140.0-195.8, 200.0-208.9, 230.0-234.9. Use additional code, if applicable, for any personal history of malignant neoplasm: V10.0-V10.9)

Terms To Know

malignant. Any condition tending to progress toward death, specifically an invasive tumor with a loss of cellular differentiation that has the ability to spread or metastasize to other areas in the body.

secondary. Second in order of occurrence or importance, or appearing during the course of another disease or condition.

CCI Version 18.3

0213T, 0216T, 0228T, 0230T, 12001-12007, 12011-12057, 13100-13153, 36000, 36400-36410, 36420-36430, 36440, 36600, 36640, 37202, 43752, 44005, 44180, 44602-44605, 44820-44850, 44950, 44970, 49000-49010, 49082-49084, 49180, 49255, 49320, 49322, 49570, 50715, 51701-51703, 57410, 57530-57545, 58140-58200, 58210, 58260-58263, 58267-58285, 58541-58544, 58548-58550, 58552, 58554, 58570-58571, 58660-58673, 58700-58740, 58805, 58900-58925, 58943, 58960, 62310-62319, 64400-64435, 64445-64450, 64479, 64483, 64490, 64493, 64505-64530, 69990, 93000-93010, 93040-93042, 93318, 94002, 94200, 94250, 94680-94690, 94770, 95812-95816, 95819, 95822, 95829, 95955, 96360, 96365, 96372, 96374-96376, 99148-99149, 99150

Note: These CCI edits are used for Medicare. Other payers may reimburse on codes listed above.

Medicare Edits

	Fac RVU	Non-Fac RVU	FUD	Status
58950	32.28	32.28	90	A

	MUE		Modifiers	
58950	1	51	N/A 62*	80

* with documentation

Medicare References: None

58951

58951 Resection (initial) of ovarian, tubal or primary peritoneal malignancy with bilateral salpingo-oophorectomy and omentectomy; with total abdominal hysterectomy, pelvic and limited para-aortic lymphadenectomy

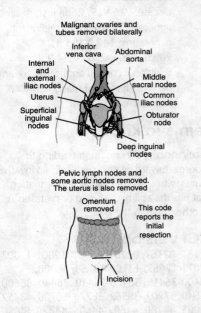

Malignant ovaries and tubes removed bilaterally

Inferior vena cava
Abdominal aorta
Internal and external iliac nodes
Middle sacral nodes
Uterus
Common iliac nodes
Superficial inguinal nodes
Obturator node
Deep inguinal nodes

Pelvic lymph nodes and some aortic nodes removed. The uterus is also removed

Omentum removed
This code reports the initial resection
Incision

Explanation

Through a full abdominal incision extending from just above the pubic hairline to the rib cage, the physician treats an ovarian, tubal, or peritoneal malignancy by taking out both tubes, both ovaries, and the omentum, which is a membrane of lymph nodes, blood vessels, and fat that forms a protective layer extending from the stomach to the transverse colon. The physician also removes the uterus, the pelvic lymph nodes, and a portion of the lymph nodes surrounding the lower aorta. The abdominal incision is closed with layered sutures. This code is to be used only for the initial surgical resection of the malignancy.

Coding Tips

The documentation or pathology report should verify a total removal of both tubes, ovaries, and the omentum with a total hysterectomy due to malignancy. The pelvic or limited para-aortic lymphadenectomies are not identified separately. If this procedure is performed with radical dissection and debulking, report 58952. If completing the hysterectomy for reasons other than malignancy, see 58150–58285 for the most appropriate choice.

ICD-9-CM Procedural

40.3   Regional lymph node excision

54.4   Excision or destruction of peritoneal tissue

65.61   Other removal of both ovaries and tubes at same operative episode

68.49   Other and unspecified total abdominal hysterectomy

Anesthesia

58951   00846

ICD-9-CM Diagnostic

158.8   Malignant neoplasm of specified parts of peritoneum

158.9   Malignant neoplasm of peritoneum, unspecified

183.0   Malignant neoplasm of ovary — (Use additional code to identify any functional activity)

183.2   Malignant neoplasm of fallopian tube

183.8   Malignant neoplasm of other specified sites of uterine adnexa

196.2   Secondary and unspecified malignant neoplasm of intra-abdominal lymph nodes

196.6   Secondary and unspecified malignant neoplasm of intrapelvic lymph nodes

198.6   Secondary malignant neoplasm of ovary

198.82 Secondary malignant neoplasm of genital organs

209.71 Secondary neuroendocrine tumor of distant lymph nodes

209.74 Secondary neuroendocrine tumor of peritoneum

235.4   Neoplasm of uncertain behavior of retroperitoneum and peritoneum

236.2   Neoplasm of uncertain behavior of ovary — (Use additional code to identify any functional activity)

236.3   Neoplasm of uncertain behavior of other and unspecified female genital organs

V84.02 Genetic susceptibility to malignant neoplasm of ovary — (Use additional code, if applicable, for any associated family history of the disease: V16-V19. Code first, if applicable, any current malignant neoplasms: 140.0-195.8, 200.0-208.9, 230.0-234.9. Use additional code, if applicable, for any personal history of malignant neoplasm: V10.0-V10.9)

V84.04 Genetic susceptibility to malignant neoplasm of endometrium — (Use additional code, if applicable, for any associated family history of the disease: V16-V19. Code first, if applicable, any current malignant neoplasms: 140.0-195.8, 200.0-208.9, 230.0-234.9. Use additional code, if applicable, for any personal history of malignant neoplasm: V10.0-V10.9)

V84.09 Genetic susceptibility to other malignant neoplasm — (Use additional code, if applicable, for any associated family history of the disease: V16-V19. Code first, if applicable, any current malignant neoplasms: 140.0-195.8, 200.0-208.9, 230.0-234.9. Use additional code, if applicable, for any personal history of malignant neoplasm: V10.0-V10.9)

Terms To Know

malignant neoplasm. Any cancerous tumor or lesion exhibiting uncontrolled tissue growth that can progressively invade other parts of the body with its disease-generating cells.

CCI Version 18.3

0213T, 0216T, 0228T, 0230T, 12001-12007, 12011-12057, 13100-13153, 36000, 36400-36410, 36420-36430, 36440, 36600, 36640, 37202, 38562, 38570-38572, 38770, 38780, 43752, 44005, 44180, 44602-44605, 44820-44850, 44950, 44970, 49000-49010, 49082-49084, 49180, 49203, 49255, 49320, 49322, 49570, 50715, 51701-51703, 57410, 57530-57545, 58100, 58120-58200, 58210, 58541-58544, 58548-58550, 58552, 58554, 58558, 58570-58573, 58660-58673, 58700-58740, 58805, 58900-58925, 58943, 58950, 58960, 62310-62319, 64400-64435, 64445-64450, 64479, 64483, 64490, 64493, 64505-64530, 69990, 93000-93010, 93040-93042, 93318, 94002, 94200, 94250, 94680-94690, 94770, 95812-95816, 95819, 95822, 95829, 95955, 96360, 96365, 96372, 96374-96376, 99148-99149, 99150

Note: These CCI edits are used for Medicare. Other payers may reimburse on codes listed above.

Medicare Edits

	Fac RVU	Non-Fac RVU	FUD	Status
58951	41.45	41.45	90	A

	MUE			Modifiers	
58951	1	51	N/A	62*	80

* with documentation

Medicare References: None

58952

58952 Resection (initial) of ovarian, tubal or primary peritoneal malignancy with bilateral salpingo-oophorectomy and omentectomy; with radical dissection for debulking (ie, radical excision or destruction, intra-abdominal or retroperitoneal tumors)

Ovary

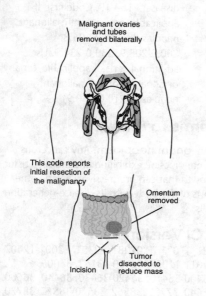

Malignant ovaries and tubes removed bilaterally

This code reports initial resection of the malignancy

Omentum removed

Incision

Tumor dissected to reduce mass

Explanation

Through a full abdominal incision extending from just above the pubic hairline to the rib cage, the physician treats an ovarian, tubal, or peritoneal malignancy by excising both tubes, both ovaries, and the omentum, which is a membrane containing fat, lymph, and blood vessels that acts as a protective layer extending from the stomach to the transverse colon. The physician also reduces the size of a tumor that has grown large enough to cause discomfort or problems. Due to the size and location, it may not be possible to remove the tumor. The abdominal incision is closed with layered sutures. This code is to be used only for the initial surgical resection of the malignancy.

Coding Tips

The documentation or pathology report should verify a total removal of both tubes, ovaries, and the omentum with radical excision of an intra-abdominal or retroperitoneal tumor due to malignancy. This procedure involves an extensive amount of work debulking the surrounding tissues and there is a large amount of clean up involved, which is not identified separately. If performed with total abdominal hysterectomy and lymphadenectomies, report 58951.

ICD-9-CM Procedural

54.4 Excision or destruction of peritoneal tissue

65.61 Other removal of both ovaries and tubes at same operative episode

Anesthesia

58952 00846

ICD-9-CM Diagnostic

158.8 Malignant neoplasm of specified parts of peritoneum

158.9 Malignant neoplasm of peritoneum, unspecified

183.0 Malignant neoplasm of ovary — (Use additional code to identify any functional activity)

183.2 Malignant neoplasm of fallopian tube

183.8 Malignant neoplasm of other specified sites of uterine adnexa

197.6 Secondary malignant neoplasm of retroperitoneum and peritoneum

198.6 Secondary malignant neoplasm of ovary

198.82 Secondary malignant neoplasm of genital organs

198.89 Secondary malignant neoplasm of other specified sites

199.0 Disseminated malignant neoplasm

199.1 Other malignant neoplasm of unspecified site

209.74 Secondary neuroendocrine tumor of peritoneum

235.4 Neoplasm of uncertain behavior of retroperitoneum and peritoneum

236.2 Neoplasm of uncertain behavior of ovary — (Use additional code to identify any functional activity)

236.3 Neoplasm of uncertain behavior of other and unspecified female genital organs

V84.02 Genetic susceptibility to malignant neoplasm of ovary — (Use additional code, if applicable, for any associated family history of the disease: V16-V19. Code first, if applicable, any current malignant neoplasms: 140.0-195.8, 200.0-208.9, 230.0-234.9. Use additional code, if applicable, for any personal history of malignant neoplasm: V10.0-V10.9)

V84.04 Genetic susceptibility to malignant neoplasm of endometrium — (Use additional code, if applicable, for any associated family history of the disease: V16-V19. Code first, if applicable, any current malignant

neoplasms: 140.0-195.8, 200.0-208.9, 230.0-234.9. Use additional code, if applicable, for any personal history of malignant neoplasm: V10.0-V10.9)

V84.09 Genetic susceptibility to other malignant neoplasm — (Use additional code, if applicable, for any associated family history of the disease: V16-V19. Code first, if applicable, any current malignant neoplasms: 140.0-195.8, 200.0-208.9, 230.0-234.9. Use additional code, if applicable, for any personal history of malignant neoplasm: V10.0-V10.9)

Terms To Know

malignant. Any condition tending to progress toward death, specifically an invasive tumor with a loss of cellular differentiation that has the ability to spread or metastasize to other areas in the body.

CCI Version 18.3

0213T, 0216T, 0228T, 0230T, 12001-12007, 12011-12057, 13100-13153, 36000, 36400-36410, 36420-36430, 36440, 36600, 36640, 37202, 38562, 38770, 38780, 43752, 44005, 44180, 44602-44605, 44820-44850, 44950, 44970, 49000-49010, 49082-49084, 49180, 49203-49204, 49215, 49255, 49320, 49322, 49570, 50715, 51701-51703, 57410, 57530-57545, 58140-58200, 58210, 58260-58263, 58267-58285, 58541-58544, 58548-58550, 58552, 58554, 58570-58573, 58660-58673, 58700-58740, 58805, 58900-58940, 58943, 58950-58951, 58957, 58960, 62310-62319, 64400-64435, 64445-64450, 64479, 64483, 64490, 64493, 64505-64530, 69990, 93000-93010, 93040-93042, 93318, 94002, 94200, 94250, 94680-94690, 94770, 95812-95816, 95819, 95822, 95829, 95955, 96360, 96365, 96372, 96374-96376, 99148-99149, 99150

Note: These CCI edits are used for Medicare. Other payers may reimburse on codes listed above.

Medicare Edits

	Fac RVU	Non-Fac RVU	FUD	Status
58952	46.84	46.84	90	A

	MUE		Modifiers		
58952	1	51	N/A	62*	80

* with documentation

Medicare References: None

58953

58953 Bilateral salpingo-oophorectomy with omentectomy, total abdominal hysterectomy and radical dissection for debulking;

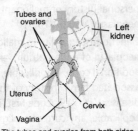

The tubes and ovaries from both sides and the uterus are removed along with the omentum (fatty layer of peritoneum covering the organs and viscera of the abdominal cavity)

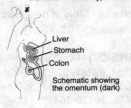

Schematic showing the omentum (dark)

Explanation

Through a full abdominal incision extending from just above the pubic hairline to the rib cage, the physician treats an ovarian malignancy. The physician makes a full abdominal incision and carries dissection down to the abdominal cavity. The physician excises the fallopian tubes, both ovaries, the uterus, and the omentum, which is a membrane containing lymph, blood vessels, and fat in a protective layer that extends from the stomach to the transverse colon. The physician removes or reduces metastatic ovarian cancer implants from the abdominal cavity. The abdominal incision is closed with layered sutures.

Coding Tips

For bilateral salpingo-oophorectomy with omentectomy, total abdominal hysterectomy and radical dissection for debulking, with pelvic lymphadenectomy and limited para-aortic lymphadenectomy, see 58954. For resection of ovarian, tubal, or primary peritoneal malignancy with bilateral salpingo-oophorectomy and omentectomy alone, see 58950; with radical dissection for debulking, without total abdominal hysterectomy, see 58952. For resection of ovarian, tubal, or primary peritoneal malignancy with bilateral salpingo-oophorectomy and omentectomy, with total abdominal hysterectomy, pelvic and

limited para-aortic lymphadenectomy, without radical dissection for debulking, see 58951.

ICD-9-CM Procedural

54.4   Excision or destruction of peritoneal tissue

68.69   Other and unspecified radical abdominal hysterectomy

Anesthesia

58953   00846

ICD-9-CM Diagnostic

158.8   Malignant neoplasm of specified parts of peritoneum

158.9   Malignant neoplasm of peritoneum, unspecified

183.0   Malignant neoplasm of ovary — (Use additional code to identify any functional activity)

183.2   Malignant neoplasm of fallopian tube

183.8   Malignant neoplasm of other specified sites of uterine adnexa

197.6   Secondary malignant neoplasm of retroperitoneum and peritoneum

198.6   Secondary malignant neoplasm of ovary

198.82 Secondary malignant neoplasm of genital organs

198.89 Secondary malignant neoplasm of other specified sites

209.74 Secondary neuroendocrine tumor of peritoneum

235.4   Neoplasm of uncertain behavior of retroperitoneum and peritoneum

236.2   Neoplasm of uncertain behavior of ovary — (Use additional code to identify any functional activity)

236.3   Neoplasm of uncertain behavior of other and unspecified female genital organs

V84.02 Genetic susceptibility to malignant neoplasm of ovary — (Use additional code, if applicable, for any associated family history of the disease: V16-V19. Code first, if applicable, any current malignant neoplasms: 140.0-195.8, 200.0-208.9, 230.0-234.9. Use additional code, if applicable, for any personal history of malignant neoplasm: V10.0-V10.9)

V84.04 Genetic susceptibility to malignant neoplasm of endometrium — (Use additional code, if applicable, for any associated family history of the disease: V16-V19. Code first, if applicable, any current malignant neoplasms: 140.0-195.8,

200.0-208.9, 230.0-234.9. Use additional code, if applicable, for any personal history of malignant neoplasm: V10.0-V10.9)

V84.09 Genetic susceptibility to other malignant neoplasm — (Use additional code, if applicable, for any associated family history of the disease: V16-V19. Code first, if applicable, any current malignant neoplasms: 140.0-195.8, 200.0-208.9, 230.0-234.9. Use additional code, if applicable, for any personal history of malignant neoplasm: V10.0-V10.9)

Terms To Know

dissection. Separating by cutting tissue or body structures apart.

salpingo-oophorectomy. Surgical removal of both the fallopian tube and ovary.

secondary. Second in order of occurrence or importance, or appearing during the course of another disease or condition.

CCI Version 18.3

0213T, 0216T, 0228T, 0230T, 12001-12007, 12011-12057, 13100-13153, 36000, 36400-36410, 36420-36430, 36440, 36600, 36640, 37202, 38562, 38770, 38780, 43752, 44005, 44180, 44602-44605, 44820-44850, 44950, 44970, 49000-49010, 49082-49084, 49180, 49203-49215, 49255, 49320, 49322, 49570, 50715, 51701-51703, 57410, 57530-57545, 58100, 58120-58145, 58150-58200, 58210, 58260-58263, 58267-58285, 58541-58544, 58548-58550, 58558, 58570-58573, 58660-58673, 58700-58740, 58805, 58822, 58900-58940, 58943, 58950-58952, 58956-58960, 62310-62319, 64400-64435, 64445-64450, 64479, 64483, 64490, 64493, 64505-64530, 69990, 93000-93010, 93040-93042, 93318, 94002, 94200, 94250, 94680-94690, 94770, 95812-95816, 95819, 95822, 95829, 95955, 96360, 96365, 96372, 96374-96376, 99148-99149, 99150, P9612

Note: These CCI edits are used for Medicare. Other payers may reimburse on codes listed above.

Medicare Edits

	Fac RVU	Non-Fac RVU	FUD	Status
58953	57.93	57.93	90	A

	MUE		Modifiers		
58953	1	51	N/A	62*	80

* with documentation

Medicare References: None

58954

58954 Bilateral salpingo-oophorectomy with omentectomy, total abdominal hysterectomy and radical dissection for debulking; with pelvic lymphadenectomy and limited para-aortic lymphadenectomy

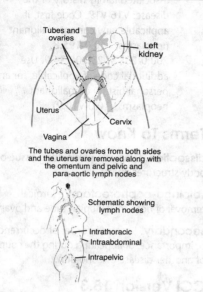

Tubes and ovaries

Left kidney

Uterus

Cervix

Vagina

The tubes and ovaries from both sides and the uterus are removed along with the omentum and pelvic and para-aortic lymph nodes

Schematic showing lymph nodes

Intrathoracic
Intraabdominal
Intrapelvic

Explanation

Through a full abdominal incision extending from just above the pubic hairline to the rib cage, the physician treats an ovarian malignancy. Additionally, the physician excises pelvic lymph nodes and partially removes para-aortic lymph nodes. The physician makes a full abdominal incision and carries dissection down to the abdominal cavity. The physician excises the fallopian tubes, both ovaries, the uterus, and the omentum, which is a membrane containing lymph, blood vessels, and fat in a protective layer that extends from the stomach to the transverse colon. The physician removes or reduces metastatic ovarian cancer implants from the abdominal cavity. The physician additionally removes pelvic lymph nodes and a portion of the lymph nodes that surrounds the lower aorta within the pelvis. The abdominal incision is closed with layered sutures.

Coding Tips

For bilateral salpingo-oophorectomy with omentectomy, total abdominal hysterectomy and radical dissection for debulking, see 58953. For resection of ovarian, tubal, or primary peritoneal malignancy with bilateral salpingo-oophorectomy and omentectomy alone, see 58950; with radical dissection for debulking without total abdominal hysterectomy, see 58952. For resection of

ovarian, tubal, or primary peritoneal malignancy with bilateral salpingo-oophorectomy and omentectomy, with total abdominal hysterectomy, pelvic and limited para-aortic lymphadenectomy, without radical dissection for debulking, see 58951.

ICD-9-CM Procedural

40.3	Regional lymph node excision
54.4	Excision or destruction of peritoneal tissue
65.61	Other removal of both ovaries and tubes at same operative episode
68.49	Other and unspecified total abdominal hysterectomy
68.69	Other and unspecified radical abdominal hysterectomy

Anesthesia

58954 00840, 00846

ICD-9-CM Diagnostic

158.8	Malignant neoplasm of specified parts of peritoneum
158.9	Malignant neoplasm of peritoneum, unspecified
183.0	Malignant neoplasm of ovary — (Use additional code to identify any functional activity)
183.2	Malignant neoplasm of fallopian tube
183.8	Malignant neoplasm of other specified sites of uterine adnexa
196.2	Secondary and unspecified malignant neoplasm of intra-abdominal lymph nodes
196.6	Secondary and unspecified malignant neoplasm of intrapelvic lymph nodes
197.6	Secondary malignant neoplasm of retroperitoneum and peritoneum
198.6	Secondary malignant neoplasm of ovary
198.82	Secondary malignant neoplasm of genital organs
198.89	Secondary malignant neoplasm of other specified sites
209.71	Secondary neuroendocrine tumor of distant lymph nodes
209.74	Secondary neuroendocrine tumor of peritoneum
235.4	Neoplasm of uncertain behavior of retroperitoneum and peritoneum
236.2	Neoplasm of uncertain behavior of ovary — (Use additional code to identify any functional activity)
236.3	Neoplasm of uncertain behavior of other and unspecified female genital organs

V84.02 Genetic susceptibility to malignant neoplasm of ovary — (Use additional code, if applicable, for any associated family history of the disease: V16-V19. Code first, if applicable, any current malignant neoplasms: 140.0-195.8, 200.0-208.9, 230.0-234.9. Use additional code, if applicable, for any personal history of malignant neoplasm: V10.0-V10.9)

V84.04 Genetic susceptibility to malignant neoplasm of endometrium — (Use additional code, if applicable, for any associated family history of the disease: V16-V19. Code first, if applicable, any current malignant neoplasms: 140.0-195.8, 200.0-208.9, 230.0-234.9. Use additional code, if applicable, for any personal history of malignant neoplasm: V10.0-V10.9)

CCI Version 18.3

0213T, 0216T, 0228T, 0230T, 12001-12007, 12011-12057, 13100-13153, 36000, 36400-36410, 36420-36430, 36440, 36600, 36640, 37202, 38562, 38570-38572, 38770, 38780, 43752, 44005, 44180, 44602-44605, 44820-44850, 44950, 44970, 49000-49010, 49082-49084, 49180, 49203-49215, 49255, 49320, 49322, 49570, 50715, 51701-51703, 57410, 57530-57545, 58100, 58120-58145, 58150-58200, 58210, 58260-58263, 58267-58285, 58541-58544, 58548-58550, 58558, 58570-58573, 58660-58673, 58700-58740, 58805, 58822, 58900-58940, 58943, 58950-58953, 58956-58960, 62310-62319, 64400-64435, 64445-64450, 64479, 64483, 64490, 64493, 64505-64530, 69990, 93000-93010, 93040-93042, 93318, 94002, 94200, 94250, 94680-94690, 94770, 95812-95816, 95819, 95822, 95829, 95955, 96360, 96365, 96372, 96374-96376, 99148-99149, 99150, P9612

Note: These CCI edits are used for Medicare. Other payers may reimburse on codes listed above.

Medicare Edits

	Fac RVU	Non-Fac RVU	FUD	Status
58954	62.78	62.78	90	A

	MUE		Modifiers		
58954	1	51	N/A	62*	80

* with documentation

Medicare References: None

Coding Companion for Ob/Gyn

58956

58956 Bilateral salpingo-oophorectomy with total omentectomy, total abdominal hysterectomy for malignancy

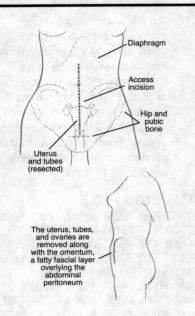

Diaphragm

Access incision

Hip and pubic bone

Uterus and tubes (resected)

The uterus, tubes, and ovaries are removed along with the omentum, a fatty fascial layer overlying the abdominal peritoneum

Explanation

The physician performs a bilateral salpingo-oophorectomy with total omentectomy and total abdominal hysterectomy to treat a malignancy. A full abdominal incision is made extending from just above the pubic hairline to the rib cage. Dissection is carried down to the abdominal cavity. The physician excises the fallopian tubes, ovaries, the uterus, and the omentum. The supporting pedicles containing the tubes, ligaments, and arteries are clamped and cut free. The uterus and cervix are removed along with a narrow rim or cuff of the vaginal lining. The vaginal defect is often left open for drainage. Attention is directed to the omentum, a membrane of lymph, blood vessels, and fat that forms a protective layer that extends from the stomach to the transverse colon. The omentum is mobilized from the stomach and colon, divided from its blood supply, and removed. The physician inspects the abdominal cavity and removes any metastatic lesions. The abdominal incision is closed with layered sutures.

Coding Tips

This is a bilateral procedure. If salpingo-oophorectomy is performed only on one side, append modifier 52. This procedure should not be reported with the following codes: 49255, 58150, 58180, 58262, 58263, 58550, 58661, 58700, 58720, 58900, 58925, 58940, 58957, or 58958.

ICD-9-CM Procedural

54.4	Excision or destruction of peritoneal tissue
65.61	Other removal of both ovaries and tubes at same operative episode
68.49	Other and unspecified total abdominal hysterectomy

Anesthesia

58956 00846

ICD-9-CM Diagnostic

158.8	Malignant neoplasm of specified parts of peritoneum
179	Malignant neoplasm of uterus, part unspecified
180.0	Malignant neoplasm of endocervix
180.1	Malignant neoplasm of exocervix
180.8	Malignant neoplasm of other specified sites of cervix
180.9	Malignant neoplasm of cervix uteri, unspecified site
182.0	Malignant neoplasm of corpus uteri, except isthmus
182.1	Malignant neoplasm of isthmus
182.8	Malignant neoplasm of other specified sites of body of uterus
183.0	Malignant neoplasm of ovary — (Use additional code to identify any functional activity)
183.2	Malignant neoplasm of fallopian tube
183.3	Malignant neoplasm of broad ligament of uterus
183.4	Malignant neoplasm of parametrium of uterus
183.5	Malignant neoplasm of round ligament of uterus
183.8	Malignant neoplasm of other specified sites of uterine adnexa
183.9	Malignant neoplasm of uterine adnexa, unspecified site
184.0	Malignant neoplasm of vagina
184.8	Malignant neoplasm of other specified sites of female genital organs
184.9	Malignant neoplasm of female genital organ, site unspecified
197.5	Secondary malignant neoplasm of large intestine and rectum
197.6	Secondary malignant neoplasm of retroperitoneum and peritoneum
198.1	Secondary malignant neoplasm of other urinary organs
198.6	Secondary malignant neoplasm of ovary
198.82	Secondary malignant neoplasm of genital organs
199.0	Disseminated malignant neoplasm
199.1	Other malignant neoplasm of unspecified site
209.74	Secondary neuroendocrine tumor of peritoneum
V84.02	Genetic susceptibility to malignant neoplasm of ovary — (Use additional code, if applicable, for any associated family history of the disease: V16-V19. Code first, if applicable, any current malignant neoplasms: 140.0-195.8, 200.0-208.9, 230.0-234.9. Use additional code, if applicable, for any personal history of malignant neoplasm: V10.0-V10.9)

CCI Version 18.3

0213T, 0216T, 0228T, 0230T, 12001-12007, 12011-12057, 13100-13153, 36000, 36400-36410, 36420-36430, 36440, 36600, 36640, 37202, 38562, 38770, 38780, 43752, 44005, 44180, 44602-44605, 44820-44850, 44950, 44970, 49000-49010, 49082-49084, 49180, 49203, 49255, 49320, 49322, 49570, 50715, 51701-51703, 57410, 57530-57545, 58100, 58120-58200, 58210, 58260-58263, 58267-58294, 58541-58550, 58552-58554, 58570-58572, 58660-58673, 58700-58740, 58805, 58822, 58900-58940, 58943, 58950-58952, 58960, 62310-62319, 64400-64435, 64445-64450, 64479, 64483, 64490, 64493, 64505-64530, 69990, 93000-93010, 93040-93042, 93318, 94002, 94200, 94250, 94680-94690, 94770, 95812-95816, 95819, 95822, 95829, 95955, 96360, 96365, 96372, 96374-96376, 99148-99149, 99150, P9612

Note: These CCI edits are used for Medicare. Other payers may reimburse on codes listed above.

Medicare Edits

	Fac RVU	Non-Fac RVU	FUD	Status
58956	39.58	39.58	90	A

	MUE		Modifiers		
58956	1	51	N/A	62*	80

* with documentation

Medicare References: None

58957-58958

58957 Resection (tumor debulking) of recurrent ovarian, tubal, primary peritoneal, uterine malignancy (intra-abdominal, retroperitoneal tumors), with omentectomy, if performed;

58958 with pelvic lymphadenectomy and limited para-aortic lymphadenectomy

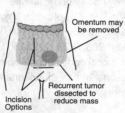

Recurrent malignancy is debulked

Omentum may be removed

Recurrent tumor dissected to reduce mass

Incision Options

In 58958, pelvic and limited para-aortic lymphadenectomy is performed

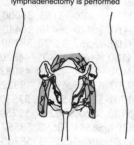

Explanation

These codes report tumor debulking in recurrent ovarian, uterine, tubal, or peritoneal malignancies. Through a full abdominal incision extending from just above the pubic hairline to the rib cage, the physician explores the abdomen, pelvis, and viscera. In addition to debulking recurrent malignancy, the physician releases intestinal adhesions or excises all or portions of the omentum, ovaries, or fallopian tubes. The physician may remove all visible tumors or only reduce their size, depending on the nature of the malignancy and the structures involved. The abdominal incision is closed with layered sutures. Report 58958 when pelvic and para-aortic lymph nodes are also removed.

Coding Tips

If significant additional time and effort is documented, append modifier 22 and submit a cover letter and operative report. This is a bilateral procedure and as such is reported once even if the procedure is performed on both sides. 58958 includes any lymphadenectomy or omentectomy the physician may perform. For initial malignancy of the ovaries, uterus, tubes, or primary peritoneal structures, see 58900–58952. For staging of tubal, ovarian, or primary peritoneal malignancy, see 58960.

ICD-9-CM Procedural

40.3 Regional lymph node excision

54.4 Excision or destruction of peritoneal tissue

Anesthesia

00840

ICD-9-CM Diagnostic

158.8 Malignant neoplasm of specified parts of peritoneum

158.9 Malignant neoplasm of peritoneum, unspecified

183.0 Malignant neoplasm of ovary — (Use additional code to identify any functional activity)

183.2 Malignant neoplasm of fallopian tube

183.8 Malignant neoplasm of other specified sites of uterine adnexa

196.2 Secondary and unspecified malignant neoplasm of intra-abdominal lymph nodes

196.6 Secondary and unspecified malignant neoplasm of intrapelvic lymph nodes

198.6 Secondary malignant neoplasm of ovary

198.82 Secondary malignant neoplasm of genital organs

209.71 Secondary neuroendocrine tumor of distant lymph nodes

209.74 Secondary neuroendocrine tumor of peritoneum

209.79 Secondary neuroendocrine tumor of other sites

235.4 Neoplasm of uncertain behavior of retroperitoneum and peritoneum

236.2 Neoplasm of uncertain behavior of ovary — (Use additional code to identify any functional activity)

236.3 Neoplasm of uncertain behavior of other and unspecified female genital organs

V84.02 Genetic susceptibility to malignant neoplasm of ovary — (Use additional code, if applicable, for any associated family history of the disease: V16-V19. Code first, if applicable, any current malignant neoplasms: 140.0-195.8, 200.0-208.9, 230.0-234.9. Use additional code, if applicable, for any personal history of malignant neoplasm: V10.0-V10.9)

V84.04 Genetic susceptibility to malignant neoplasm of endometrium — (Use additional code, if applicable, for any associated family history of the disease: V16-V19. Code first, if applicable, any current malignant neoplasms: 140.0-195.8, 200.0-208.9, 230.0-234.9. Use additional code, if applicable, for any personal history of malignant neoplasm: V10.0-V10.9)

V84.09 Genetic susceptibility to other malignant neoplasm — (Use additional code, if applicable, for any associated family history of the disease: V16-V19. Code first, if applicable, any current malignant neoplasms: 140.0-195.8, 200.0-208.9, 230.0-234.9. Use additional code, if applicable, for any personal history of malignant neoplasm: V10.0-V10.9)

CCI Version 18.3

0213T, 0216T, 0228T, 0230T, 12001-12007, 12011-12057, 13100-13153, 36000, 36400-36410, 36420-36430, 36440, 36600, 36640, 37202, 38570-38572, 38770, 38780, 43752, 44005, 44180, 44602-44605, 44820-44850, 44950, 44970, 49000-49010, 49082-49084, 49180, 49203-49204, 49215, 49255, 49320, 49570, 50715, 51701-51703, 57410, 58541-58544, 58548, 58570-58573, 58660-58673, 58700-58740, 58900-58940, 58943, 58960, 62310-62319, 64400-64435, 64445-64450, 64479, 64483, 64490, 64493, 64505-64530, 69990, 93000-93010, 93040-93042, 93318, 94002, 94200, 94250, 94680-94690, 94770, 95812-95816, 95819, 95822, 95829, 95955, 96360, 96365, 96372, 96374-96376, 99148-99149, 99150

Also not with 58957: 58950-58951, 58956

Also not with 58958: 58950-58952, 58956-58957

Note: These CCI edits are used for Medicare. Other payers may reimburse on codes listed above.

Medicare Edits

	Fac RVU	Non-Fac RVU	FUD	Status
58957	45.22	45.22	90	A
58958	49.69	49.69	90	A

	MUE		Modifiers		
58957	1	51	N/A	62*	80
58958	1	51	N/A	62*	80

* with documentation

Medicare References: None

58960

58960 Laparotomy, for staging or restaging of ovarian, tubal, or primary peritoneal malignancy (second look), with or without omentectomy, peritoneal washing, biopsy of abdominal and pelvic peritoneum, diaphragmatic assessment with pelvic and limited para-aortic lymphadenectomy

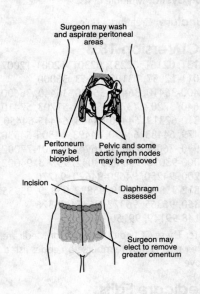

Surgeon may wash and aspirate peritoneal areas

Peritoneum may be biopsied

Pelvic and some aortic lymph nodes may be removed

Incision

Diaphragm assessed

Surgeon may elect to remove greater omentum

Explanation

This procedure is the second operation to check for a recurrence of the ovarian malignancy. Through a full abdominal incision extending from just above the pubic hairline to the rib cage, the physician may elect to remove the omentum, a membrane of lymph, blood vessels, and fat that forms a protective layer that extends from the stomach to the transverse colon. The physician may flush the lining of the abdominal cavity (peritoneum) and remove the liquid to check for cancerous cells. A tissue sample of the abdominal and pelvic peritoneum may be taken. The physician also may examine and take tissue samples of the diaphragm. The pelvic lymph nodes are removed and a portion of the lymph nodes that surrounds the lower aorta within the pelvis is removed. The abdominal incision is closed with layered sutures.

Coding Tips

A prior surgery for ovarian malignancy should be documented. For initial treatment and guidelines, see 58950–58952.

ICD-9-CM Procedural

40.3   Regional lymph node excision

54.11   Exploratory laparotomy

54.12   Reopening of recent laparotomy site

54.23   Biopsy of peritoneum

Anesthesia

58960   00840

ICD-9-CM Diagnostic

183.0   Malignant neoplasm of ovary — (Use additional code to identify any functional activity)

183.8   Malignant neoplasm of other specified sites of uterine adnexa

196.6   Secondary and unspecified malignant neoplasm of intrapelvic lymph nodes

197.6   Secondary malignant neoplasm of retroperitoneum and peritoneum

198.6   Secondary malignant neoplasm of ovary

198.89   Secondary malignant neoplasm of other specified sites

209.71   Secondary neuroendocrine tumor of distant lymph nodes

209.74   Secondary neuroendocrine tumor of peritoneum

209.79   Secondary neuroendocrine tumor of other sites

236.2   Neoplasm of uncertain behavior of ovary — (Use additional code to identify any functional activity)

V10.43   Personal history of malignant neoplasm of ovary

V84.02   Genetic susceptibility to malignant neoplasm of ovary — (Use additional code, if applicable, for any associated family history of the disease: V16-V19. Code first, if applicable, any current malignant neoplasms: 140.0-195.8, 200.0-208.9, 230.0-234.9. Use additional code, if applicable, for any personal history of malignant neoplasm: V10.0-V10.9)

V84.04   Genetic susceptibility to malignant neoplasm of endometrium — (Use additional code, if applicable, for any associated family history of the disease: V16-V19. Code first, if applicable, any current malignant neoplasms: 140.0-195.8, 200.0-208.9, 230.0-234.9. Use additional code, if applicable, for any personal history of malignant neoplasm: V10.0-V10.9)

V84.09   Genetic susceptibility to other malignant neoplasm — (Use additional code, if applicable, for any associated family history of the disease: V16-V19. Code first, if applicable, any current malignant

neoplasms: 140.0-195.8, 200.0-208.9, 230.0-234.9. Use additional code, if applicable, for any personal history of malignant neoplasm: V10.0-V10.9)

Terms To Know

malignant. Any condition tending to progress toward death, specifically an invasive tumor with a loss of cellular differentiation that has the ability to spread or metastasize to other areas in the body.

omentum. Fold of peritoneal tissue suspended between the stomach and neighboring visceral organs of the abdominal cavity.

peritoneum. Strong, continuous membrane that forms the lining of the abdominal and pelvic cavity. The parietal peritoneum, or outer layer, is attached to the abdominopelvic walls and the visceral peritoneum, or inner layer, surrounds the organs inside the abdominal cavity.

CCI Version 18.3

0213T, 0216T, 0228T, 0230T, 12001-12007, 12011-12057, 13100-13153, 36000, 36400-36410, 36420-36430, 36440, 36600, 36640, 37202, 38562, 38571-38572, 38770, 38780, 43752, 44005, 44180, 44602-44605, 44820-44850, 44950, 44970, 49000-49010, 49255, 49320, 49570, 50715, 51701-51703, 57410, 58548, 58660, 58720, 58805, 58900, 62310-62319, 64400-64435, 64445-64450, 64479, 64483, 64490, 64493, 64505-64530, 69990, 93000-93010, 93040-93042, 93318, 94002, 94200, 94250, 94680-94690, 94770, 95812-95816, 95819, 95822, 95829, 95955, 96360, 96365, 96372, 96374-96376, 99148-99149, 99150

Note: These CCI edits are used for Medicare. Other payers may reimburse on codes listed above.

Medicare Edits

	Fac RVU	Non-Fac RVU	FUD	Status
58960	27.68	27.68	90	A

	MUE		Modifiers		
58960	1	51	N/A	62*	80

* with documentation

Medicare References: None

58970

58970 Follicle puncture for oocyte retrieval, any method

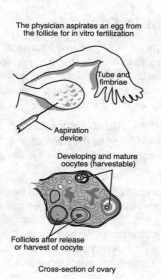

The physician aspirates an egg from the follicle for in vitro fertilization

Tube and fimbriae

Aspiration device

Developing and mature oocytes (harvestable)

Follicles after release or harvest of oocyte

Cross-section of ovary

Explanation

The physician aspirates a mature or nearly mature egg from its follicle for in vitro fertilization. Visualization of the aspiration may be done laparoscopically or by ultrasound. The laparoscopic method uses three puncture sites in the lower abdomen—one for the laparoscope, one for the holding forceps, and one for the aspirating needle. The ultrasound guided technique involves using a transabdominal ultrasound transducer for guidance. The aspirating needle is passed through the bladder wall to the ovary or through the urethra and into the pelvic cavity. Another ultrasound method uses transvaginal ultrasound and transvaginal needle aspiration of the ovary. In all methods, the ovary and preovulatory follicle are visualized and punctured with a needle to withdraw the follicular fluid containing the egg.

Coding Tips

This procedure only reports the retrieval of an oocyte. This code includes any method of retrieval performed by the physician. For culture and fertilization of an oocyte, report 89250. For assisted oocyte fertilization by microtechnique, see 89252. For subsequent intrauterine embryo transfer, see 58974. For gamete, zygote, or embryo intrafallopian transfer, see 58976. When 58970 is performed with another separately identifiable procedure, the highest dollar value code is listed as the primary procedure and subsequent procedures are appended with modifier 51. For ultrasonic

guidance (supervision and interpretation), see 76948.

ICD-9-CM Procedural

65.99   Other operations on ovary

Anesthesia

58970   00840

ICD-9-CM Diagnostic

256.4   Polycystic ovaries

614.5   Acute or unspecified pelvic peritonitis, female — (Use additional code to identify organism: 041.00-041.09, 041.10-041.19)

614.6   Pelvic peritoneal adhesions, female (postoperative) (postinfection) — (Use additional code to identify organism: 041.00-041.09, 041.10-041.19) (Use additional code to identify any associated infertility: 628.2)

617.0   Endometriosis of uterus

617.3   Endometriosis of pelvic peritoneum

628.0   Female infertility associated with anovulation — (Use additional code for any associated Stein-Leventhal syndrome: 256.4)

628.1   Female infertility of pituitary-hypothalamic origin — (Code first underlying cause: 253.0-253.4, 253.8)

628.2   Female infertility of tubal origin — (Use additional code for any associated peritubal adhesions: 614.6)

628.3   Female infertility of uterine origin — (Use additional code for any associated tuberculous endometriosis: 016.7)

628.4   Female infertility of cervical or vaginal origin

628.8   Female infertility of other specified origin

628.9   Female infertility of unspecified origin

V26.81   Encounter for assisted reproductive fertility procedure cycle

V26.82   Encounter for fertility preservation procedure

V26.89   Other specified procreative management

V59.70   Egg (oocyte) (ovum) donor, unspecified

V59.71   Egg (oocyte) (ovum) donor, under age 35, anonymous recipient

V59.72   Egg (oocyte) (ovum) donor, under age 35, designated recipient

V59.73   Egg (oocyte) (ovum) donor, age 35 and over, anonymous recipient

V59.74   Egg (oocyte) (ovum) donor, age 35 and over, designated recipient

Terms To Know

aspirate. To withdraw fluid or air from a body cavity by suction.

cyst. Elevated encapsulated mass containing fluid, semisolid, or solid material with a membranous lining.

polycystic. Multiple cysts.

puncture. Creating a hole.

CCI Version 18.3

0213T, 0216T, 0228T, 0230T, 12001-12007, 12011-12057, 13100-13153, 36000, 36400-36410, 36420-36430, 36440, 36600, 36640, 37202, 43752, 51701-51703, 57410, 62310-62319, 64400-64435, 64445-64450, 64479, 64483, 64490, 64493, 64505-64530, 69990, 76000-76001, 76942, 77001-77002, 93000-93010, 93040-93042, 93318, 94002, 94200, 94250, 94680-94690, 94770, 95812-95816, 95819, 95822, 95829, 95955, 96360, 96365, 96372, 96374-96376, 99148-99149, 99150

Note: These CCI edits are used for Medicare. Other payers may reimburse on codes listed above.

Medicare Edits

	Fac RVU	Non-Fac RVU	FUD	Status
58970	5.65	6.32	0	A

	MUE		Modifiers		
58970	1	51	N/A	N/A	80*

* with documentation

Medicare References: None

Coding Companion for Ob/Gyn

In Vitro

58974

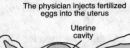

58974 Embryo transfer, intrauterine

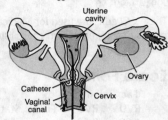

The physician injects fertilized eggs into the uterus

Uterine cavity

Ovary

Catheter

Cervix

Vaginal canal

Explanation

The physician places fertilized eggs in the uterus after the eggs have undergone 48 to 72 hours of laboratory culture. The embryos are aspirated into a small catheter. The catheter is passed through the cervical os and into the uterus. The eggs are injected into the uterus.

Coding Tips

This code includes only intrauterine transfer. For gamete, zygote, or embryo intrafallopian transfer, any method, see 58976. For preparation of embryo for transfer, see 89255. For preparation of cryopreserved embryos for transfer, see 89256. For follicle puncture for oocyte retrieval, any method, see 58970. Because this procedure is usually not done out of medical necessity, the patient may be responsible for charges. Verify with the insurance carrier for coverage.

ICD-9-CM Procedural

71.9   Other operations on female genital organs

Anesthesia

58974   00940

ICD-9-CM Diagnostic

256.39 Other ovarian failure — (Use additional code for states associated with natural menopause: 627.2)

256.4   Polycystic ovaries

256.8   Other ovarian dysfunction

614.6   Pelvic peritoneal adhesions, female (postoperative) (postinfection) — (Use additional code to identify organism: 041.00-041.09, 041.10-041.19) (Use additional code to identify any associated infertility: 628.2)

628.0   Female infertility associated with anovulation — (Use additional code for any associated Stein-Leventhal syndrome: 256.4)

628.1   Female infertility of pituitary-hypothalamic origin — (Code first underlying cause: 253.0-253.4, 253.8)

628.2   Female infertility of tubal origin — (Use additional code for any associated peritubal adhesions: 614.6)

628.3   Female infertility of uterine origin — (Use additional code for any associated tuberculous endometriosis: 016.7)

628.4   Female infertility of cervical or vaginal origin

628.8   Female infertility of other specified origin

628.9   Female infertility of unspecified origin

V26.81 Encounter for assisted reproductive fertility procedure cycle

V26.89 Other specified procreative management

Terms To Know

adhesion. Abnormal fibrous connection between two structures, soft tissue or bony structures, that may occur as the result of surgery, infection, or trauma.

anovulation. Abnormal condition in which an ovum is not released each month. Anovulation is a prime factor in female infertility.

embryo. Developing cells of a new organism that will become a fetus; the period defined from the fourth day after fertilization to the end of the eighth week.

peritoneum. Strong, continuous membrane that forms the lining of the abdominal and pelvic cavity. The parietal peritoneum, or outer layer, is attached to the abdominopelvic walls and the visceral peritoneum, or inner layer, surrounds the organs inside the abdominal cavity.

CCI Version 18.3

0213T, 0216T, 0228T, 0230T, 12001-12007, 12011-12057, 13100-13153, 36000, 36400-36410, 36420-36430, 36440, 36600, 36640, 37202, 43752, 51701-51703, 57410, 62310-62319, 64400-64435, 64445-64450,

64479, 64483, 64490, 64493, 64505-64530, 69990, 93000-93010, 93040-93042, 93318, 94002, 94200, 94250, 94680-94690, 94770, 95812-95816, 95819, 95822, 95829, 95955, 96360, 96365, 96372, 96374-96376, 99148-99149, 99150

Note: These CCI edits are used for Medicare. Other payers may reimburse on codes listed above.

Medicare Edits

	Fac RVU	Non-Fac RVU	FUD	Status
58974	0.0	0.0	0	C

	MUE		Modifiers	
58974	1	51	N/A 62*	80

* with documentation

Medicare References: None

Coding Companion for Ob/Gyn

58976

58976 Gamete, zygote, or embryo intrafallopian transfer, any method

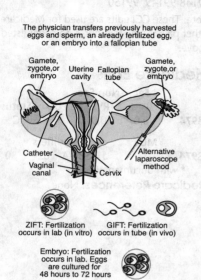

The physician transfers previously harvested eggs and sperm, an already fertilized egg, or an embryo into a fallopian tube

Gamete, zygote, or embryo

Uterine cavity

Fallopian tube

Gamete, zygote, or embryo

Catheter

Vaginal canal

Cervix

Alternative laparoscope method

ZIFT: Fertilization occurs in lab (in vitro)

GIFT: Fertilization occurs in tube (in vivo)

Embryo: Fertilization occurs in lab. Eggs are cultured for 48 hours to 72 hours

Explanation

In gamete intrafallopian transfer (GIFT), the physician mixes previously captured eggs with sperm and draws the mixture into a catheter. The catheter is passed through the cervix and uterus and into the tubes or passed through an abdominal incision and directly into the fimbrial end of the fallopian tube. The physician deposits the eggs and sperm in the tubes, permitting fertilization. In a zygote intrafallopian transfer (ZIFT), a physician draws an already fertilized egg into a catheter. The catheter is passed through the cervix and uterus and into the tube where the egg is deposited. GIFT is a one-step procedure while ZIFT is a two-step process. In ZIFT, the egg is collected and fertilized and transferred to the fallopian tube at a later time. GIFT and ZIFT can be done laparoscopically or hysteroscopically.

Coding Tips

For follicle puncture for oocyte retrieval, any method, see 58970. For culture and fertilization of an oocyte, see 89250. For embryo transfer, intrauterine, see 58974. This code can be reported more than once to reflect additional transfers. When 58976 is performed with another separately identifiable procedure, the highest dollar value code is listed as the primary procedure and subsequent procedures are appended with modifier 51.

ICD-9-CM Procedural

71.9 Other operations on female genital organs

Anesthesia

58976 00840

ICD-9-CM Diagnostic

256.39 Other ovarian failure — (Use additional code for states associated with natural menopause: 627.2)

256.4 Polycystic ovaries

617.1 Endometriosis of ovary

628.0 Female infertility associated with anovulation — (Use additional code for any associated Stein-Leventhal syndrome: 256.4)

628.1 Female infertility of pituitary-hypothalamic origin — (Code first underlying cause: 253.0-253.4, 253.8)

628.2 Female infertility of tubal origin — (Use additional code for any associated peritubal adhesions: 614.6)

628.8 Female infertility of other specified origin

628.9 Female infertility of unspecified origin

V26.81 Encounter for assisted reproductive fertility procedure cycle

V26.89 Other specified procreative management

Terms To Know

anovulation. Abnormal condition in which an ovum is not released each month. Anovulation is a prime factor in female infertility.

cyst. Elevated encapsulated mass containing fluid, semisolid, or solid material with a membranous lining.

embryo. Developing cells of a new organism that will become a fetus; the period defined from the fourth day after fertilization to the end of the eighth week.

endometriosis. Aberrant uterine mucosal tissue appearing in areas of the pelvic cavity outside of its normal location, lining the uterus and inflaming surrounding tissues, and can result in infertility and spontaneous abortion.

gamete. Unfertilized male or female reproductive cell; an ovum or a spermatozoon.

polycystic. Multiple cysts.

zygote. Fertilized ovum or the cell created after the union of a male and female gamete.

CCI Version 18.3

0213T, 0216T, 0228T, 0230T, 12001-12007, 12011-12057, 13100-13153, 36000, 36400-36410, 36420-36430, 36440, 36600, 36640, 37202, 43752, 51701-51703, 57410, 62310-62319, 64400-64435, 64445-64450, 64479, 64483, 64490, 64493, 64505-64530, 69990, 93000-93010, 93040-93042, 93318, 94002, 94200, 94250, 94680-94690, 94770, 95812-95816, 95819, 95822, 95829, 95955, 96360, 96365, 96372, 96374-96376, 99148-99149, 99150

Note: These CCI edits are used for Medicare. Other payers may reimburse on codes listed above.

Medicare Edits

	Fac RVU	Non-Fac RVU	FUD	Status
58976	6.09	7.09	0	A

	MUE		Modifiers	
58976	2	51	N/A	62*	80

* with documentation

Medicare References: None

Coding Companion for Ob/Gyn

In Vitro

59000

59000 Amniocentesis; diagnostic

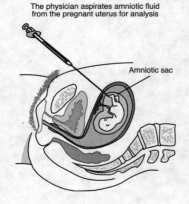

The physician aspirates amniotic fluid from the pregnant uterus for analysis

Amniotic sac

Explanation

The physician aspirates fluid from the amniotic sac for diagnostic purposes. Using separately reportable ultrasonic guidance, the physician inserts an amniocentesis needle through the abdominal wall into the interior of the pregnant uterus and directly into the amniotic sac to collect amniotic fluid for separately reportable analysis.

Coding Tips

For radiological supervision and interpretation, see 76946. For L/S ratio testing, see 83661. For chromosome analysis, see 88267 and 88269. For alpha-fetoprotein by amniotic fluid specimen, see 82106. For amniotic fluid scan (spectrophotometric), see 82143.

ICD-9-CM Procedural

75.1   Diagnostic amniocentesis

Anesthesia

59000   00842

ICD-9-CM Diagnostic

642.03 Benign essential hypertension antepartum
644.03 Threatened premature labor, antepartum
648.03 Maternal diabetes mellitus, antepartum — (Use additional code(s) to identify the condition)
651.03 Twin pregnancy, antepartum
651.13 Triplet pregnancy, antepartum
651.23 Quadruplet pregnancy, antepartum

651.33 Twin pregnancy with fetal loss and retention of one fetus, antepartum
651.43 Triplet pregnancy with fetal loss and retention of one or more, antepartum
651.73 Multiple gestation following (elective) fetal reduction, antepartum condition or complication
655.03 Central nervous system malformation in fetus, antepartum
655.13 Chromosomal abnormality in fetus, affecting management of mother, antepartum
655.23 Hereditary disease in family possibly affecting fetus, affecting management of mother, antepartum condition or complication
655.33 Suspected damage to fetus from viral disease in mother, affecting management of mother, antepartum condition or complication
655.53 Suspected damage to fetus from drugs, affecting management of mother, antepartum
655.73 Decreased fetal movements, affecting management of mother, antepartum condition or complication
656.13 Rhesus isoimmunization affecting management of mother, antepartum condition
656.23 Isoimmunization from other and unspecified blood-group incompatibility, affecting management of mother, antepartum
656.53 Poor fetal growth, affecting management of mother, antepartum condition or complication
657.03 Polyhydramnios, antepartum complication
658.43 Infection of amniotic cavity, antepartum
659.53 Elderly primigravida, antepartum
659.63 Elderly multigravida, with antepartum condition or complication
758.0   Down's syndrome — (Use additional codes for conditions associated with the chromosomal anomalies)
758.31 Cri-du-chat syndrome — (Use additional codes for conditions associated with the chromosomal anomalies)
758.32 Velo-cardio-facial syndrome — (Use additional codes for conditions associated with the chromosomal anomalies)
758.33 Autosomal deletion syndromes, other microdeletions — (Use additional codes for conditions associated with the chromosomal anomalies)

758.39 Autosomal deletion syndromes, other autosomal deletions — (Use additional codes for conditions associated with the chromosomal anomalies)
758.4   Balanced autosomal translocation in normal individual — (Use additional codes for conditions associated with the chromosomal anomalies)
758.7   Klinefelter's syndrome — (Use additional codes for conditions associated with the chromosomal anomalies)
762.7   Fetus or newborn affected by chorioamnionitis — (Use additional code(s) to further specify condition)
792.3   Nonspecific abnormal finding in amniotic fluid
V18.4   Family history of intellectual disabilities
V23.81 Supervision of high-risk pregnancy of elderly primigravida
V23.82 Supervision of high-risk pregnancy of elderly multigravida
V28.0   Screening for chromosomal anomalies by amniocentesis
V28.1   Screening for raised alpha-fetoprotein levels in amniotic fluid
V28.5   Antenatal screening for isoimmunization

Terms To Know

antepartum. Period of pregnancy between conception and the onset of labor.

CCI Version 18.3

0213T, 0216T, 0228T, 0230T, 12001-12007, 12011-12057, 13100-13153, 36000, 36400-36410, 36420-36430, 36440, 36600, 36640, 37202, 43752, 51701-51703, 57410, 62310-62319, 64400-64435, 64445-64450, 64479, 64483, 64490, 64493, 64505-64530, 69990, 76000-76001, 76942, 77001-77002, 93000-93010, 93040-93042, 93318, 94002, 94200, 94250, 94680-94690, 94770, 95812-95816, 95819, 95822, 95829, 95955, 96360, 96365, 96372, 96374-96376, 99148-99149, 99150

Note: These CCI edits are used for Medicare. Other payers may reimburse on codes listed above.

Medicare Edits

	Fac RVU	Non-Fac RVU	FUD	Status
59000	2.44	3.8	0	A

	MUE		Modifiers		
59000	-	51	N/A	N/A	N/A

* with documentation

Medicare References: None

59001

59001 Amniocentesis; therapeutic amniotic fluid reduction (includes ultrasound guidance)

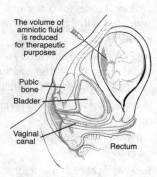

The volume of amniotic fluid is reduced for therapeutic purposes

Pubic bone

Bladder

Vaginal canal

Rectum

Explanation

The physician performs a therapeutic amniotic fluid reduction. Using separately reportable ultrasonic guidance, the physician inserts an 18- or 20-guage amniocentesis needle through the abdominal wall into the interior of the pregnant uterus and directly into the amniotic sac to remove excess levels of amniotic fluid (amnioreduction). Serial amniotic fluid volume reduction may be accomplished on an ongoing basis by repeating the procedure.

Coding Tips

Note that this amniocentesis procedure is for the therapeutic purpose of reducing excess amniotic fluid only. For an amniocentesis for diagnostic purposes, see 59000.

ICD-9-CM Procedural

75.99   Other obstetric operations

Anesthesia

59001   00842

ICD-9-CM Diagnostic

657.00 Polyhydramnios, unspecified as to episode of care

657.01 Polyhydramnios, with delivery

657.03 Polyhydramnios, antepartum complication

Terms To Know

amniocentesis. Surgical puncture through the abdominal wall, with a specialized needle and under ultrasonic guidance, into the interior of the pregnant uterus and directly into the amniotic sac to collect fluid for diagnostic analysis or therapeutic reduction of fluid levels.

polyhydramnios. Excess amniotic fluid surrounding the fetus, typically defined as a total fluid volume of greater than 24.0 cc.

therapeutic. Act meant to alleviate a medical or mental condition.

ultrasound. Imaging using ultra-high sound frequency bounced off body structures.

CCI Version 18.3

0213T, 0216T, 0228T, 0230T, 12001-12007, 12011-12057, 13100-13153, 36000, 36400-36410, 36420-36430, 36440, 36600, 36640, 37202, 43752, 51701-51703, 57410, 59000, 62310-62319, 64400-64435, 64445-64450, 64479, 64483, 64490, 64493, 64505-64530, 69990, 76941-76942, 76945-76946, 93000-93010, 93040-93042, 93318, 94002, 94200, 94250, 94680-94690, 94770, 95812-95816, 95819, 95822, 95829, 95955, 96360, 96365, 96372, 96374-96376, 99148-99149, 99150

Note: These CCI edits are used for Medicare. Other payers may reimburse on codes listed above.

Medicare Edits

	Fac RVU	Non-Fac RVU	FUD	Status
59001	5.46	5.46	0	A

	MUE		Modifiers		
59001	-	51	N/A	N/A	N/A

* with documentation

Medicare References: None

Maternity Care

59012

59012 Cordocentesis (intrauterine), any method

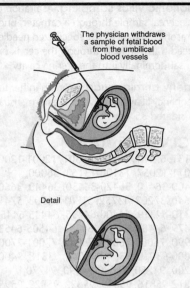

The physician withdraws a sample of fetal blood from the umbilical blood vessels

Detail

Explanation

The physician removes blood from the fetal umbilical cord for diagnostic purposes. Using separately reportable ultrasonic guidance, the physician inserts an amniocentesis needle through the abdominal wall into the cavity of the pregnant uterus and into the umbilical vessels to obtain fetal blood. This may be accomplished with a transplacental or transamniotic approach.

Coding Tips

For radiological supervision and interpretation, see 76941. For diagnostic amniocentesis, see 59000. For chorionic villus sampling, see 59015. For fetal hemoglobin test, see 83030 and 83033. For fetal hemoglobin or RBCs for fetomaternal hemorrhage, see 85460–85461.

ICD-9-CM Procedural

75.35   Other diagnostic procedures on fetus and amnion

Anesthesia

59012   00842

ICD-9-CM Diagnostic

646.13   Edema or excessive weight gain, antepartum — (Use additional code to further specify complication)

646.83   Other specified complication, antepartum — (Use additional code to further specify complication)

655.13   Chromosomal abnormality in fetus, affecting management of mother, antepartum

655.23   Hereditary disease in family possibly affecting fetus, affecting management of mother, antepartum condition or complication

655.33   Suspected damage to fetus from viral disease in mother, affecting management of mother, antepartum condition or complication

655.43   Suspected damage to fetus from other disease in mother, affecting management of mother, antepartum condition or complication

656.03   Fetal-maternal hemorrhage, antepartum condition or complication

658.43   Infection of amniotic cavity, antepartum

659.53   Elderly primigravida, antepartum

678.03   Fetal hematologic conditions, antepartum condition or complication

678.13   Fetal conjoined twins, antepartum condition or complication

679.03   Maternal complications from in utero procedure, antepartum condition or complication

759.83   Fragile X syndrome

762.7   Fetus or newborn affected by chorioamnionitis — (Use additional code(s) to further specify condition)

762.8   Fetus or newborn affected by other specified abnormalities of chorion and amnion — (Use additional code(s) to further specify condition)

772.0   Fetal blood loss affecting newborn — (Use additional code(s) to further specify condition)

V15.21   Personal history of undergoing in utero procedure during pregnancy

V15.29   Personal history of surgery to other organs

V23.81   Supervision of high-risk pregnancy of elderly primigravida

V23.82   Supervision of high-risk pregnancy of elderly multigravida

V23.85   Supervision of high risk pregnancy, pregnancy resulting from assisted reproductive technology

V23.86   Supervision of high risk pregnancy, pregnancy with history of in utero procedure during previous pregnancy

V89.01   Suspected problem with amniotic cavity and membrane not found

V89.02   Suspected placental problem not found

V89.03   Suspected fetal anomaly not found

V89.04   Suspected problem with fetal growth not found

V89.09   Other suspected maternal and fetal condition not found

Terms To Know

elderly primigravida. Woman in her first pregnancy at an age beyond the norm, usually considered 35 years or older.

ultrasound. Imaging using ultra-high sound frequency bounced off body structures.

CCI Version 18.3

0213T, 0216T, 0228T, 0230T, 12001-12007, 12011-12057, 13100-13153, 36000, 36400-36410, 36420-36430, 36440, 36600, 36640, 37202, 43752, 51701-51703, 57410, 62310-62319, 64400-64435, 64445-64450, 64479, 64483, 64490, 64493, 64505-64530, 69990, 76000-76001, 76942, 77001-77002, 93000-93010, 93040-93042, 93318, 94002, 94200, 94250, 94680-94690, 94770, 95812-95816, 95819, 95822, 95829, 95955, 96360, 96365, 96372, 96374-96376, 99148-99149, 99150

Note: These CCI edits are used for Medicare. Other payers may reimburse on codes listed above.

Medicare Edits

	Fac RVU	Non-Fac RVU	FUD	Status
59012	6.05	6.05	0	A

	MUE		Modifiers		
59012	-	51	N/A	N/A	80*

* with documentation

Medicare References: None

© 2012 OptumInsight, Inc.

59015

59015 Chorionic villus sampling, any method

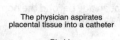

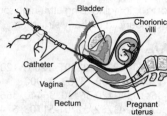

The physician aspirates placental tissue into a catheter

Bladder
Chorionic villi
Catheter
Vagina
Rectum
Pregnant uterus

Explanation

The physician samples tissue from the placenta for diagnostic purposes. This procedure uses ultrasonic guidance and can be done by any one of three methods. In the transcervical method, the physician inserts a catheter through the cervix and into the uterine cavity toward the placental site. A sample of the placenta (chorionic villus) is aspirated to obtain placental cells for analysis for chromosomal abnormalities. The procedure may also be performed transvaginally or transabdominally.

Coding Tips

For radiological supervision and interpretation, see 76945. For diagnostic amniocentesis, see 59000. For cordocentesis (intrauterine), see 59012. For chromosome analysis, see 88267.

ICD-9-CM Procedural

75.35 Other diagnostic procedures on fetus and amnion

Anesthesia

59015 00842

ICD-9-CM Diagnostic

646.03 Papyraceous fetus, antepartum — (Use additional code to further specify complication)

655.13 Chromosomal abnormality in fetus, affecting management of mother, antepartum

655.23 Hereditary disease in family possibly affecting fetus, affecting management of mother, antepartum condition or complication

655.33 Suspected damage to fetus from viral disease in mother, affecting management of mother, antepartum condition or complication

655.43 Suspected damage to fetus from other disease in mother, affecting management of mother, antepartum condition or complication

655.83 Other known or suspected fetal abnormality, not elsewhere classified, affecting management of mother, antepartum condition or complication

655.93 Unspecified fetal abnormality affecting management of mother, antepartum condition or complication

659.53 Elderly primigravida, antepartum

659.63 Elderly multigravida, with antepartum condition or complication

678.03 Fetal hematologic conditions, antepartum condition or complication

678.13 Fetal conjoined twins, antepartum condition or complication

V13.69 Personal history of other (corrected) congenital malformations

V15.21 Personal history of undergoing in utero procedure during pregnancy

V15.29 Personal history of surgery to other organs

V19.5 Family history of congenital anomalies

V23.81 Supervision of high-risk pregnancy of elderly primigravida

V23.85 Supervision of high risk pregnancy, pregnancy resulting from assisted reproductive technology

V23.86 Supervision of high risk pregnancy, pregnancy with history of in utero procedure during previous pregnancy

V23.89 Supervision of other high-risk pregnancy

V28.81 Encounter for fetal anatomic survey

V28.89 Other specified antenatal screening

V89.02 Suspected placental problem not found

V89.03 Suspected fetal anomaly not found

V89.09 Other suspected maternal and fetal condition not found

Terms To Know

analysis. Study of body fluid, tissue, section, or parts.

aspiration. Drawing fluid out by suction.

catheter. Flexible tube inserted into an area of the body for introducing or withdrawing fluid.

chorionic villus sampling. Aspiration of a placental sample through a catheter, under ultrasonic guidance. The specialized needle is placed transvaginally through the cervix or transabdominally into the uterine cavity.

elderly primigravida. Woman in her first pregnancy at an age beyond the norm, usually considered 35 years or older.

CCI Version 18.3

0213T, 0216T, 0228T, 0230T, 12001-12007, 12011-12057, 13100-13153, 36000, 36400-36410, 36420-36430, 36440, 36600, 36640, 37202, 43752, 51701-51703, 57410, 62310-62319, 64400-64435, 64445-64450, 64479, 64483, 64490, 64493, 64505-64530, 69990, 76000-76001, 76942, 77001-77002, 93000-93010, 93040-93042, 93318, 94002, 94200, 94250, 94680-94690, 94770, 95812-95816, 95819, 95822, 95829, 95955, 96360, 96365, 96372, 96374-96376, 99148-99149, 99150

Note: These CCI edits are used for Medicare. Other payers may reimburse on codes listed above.

Medicare Edits

	Fac RVU	Non-Fac RVU	FUD	Status
59015	3.99	4.68	0	A

	MUE		Modifiers		
59015	-	51	N/A	N/A	80*

* with documentation

Medicare References: None

Maternity Care

59020

59020 Fetal contraction stress test

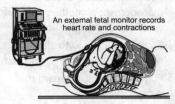

The physician administers an intravenous injection to induce contractions (stress)

An external fetal monitor records heart rate and contractions

Explanation

The physician evaluates fetal response to induced contractions in the mother. The physician applies external fetal monitors to the maternal abdominal wall. Pitocin is given intravenously to the mother to cause uterine contractions. The fetal heart rate and uterine contractions are monitored and recorded for 20 minutes to determine the effect of contractions on the fetus. This procedure is usually performed during the third trimester.

Coding Tips

For fetal non-stress test, see 59025; fetal scalp blood sampling, see 59030.

ICD-9-CM Procedural

75.34   Other fetal monitoring

Anesthesia

59020   N/A

ICD-9-CM Diagnostic

642.03 Benign essential hypertension antepartum

642.13 Hypertension secondary to renal disease, antepartum

642.23 Other pre-existing hypertension, antepartum

642.33 Transient hypertension of pregnancy, antepartum

642.43 Mild or unspecified pre-eclampsia, antepartum

642.53 Severe pre-eclampsia, antepartum

642.73 Pre-eclampsia or eclampsia superimposed on pre-existing hypertension, antepartum

642.93 Unspecified hypertension antepartum

643.13 Hyperemesis gravidarum with metabolic disturbance, antepartum

643.23 Late vomiting of pregnancy, antepartum

645.13 Post term pregnancy, antepartum condition or complication

645.23 Prolonged pregnancy, antepartum condition or complication

646.13 Edema or excessive weight gain, antepartum — (Use additional code to further specify complication)

648.03 Maternal diabetes mellitus, antepartum — (Use additional code(s) to identify the condition)

648.53 Maternal congenital cardiovascular disorders, antepartum — (Use additional code(s) to identify the condition)

648.83 Abnormal maternal glucose tolerance, antepartum — (Use additional code(s) to identify the condition. Use additional code, if applicable, for associated long-term (current) insulin use: V58.67)

649.13 Obesity complicating pregnancy, childbirth, or the puerperium, antepartum condition or complication — (Use additional code to identify the obesity: 278.00-278.01)

649.23 Bariatric surgery status complicating pregnancy, childbirth, or the puerperium, antepartum condition or complication

649.63 Uterine size date discrepancy, antepartum condition or complication

651.03 Twin pregnancy, antepartum

651.13 Triplet pregnancy, antepartum

651.23 Quadruplet pregnancy, antepartum

651.33 Twin pregnancy with fetal loss and retention of one fetus, antepartum

651.43 Triplet pregnancy with fetal loss and retention of one or more, antepartum

651.53 Quadruplet pregnancy with fetal loss and retention of one or more, antepartum

651.73 Multiple gestation following (elective) fetal reduction, antepartum condition or complication

654.23 Previous cesarean delivery, antepartum condition or complication — (Code first any associated obstructed labor, 660.2)

655.23 Hereditary disease in family possibly affecting fetus, affecting management of mother, antepartum condition or complication

655.33 Suspected damage to fetus from viral disease in mother, affecting management of mother, antepartum condition or complication

656.03 Fetal-maternal hemorrhage, antepartum condition or complication

656.33 Fetal distress affecting management of mother, antepartum

656.53 Poor fetal growth, affecting management of mother, antepartum condition or complication

656.63 Excessive fetal growth affecting management of mother, antepartum

657.03 Polyhydramnios, antepartum complication

658.03 Oligohydramnios, antepartum

659.73 Abnormality in fetal heart rate or rhythm, antepartum condition or complication

V23.81 Supervision of high-risk pregnancy of elderly primigravida

V23.82 Supervision of high-risk pregnancy of elderly multigravida

V23.83 Supervision of high-risk pregnancy of young primigravida

V23.84 Supervision of high-risk pregnancy of young multigravida

CCI Version 18.3

0213T, 0216T, 0228T, 0230T, 12001-12007, 12011-12057, 13100-13153, 36000, 36400-36410, 36420-36430, 36440, 36600, 36640, 37202, 43752, 51701-51703, 57410, 62310-62319, 64400-64435, 64445-64450, 64479, 64483, 64490, 64493, 64505-64530, 69990, 93000-93010, 93040-93042, 93318, 94002, 94200, 94250, 94680-94690, 94770, 95812-95816, 95819, 95822, 95829, 95955, 96360, 96365, 96372, 96374-96376, 99148-99149, 99150

Note: These CCI edits are used for Medicare. Other payers may reimburse on codes listed above.

Medicare Edits

	Fac RVU	Non-Fac RVU	FUD	Status
59020	2.1	2.1	0	A

	MUE				Modifiers
59020	1	N/A	N/A	N/A	80*

* with documentation

Medicare References: None

59025

59025 Fetal non-stress test

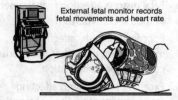

External fetal monitor records
fetal movements and heart rate

Explanation

The physician evaluates fetal heart rate response to its own activity. The patient reports fetal movements as an external monitor records fetal heart rate changes. The procedure is noninvasive and takes 20 to 40 minutes to perform. If the fetus is not active, an acoustic device may be used to stimulate activity.

Coding Tips

Check with third-party payers to see if one fetal non-stress test is included in the total obstetrical package. For patients with conditions complicating pregnancy, 59025 is typically performed weekly for the last six weeks of gestation. The non-stress test is usually the primary means of surveillance for most conditions that place the fetus at high risk for placental insufficiency. Procedure 59025 has both a technical and professional component. To claim only the professional component, append modifier 26. To claim only the technical component, append modifier TC. To claim the complete procedure (i.e., both the professional and technical components), submit without a modifier. For fetal contraction stress test, see 59020.

ICD-9-CM Procedural

75.34   Other fetal monitoring

Anesthesia

59025   N/A

ICD-9-CM Diagnostic

641.03   Placenta previa without hemorrhage, antepartum

642.03   Benign essential hypertension antepartum

642.33   Transient hypertension of pregnancy, antepartum

642.43   Mild or unspecified pre-eclampsia, antepartum

642.53   Severe pre-eclampsia, antepartum

642.73   Pre-eclampsia or eclampsia superimposed on pre-existing hypertension, antepartum

643.13   Hyperemesis gravidarum with metabolic disturbance, antepartum

644.03   Threatened premature labor, antepartum

645.13   Post term pregnancy, antepartum condition or complication

646.13   Edema or excessive weight gain, antepartum — (Use additional code to further specify complication)

648.03   Maternal diabetes mellitus, antepartum — (Use additional code(s) to identify the condition)

648.23   Maternal anemia, antepartum — (Use additional code(s) to identify the condition)

648.63   Other maternal cardiovascular diseases, antepartum — (Use additional code(s) to identify the condition)

648.83   Abnormal maternal glucose tolerance, antepartum — (Use additional code(s) to identify the condition. Use additional code, if applicable, for associated long-term (current) insulin use: V58.67)

649.13   Obesity complicating pregnancy, childbirth, or the puerperium, antepartum condition or complication — (Use additional code to identify the obesity: 278.00-278.01)

649.23   Bariatric surgery status complicating pregnancy, childbirth, or the puerperium, antepartum condition or complication

649.63   Uterine size date discrepancy, antepartum condition or complication

651.03   Twin pregnancy, antepartum

651.33   Twin pregnancy with fetal loss and retention of one fetus, antepartum

651.73   Multiple gestation following (elective) fetal reduction, antepartum condition or complication

655.23   Hereditary disease in family possibly affecting fetus, affecting management of mother, antepartum condition or complication

656.23   Isoimmunization from other and unspecified blood-group incompatibility, affecting management of mother, antepartum

656.33   Fetal distress affecting management of mother, antepartum

656.53   Poor fetal growth, affecting management of mother, antepartum condition or complication

656.63   Excessive fetal growth affecting management of mother, antepartum

657.03   Polyhydramnios, antepartum complication

658.03   Oligohydramnios, antepartum

658.13   Premature rupture of membranes in pregnancy, antepartum

658.23   Delayed delivery after spontaneous or unspecified rupture of membranes, antepartum

658.33   Delayed delivery after artificial rupture of membranes, antepartum

659.03   Failed mechanical induction of labor, antepartum

659.63   Elderly multigravida, with antepartum condition or complication

659.73   Abnormality in fetal heart rate or rhythm, antepartum condition or complication

CCI Version 18.3

0213T, 0216T, 0228T, 0230T, 12001-12007, 12011-12057, 13100-13153, 36000, 36400-36410, 36420-36430, 36440, 36600, 36640, 37202, 43752, 51701-51703, 57410, 62310-62319, 64400-64435, 64445-64450, 64479, 64483, 64490, 64493, 64505-64530, 69990, 93000-93010, 93040-93042, 93318, 94002, 94200, 94250, 94680-94690, 94770, 95812-95816, 95819, 95822, 95829, 95955, 99148-99149, 99150

Note: These CCI edits are used for Medicare. Other payers may reimburse on codes listed above.

Medicare Edits

	Fac RVU	Non-Fac RVU	FUD	Status
59025	1.42	1.42	0	A

	MUE			Modifiers	
59025	1	N/A	N/A	N/A	80*

* with documentation

Medicare References: None

59030

59030 Fetal scalp blood sampling

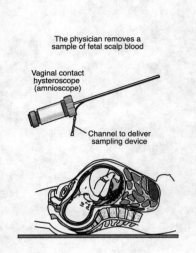

The physician removes a sample of fetal scalp blood

Vaginal contact hysteroscope (amnioscope)

Channel to deliver sampling device

Explanation

The physician samples fetal scalp blood during active labor for diagnostic purposes. This test, which assesses fetal distress during labor, must be done when the cervix is dilated more than 2 cm and the fetal vertex is low in the pelvis. The physician breaks the amniotic sac in patients whose water has not broken spontaneously and inserts an amnioscope through the vagina. An incision is made in the scalp with a narrow blade that penetrates no more than 2 mm. Blood is aspirated into a tube.

Coding Tips

Note that 59030 can be reported in addition to the maternity package.

ICD-9-CM Procedural

75.33 Fetal blood sampling and biopsy

Anesthesia

59030 N/A

ICD-9-CM Diagnostic

642.41 Mild or unspecified pre-eclampsia, with delivery

642.43 Mild or unspecified pre-eclampsia, antepartum

642.51 Severe pre-eclampsia, with delivery

642.53 Severe pre-eclampsia, antepartum

642.61 Eclampsia, with delivery

642.63 Eclampsia, antepartum

642.71 Pre-eclampsia or eclampsia superimposed on pre-existing hypertension, with delivery

642.73 Pre-eclampsia or eclampsia superimposed on pre-existing hypertension, antepartum

648.01 Maternal diabetes mellitus with delivery — (Use additional code(s) to identify the condition)

648.03 Maternal diabetes mellitus, antepartum — (Use additional code(s) to identify the condition)

649.23 Bariatric surgery status complicating pregnancy, childbirth, or the puerperium, antepartum condition or complication

649.33 Coagulation defects complicating pregnancy, childbirth, or the puerperium, antepartum condition or complication — (Use additional code to identify the specific coagulation defect: 286.0-286.9, 287.0-287.9, 289.0-289.9)

649.43 Epilepsy complicating pregnancy, childbirth, or the puerperium, antepartum condition or complication — (Use additional code to identify the specific type of epilepsy: 345.00-345.91)

649.53 Spotting complicating pregnancy, antepartum condition or complication

656.11 Rhesus isoimmunization affecting management of mother, delivered

656.13 Rhesus isoimmunization affecting management of mother, antepartum condition

656.31 Fetal distress affecting management of mother, delivered

656.33 Fetal distress affecting management of mother, antepartum

656.71 Other placental conditions affecting management of mother, delivered

656.73 Other placental conditions affecting management of mother, antepartum

658.31 Delayed delivery after artificial rupture of membranes, delivered

658.33 Delayed delivery after artificial rupture of membranes, antepartum

659.71 Abnormality in fetal heart rate or rhythm, delivered, with or without mention of antepartum condition

659.73 Abnormality in fetal heart rate or rhythm, antepartum condition or complication

661.01 Primary uterine inertia, with delivery

661.03 Primary uterine inertia, antepartum

661.11 Secondary uterine inertia, with delivery

661.13 Secondary uterine inertia, antepartum

661.21 Other and unspecified uterine inertia, with delivery

661.23 Other and unspecified uterine inertia, antepartum

661.41 Hypertonic, incoordinate, or prolonged uterine contractions, with delivery

661.43 Hypertonic, incoordinate, or prolonged uterine contractions, antepartum

662.01 Prolonged first stage of labor, delivered

662.03 Prolonged first stage of labor, antepartum

662.11 Unspecified prolonged labor, delivered

662.13 Unspecified prolonged labor, antepartum

662.21 Prolonged second stage of labor, delivered

662.23 Prolonged second stage of labor, antepartum

CCI Version 18.3

0213T, 0216T, 0228T, 0230T, 12001-12007, 12011-12057, 13100-13153, 36000, 36400-36410, 36420-36430, 36440, 36600, 36640, 37202, 43752, 51701-51702, 57410, 62310-62319, 64400-64435, 64445-64450, 64479, 64483, 64490, 64493, 64505-64530, 69990, 93000-93010, 93040-93042, 93318, 94002, 94200, 94250, 94680-94690, 94770, 95812-95816, 95819, 95822, 95829, 95955, 96360, 96365, 96372, 96374-96376, 99148-99149, 99150

Note: These CCI edits are used for Medicare. Other payers may reimburse on codes listed above.

Medicare Edits

	Fac RVU	Non-Fac RVU	FUD	Status
59030	2.91	2.91	0	A

	MUE		Modifiers		
59030	-	51	N/A	N/A	80*

* with documentation

Medicare References: None

59050-59051

59050 Fetal monitoring during labor by consulting physician (ie, non-attending physician) with written report; supervision and interpretation

59051 interpretation only

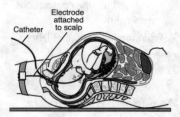

In 59050, a non-attending physician supervises the internal monitoring of the fetus during labor and provides a written analysis and interpretive report. In 59051, only the analysis and interpretive report is provided

Explanation

In 59050, a consultant other than the attending physician attaches an electrode directly to the presenting fetus' scalp via the cervix. The electrocardiographic impulses are transmitted to a cardiotachometer which converts the fetal electrocardiographic pattern into recorded electronic impulses. A catheter is inserted through the dilated cervix into the amniotic sac to measure and record the intervals between contractions. The procedure is supervised during labor until delivery. The recordings are analyzed and accompanied by an interpretive written report. In 59051, the consultant initiates the monitoring, provides the analysis and interpretive report, but does not supervise the patient during labor.

Coding Tips

These codes are to be used by the consulting (non-attending) physician only. They are part of the maternity package when performed by the attending physician.

ICD-9-CM Procedural

75.34   Other fetal monitoring

Anesthesia

N/A

ICD-9-CM Diagnostic

The application of this code is too broad to adequately present ICD-9-CM diagnostic code links here. Refer to your ICD-9-CM book.

Terms To Know

eclampsia. Tetany and toxemia producing seizure activity or coma in a pregnant patient who most often has presented with prior preeclampsia (i.e., hypertension, albuminuria, and edema).

internal os. Opening through the cervix into the uterus.

placenta previa. Implantation of the placenta in the lower segment of the uterus, over or near the internal cervical os. In total previa, the cervical os is completely covered by the placenta; in partial previa, only a portion is covered.

preeclampsia. Complication of pregnancy manifesting in the development of borderline hypertension, protein in the urine, and unresponsive swelling between the 20th week of pregnancy and the end of the first week following birth in mild to moderate cases. Severe preeclampsia presents with hypertension (blood pressure greater than 150/100), associated with marked swelling, proteinuria, abdominal pain, and/or visual changes.

CCI Version 18.3

0213T, 0216T, 36000, 36410, 37202, 57410, 62318-62319, 64415-64417, 64450, 64490, 64493, 69990, 96360, 96365

Also not with 59050: 51701-51702, 59051

Also not with 59051: 51701-51703

Note: These CCI edits are used for Medicare. Other payers may reimburse on codes listed above.

Medicare Edits

	Fac RVU	Non-Fac RVU	FUD	Status
59050	1.53	1.53	N/A	A
59051	1.27	1.27	N/A	A

	MUE		Modifiers		
59050	1	N/A	N/A	N/A	80*
59051	1	N/A	N/A	N/A	80*

* with documentation

Medicare References: None

Coding Companion for Ob/Gyn

Maternity Care

59070

59070 Transabdominal amnioinfusion, including ultrasound guidance

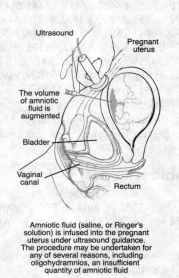

Amniotic fluid (saline, or Ringer's solution) is infused into the pregnant uterus under ultrasound guidance. The procedure may be undertaken for any of several reasons, including oligohydramnios, an insufficient quantity of amniotic fluid

Explanation

The physician infuses an abnormally underhydrated amniotic sac with fluid. This may be done as a prophylactic measure for the fetus or to enhance sonographic imaging. An amniocentesis needle is placed through the mother's abdomen and advanced between extremities of the fetus under separately reportable ultrasound guidance. Normal sterile saline is infused into the uterus until the fetal anatomy is adequately visualized. The needle is removed and a detailed ultrasound is carried out.

Coding Tips

This procedure includes the radiology services of ultrasound guidance. This procedure may be necessary before more invasive procedures, such as fetal shunt placement, can be done. For fetal shunt placement, see 59076.

ICD-9-CM Procedural

75.37 Amnioinfusion

Anesthesia

59070 00800, 00842

ICD-9-CM Diagnostic

656.83 Other specified fetal and placental problems affecting management of mother, antepartum

658.03 Oligohydramnios, antepartum

658.43 Infection of amniotic cavity, antepartum

659.73 Abnormality in fetal heart rate or rhythm, antepartum condition or complication

663.13 Cord around neck, with compression, complicating labor and delivery, antepartum

663.23 Other and unspecified cord entanglement, with compression, complicating labor and delivery, antepartum

V89.01 Suspected problem with amniotic cavity and membrane not found

V89.09 Other suspected maternal and fetal condition not found

Terms To Know

hypoplasia. Condition in which there is underdevelopment of an organ or tissue.

meconium. First stool passed by a fetus, sometimes while still in the uterus. In this event, the meconium combines with the maternal amniotic fluid. Complications may occur if meconium is aspirated by the fetus while in utero or at the time of birth.

oligohydramnios. Condition of less than the normal amount of amniotic fluid present, occurring most frequently in the last trimester.

prolapse. Falling, sliding, or sinking of an organ from its normal location in the body.

ultrasound. Imaging using ultra-high sound frequency bounced off body structures.

CCI Version 18.3

0213T, 0216T, 0228T, 0230T, 12001-12007, 12011-12057, 13100-13153, 36000, 36400-36410, 36420-36430, 36440, 36600, 36640, 37202, 43752, 51701-51703, 57410, 62310-62319, 64400-64435, 64445-64450, 64479, 64483, 64490, 64493, 64505-64530, 69990, 76941-76942, 76945-76946, 76998, 93000-93010, 93040-93042, 93318, 94002, 94200, 94250, 94680-94690, 94770, 95812-95816, 95819, 95822, 95829, 95955, 96360, 96365, 96372, 96374-96376, 99148-99149, 99150, J0670, J2001

Note: These CCI edits are used for Medicare. Other payers may reimburse on codes listed above.

Medicare Edits

	Fac RVU	Non-Fac RVU	FUD	Status
59070	9.42	12.38	0	A

	MUE				Modifiers	
59070	-		51	N/A	N/A	80

* with documentation

Medicare References: None

59072

59072 Fetal umbilical cord occlusion, including ultrasound guidance

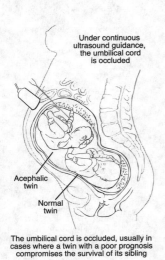

Under continuous ultrasound guidance, the umbilical cord is occluded

Acephalic twin

Normal twin

The umbilical cord is occluded, usually in cases where a twin with a poor prognosis compromises the survival of its sibling

Explanation

Fetal umbilical cord occlusion is carried out in cases of complicated monochorionic multiple gestation pregnancies or in cases to terminate a pregnancy due to a birth defect. Ultrasound is used to locate access to the umbilical cord, avoiding the placenta. Using ultrasound guidance, small forceps are advanced into the uterus and the cord of the affected fetus is identified and grasped. The umbilical cord may be ligated, occluded, or compressed. Complete absence of flow through the cord is confirmed and the instruments are removed.

Coding Tips

This procedure includes ultrasound guidance.

ICD-9-CM Procedural

75.35 Other diagnostic procedures on fetus and amnion

Anesthesia

59072 00800

ICD-9-CM Diagnostic

649.70 Cervical shortening, unspecified as to episode of care or not applicable

649.71 Cervical shortening, delivered, with or without mention of antepartum condition

649.73 Cervical shortening, antepartum condition or complication

651.03 Twin pregnancy, antepartum

651.13 Triplet pregnancy, antepartum

651.23 Quadruplet pregnancy, antepartum

651.73 Multiple gestation following (elective) fetal reduction, antepartum condition or complication

651.83 Other specified multiple gestation, antepartum

653.73 Other fetal abnormality causing disproportion, antepartum — (Code first any associated obstructed labor, 660.1)

657.03 Polyhydramnios, antepartum complication

658.03 Oligohydramnios, antepartum

658.83 Other problem associated with amniotic cavity and membranes, antepartum

678.03 Fetal hematologic conditions, antepartum condition or complication

678.13 Fetal conjoined twins, antepartum condition or complication

679.03 Maternal complications from in utero procedure, antepartum condition or complication

V15.29 Personal history of surgery to other organs

V23.85 Supervision of high risk pregnancy, pregnancy resulting from assisted reproductive technology

V23.86 Supervision of high risk pregnancy, pregnancy with history of in utero procedure during previous pregnancy

V89.03 Suspected fetal anomaly not found

V89.09 Other suspected maternal and fetal condition not found

Terms To Know

fetus. Unborn offspring past the embryonic stage that has developed major structures. It is the period defined from nine weeks after fertilization until birth.

ligation. Tying off a blood vessel or duct with a suture or a soft, thin wire.

occlusion. Constriction, closure, or blockage of a passage.

oligohydramnios. Condition of less than the normal amount of amniotic fluid present, occurring most frequently in the last trimester.

polyhydramnios. Excess amniotic fluid surrounding the fetus, typically defined as a total fluid volume of greater than 24.0 cc.

ultrasound. Imaging using ultra-high sound frequency bounced off body structures.

CCI Version 18.3

0213T, 0216T, 0228T, 0230T, 12001-12007, 12011-12057, 13100-13153, 36000, 36400-36410, 36420-36430, 36440, 36600, 36640, 37202, 43752, 51701-51703, 57410, 62310-62319, 64400-64435, 64445-64450, 64479, 64483, 64490, 64493, 64505-64530, 69990, 76941-76942, 76945-76946, 76998, 93000-93010, 93040-93042, 93318, 94002, 94200, 94250, 94680-94690, 94770, 95812-95816, 95819, 95822, 95829, 95955, 96360, 96365, 96372, 96374-96376, 99148-99149, 99150

Note: These CCI edits are used for Medicare. Other payers may reimburse on codes listed above.

Medicare Edits

	Fac RVU	Non-Fac RVU	FUD	Status
59072	15.66	15.66	0	A

	MUE		Modifiers		
59072	-	51	N/A	N/A	N/A

* with documentation

Medicare References: None

59074

59074 Fetal fluid drainage (eg, vesicocentesis, thoracocentesis, paracentesis), including ultrasound guidance

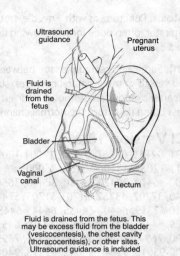

Fluid is drained from the fetus. This may be excess fluid from the bladder (vesicocentesis), the chest cavity (thoracocentesis), or other sites. Ultrasound guidance is included

Explanation

Fetal fluid drainage is done in cases of pleural effusions or pulmonary cysts, and especially in fetal megavesica, a rare syndrome caused by functional obstruction of the fetal urethra. The fetus' bladder is enlarged. Oligohydramnios, dilation of the lower and upper urinary tract, and hydronephrosis may also be present. Pulmonary hypoplasia can result from this and lead to hypoplastic abdominal musculature, urinary tract anomalies, and cryptorchidism. The fetal urinary bladder is emptied by transabdominal intrauterine vesicocentesis. Under continual ultrasound guidance, a 20-22 gauge needle is inserted through the mother's abdomen and advanced into the fetus' bladder. Fetal urine is aspirated and sent to the lab for analysis of urinary electrolytes and to determine renal function. The needle is removed and the patient kept for monitoring for up to another hour to check for refilling in the bladder. Similar fluid drainage is done by transabdominal intrauterine thoracocentesis for fetal pleural effusion.

Coding Tips

This procedure includes ultrasound guidance.

ICD-9-CM Procedural

75.35 Other diagnostic procedures on fetus and amnion

Anesthesia

59074 00800

ICD-9-CM Diagnostic

078.5 Cytomegaloviral disease — (Use additional code to identify manifestation: 484.1, 573.1)

647.63 Other maternal viral disease, antepartum — (Use additional code to further specify complication)

653.73 Other fetal abnormality causing disproportion, antepartum — (Code first any associated obstructed labor, 660.1)

655.33 Suspected damage to fetus from viral disease in mother, affecting management of mother, antepartum condition or complication

655.83 Other known or suspected fetal abnormality, not elsewhere classified, affecting management of mother, antepartum condition or complication

656.83 Other specified fetal and placental problems affecting management of mother, antepartum

657.03 Polyhydramnios, antepartum complication

679.03 Maternal complications from in utero procedure, antepartum condition or complication

V15.21 Personal history of undergoing in utero procedure during pregnancy

V15.29 Personal history of surgery to other organs

V23.85 Supervision of high risk pregnancy, pregnancy resulting from assisted reproductive technology

V23.86 Supervision of high risk pregnancy, pregnancy with history of in utero procedure during previous pregnancy

V89.01 Suspected problem with amniotic cavity and membrane not found

V89.03 Suspected fetal anomaly not found

V89.09 Other suspected maternal and fetal condition not found

Terms To Know

aspirate. To withdraw fluid or air from a body cavity by suction.

centesis. Puncture, as with a needle, trocar, or aspirator, often done for withdrawing fluid from a cavity.

fetus. Unborn offspring past the embryonic stage that has developed major structures. It is the period defined from nine weeks after fertilization until birth.

hydronephrosis. Distension of the kidney caused by an accumulation of urine that cannot flow out due to an obstruction that may be caused by conditions such as kidney stones or vesicoureteral reflux.

oligohydramnios. Condition of less than the normal amount of amniotic fluid present, occurring most frequently in the last trimester.

polyhydramnios. Excess amniotic fluid surrounding the fetus, typically defined as a total fluid volume of greater than 24.0 cc.

ultrasound. Imaging using ultra-high sound frequency bounced off body structures.

CCI Version 18.3

0213T, 0216T, 0228T, 0230T, 12001-12007, 12011-12057, 13100-13153, 36000, 36400-36410, 36420-36430, 36440, 36600, 36640, 37202, 43752, 51701-51703, 57410, 62310-62319, 64400-64435, 64445-64450, 64479, 64483, 64490, 64493, 64505-64530, 69990, 76941-76942, 76945-76946, 76998, 93000-93010, 93040-93042, 93318, 94002, 94200, 94250, 94680-94690, 94770, 95812-95816, 95819, 95822, 95829, 95955, 96360, 96365, 96372, 96374-96376, 99148-99149, 99150, J0670, J2001

Note: These CCI edits are used for Medicare. Other payers may reimburse on codes listed above.

Medicare Edits

	Fac RVU	Non-Fac RVU	FUD	Status
59074	9.58	12.65	0	A

	MUE		Modifiers		
59074	-	51	N/A	N/A	80

* with documentation

Medicare References: None

Coding Companion for Ob/Gyn

© 2012 OptumInsight, Inc.

Maternity Care

59076

59076 Fetal shunt placement, including ultrasound guidance

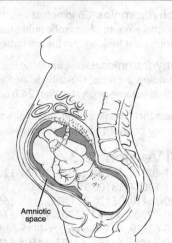

Amniotic space

A shunt is placed from an area in the fetus that requires drainage (e.g., bladder) to the amniotic space surrounding the fetus

Explanation

Fetal shunt placement is performed for pleural or vesical amniotic shunting in cases of pleural effusion, pulmonary cysts, or fetal megavesica, where the bladder is enlarged because of urethra blockage. Shunting is done to supply continuous drainage when reaccumulation of fluid is not successfully treated by isolated vesicocentesis or thoracocentesis. Fluids can be drained into the amniotic cavity through a double pigtailed catheter. The entry site on the mother's abdomen is cleansed with antiseptic solution and local anesthetic is infiltrated down to the myometrium. Under ultrasound guidance, a metal cannula with a trocar is introduced transabdominally into the amniotic cavity and inserted through the fetal chest wall in the midthoracic region, into the effusion or cyst (if megavesical fluid accumulation is the problem, the shunt is placed into the bladder). The trocar is removed and the catheter is inserted into the cannula. A short introducer rod is used to place the proximal half of the catheter into the effusion or cyst. The cannula is gradually removed into the amniotic cavity where the other half of the catheter is pushed by a longer introducer. There is now a conduit for fluid drainage into the amniotic space. Placement of the shunt is confirmed, the instruments are removed, and the patient is monitored for one to two hours. Follow-up ultrasound scans are performed at weekly intervals to check drainage and determine if the effusions reaccumulate, in which case another shunt

may be inserted. The drains are immediately clamped and removed after delivery.

Coding Tips

This procedure includes ultrasound guidance.

ICD-9-CM Procedural

75.35   Other diagnostic procedures on fetus and amnion

Anesthesia

59076   00800

ICD-9-CM Diagnostic

078.5   Cytomegaloviral disease — (Use additional code to identify manifestation: 484.1, 573.1)

647.63   Other maternal viral disease, antepartum — (Use additional code to further specify complication)

653.73   Other fetal abnormality causing disproportion, antepartum — (Code first any associated obstructed labor, 660.1)

655.33   Suspected damage to fetus from viral disease in mother, affecting management of mother, antepartum condition or complication

655.83   Other known or suspected fetal abnormality, not elsewhere classified, affecting management of mother, antepartum condition or complication

656.83   Other specified fetal and placental problems affecting management of mother, antepartum

657.03   Polyhydramnios, antepartum complication

679.03   Maternal complications from in utero procedure, antepartum condition or complication

V15.21   Personal history of undergoing in utero procedure during pregnancy

V15.29   Personal history of surgery to other organs

V23.85   Supervision of high risk pregnancy, pregnancy resulting from assisted reproductive technology

V23.86   Supervision of high risk pregnancy, pregnancy with history of in utero procedure during previous pregnancy

V89.01   Suspected problem with amniotic cavity and membrane not found

V89.03   Suspected fetal anomaly not found

V89.09   Other suspected maternal and fetal condition not found

Terms To Know

cannula. Tube inserted into a blood vessel, duct, or body cavity to facilitate passage.

catheter. Flexible tube inserted into an area of the body for introducing or withdrawing fluid.

centesis. Puncture, as with a needle, trocar, or aspirator, often done for withdrawing fluid from a cavity.

shunt. Surgically created passage between blood vessels or other natural passages, such as an arteriovenous anastomosis, to divert or bypass blood flow from the normal channel.

CCI Version 18.3

0213T, 0216T, 0228T, 0230T, 12001-12007, 12011-12057, 13100-13153, 36000, 36400-36410, 36420-36430, 36440, 36600, 36640, 37202, 43752, 51701-51703, 57410, 62310-62319, 64400-64435, 64445-64450, 64479, 64483, 64490, 64493, 64505-64530, 69990, 76941-76942, 76945-76946, 76998, 93000-93010, 93040-93042, 93318, 94002, 94200, 94250, 94680-94690, 94770, 95812-95816, 95819, 95822, 95829, 95955, 96360, 96365, 96372, 96374-96376, 99148-99149, 99150

Note: These CCI edits are used for Medicare. Other payers may reimburse on codes listed above.

Medicare Edits

	Fac RVU	Non-Fac RVU	FUD	Status
59076	15.58	15.58	0	A

	MUE			Modifiers	
59076	-	51	N/A	N/A	80

* with documentation

Medicare References: None

Maternity Care

59100

59100 Hysterotomy, abdominal (eg, for hydatidiform mole, abortion)

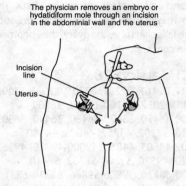

The physician removes an embryo or hydatidiform mole through an incision in the abdominal wall and the uterus

Incision line

Uterus

Explanation

The physician removes an embryo or hydatidiform mole through an incision in the abdominal wall and uterus. The surgery is similar to a cesarean section but the abdominal and uterine incisions are smaller. The lower abdominal wall is opened with a vertical or horizontal incision and the uterus is entered through the lower uterine segment. The physician removes the embryo or hydatidiform mole and may also remove any remaining membranes and placenta from the uterine cavity. Curettage of the uterine cavity may also be performed. The abdominal and uterine incisions are closed by suturing.

Coding Tips

Hysterotomy for abortion or for hydatidiform molar pregnancy is rarely performed. Suction curettage has replaced hysterotomy as the method of choice in the treatment of hydatidiform mole. For treatment of hydatidiform mole by suction curettage, see 59870. When tubal ligation is performed at the same time as hysterotomy, see 58611 in addition to 59100. Because 58611 is a subsidiary or "in addition to" code, reimbursement reduction and modifier 51 do not apply.

ICD-9-CM Procedural

68.0   Hysterotomy
74.91   Hysterotomy to terminate pregnancy
75.33   Fetal blood sampling and biopsy

Anesthesia
59100   00840

ICD-9-CM Diagnostic

630   Hydatidiform mole — (Use additional code from category 639 to identify any associated complications)
631.8   Other abnormal products of conception
632   Missed abortion — (Use additional code from category 639 to identify any associated complications)
655.01   Central nervous system malformation in fetus, with delivery
655.03   Central nervous system malformation in fetus, antepartum
655.11   Chromosomal abnormality in fetus, affecting management of mother, with delivery
655.13   Chromosomal abnormality in fetus, affecting management of mother, antepartum
655.21   Hereditary disease in family possibly affecting fetus, affecting management of mother, with delivery
655.23   Hereditary disease in family possibly affecting fetus, affecting management of mother, antepartum condition or complication
655.31   Suspected damage to fetus from viral disease in mother, affecting management of mother, with delivery
655.33   Suspected damage to fetus from viral disease in mother, affecting management of mother, antepartum condition or complication
655.41   Suspected damage to fetus from other disease in mother, affecting management of mother, with delivery
655.43   Suspected damage to fetus from other disease in mother, affecting management of mother, antepartum condition or complication
655.51   Suspected damage to fetus from drugs, affecting management of mother, delivered
655.53   Suspected damage to fetus from drugs, affecting management of mother, antepartum
655.61   Suspected damage to fetus from radiation, affecting management of mother, delivered
655.63   Suspected damage to fetus from radiation, affecting management of mother, antepartum condition or complication

655.71   Decreased fetal movements, affecting management of mother, delivered
655.73   Decreased fetal movements, affecting management of mother, antepartum condition or complication
655.81   Other known or suspected fetal abnormality, not elsewhere classified, affecting management of mother, delivery
655.83   Other known or suspected fetal abnormality, not elsewhere classified, affecting management of mother, antepartum condition or complication
656.41   Intrauterine death affecting management of mother, delivered
656.43   Intrauterine death affecting management of mother, antepartum
659.51   Elderly primigravida, delivered
659.53   Elderly primigravida, antepartum
659.61   Elderly multigravida, delivered, with mention of antepartum condition
659.63   Elderly multigravida, with antepartum condition or complication
678.13   Fetal conjoined twins, antepartum condition or complication
V13.1   Personal history of trophoblastic disease
V19.5   Family history of congenital anomalies
V23.1   Pregnancy with history of trophoblastic disease

CCI Version 18.3

0213T, 0216T, 0228T, 0230T, 12001-12007, 12011-12057, 13100-13153, 36000, 36400-36410, 36420-36430, 36440, 36600, 36640, 37202, 43752, 44005, 44180, 44602-44605, 44850, 49000-49010, 49255, 49320, 49570, 51701-51703, 57410, 59856-59857❖, 62310-62319, 64400-64435, 64445-64450, 64479, 64483, 64490, 64493, 64505-64530, 69990, 93000-93010, 93040-93042, 93318, 94002, 94200, 94250, 94680-94690, 94770, 95812-95816, 95819, 95822, 95829, 95955, 96360, 96365, 96372, 96374-96376, 99148-99149, 99150

Note: These CCI edits are used for Medicare. Other payers may reimburse on codes listed above.

Medicare Edits

	Fac RVU	Non-Fac RVU	FUD	Status
59100	25.06	25.06	90	A

	MUE			Modifiers	
59100	1	51	N/A	62*	80

* with documentation

Medicare References: None

Maternity Care

59120-59121

59120 Surgical treatment of ectopic pregnancy; tubal or ovarian, requiring salpingectomy and/or oophorectomy, abdominal or vaginal approach

59121 tubal or ovarian, without salpingectomy and/or oophorectomy

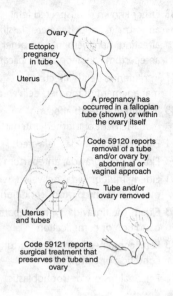

Ovary

Ectopic pregnancy in tube

Uterus

A pregnancy has occurred in a fallopian tube (shown) or within the ovary itself

Code 59120 reports removal of a tube and/or ovary by abdominal or vaginal approach

Tube and/or ovary removed

Uterus and tubes

Code 59121 reports surgical treatment that preserves the tube and ovary

Explanation

The physician treats a tubal or ovarian ectopic pregnancy by removing the fallopian tube and/or ovary. Through the vagina or through an incision in the lower abdomen, the physician explores the pelvic cavity, inspects the gestation site for bleeding, and removes all products of conception, clots, and free blood. If the tube is affected, it may be excised by cutting a small wedge of the uterine wall at the junction of the fallopian tube and body of the uterus. If the ovary is affected, it may be removed. Lysis of adhesions may be indicated and the pelvis lavaged with saline solution. If an abdominal approach is used, the incision is closed with sutures.

Coding Tips

For surgical treatment of other ectopic pregnancies, see 59130–59140. For laparoscopic treatment of an ectopic pregnancy, see 59150 and 59151. Complications such as control of hemorrhage resulting from the ectopic pregnancy are not included and are reported separately.

ICD-9-CM Procedural

65.22 Wedge resection of ovary
65.39 Other unilateral oophorectomy
65.49 Other unilateral salpingo-oophorectomy
66.01 Salpingotomy
66.62 Salpingectomy with removal of tubal pregnancy

Anesthesia

00840

ICD-9-CM Diagnostic

633.10 Tubal pregnancy without intrauterine pregnancy — (Use additional code from category 639 to identify any associated complications)

633.11 Tubal pregnancy with intrauterine pregnancy — (Use additional code from category 639 to identify any associated complications)

633.20 Ovarian pregnancy without intrauterine pregnancy — (Use additional code from category 639 to identify any associated complications)

633.21 Ovarian pregnancy with intrauterine pregnancy — (Use additional code from category 639 to identify any associated complications)

633.80 Other ectopic pregnancy without intrauterine pregnancy — (Use additional code from category 639 to identify any associated complications)

633.81 Other ectopic pregnancy with intrauterine pregnancy — (Use additional code from category 639 to identify any associated complications)

633.90 Unspecified ectopic pregnancy without intrauterine pregnancy — (Use additional code from category 639 to identify any associated complications)

633.91 Unspecified ectopic pregnancy with intrauterine pregnancy — (Use additional code from category 639 to identify any associated complications)

639.0 Genital tract and pelvic infection following abortion or ectopic and molar pregnancies

639.1 Delayed or excessive hemorrhage following abortion or ectopic and molar pregnancies

639.2 Damage to pelvic organs and tissues following abortion or ectopic and molar pregnancies

639.8 Other specified complication following abortion or ectopic and molar pregnancies

639.9 Unspecified complication following abortion or ectopic and molar pregnancies

789.00 Abdominal pain, unspecified site
789.03 Abdominal pain, right lower quadrant
789.04 Abdominal pain, left lower quadrant
V64.41 Laparoscopic surgical procedure converted to open procedure

Terms To Know

ectopic pregnancy. Fertilized ovum that implants and develops outside the uterus. The ovum may implant itself in different sites, such as the fallopian tube, the ovary, the abdomen, or the cervix.

CCI Version 18.3

0213T, 0216T, 0228T, 0230T, 12001-12007, 12011-12057, 13100-13153, 36000, 36400-36410, 36420-36430, 36440, 36600, 36640, 37202, 43752, 44005, 44180, 44602-44605, 44850, 49000-49010, 49255, 49320, 49570, 51701-51703, 57410, 58700-58720, 59856-59866, 62310-62319, 64400-64435, 64445-64450, 64479, 64483, 64490, 64493, 64505-64530, 69990, 93000-93010, 93040-93042, 93318, 94002, 94200, 94250, 94680-94690, 94770, 95812-95816, 95819, 95822, 95829, 95955, 96360, 96365, 96372, 96374-96376, 99148-99149, 99150

Note: These CCI edits are used for Medicare. Other payers may reimburse on codes listed above.

Medicare Edits

	Fac RVU	Non-Fac RVU	FUD	Status
59120	23.92	23.92	90	A
59121	23.94	23.94	90	A

	MUE		Modifiers		
59120	1	51	N/A	62*	80
59121	1	51	N/A	62*	80

* with documentation

Medicare References: 100-3,230.3

Coding Companion for Ob/Gyn

Maternity Care

59130

59130 Surgical treatment of ectopic pregnancy; abdominal pregnancy

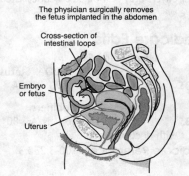

The physician surgically removes the fetus implanted in the abdomen

Cross-section of intestinal loops

Embryo or fetus

Uterus

Explanation

The physician removes an embryo or fetus implanted in the abdomen. The fertilized ovum may have implanted directly in the abdomen (primary) or it may have implanted after escaping from the tube through a rupture or through the fimbriated end (secondary). After making an abdominal incision, the physician surgically removes the fetus from the abdomen. The membranes are also removed and the cord is ligated near the placenta. The placenta is usually not removed unless attached to the fallopian tube, ovary, or uterine broad ligament. Abdominal lavage may also be indicated. The abdominal incision is then closed with sutures. Although this procedure is rare, it can be done any time during gestation, even at or near term.

Coding Tips

For surgical treatment of other ectopic pregnancies, see 59120, 59121, and 59135–59140. For laparoscopic treatment of an ectopic pregnancy, see 59150 and 59151. Complications such as control of hemorrhage resulting from the ectopic pregnancy are not included and are reported separately.

ICD-9-CM Procedural

74.3   Removal of extratubal ectopic pregnancy

75.99   Other obstetric operations

Anesthesia

59130   00840

ICD-9-CM Diagnostic

633.00   Abdominal pregnancy without intrauterine pregnancy — (Use additional code from category 639 to identify any associated complications)

633.01   Abdominal pregnancy with intrauterine pregnancy — (Use additional code from category 639 to identify any associated complications)

633.80   Other ectopic pregnancy without intrauterine pregnancy — (Use additional code from category 639 to identify any associated complications)

633.81   Other ectopic pregnancy with intrauterine pregnancy — (Use additional code from category 639 to identify any associated complications)

639.0   Genital tract and pelvic infection following abortion or ectopic and molar pregnancies

639.1   Delayed or excessive hemorrhage following abortion or ectopic and molar pregnancies

639.2   Damage to pelvic organs and tissues following abortion or ectopic and molar pregnancies

639.8   Other specified complication following abortion or ectopic and molar pregnancies

639.9   Unspecified complication following abortion or ectopic and molar pregnancies

Terms To Know

ectopic pregnancy. Fertilized ovum that implants and develops outside the uterus. The ovum may implant itself in different sites, such as the fallopian tube, the ovary, the abdomen, or the cervix.

embryo. Developing cells of a new organism that will become a fetus; the period defined from the fourth day after fertilization to the end of the eighth week.

fetus. Unborn offspring past the embryonic stage that has developed major structures. It is the period defined from nine weeks after fertilization until birth.

lavage. Washing.

ligate. To tie off a blood vessel or duct with a suture or a soft, thin wire (ligature wire).

CCI Version 18.3

0213T, 0216T, 0228T, 0230T, 12001-12007, 12011-12057, 13100-13153, 36000,

36400-36410, 36420-36430, 36440, 36600, 36640, 37202, 43752, 44005, 44180, 44602-44605, 44820-44850, 49000-49002, 49255, 49320, 49570, 51701-51703, 57410, 59857-59866, 62310-62319, 64400-64435, 64445-64450, 64479, 64483, 64490, 64493, 64505-64530, 69990, 93000-93010, 93040-93042, 93318, 94002, 94200, 94250, 94680-94690, 94770, 95812-95816, 95819, 95822, 95829, 95955, 96360, 96365, 96372, 96374-96376, 99148-99149, 99150

Note: These CCI edits are used for Medicare. Other payers may reimburse on codes listed above.

Medicare Edits

	Fac RVU	Non-Fac RVU	FUD	Status
59130	24.46	24.46	90	A

	MUE		Modifiers		
59130	1	51	N/A	N/A	80*

* with documentation

Medicare References: None

Coding Companion for Ob/Gyn

59135

59135 Surgical treatment of ectopic pregnancy; interstitial, uterine pregnancy requiring total hysterectomy

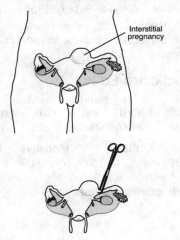

The physician removes the uterus and cervix, and may elect to remove tubes and/or ovaries

Interstitial pregnancy

Explanation

The physician treats an interstitial pregnancy where the fertilized ovum has implanted in the portion of the tube that transverses the uterine wall by removing the uterus and cervix. Through an incision extending from just above the pubic hairline to the rib cage, the physician clamps and cuts free the supporting pedicles containing the tubes, ligaments, and arteries. The physician removes the uterus and cervix and may elect to remove the tubes and/or ovaries. Abdominal or pelvic lavage may also be indicated. The abdominal incision is closed with sutures.

Coding Tips

For surgical treatment of other ectopic pregnancies, see 59120–59130, 59136, and 59140. For laparoscopic treatment of an ectopic pregnancy, see 59150 and 59151. Complications such as control of hemorrhage resulting from the ectopic pregnancy are not included and are reported separately.

ICD-9-CM Procedural

68.39 Other and unspecified subtotal abdominal hysterectomy

68.49 Other and unspecified total abdominal hysterectomy

74.3 Removal of extratubal ectopic pregnancy

Anesthesia

59135 00840

ICD-9-CM Diagnostic

633.80 Other ectopic pregnancy without intrauterine pregnancy — (Use additional code from category 639 to identify any associated complications)

633.81 Other ectopic pregnancy with intrauterine pregnancy — (Use additional code from category 639 to identify any associated complications)

633.90 Unspecified ectopic pregnancy without intrauterine pregnancy — (Use additional code from category 639 to identify any associated complications)

633.91 Unspecified ectopic pregnancy with intrauterine pregnancy — (Use additional code from category 639 to identify any associated complications)

639.0 Genital tract and pelvic infection following abortion or ectopic and molar pregnancies

639.1 Delayed or excessive hemorrhage following abortion or ectopic and molar pregnancies

639.2 Damage to pelvic organs and tissues following abortion or ectopic and molar pregnancies

639.8 Other specified complication following abortion or ectopic and molar pregnancies

639.9 Unspecified complication following abortion or ectopic and molar pregnancies

Terms To Know

ectopic pregnancy. Fertilized ovum that implants and develops outside the uterus. The ovum may implant itself in different sites, such as the fallopian tube, the ovary, the abdomen, or the cervix.

hydatidiform mole. Trophoblastic neoplasm that mimics pregnancy by proliferating from a pathologic ovum and resulting only in a mass of cysts resembling grapes, 80 percent of which are benign, but require surgical removal. Hydatidiform moles can be complete, in which there is no fetal tissue, or partial, in which fetal tissue is frequently present.

CCI Version 18.3

0213T, 0216T, 0228T, 0230T, 12001-12007, 12011-12057, 13100-13153, 36000, 36400-36410, 36420-36430, 36440, 36600, 36640, 37202, 43752, 44005, 44180, 44602-44605, 44820-44850, 49000-49010,

49255, 49320, 49570, 51701-51703, 57410, 59866, 62310-62319, 64400-64435, 64445-64450, 64479, 64483, 64490, 64493, 64505-64530, 69990, 93000-93010, 93040-93042, 93318, 94002, 94200, 94250, 94680-94690, 94770, 95812-95816, 95819, 95822, 95829, 95955, 96360, 96365, 96372, 96374-96376, 99148-99149, 99150

Note: These CCI edits are used for Medicare. Other payers may reimburse on codes listed above.

Medicare Edits

	Fac RVU	Non-Fac RVU	FUD	Status
59135	24.87	24.87	90	A

	MUE		Modifiers	
59135	1	51 N/A	N/A	80*

* with documentation

Medicare References: 100-3, 230.3

Maternity Care

59136

59136 Surgical treatment of ectopic pregnancy; interstitial, uterine pregnancy with partial resection of uterus

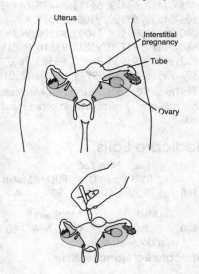

The physician resects the uterus to remove an interstitial ectopic pregnancy

Uterus

Interstitial pregnancy

Tube

Ovary

Explanation

The physician treats an interstitial ectopic pregnancy where the fertilized ovum has implanted in the portion of the tube that transverses the uterine wall by partially resecting the uterus. Through an incision extending from just above the pubic hairline to the rib cage, the physician resects and reconstructs the uterine wall. The physician may also remove a portion or all of the fallopian tube. Abdominal or pelvic lavage may be indicated. The abdominal incision is closed with sutures.

Coding Tips

For surgical treatment of other ectopic pregnancies, see 59120–59135 and 59140. For laparoscopic treatment of an ectopic pregnancy, see 59150 and 59151. Complications such as control of hemorrhage resulting from the ectopic pregnancy are not included and are reported separately.

ICD-9-CM Procedural

68.39 Other and unspecified subtotal abdominal hysterectomy

68.49 Other and unspecified total abdominal hysterectomy

74.3 Removal of extratubal ectopic pregnancy

Anesthesia

59136 00840

ICD-9-CM Diagnostic

633.80 Other ectopic pregnancy without intrauterine pregnancy — (Use additional code from category 639 to identify any associated complications)

633.81 Other ectopic pregnancy with intrauterine pregnancy — (Use additional code from category 639 to identify any associated complications)

633.90 Unspecified ectopic pregnancy without intrauterine pregnancy — (Use additional code from category 639 to identify any associated complications)

633.91 Unspecified ectopic pregnancy with intrauterine pregnancy — (Use additional code from category 639 to identify any associated complications)

639.0 Genital tract and pelvic infection following abortion or ectopic and molar pregnancies

639.1 Delayed or excessive hemorrhage following abortion or ectopic and molar pregnancies

639.2 Damage to pelvic organs and tissues following abortion or ectopic and molar pregnancies

639.8 Other specified complication following abortion or ectopic and molar pregnancies

639.9 Unspecified complication following abortion or ectopic and molar pregnancies

Terms To Know

ectopic pregnancy. Fertilized ovum that implants and develops outside the uterus. The ovum may implant itself in different sites, such as the fallopian tube, the ovary, the abdomen, or the cervix.

incision. Act of cutting into tissue or an organ.

lavage. Washing.

reconstruct. Tissue rebuilding.

resection. Surgical removal of a part or all of an organ or body part.

suture. Numerous stitching techniques employed in wound closure: 1) Buried suture: Continuous or interrupted suture placed under the skin for a layered closure. 2) Continuous suture: Running stitch with tension evenly distributed across a single strand to provide a leakproof closure line. 3) Interrupted suture: Series of single stitches with tension isolated at each stitch, in which all stitches are not affected if one becomes loose, and the isolated sutures cannot act as a wick to transport an infection. 4) Purse-string suture: Continuous suture placed around a tubular structure and tightened, to reduce or close the lumen. 5) Retention suture: Secondary stitching that bridges the primary suture, providing support for the primary repair; a plastic or rubber bolster may be placed over the primary repair and under the retention sutures.

CCI Version 18.3

0213T, 0216T, 0228T, 0230T, 12001-12007, 12011-12057, 13100-13153, 36000, 36400-36410, 36420-36430, 36440, 36600, 36640, 37202, 43752, 44005, 44180, 44602-44605, 44820-44850, 49000-49010, 49255, 49320, 49570, 51701-51703, 57410, 59857-59866, 62310-62319, 64400-64435, 64445-64450, 64479, 64483, 64490, 64493, 64505-64530, 69990, 93000-93010, 93040-93042, 93318, 94002, 94200, 94250, 94680-94690, 94770, 95812-95816, 95819, 95822, 95829, 95955, 96360, 96365, 96372, 96374-96376, 99148-99149, 99150

Note: These CCI edits are used for Medicare. Other payers may reimburse on codes listed above.

Medicare Edits

	Fac RVU	Non-Fac RVU	FUD	Status
59136	26.26	26.26	90	A

	MUE		Modifiers		
59136	1	51	N/A	N/A	80

* with documentation

Medicare References: 100-3,230.3

Coding Companion for Ob/Gyn

59140

59140 Surgical treatment of ectopic pregnancy; cervical, with evacuation

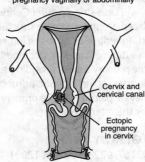

The physician removes a cervical ectopic pregnancy vaginally or abdominally

Cervix and cervical canal

Ectopic pregnancy in cervix

Explanation

The physician treats an ectopic pregnancy where the embryo has implanted in the cervix. If the pregnancy is less than 12 weeks gestation, the physician usually removes the embryo through the vagina. The physician ligates the hypogastric arteries or the cervical branches of the uterus to control bleeding. Curettage of the endocervix and endometrium may stop heavy bleeding. Sutures and gauze packing may also be necessary. If later than 12 weeks gestation, the physician may treat the cervical pregnancy by performing an abdominal hysterectomy. Through a horizontal incision just within the pubic hairline, the physician clamps and cuts free the supporting pedicles containing the tubes, ligaments, and arteries. The uterus is removed above the cervix, and the incision is closed by suturing.

Coding Tips

For surgical treatment of other ectopic pregnancies, see 59120–59136. For laparoscopic treatment of an ectopic pregnancy, see 59150 and 59151. Complications such as control of hemorrhage resulting from the ectopic pregnancy are not included and are reported separately.

ICD-9-CM Procedural

68.39   Other and unspecified subtotal abdominal hysterectomy

68.49   Other and unspecified total abdominal hysterectomy

74.3   Removal of extratubal ectopic pregnancy

Anesthesia

59140   00940

ICD-9-CM Diagnostic

633.80   Other ectopic pregnancy without intrauterine pregnancy — (Use additional code from category 639 to identify any associated complications)

633.81   Other ectopic pregnancy with intrauterine pregnancy — (Use additional code from category 639 to identify any associated complications)

633.90   Unspecified ectopic pregnancy without intrauterine pregnancy — (Use additional code from category 639 to identify any associated complications)

633.91   Unspecified ectopic pregnancy with intrauterine pregnancy — (Use additional code from category 639 to identify any associated complications)

639.0   Genital tract and pelvic infection following abortion or ectopic and molar pregnancies

639.1   Delayed or excessive hemorrhage following abortion or ectopic and molar pregnancies

639.2   Damage to pelvic organs and tissues following abortion or ectopic and molar pregnancies

639.8   Other specified complication following abortion or ectopic and molar pregnancies

639.9   Unspecified complication following abortion or ectopic and molar pregnancies

Terms To Know

ectopic pregnancy. Fertilized ovum that implants and develops outside the uterus. The ovum may implant itself in different sites, such as the fallopian tube, the ovary, the abdomen, or the cervix.

hydatidiform mole. Trophoblastic neoplasm that mimics pregnancy by proliferating from a pathologic ovum and resulting only in a mass of cysts resembling grapes, 80 percent of which are benign, but require surgical removal. Hydatidiform moles can be complete, in which there is no fetal tissue, or partial, in which fetal tissue is frequently present.

CCI Version 18.3

0213T, 0216T, 0228T, 0230T, 12001-12007, 12011-12057, 13100-13153, 36000, 36400-36410, 36420-36430, 36440, 36600, 36640, 37202, 43752, 44005, 44180, 44602-44605, 44850, 49000-49010, 49255, 49320, 49570, 51701-51703, 57410, 59856-59866, 62310-62319, 64400-64435, 64445-64450, 64479, 64483, 64490, 64493, 64505-64530, 69990, 93000-93010, 93040-93042, 93318, 94002, 94200, 94250, 94680-94690, 94770, 95812-95816, 95819, 95822, 95829, 95955, 96360, 96365, 96372, 96374-96376, 99148-99149, 99150, J2001

Note: These CCI edits are used for Medicare. Other payers may reimburse on codes listed above.

Medicare Edits

	Fac RVU	Non-Fac RVU	FUD	Status
59140	10.72	10.72	90	A

	MUE		Modifiers		
59140	1	51	N/A	N/A	80

* with documentation

Medicare References: None

59150

59150 Laparoscopic treatment of ectopic pregnancy; without salpingectomy and/or oophorectomy

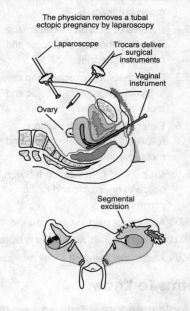

The physician removes a tubal ectopic pregnancy by laparoscopy

Laparoscope

Trocars deliver surgical instruments

Vaginal instrument

Ovary

Segmental excision

Explanation

The physician treats an ectopic pregnancy by laparoscopy without salpingectomy and/or oophorectomy. The physician inserts an instrument through the vagina to grasp the cervix while passing another instrument through the cervix and into the uterus to manipulate the uterus. Next, the physician makes a 1 cm incision in the umbilicus through which the abdomen is inflated and a fiberoptic laparoscope is inserted. A second incision is made on the left or right side of the abdomen. After locating the site of the gestation, another small incision is made above the site. Instruments are passed into the abdomen through the incisions. The physician removes the ectopic pregnancy by making an incision in the tube or ovary or by segmental excision. The abdominal incisions are closed with sutures.

Coding Tips

If significant additional time and effort is documented, append modifier 22 and submit a cover letter and operative report. This code includes diagnostic laparoscopy performed by the physician. This code is appropriate for reporting this procedure when performed with any technique or combination of techniques (e.g., laser, hot cautery). For failed laparoscopic procedures followed by an open procedure, code the open procedure as the primary procedure and a diagnostic laparoscopy as a secondary procedure with modifier 51. For laparoscopic treatment of an

ectopic pregnancy, with salpingectomy and/or oophorectomy, see 59151.

ICD-9-CM Procedural

66.01 Salpingotomy
74.3 Removal of extratubal ectopic pregnancy

Anesthesia
59150 00840

ICD-9-CM Diagnostic

633.00 Abdominal pregnancy without intrauterine pregnancy — (Use additional code from category 639 to identify any associated complications)
633.01 Abdominal pregnancy with intrauterine pregnancy — (Use additional code from category 639 to identify any associated complications)
633.10 Tubal pregnancy without intrauterine pregnancy — (Use additional code from category 639 to identify any associated complications)
633.11 Tubal pregnancy with intrauterine pregnancy — (Use additional code from category 639 to identify any associated complications)
633.20 Ovarian pregnancy without intrauterine pregnancy — (Use additional code from category 639 to identify any associated complications)
633.21 Ovarian pregnancy with intrauterine pregnancy — (Use additional code from category 639 to identify any associated complications)
633.80 Other ectopic pregnancy without intrauterine pregnancy — (Use additional code from category 639 to identify any associated complications)
633.81 Other ectopic pregnancy with intrauterine pregnancy — (Use additional code from category 639 to identify any associated complications)
633.90 Unspecified ectopic pregnancy without intrauterine pregnancy — (Use additional code from category 639 to identify any associated complications)
633.91 Unspecified ectopic pregnancy with intrauterine pregnancy — (Use additional code from category 639 to identify any associated complications)
639.0 Genital tract and pelvic infection following abortion or ectopic and molar pregnancies

639.1 Delayed or excessive hemorrhage following abortion or ectopic and molar pregnancies
639.2 Damage to pelvic organs and tissues following abortion or ectopic and molar pregnancies
639.8 Other specified complication following abortion or ectopic and molar pregnancies
639.9 Unspecified complication following abortion or ectopic and molar pregnancies
789.00 Abdominal pain, unspecified site
789.03 Abdominal pain, right lower quadrant
789.04 Abdominal pain, left lower quadrant

Terms To Know

ectopic pregnancy. Fertilized ovum that implants and develops outside the uterus. The ovum may implant itself in different sites, such as the fallopian tube, the ovary, the abdomen, or the cervix.

CCI Version 18.3

0213T, 0216T, 0228T, 0230T, 12001-12007, 12011-12057, 13100-13153, 36000, 36400-36410, 36420-36430, 36440, 36600, 36640, 37202, 43752, 51701-51703, 57410, 58700-58720, 59856-59866, 62310-62319, 64400-64435, 64445-64450, 64479, 64483, 64490, 64493, 64505-64530, 69990, 93000-93010, 93040-93042, 93318, 94002, 94200, 94250, 94680-94690, 94770, 95812-95816, 95819, 95822, 95829, 95955, 96360, 96365, 96372, 96374-96376, 99148-99149, 99150

Note: These CCI edits are used for Medicare. Other payers may reimburse on codes listed above.

Medicare Edits

	Fac RVU	Non-Fac RVU	FUD	Status
59150	23.15	23.15	90	A

	MUE		Modifiers		
59150	1	51	N/A	N/A	80

* with documentation

Medicare References: None

59151

59151 Laparoscopic treatment of ectopic pregnancy; with salpingectomy and/or oophorectomy

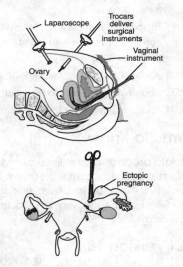

The physician removes a fallopian tube to treat ectopic pregnancy; ovary may also be removed

Explanation

The physician treats an ectopic pregnancy by laparoscopy with salpingectomy and/or oophorectomy. The physician inserts an instrument through the vagina to grasp the cervix while passing another instrument through the cervix and into the uterus to manipulate the uterus. Next, the physician makes a 1 cm incision in the umbilicus through which the abdomen is inflated and a fiberoptic laparoscope is inserted. A second incision is made on the left or right side of the abdomen. After locating the site of the gestation, another small incision is made above the site. Instruments are passed into the abdomen through the incisions. The physician removes the tube and/or ovary containing the embryo and closes the abdominal incisions with sutures.

Coding Tips

A diagnostic laparoscopy is included in this procedure and should not be reported separately. This code is appropriate for reporting this procedure when performed with any technique or combination of techniques (e.g., laser, hot cautery). If significant additional time and effort is documented, append modifier 22 and submit a cover letter and operative report. For laparoscopic treatment of an ectopic pregnancy, without salpingectomy and/or oophorectomy, see 59150.

ICD-9-CM Procedural

65.01	Laparoscopic oophorotomy
65.31	Laparoscopic unilateral oophorectomy
65.41	Laparoscopic unilateral salpingo-oophorectomy
65.54	Laparoscopic removal of remaining ovary
65.63	Laparoscopic removal of both ovaries and tubes at same operative episode
65.64	Laparoscopic removal of remaining ovary and tube
66.4	Total unilateral salpingectomy
66.62	Salpingectomy with removal of tubal pregnancy

Anesthesia

59151 00840

ICD-9-CM Diagnostic

633.00	Abdominal pregnancy without intrauterine pregnancy — (Use additional code from category 639 to identify any associated complications)
633.01	Abdominal pregnancy with intrauterine pregnancy — (Use additional code from category 639 to identify any associated complications)
633.10	Tubal pregnancy without intrauterine pregnancy — (Use additional code from category 639 to identify any associated complications)
633.11	Tubal pregnancy with intrauterine pregnancy — (Use additional code from category 639 to identify any associated complications)
633.20	Ovarian pregnancy without intrauterine pregnancy — (Use additional code from category 639 to identify any associated complications)
633.21	Ovarian pregnancy with intrauterine pregnancy — (Use additional code from category 639 to identify any associated complications)
633.80	Other ectopic pregnancy without intrauterine pregnancy — (Use additional code from category 639 to identify any associated complications)
633.81	Other ectopic pregnancy with intrauterine pregnancy — (Use additional code from category 639 to identify any associated complications)
633.90	Unspecified ectopic pregnancy without intrauterine pregnancy — (Use additional code from category 639 to identify any associated complications)
633.91	Unspecified ectopic pregnancy with intrauterine pregnancy — (Use additional code from category 639 to identify any associated complications)
639.0	Genital tract and pelvic infection following abortion or ectopic and molar pregnancies
639.1	Delayed or excessive hemorrhage following abortion or ectopic and molar pregnancies
639.2	Damage to pelvic organs and tissues following abortion or ectopic and molar pregnancies
639.8	Other specified complication following abortion or ectopic and molar pregnancies
639.9	Unspecified complication following abortion or ectopic and molar pregnancies
789.00	Abdominal pain, unspecified site
789.03	Abdominal pain, right lower quadrant
789.04	Abdominal pain, left lower quadrant

Terms To Know

ectopic pregnancy. Fertilized ovum that implants and develops outside the uterus. The ovum may implant itself in different sites, such as the fallopian tube, the ovary, the abdomen, or the cervix.

CCI Version 18.3

0213T, 0216T, 0228T, 0230T, 12001-12007, 12011-12057, 13100-13153, 36000, 36400-36410, 36420-36430, 36440, 36600, 36640, 37202, 43752, 51701-51703, 57410, 58700-58720, 59150, 59866, 62310-62319, 64400-64435, 64445-64450, 64479, 64483, 64490, 64493, 64505-64530, 69990, 93000-93010, 93040-93042, 93318, 94002, 94200, 94250, 94680-94690, 94770, 95812-95816, 95819, 95822, 95829, 95955, 96360, 96365, 96372, 96374-96376, 99148-99149, 99150

Note: These CCI edits are used for Medicare. Other payers may reimburse on codes listed above.

Medicare Edits

	Fac RVU	Non-Fac RVU	FUD	Status
59151	22.53	22.53	90	A

	MUE			Modifiers	
59151	1	51	N/A	N/A	80

* with documentation

Medicare References: 100-3,230.3

59160

59160 Curettage, postpartum

The physician scrapes the endometrial lining of the uterus following childbirth

Postpartum uterus

Curette

Uterus

Endometrial lining

Curette

Explanation

The physician scrapes the endometrial lining of the uterus following childbirth. The physician passes a curette through the cervix and endocervical canal, and into the uterus. Due to the large, soft postpartum uterus that is especially susceptible to perforation, a large blunt curette, also known as a "banjo" curette, is preferable to the suction curette. The physician gently scrapes the endometrial lining of the uterus to control bleeding, treat obstetric lacerations, or remove any remaining placental tissue.

Coding Tips

Because the postpartum uterus has been previously dilated during delivery of the newborn, dilation is not required for this surgery. This code is only to be used for postpartum curettage. For dilation and curettage, diagnostic and/or therapeutic (nonobstetrical), see 58120.

ICD-9-CM Procedural

69.02 Dilation and curettage following delivery or abortion
69.52 Aspiration curettage following delivery or abortion

Anesthesia

59160 00940

ICD-9-CM Diagnostic

666.00 Third-stage postpartum hemorrhage, unspecified as to episode of care

666.02 Third-stage postpartum hemorrhage, with delivery
666.04 Third-stage postpartum hemorrhage, postpartum condition or complication
666.10 Other immediate postpartum hemorrhage, unspecified as to episode of care
666.12 Other immediate postpartum hemorrhage, with delivery
666.14 Other immediate postpartum hemorrhage, postpartum condition or complication
666.20 Delayed and secondary postpartum hemorrhage, unspecified as to episode of care
666.22 Delayed and secondary postpartum hemorrhage, with delivery
666.24 Delayed and secondary postpartum hemorrhage, postpartum condition or complication
666.30 Postpartum coagulation defects, unspecified as to episode of care
666.32 Postpartum coagulation defects, with delivery
666.34 Postpartum coagulation defects, postpartum condition or complication
667.00 Retained placenta without hemorrhage, unspecified as to episode of care
667.02 Retained placenta without hemorrhage, with delivery, with mention of postpartum complication
667.04 Retained placenta without hemorrhage, postpartum condition or complication
667.10 Retained portions of placenta or membranes, without hemorrhage, unspecified as to episode of care
667.12 Retained portions of placenta or membranes, without hemorrhage, delivered, with mention of postpartum complication
667.14 Retained portions of placenta or membranes, without hemorrhage, postpartum condition or complication

Terms To Know

curettage. Removal of tissue by scraping.

hemorrhage. Internal or external bleeding with loss of significant amounts of blood.

postpartum. Period of time following childbirth.

CCI Version 18.3

0213T, 0216T, 0228T, 0230T, 12001-12007, 12011-12057, 13100-13153, 36000, 36400-36410, 36420-36430, 36440, 36600, 36640, 37202, 43752, 51701-51703, 57410, 59856-59857❖, 62310-62319, 64400-64435, 64445-64450, 64479, 64483, 64490, 64493, 64505-64530, 69990, 93000-93010, 93040-93042, 93318, 94002, 94200, 94250, 94680-94690, 94770, 95812-95816, 95819, 95822, 95829, 95955, 96360, 96365, 96372, 96374-96376, 99148-99149, 99150, J2001

Note: These CCI edits are used for Medicare. Other payers may reimburse on codes listed above.

Medicare Edits

	Fac RVU	Non-Fac RVU	FUD	Status
59160	5.26	6.19	10	A

	MUE		Modifiers		
59160	1	51	N/A	N/A	80*

* with documentation

Medicare References: None

Coding Companion for Ob/Gyn

59200

59200 Insertion of cervical dilator (eg, laminaria, prostaglandin) (separate procedure)

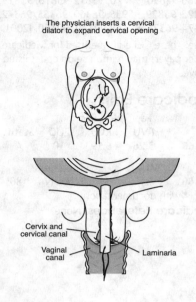

The physician inserts a cervical dilator to expand cervical opening

Cervix and cervical canal

Vaginal canal

Laminaria

Explanation

The physician inserts a cervical dilator, such as a laminaria or prostaglandin, into the endocervix to chemically stimulate and dilate the cervical canal. Using a speculum, the physician views the cervix then uses a tool to grasp it and pull it down. A laminaria, which is a sterile applicator made of kelp or synthetic material, may be placed in the cervical canal where it absorbs moisture, swells, and gradually dilates the cervix prior to inducing labor. Or the physician may insert prostaglandin in the form of gel or suppositories into the cervix in order to prime it six to 12 hours before induction.

Coding Tips

This separate procedure by definition is usually a component of a more complex service and is not identified separately. When performed alone or with other unrelated procedures/services it may be reported. If performed alone, list the code; if performed with other procedures/services, list the code and append modifier 59. For introduction of a hypertonic solution and/or prostaglandin to initiate labor, see 59850–59857.

ICD-9-CM Procedural

69.93   Insertion of laminaria
73.1   Other surgical induction of labor

Anesthesia

59200   00940

ICD-9-CM Diagnostic

645.11   Post term pregnancy, delivered, with or without mention of antepartum condition
645.13   Post term pregnancy, antepartum condition or complication
645.21   Prolonged pregnancy, delivered, with or without mention of antepartum condition
645.23   Prolonged pregnancy, antepartum condition or complication
656.40   Intrauterine death affecting management of mother, unspecified as to episode of care
656.41   Intrauterine death affecting management of mother, delivered
656.43   Intrauterine death affecting management of mother, antepartum
658.10   Premature rupture of membranes in pregnancy, unspecified as to episode of care
658.11   Premature rupture of membranes in pregnancy, delivered
658.13   Premature rupture of membranes in pregnancy, antepartum
658.20   Delayed delivery after spontaneous or unspecified rupture of membranes, unspecified as to episode of care
658.21   Delayed delivery after spontaneous or unspecified rupture of membranes, delivered
658.23   Delayed delivery after spontaneous or unspecified rupture of membranes, antepartum
658.30   Delayed delivery after artificial rupture of membranes, unspecified as to episode of care
658.31   Delayed delivery after artificial rupture of membranes, delivered
658.33   Delayed delivery after artificial rupture of membranes, antepartum
658.90   Unspecified problem associated with amniotic cavity and membranes, unspecified as to episode of care
658.91   Unspecified problem associated with amniotic cavity and membranes, delivered
658.93   Unspecified problem associated with amniotic cavity and membranes, antepartum
659.10   Failed medical or unspecified induction of labor, unspecified as to episode of care
659.11   Failed medical or unspecified induction of labor, delivered
659.13   Failed medical or unspecified induction of labor, antepartum
661.00   Primary uterine inertia, unspecified as to episode of care
661.01   Primary uterine inertia, with delivery
661.03   Primary uterine inertia, antepartum
661.10   Secondary uterine inertia, unspecified as to episode of care
661.13   Secondary uterine inertia, antepartum
661.20   Other and unspecified uterine inertia, unspecified as to episode of care
661.23   Other and unspecified uterine inertia, antepartum
661.40   Hypertonic, incoordinate, or prolonged uterine contractions, unspecified as to episode of care
661.41   Hypertonic, incoordinate, or prolonged uterine contractions, with delivery
661.43   Hypertonic, incoordinate, or prolonged uterine contractions, antepartum
661.90   Unspecified abnormality of labor, unspecified as to episode of care
661.91   Unspecified abnormality of labor, with delivery
661.93   Unspecified abnormality of labor, antepartum
662.00   Prolonged first stage of labor, unspecified as to episode of care
662.03   Prolonged first stage of labor, antepartum

CCI Version 18.3

0213T, 0216T, 0228T, 0230T, 12001-12007, 12011-12057, 13100-13153, 36000, 36400-36410, 36420-36430, 36440, 36600, 36640, 37202, 43752, 51701-51703, 57410, 62310-62319, 64400-64435, 64445-64450, 64479, 64483, 64490, 64493, 64505-64530, 69990, 93000-93010, 93040-93042, 93318, 94002, 94200, 94250, 94680-94690, 94770, 95812-95816, 95819, 95822, 95829, 95955, 96360, 96365, 96372, 96374-96376, 99148-99149, 99150, J2001

Note: These CCI edits are used for Medicare. Other payers may reimburse on codes listed above.

Medicare Edits

	Fac RVU	Non-Fac RVU	FUD	Status
59200	1.36	2.19	0	A

	MUE		Modifiers		
59200	1	51	N/A	N/A	N/A

* with documentation

Medicare References: None

59300

59300 Episiotomy or vaginal repair, by other than attending

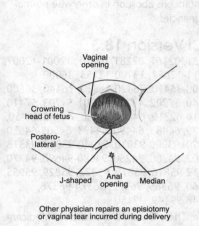

Other physician repairs an episiotomy or vaginal tear incurred during delivery

Explanation

A qualified health care provider, other than the provider who performed the delivery, repairs an episiotomy, vaginal tear, or laceration using sutures.

Coding Tips

This code has been revised for 2013 in the official CPT description. This code is for use by the (non-attending) provider only. For tracheloplasty, see 57700. Local anesthesia is included in this service. However, this procedure may be performed under general anesthesia, depending on the age and/or condition of the patient. Surgical trays, A4550, are not separately reimbursed by Medicare; however, other third-party payers may cover them. Check with the specific payer to determine coverage.

ICD-9-CM Procedural

73.6 Episiotomy
75.69 Repair of other current obstetric laceration

Anesthesia

59300 00940

ICD-9-CM Diagnostic

664.01 First-degree perineal laceration, with delivery
664.04 First-degree perineal laceration, postpartum condition or complication
664.11 Second-degree perineal laceration, with delivery
664.14 Second-degree perineal laceration, postpartum condition or complication
664.21 Third-degree perineal laceration, with delivery
664.24 Third-degree perineal laceration, postpartum condition or complication
664.31 Fourth-degree perineal laceration, with delivery
664.34 Fourth-degree perineal laceration, postpartum condition or complication
664.41 Unspecified perineal laceration, with delivery
664.44 Unspecified perineal laceration, postpartum condition or complication
665.41 High vaginal laceration, with delivery
665.44 High vaginal laceration, postpartum condition or complication

Terms To Know

delivery trauma. Perineal tears are classified by degree of tissue involvement, with or without an episiotomy: first-degree lacerations are superficial and involve vaginal mucosa and perineal skin in the fourchette; second-degree lacerations involve the pelvic floor and muscles; third-degree lacerations affect the anal sphincter; fourth-degree lacerations extend to the anal or rectal mucosa.

episiotomy. Deliberate incision in the perineal tissue to facilitate delivery of the fetus and avoid traumatic tearing. In a midline or median episiotomy, the incision is made from the vagina straight down toward the anus. In a mediolateral episiotomy, the incision slants to one side.

incision. Act of cutting into tissue or an organ.

laceration. Tearing injury; a torn, ragged-edged wound.

perineal. Pertaining to the pelvic floor area between the thighs; the diamond-shaped area bordered by the pubic symphysis in front, the ischial tuberosities on the sides, and the coccyx in back.

repair. Surgical closure of a wound. The wound may be a result of injury/trauma or it may be a surgically created defect. Repairs are divided into three categories: simple, intermediate, and complex.

CCI Version 18.3

0213T, 0216T, 0228T, 0230T, 12001-12007, 12011-12057, 13100-13153, 36000, 36400-36410, 36420-36430, 36440, 36600, 36640, 37202, 43752, 51701-51703, 57410, 62310-62319, 64400-64435, 64445-64450, 64479, 64483, 64490, 64493, 64505-64530, 69990, 93000-93010, 93040-93042, 93318, 94002, 94200, 94250, 94680-94690, 94770, 95812-95816, 95819, 95822, 95829, 95955, 96360, 96365, 96372, 96374-96376, 99148-99149, 99150, J0670, J2001

Note: These CCI edits are used for Medicare. Other payers may reimburse on codes listed above.

Medicare Edits

	Fac RVU	Non-Fac RVU	FUD	Status
59300	4.45	5.78	0	A

	MUE		Modifiers			
59300	1		51	N/A	N/A	80*

* with documentation

Medicare References: None

Coding Companion for Ob/Gyn

59320

59320 Cerclage of cervix, during pregnancy; vaginal

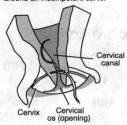

Using a vaginal approach, the physician threads and tightens suture material around an incompetent cervix

Cervical canal

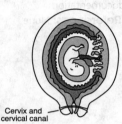

Cervix

Cervical os (opening)

Cervix and cervical canal

Explanation

The physician threads suture material or wraps banding around the cervix to close an incompetent cervix. An incompetent cervix is one that dilates during the second trimester and will eventually allow the pregnancy to fall out. After inserting a speculum into the vagina to view the cervix, heavy suture material or wire is threaded around the cervix using purse-string sutures. The sutures are pulled tight to make the opening smaller and prevent spontaneous abortion.

Coding Tips

For cerclage of cervix, during pregnancy, abdominal, see 59325. For nonobstetric cerclage, see 57700.

ICD-9-CM Procedural

67.51   Transabdominal cerclage of cervix

67.59   Other repair of cervical os

Anesthesia

59320   00948

ICD-9-CM Diagnostic

622.3   Old laceration of cervix

654.50 Cervical incompetence, unspecified as to episode of care in pregnancy — (Code first any associated obstructed labor, 660.2)

654.53 Cervical incompetence, antepartum condition or complication — (Code

first any associated obstructed labor, 660.2)

654.60 Other congenital or acquired abnormality of cervix, unspecified as to episode of care in pregnancy — (Code first any associated obstructed labor, 660.2)

654.63 Other congenital or acquired abnormality of cervix, antepartum condition or complication — (Code first any associated obstructed labor, 660.2)

654.90 Other and unspecified abnormality of organs and soft tissues of pelvis, unspecified as to episode of care in pregnancy — (Code first any associated obstructed labor, 660.2)

654.93 Other and unspecified abnormality of organs and soft tissues of pelvis, antepartum condition or complication — (Code first any associated obstructed labor, 660.2)

V23.2   Pregnancy with history of abortion

V23.81 Supervision of high-risk pregnancy of elderly primigravida

V23.82 Supervision of high-risk pregnancy of elderly multigravida

V23.83 Supervision of high-risk pregnancy of young primigravida

V23.84 Supervision of high-risk pregnancy of young multigravida

V23.89 Supervision of other high-risk pregnancy

Terms To Know

cerclage. Looping or encircling an organ or tissue with wire or ligature for positional support.

elderly primigravida. Woman in her first pregnancy at an age beyond the norm, usually considered 35 years or older.

internal os. Opening through the cervix into the uterus.

McDonald operation. Surgical procedure in which the opening of the cervix is decreased via pursestring sutures around the bottom of the cervix.

multigravida. Female who has had two or more pregnancies. Women in this category are considered to be at high risk during pregnancy.

obstetric cerclage. Surgical procedure that encircles an incompetent cervix with suture material for support in an attempt to retain a pregnancy, usually performed between 12 and 14 weeks' gestation and often employed in patients with a history of spontaneous abortion in otherwise normal pregnancies.

CCI Version 18.3

0213T, 0216T, 0228T, 0230T, 12001-12007, 12011-12057, 13100-13153, 36000, 36400-36410, 36420-36430, 36440, 36600, 36640, 37202, 43752, 51701-51703, 57410, 62310-62319, 64400-64435, 64445-64450, 64479, 64483, 64490, 64493, 64505-64530, 69990, 93000-93010, 93040-93042, 93318, 94002, 94200, 94250, 94680-94690, 94770, 95812-95816, 95819, 95822, 95829, 95955, 96360, 96365, 96372, 96374-96376, 99148-99149, 99150

Note: These CCI edits are used for Medicare. Other payers may reimburse on codes listed above.

Medicare Edits

	Fac RVU	Non-Fac RVU	FUD	Status
59320	4.59	4.59	0	A

	MUE		Modifiers		
59320	1	51	N/A	N/A	80*

* with documentation

Medicare References: None

59325

59325 Cerclage of cervix, during pregnancy; abdominal

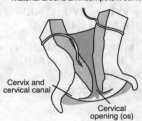

Using an abdominal surgical approach, the physician wraps and tightens banding material around an incompetent cervix

Cervix and cervical canal

Cervical opening (os)

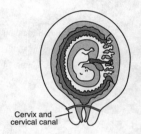

Cervix and cervical canal

Explanation

Through a small abdominal incision just above the pubic hairline, the physician places a band around the cervix at the level of the internal os (opening) to make the cervical opening smaller and prevent spontaneous abortion from an incompetent cervix. An incompetent cervix is one that dilates during the second trimester and will eventually allow the pregnancy to fall out. The abdominal incision is then closed with sutures.

Coding Tips

Intra-abdominal cerclage is rare and only indicated in such instances as traumatic cervical laceration, congenital shortening of the cervix, previous failed vaginal cerclage, and advanced cervical effacement. For vaginal cerclage of the cervix during pregnancy, see 59320. For nonobstetric cerclage, see 57700.

ICD-9-CM Procedural

67.51 Transabdominal cerclage of cervix

Anesthesia

59325 00840

ICD-9-CM Diagnostic

622.3 Old laceration of cervix

654.50 Cervical incompetence, unspecified as to episode of care in pregnancy — (Code first any associated obstructed labor, 660.2)

654.53 Cervical incompetence, antepartum condition or complication — (Code first any associated obstructed labor, 660.2)

654.60 Other congenital or acquired abnormality of cervix, unspecified as to episode of care in pregnancy — (Code first any associated obstructed labor, 660.2)

654.63 Other congenital or acquired abnormality of cervix, antepartum condition or complication — (Code first any associated obstructed labor, 660.2)

654.90 Other and unspecified abnormality of organs and soft tissues of pelvis, unspecified as to episode of care in pregnancy — (Code first any associated obstructed labor, 660.2)

654.93 Other and unspecified abnormality of organs and soft tissues of pelvis, antepartum condition or complication — (Code first any associated obstructed labor, 660.2)

V23.2 Pregnancy with history of abortion

V23.81 Supervision of high-risk pregnancy of elderly primigravida

V23.82 Supervision of high-risk pregnancy of elderly multigravida

V23.83 Supervision of high-risk pregnancy of young primigravida

V23.84 Supervision of high-risk pregnancy of young multigravida

V23.89 Supervision of other high-risk pregnancy

Terms To Know

cerclage. Looping or encircling an organ or tissue with wire or ligature for positional support.

elderly primigravida. Woman in her first pregnancy at an age beyond the norm, usually considered 35 years or older.

internal os. Opening through the cervix into the uterus.

McDonald operation. Surgical procedure in which the opening of the cervix is decreased via pursestring sutures around the bottom of the cervix.

multigravida. Female who has had two or more pregnancies. Women in this category are considered to be at high risk during pregnancy.

obstetric cerclage. Surgical procedure that encircles an incompetent cervix with suture material for support in an attempt to retain a pregnancy, usually performed between 12 and 14 weeks' gestation and often employed in patients with a history of spontaneous abortion in otherwise normal pregnancies.

CCI Version 18.3

0213T, 0216T, 0228T, 0230T, 12001-12007, 12011-12057, 13100-13153, 36000, 36400-36410, 36420-36430, 36440, 36600, 36640, 37202, 43752, 44005, 44180, 44602-44605, 44820-44850, 49000-49010, 49255, 49320, 49570, 51701-51703, 57410, 62310-62319, 64400-64435, 64445-64450, 64479, 64483, 64490, 64493, 64505-64530, 69990, 93000-93010, 93040-93042, 93318, 94002, 94200, 94250, 94680-94690, 94770, 95812-95816, 95819, 95822, 95829, 95955, 96360, 96365, 96372, 96374-96376, 99148-99149, 99150

Note: These CCI edits are used for Medicare. Other payers may reimburse on codes listed above.

Medicare Edits

	Fac RVU	Non-Fac RVU	FUD	Status
59325	6.45	6.45	0	A

	MUE		Modifiers		
59325	1	51	N/A	N/A	80*

* with documentation

Medicare References: None

59350

59350 Hysterorrhaphy of ruptured uterus

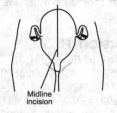

The physician uses layered sutures to repair a uterus ruptured or lacerated during pregnancy

Midline incision

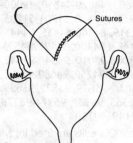

Sutures

Explanation

The physician repairs a uterus that is lacerated or ruptured during pregnancy. A large incision is made in the abdomen and the uterus is sutured in layers. The abdominal incision is closed with sutures.

Coding Tips

For nonobstetric hysterorrhaphy, see 58520. For hysteroplasty, repair of uterine anomaly, see 58540.

ICD-9-CM Procedural

69.41   Suture of laceration of uterus

75.50   Repair of current obstetric laceration of uterus, not otherwise specified

75.52   Repair of current obstetric laceration of corpus uteri

Anesthesia

59350   00840

ICD-9-CM Diagnostic

654.20 Previous cesarean delivery, unspecified as to episode of care or not applicable — (Code first any associated obstructed labor, 660.2)

654.21 Previous cesarean delivery, delivered, with or without mention of antepartum condition — (Code first any associated obstructed labor, 660.2)

654.23 Previous cesarean delivery, antepartum condition or complication

— (Code first any associated obstructed labor, 660.2)

665.00 Rupture of uterus before onset of labor, unspecified as to episode of care

665.01 Rupture of uterus before onset of labor, with delivery

665.03 Rupture of uterus before onset of labor, antepartum

665.10 Rupture of uterus during labor, unspecified as to episode

665.11 Rupture of uterus during labor, with delivery

Terms To Know

delivery. Expulsion or extraction of a child and the afterbirth.

incision. Act of cutting into tissue or an organ.

laceration. Tearing injury; a torn, ragged-edged wound.

repair. Surgical closure of a wound. The wound may be a result of injury/trauma or it may be a surgically created defect. Repairs are divided into three categories: simple, intermediate, and complex.

rupture. Tearing or breaking open of tissue.

suture. Numerous stitching techniques employed in wound closure: 1) Buried suture: Continuous or interrupted suture placed under the skin for a layered closure. 2) Continuous suture: Running stitch with tension evenly distributed across a single strand to provide a leakproof closure line. 3) Interrupted suture: Series of single stitches with tension isolated at each stitch, in which all stitches are not affected if one becomes loose, and the isolated sutures cannot act as a wick to transport an infection. 4) Purse-string suture: Continuous suture placed around a tubular structure and tightened, to reduce or close the lumen. 5) Retention suture: Secondary stitching that bridges the primary suture, providing support for the primary repair; a plastic or rubber bolster may be placed over the primary repair and under the retention sutures.

CCI Version 18.3

0213T, 0216T, 0228T, 0230T, 12001-12007, 12011-12057, 13100-13153, 36000, 36400-36410, 36420-36430, 36440, 36600, 36640, 37202, 43752, 44005, 44180, 44602-44605, 44820-44850, 49000-49010, 49255, 49320, 49570, 51701-51703, 57410, 59866, 62310-62319, 64400-64435, 64445-64450, 64479, 64483, 64490, 64493, 64505-64530, 69990, 93000-93010, 93040-93042, 93318, 94002, 94200, 94250, 94680-94690, 94770, 95812-95816, 95819,

95822, 95829, 95955, 96360, 96365, 96372, 96374-96376, 99148-99149, 99150

Note: These CCI edits are used for Medicare. Other payers may reimburse on codes listed above.

Medicare Edits

	Fac RVU	Non-Fac RVU	FUD	Status
59350	8.45	8.45	0	A

	MUE				Modifiers	
59350	1	51	N/A	N/A	80	

* with documentation

Medicare References: None

59400

59400 Routine obstetric care including antepartum care, vaginal delivery (with or without episiotomy, and/or forceps) and postpartum care

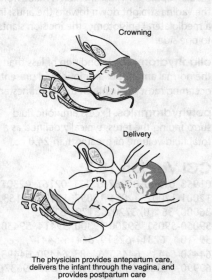

Crowning

Delivery

The physician provides antepartum care, delivers the infant through the vagina, and provides postpartum care

Explanation

The physician delivers an infant and placenta through the uterus and vagina. The physician may elect to assist the delivery with the use of forceps, vacuum extraction, or rupture of membranes. The physician may also elect to do an episiotomy, which is an incision in the perineum to widen the external opening. Episiotomy and laceration repair are included as well. This procedure covers both antepartum and postpartum care. Antepartum or prenatal care includes the initial and subsequent histories, physical examinations, recording of weight, blood pressures, fetal heart tones, and routine chemical urinalysis. It includes monthly visits up to 28 weeks gestation, biweekly visits to 36 weeks gestation, and weekly visits until delivery. Postpartum care includes hospital and office visits following delivery.

Coding Tips

Note that 59400 includes total OB care; if services provided do not match the code description of total OB care, use the appropriate stand-alone code (e.g., antepartum care, 59425–59426). If care rendered was less than the listed service (i.e., the one that most closely describes the service performed), append modifier 52 and reduce the cost of the service. See notes in CPT for directions in the use of the maternity care and delivery codes. For vaginal delivery only,

without antepartum or postpartum care, see 59409. For vaginal delivery only, including postpartum care, see 59410. For cesarean delivery, including antepartum and postpartum care, see 59510.

ICD-9-CM Procedural

72.0	Low forceps operation
72.1	Low forceps operation with episiotomy
72.21	Mid forceps operation with episiotomy
72.29	Other mid forceps operation
72.31	High forceps operation with episiotomy
72.39	Other high forceps operation
72.4	Forceps rotation of fetal head
72.51	Partial breech extraction with forceps to aftercoming head
72.52	Other partial breech extraction
72.53	Total breech extraction with forceps to aftercoming head
72.54	Other total breech extraction
72.6	Forceps application to aftercoming head
72.71	Vacuum extraction with episiotomy
72.79	Other vacuum extraction
72.8	Other specified instrumental delivery
72.9	Unspecified instrumental delivery
73.01	Induction of labor by artificial rupture of membranes
73.09	Other artificial rupture of membranes
73.4	Medical induction of labor
73.59	Other manually assisted delivery
73.6	Episiotomy

Anesthesia

59400 01967

ICD-9-CM Diagnostic

The application of this code is too broad to adequately present ICD-9-CM diagnostic code links here. Refer to your ICD-9-CM book.

Terms To Know

eclampsia. Tetany and toxemia producing seizure activity or coma in a pregnant patient who most often has presented with prior preeclampsia (i.e., hypertension, albuminuria, and edema).

elderly primigravida. Woman in her first pregnancy at an age beyond the norm, usually considered 35 years or older.

episiotomy. Deliberate incision in the perineal tissue to facilitate delivery of the fetus and avoid traumatic tearing. In a midline or median episiotomy, the incision is made from the vagina straight down toward the anus. In a mediolateral episiotomy, the incision slants to one side.

multigravida. Female who has had two or more pregnancies. Women in this category are considered to be at high risk during pregnancy.

placenta previa. Implantation of the placenta in the lower segment of the uterus, over or near the internal cervical os. In total previa, the cervical os is completely covered by the placenta; in partial previa, only a portion is covered.

preeclampsia. Complication of pregnancy manifesting in the development of borderline hypertension, protein in the urine, and unresponsive swelling between the 20th week of pregnancy and the end of the first week following birth in mild to moderate cases. Severe preeclampsia presents with hypertension (blood pressure greater than 150/100), associated with marked swelling, proteinuria, abdominal pain, and/or visual changes.

CCI Version 18.3

01958, 01960, 01967, 0213T, 0216T, 0230T, 12001-12007, 12011-12057, 13100-13153, 36000, 36410, 37202, 51701-51702, 57720, 58800, 59050-59051, 59200-59300, 59414, 59610❖, 62311-62319, 64415-64417, 64430-64435, 64450, 64483, 64490, 64493, 69990, 81000, 81002, 96360, 96365, 96372, 96374-96376, 99201-99239, 99304-99310, 99315-99318, 99324-99328, 99334-99337, 99341-99350

Note: These CCI edits are used for Medicare. Other payers may reimburse on codes listed above.

Medicare Edits

	Fac RVU	Non-Fac RVU	FUD	Status
59400	62.3	62.3	N/A	A

	MUE		Modifiers		
59400	1	51	N/A	N/A	N/A

* with documentation

Medicare References: 100-2,15,20.1; 100-2,15,180

Coding Companion for Ob/Gyn

59409-59410

59409 Vaginal delivery only (with or without episiotomy and/or forceps);

59410 including postpartum care

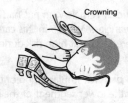
Crowning

The physician delivers the infant through the vagina

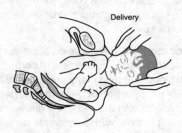
Delivery

59409 includes only delivery; 59410 includes delivery and postpartum care

Explanation

The physician delivers an infant and placenta through the uterus and vagina. The physician may elect to assist the delivery with the use of forceps, vacuum extraction, or rupture of membranes. The physician may also elect to do an episiotomy, which is an incision in the perineum to widen the external opening. Episiotomy and laceration repair are included as well. Code 59409 represents the vaginal delivery only and does not include antepartum or postpartum care. Code 59410 covers the vaginal delivery with postpartum care, which includes hospital and office visits following delivery.

Coding Tips

If services provided do not match the code description of vaginal delivery only (59409) or vaginal delivery with postpartum care (59410), use the appropriate stand-alone code (e.g., postpartum care only, 59430, or total OB care, 59400). If care rendered was less than the listed service (i.e., the one that most closely describes the service performed), append modifier 52 and reduce the cost of the service. See notes in CPT for directions on the use of the maternity care and delivery codes. For a vaginal delivery with routine obstetric care including antepartum and postpartum care, see 59400. For cesarean delivery only, see 59514. For cesarean delivery including postpartum care, see 59515. For vaginal delivery after previous cesarean section, see 59610–59614.

ICD-9-CM Procedural

72.0	Low forceps operation
72.1	Low forceps operation with episiotomy
72.21	Mid forceps operation with episiotomy
72.29	Other mid forceps operation
72.31	High forceps operation with episiotomy
72.39	Other high forceps operation
72.4	Forceps rotation of fetal head
72.51	Partial breech extraction with forceps to aftercoming head
72.52	Other partial breech extraction
72.53	Total breech extraction with forceps to aftercoming head
72.54	Other total breech extraction
72.6	Forceps application to aftercoming head
72.71	Vacuum extraction with episiotomy
72.79	Other vacuum extraction
72.8	Other specified instrumental delivery
72.9	Unspecified instrumental delivery
73.01	Induction of labor by artificial rupture of membranes
73.09	Other artificial rupture of membranes
73.4	Medical induction of labor
73.59	Other manually assisted delivery
73.6	Episiotomy

Anesthesia

59409 01960, 01967
59410 01967

ICD-9-CM Diagnostic

The application of this code is too broad to adequately present ICD-9-CM diagnostic code links here. Refer to your ICD-9-CM book.

Terms To Know

delivery trauma. Perineal tears are classified by degree of tissue involvement, with or without an episiotomy: first-degree lacerations are superficial and involve vaginal mucosa and perineal skin in the fourchette; second-degree lacerations involve the pelvic floor and muscles; third-degree lacerations affect the anal sphincter; fourth-degree lacerations extend to the anal or rectal mucosa.

eclampsia. Tetany and toxemia producing seizure activity or coma in a pregnant patient who most often has presented with prior preeclampsia (i.e., hypertension, albuminuria, and edema).

elderly primigravida. Woman in her first pregnancy at an age beyond the norm, usually considered 35 years or older.

episiotomy. Deliberate incision in the perineal tissue to facilitate delivery of the fetus and avoid traumatic tearing. In a midline or median episiotomy, the incision is made from the vagina straight down toward the anus. In a mediolateral episiotomy, the incision slants to one side.

oligohydramnios. Condition of less than the normal amount of amniotic fluid present, occurring most frequently in the last trimester.

polyhydramnios. Excess amniotic fluid surrounding the fetus, typically defined as a total fluid volume of greater than 24.0 cc.

CCI Version 18.3

01958, 01960, 01967, 0213T, 0216T, 0230T, 12001-12007, 12011-12057, 13100-13153, 36000, 36410, 37202, 51701-51702, 59050-59051, 59200-59300, 59414, 59430, 59610❖, 62311-62319, 64415-64417, 64430-64435, 64450, 64483, 64490, 64493, 69990, 96360, 96365, 96372, 96374-96376

Also not with 59410: 57720, 59409, 99201-99239, 99304-99310, 99315-99318, 99324-99328, 99334-99337, 99341-99350

Note: These CCI edits are used for Medicare. Other payers may reimburse on codes listed above.

Medicare Edits

	Fac RVU	Non-Fac RVU	FUD	Status
59409	24.5	24.5	N/A	A
59410	31.14	31.14	N/A	A

	MUE		Modifiers		
59409	-	51	N/A	N/A	80*
59410	1	51	N/A	N/A	N/A

* with documentation

Medicare References: 100-2,15,20.1; 100-2,15,180

59412

59412 External cephalic version, with or without tocolysis

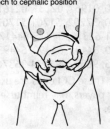

The physician turns the fetus from breech to cephalic position

Explanation

The physician turns the fetus from a breech presenting position to a cephalic presenting position. External cephalic version is performed by manipulating the fetus from the outside of the abdominal wall. The physician places both hands on the patient's abdomen and locates each pole of the fetus by palpation. The fetus is shifted so that the breech or rear end of the fetus is moved upward and the head downward. The physician may elect to use tocolytic drug therapy to suppress uterine contractions during the manipulation.

Coding Tips

This code may be used for manipulation prior to or during delivery. It may be reported in addition to any of the delivery codes (59400–59622). Procedure 59412 has not been designated in CPT as an "add-on" code or exempt from modifier 51. However, this procedure is not billed as a stand-alone service and it is recommended that it be reported using "add-on" reporting guidelines when the same physician performs the service/procedure on the same date of service as other related services/procedures.

ICD-9-CM Procedural

73.21 Internal and combined version without extraction

73.22 Internal and combined version with extraction

73.51 Manual rotation of fetal head

73.59 Other manually assisted delivery

73.91 External version to assist delivery

Anesthesia

59412 01958

ICD-9-CM Diagnostic

652.10 Breech or other malpresentation successfully converted to cephalic presentation, unspecified as to episode of care — (Code first any associated obstructed labor, 660.0)

652.11 Breech or other malpresentation successfully converted to cephalic presentation, delivered — (Code first any associated obstructed labor, 660.0)

652.13 Breech or other malpresentation successfully converted to cephalic presentation, antepartum — (Code first any associated obstructed labor, 660.0)

652.21 Breech presentation without mention of version, delivered — (Code first any associated obstructed labor, 660.0)

652.23 Breech presentation without mention of version, antepartum — (Code first any associated obstructed labor, 660.0)

Terms To Know

breech presentation. Abnormal condition in which the fetal buttocks present first. In frank breech, the legs of the fetus extend over the abdomen and thorax so that the feet lie beside the face. In complete breech, the legs are flexed and crossed, while incomplete breech presents with one or both lower legs and feet prolapsed into the vagina.

cephalad. Toward the head.

tocolytic. Drug administered during pregnancy in order to relax the uterus and reduce or halt contractions, administered primarily to stop premature labor.

CCI Version 18.3

01958, 01960, 01967, 0213T, 0216T, 0230T, 36000, 36410, 37202, 51701-51702, 62311-62319, 64415-64417, 64430-64435, 64450, 64483, 64490, 64493, 69990, 96360, 96365, 96372, 96374-96376

Note: These CCI edits are used for Medicare. Other payers may reimburse on codes listed above.

Medicare Edits

	Fac RVU	Non-Fac RVU	FUD	Status
59412	3.12	3.12	N/A	A

	MUE		Modifiers			
59412	2	N/A	N/A	N/A	N/A	80*

* with documentation

Medicare References: None

59414

59414   Delivery of placenta (separate procedure)

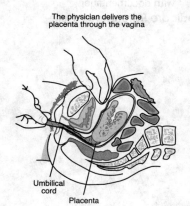

The physician delivers the placenta through the vagina

Umbilical cord

Placenta

Explanation

The physician removes a retained placenta following delivery of the fetus, usually unattended, and after separation of the placenta from its intrauterine attachment. The physician places abdominal pressure just above the symphysis to elevate the uterus into the abdomen and prevent inversion of the uterus. This also helps move the placenta downward into the vagina. The umbilical cord is very gently pulled to help guide the placenta out of the birth canal. If the placenta cannot be removed by this technique or there is brisk bleeding, manual removal of the placenta may be indicated. Manual removal requires adequate analgesia or anesthesia. It is accomplished by grasping the fundus of the uterus with a hand on the abdomen. The other hand, wearing an elbow-length glove, is passed through the vagina into the uterus to separate the placenta and remove it.

Coding Tips

This separate procedure by definition is usually a component of a more complex service and is not identified separately. When performed alone or with other unrelated procedures/services it may be reported. If performed alone, list the code; if performed with other procedures/services, list the code and append modifier 59. Complications (e.g., control of hemorrhage) are not included in 59414 and are reported separately. For postpartum curettage, see 59160.

ICD-9-CM Procedural

73.59   Other manually assisted delivery

75.4   Manual removal of retained placenta

Anesthesia

59414   00940

ICD-9-CM Diagnostic

666.02   Third-stage postpartum hemorrhage, with delivery

666.04   Third-stage postpartum hemorrhage, postpartum condition or complication

666.22   Delayed and secondary postpartum hemorrhage, with delivery

666.24   Delayed and secondary postpartum hemorrhage, postpartum condition or complication

667.02   Retained placenta without hemorrhage, with delivery, with mention of postpartum complication

667.04   Retained placenta without hemorrhage, postpartum condition or complication

667.12   Retained portions of placenta or membranes, without hemorrhage, delivered, with mention of postpartum complication

667.14   Retained portions of placenta or membranes, without hemorrhage, postpartum condition or complication

V27.0   Outcome of delivery, single liveborn — (This code is intended for the coding of the outcome of delivery on the mother's record)

V27.1   Outcome of delivery, single stillborn — (This code is intended for the coding of the outcome of delivery on the mother's record)

V27.2   Outcome of delivery, twins, both liveborn — (This code is intended for the coding of the outcome of delivery on the mother's record)

V27.3   Outcome of delivery, twins, one liveborn and one stillborn — (This code is intended for the coding of the outcome of delivery on the mother's record)

V27.4   Outcome of delivery, twins, both stillborn — (This code is intended for the coding of the outcome of delivery on the mother's record)

Terms To Know

placenta. Temporary organ within the uterus during pregnancy, joining the mother and fetus. It is attached to the fetus via the umbilical cord and provides oxygen and nutrients and helps to eliminate carbon dioxide and waste through the selective exchange of soluble substances carried via the blood. The placenta is expelled from the uterus after the baby is delivered, and is then termed the afterbirth.

secundines. Placenta and membranes; the afterbirth.

CCI Version 18.3

01960, 01967, 0213T, 0216T, 0230T, 36000, 36410, 37202, 51701-51702, 59430, 62311-62319, 64415-64417, 64430-64435, 64450, 64483, 64490, 64493, 69990, 96360, 96365, 96372, 96374-96376

Note: These CCI edits are used for Medicare. Other payers may reimburse on codes listed above.

Medicare Edits

	Fac RVU	Non-Fac RVU	FUD	Status
59414	2.76	2.76	N/A	A

	MUE		Modifiers		
59414	1	51	N/A	N/A	80*

* with documentation

Medicare References: None

59425-59426

59425 Antepartum care only; 4-6 visits
59426   7 or more visits

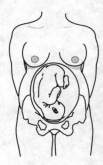

The physician provides antepartum care only

Explanation

Antepartum or prenatal care includes the initial and subsequent histories, physical examinations, recording of weight, blood pressures, fetal heart tones, and routine chemical urinalysis. It includes monthly visits up to 28 weeks gestation, biweekly visits to 36 weeks gestation, and weekly visits until delivery. 59425 includes four to six visits. 59426 covers seven or more visits.

Coding Tips

For one to three antepartum care visits, see the appropriate E/M code. Medical visits not related to maternity care, but within the antepartum time, may be reported separately.

ICD-9-CM Procedural

89.04   Other interview and evaluation
89.26   Gynecological examination

Anesthesia

N/A

ICD-9-CM Diagnostic

The application of this code is too broad to adequately present ICD-9-CM diagnostic code links here. Refer to your ICD-9-CM book.

Terms To Know

eclampsia. Tetany and toxemia producing seizure activity or coma in a pregnant patient who most often has presented with prior preeclampsia (i.e., hypertension, albuminuria, and edema). Eclampsia most commonly occurs during the third trimester or within the first 48 hours following birth.

elderly primigravida. Woman in her first pregnancy at an age beyond the norm, usually considered 35 years or older.

multigravida. Female who has had two or more pregnancies. Women in this category are considered to be at high risk during pregnancy.

oligohydramnios. Condition of less than the normal amount of amniotic fluid present, occurring most frequently in the last trimester.

placenta previa. Implantation of the placenta in the lower segment of the uterus, over or near the internal cervical os. In total previa, the cervical os is completely covered by the placenta; in partial previa, only a portion is covered.

polyhydramnios. Excess amniotic fluid surrounding the fetus, typically defined as a total fluid volume of greater than 24.0 cc.

preeclampsia. Complication of pregnancy manifesting in the development of borderline hypertension, protein in the urine, and unresponsive swelling between the 20th week of pregnancy and the end of the first week following birth in mild to moderate cases. Severe preeclampsia presents with hypertension, associated with marked swelling, proteinuria, abdominal pain, and/or visual changes.

CCI Version 18.3

0213T, 0216T, 36000, 36410, 37202, 59610❖, 62318-62319, 64415-64417, 64450, 64490, 64493, 69990, 81000, 81002, 96360, 96365, 96372, 96374-96376, 99201-99215

Also not with 59425: 59426❖

Note: These CCI edits are used for Medicare. Other payers may reimburse on codes listed above.

Medicare Edits

	Fac RVU	Non-Fac RVU	FUD	Status
59425	10.71	13.63	N/A	A
59426	18.89	24.38	N/A	A

	MUE				Modifiers
59425	1	N/A	N/A	N/A	80*
59426	1	N/A	N/A	N/A	80*

    * with documentation

Medicare References: 100-2,15,20.1; 100-2,15,180

Coding Companion for Ob/Gyn

59430

59430 Postpartum care only (separate procedure)

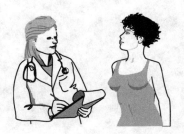

The physician provides postpartum care

Explanation

Postpartum care includes hospital and office visits following vaginal or cesarean section delivery.

Coding Tips

This separate procedure by definition is usually a component of a more complex service and is not identified separately. When performed alone or with other unrelated procedures/services it may be reported. If performed alone, list the code; if performed with other procedures/services, list the code and append modifier 59. If services provided do not match the code description of postpartum care only, use the appropriate stand-alone code (e.g., vaginal delivery with postpartum care, 59410, or total OB care, 59400). If care rendered was less than the listed service (i.e., the one that most closely describes the service performed), append modifier 52 and reduce the cost of the service. See notes in CPT for directions in the use of the maternity care and delivery codes. For antepartum care, four or more visits, see 59425 and 59426.

ICD-9-CM Procedural

89.04   Other interview and evaluation

89.26   Gynecological examination

Anesthesia

59430   N/A

ICD-9-CM Diagnostic

V24.0   Postpartum care and examination immediately after delivery

V24.1   Postpartum care and examination of lactating mother

V24.2   Routine postpartum follow-up

V72.31   Routine gynecological examination — (Use additional code(s) to identify any special screening examination(s) performed: V73.0-V82.9)

Terms To Know

cesarean section. Delivery of fetus by incision made in the upper part of the uterus, or corpus uteri, via an abdominal peritoneal approach when a vaginal delivery is not possible or advisable; often referred to as a classic c-section. Low cervical approach is a type of c-section by an incision in the lower segment of the uterus, either through a transperitoneal incision or extraperitoneally with the peritoneal fold being displaced upwards.

delivery. Expulsion or extraction of a child and the afterbirth.

postpartum. Period of time following childbirth.

CCI Version 18.3

0213T, 0216T, 36000, 36410, 37202, 49010, 62318-62319, 64415-64417, 64450, 64490, 64493, 69990, 96360, 96365, 96372, 96374-96376, 99201-99215

Note: These CCI edits are used for Medicare. Other payers may reimburse on codes listed above.

Medicare Edits

	Fac RVU	Non-Fac RVU	FUD	Status
59430	4.21	5.32	N/A	A

	MUE		Modifiers		
59430	1	51	N/A	N/A	N/A

* with documentation

Medicare References: 100-2,15,20.1; 100-2,15,180

59510

59510 Routine obstetric care including antepartum care, cesarean delivery, and postpartum care

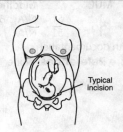

Typical incision

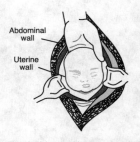

Abdominal wall

Uterine wall

The physician provides antepartum care, delivers the infant through an abdominal incision, and provides postpartum care

Explanation

The physician delivers an infant through a horizontal or vertical incision in the abdomen and uterus. Once the incisions are made, the infant is delivered and the placenta separated and removed. The uterine and abdominal incisions are closed with sutures. This procedure includes both antepartum and postpartum care. Antepartum or prenatal care includes the initial and subsequent histories, physical examinations, recording of weight, blood pressures, fetal heart tones, and routine chemical urinalysis. It includes monthly visits up to 28 weeks gestation, biweekly visits to 36 weeks gestation, and weekly visits until delivery. Postpartum care includes hospital and office visits following delivery.

Coding Tips

If services provided do not match the code description of cesarean delivery, including antepartum and postpartum care, use the appropriate stand-alone code (e.g., antepartum care, 59425–59426, or cesarean delivery only, 59514). If care rendered was less than the listed service (i.e., the one that most closely describes the service performed), append modifier 52 and reduce the cost of the service. See notes in CPT for directions in the use of the maternity care and delivery codes. For standby attendance for infant, see 99360. For cesarean delivery only, see 59514. For cesarean delivery including postpartum care, see 59515. Note that codes 59618–59622 report a cesarean delivery

following attempted vaginal delivery after a previous cesarean section.

ICD-9-CM Procedural

73.3	Failed forceps
74.0	Classical cesarean section
74.1	Low cervical cesarean section
74.2	Extraperitoneal cesarean section
74.4	Cesarean section of other specified type

Anesthesia

59510 01961, 01968

ICD-9-CM Diagnostic

The application of this code is too broad to adequately present ICD-9-CM diagnostic code links here. Refer to your ICD-9-CM book.

Terms To Know

elderly primigravida. Woman in her first pregnancy at an age beyond the norm, usually considered 35 years or older.

placenta previa. Implantation of the placenta in the lower segment of the uterus, over or near the internal cervical os. In total previa, the cervical os is completely covered by the placenta; in partial previa, only a portion is covered.

preeclampsia. Complication of pregnancy manifesting in the development of borderline hypertension, protein in the urine, and unresponsive swelling between the 20th week of pregnancy and the end of the first week following birth in mild to moderate cases. Severe preeclampsia presents with hypertension, associated with marked swelling, proteinuria, abdominal pain, and/or visual changes.

CCI Version 18.3

01958, 01961, 01968, 0213T, 0216T, 0230T, 12001-12007, 12011-12057, 13100-13153, 36000, 36410, 37202, 44005, 44180, 44602-44605, 44820-44850, 49000-49010, 49255, 49570, 51701-51702, 59050-59051, 59300, 59414, 59430, 62311-62319, 64415-64417, 64430-64435, 64450, 64483, 64490, 64493, 69990, 81000, 81002, 96360, 96365, 96372, 96374-96376, 99201-99239, 99304-99310, 99315-99318, 99324-99328, 99334-99337, 99341-99350

Note: These CCI edits are used for Medicare. Other payers may reimburse on codes listed above.

Medicare Edits

	Fac RVU	Non-Fac RVU	FUD	Status
59510	69.08	69.08	N/A	A

	MUE		Modifiers		
59510	1	51	N/A	N/A	N/A

* with documentation

Medicare References: None

59514-59515

59514 Cesarean delivery only;
59515   including postpartum care

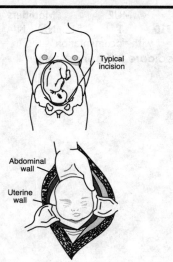

Typical incision

Abdominal wall

Uterine wall

The physician delivers the infant through an abdominal incision

59414 includes only delivery; 59415 includes delivery and postpartum care

Explanation

The physician delivers an infant through a horizontal or vertical incision in the abdomen and uterus. Once the incisions are made, the infant is delivered and the placenta separated and removed. The uterine and abdominal incisions are closed with sutures. Code 59514 represents the cesarean delivery only and does not include antepartum or postpartum care. Code 59515 covers the cesarean delivery with postpartum care, which includes hospital and office visits following delivery.

Coding Tips

If services provided do not match the code description of cesarean delivery only (59514) or cesarean delivery with postpartum care (59515), use the appropriate stand-alone code (e.g., antepartum care, 59425–59426, or total cesarean care, 59510). If care rendered was less than the listed service (i.e., the one that most closely describes the service performed), append modifier 52 and reduce the cost of the service. See notes in CPT for directions in the use of the maternity care and delivery codes. For cesarean delivery including antepartum and postpartum care, see 59510. For cesarean delivery following attempted vaginal delivery after a previous cesarean section, see 59618–59622.

ICD-9-CM Procedural

73.3   Failed forceps
74.0   Classical cesarean section
74.1   Low cervical cesarean section
74.2   Extraperitoneal cesarean section
74.4   Cesarean section of other specified type

Anesthesia
01961, 01968

ICD-9-CM Diagnostic

The application of this code is too broad to adequately present ICD-9-CM diagnostic code links here. Refer to your ICD-9-CM book.

Terms To Know

eclampsia. Tetany and toxemia producing seizure activity or coma in a pregnant patient who most often has presented with prior preeclampsia (i.e., hypertension, albuminuria, and edema). Eclampsia most commonly occurs during the third trimester or within the first 48 hours following birth.

multiparity. Condition of having had two or more pregnancies that resulted in viable fetuses; producing more than one fetus or offspring in the same gestation.

preeclampsia. Complication of pregnancy manifesting in the development of borderline hypertension, protein in the urine, and unresponsive swelling between the 20th week of pregnancy and the end of the first week following birth in mild to moderate cases. Severe preeclampsia presents with hypertension, associated with marked swelling, proteinuria, abdominal pain, and/or visual changes.

secundines. Placenta and membranes; the afterbirth.

CCI Version 18.3

01961, 01968, 0213T, 0216T, 0230T, 12001-12007, 12011-12057, 13100-13153, 36000, 36410, 37202, 44005, 44180, 44602-44605, 44820-44850, 49000-49010, 49255, 49570, 51701-51702, 59050-59051, 59300, 59414, 62311-62319, 64415-64417, 64430-64435, 64450, 64483, 64490, 64493, 69990, 96360, 96365, 96372, 96374-96376

Also not with 59514: 01958

Also not with 59515: 59430, 59514, 99201-99239, 99304-99310, 99315-99318, 99324-99328, 99334-99337, 99341-99350

Note: These CCI edits are used for Medicare. Other payers may reimburse on codes listed above.

Medicare Edits

	Fac RVU	Non-Fac RVU	FUD	Status
59514	27.67	27.67	N/A	A
59515	37.72	37.72	N/A	A

	MUE		Modifiers		
59514	1	51	N/A	62*	80
59515	1	51	N/A	N/A	N/A

* with documentation

Medicare References: None

59525

59525 Subtotal or total hysterectomy after cesarean delivery (List separately in addition to code for primary procedure)

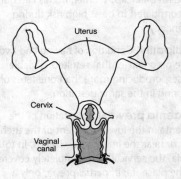

The physician removes the uterus, with or without removing the cervix, and leaving any combination of tubes and ovaries

Explanation

The physician performs a hysterectomy immediately following cesarean delivery. Through the abdominal incision, the physician clamps and cuts free the supporting pedicles containing the tubes, ligaments, and arteries. The uterus is removed and the physician may elect to remove the cervix as well. In a subtotal hysterectomy, just the uterus is removed. In a total hysterectomy, both the uterus and cervix are removed. The abdominal incision is closed with sutures.

Coding Tips

As an "add-on" code, 59525 is not subject to multiple procedure rules. No reimbursement reduction or modifier 51 is applied. "Add-on" codes describe additional intra-service work associated with the primary procedure. They are performed by the same physician on the same date of service as the primary service/procedure, and must never be reported as a stand-alone code. For total or subtotal abdominal hysterectomy not performed immediately following cesarean delivery, see 58150–58240. For physician standby attendance for cesarean/high risk delivery for newborn care, see 99360.

ICD-9-CM Procedural

68.39 Other and unspecified subtotal abdominal hysterectomy

68.49 Other and unspecified total abdominal hysterectomy

68.9 Other and unspecified hysterectomy

Anesthesia

59525 01963, 01969

ICD-9-CM Diagnostic

180.0 Malignant neoplasm of endocervix

180.1 Malignant neoplasm of exocervix

182.0 Malignant neoplasm of corpus uteri, except isthmus

182.8 Malignant neoplasm of other specified sites of body of uterus

183.2 Malignant neoplasm of fallopian tube

183.3 Malignant neoplasm of broad ligament of uterus

183.4 Malignant neoplasm of parametrium of uterus

614.7 Other chronic pelvic peritonitis, female — (Use additional code to identify organism: 041.00-041.09, 041.10-041.19)

614.8 Other specified inflammatory disease of female pelvic organs and tissues — (Use additional code to identify organism: 041.00-041.09, 041.10-041.19)

615.0 Acute inflammatory disease of uterus, except cervix — (Use additional code to identify organism: 041.00-041.09, 041.10-041.19)

615.1 Chronic inflammatory disease of uterus, except cervix — (Use additional code to identify organism: 041.00-041.09, 041.10-041.19)

615.9 Unspecified inflammatory disease of uterus — (Use additional code to identify organism: 041.00-041.09, 041.10-041.19)

617.0 Endometriosis of uterus

626.8 Other disorder of menstruation and other abnormal bleeding from female genital tract

654.11 Tumors of body of uterus, delivered — (Code first any associated obstructed labor, 660.2)

654.31 Retroverted and incarcerated gravid uterus, delivered — (Code first any associated obstructed labor, 660.2)

665.01 Rupture of uterus before onset of labor, with delivery

665.11 Rupture of uterus during labor, with delivery

666.12 Other immediate postpartum hemorrhage, with delivery

Terms To Know

broad ligament. Fold of peritoneum extending from the side of the uterus to the wall of the pelvis.

endocervix. Region of the cervix uteri that opens into the uterus or the mucous membrane lining the cervical canal.

exocervix. Region of the cervix uteri that protrudes into the vagina.

malignant neoplasm. Any cancerous tumor or lesion exhibiting uncontrolled tissue growth that can progressively invade other parts of the body with its disease-generating cells.

parametrium. Connective tissue between the uterus and the broad ligament.

uterine isthmus. Narrow portion of the uterus between the cervix and the main body of the uterus.

CCI Version 18.3

01962-01963, 01969, 0230T, 44602-44605, 44820-44850, 49000-49010, 49255, 49570, 59430, 59857❖, 62311, 64430-64435, 64483

Note: These CCI edits are used for Medicare. Other payers may reimburse on codes listed above.

Medicare Edits

	Fac RVU	Non-Fac RVU	FUD	Status
59525	14.64	14.64	N/A	A

	MUE			Modifiers	
59525	1	N/A	N/A	62*	80

* with documentation

Medicare References: None

© 2012 OptumInsight, Inc.

Maternity Care

59610

59610 Routine obstetric care including antepartum care, vaginal delivery (with or without episiotomy, and/or forceps) and postpartum care, after previous cesarean delivery

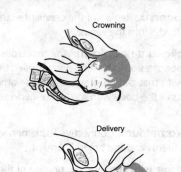

Crowning

Delivery

The physician provides antepartum care, successfully delivers the infant through the vagina, after a previous cesarean delivery, and provides postpartum care

Explanation

The physician delivers an infant and placenta through the vagina. The patient has previously delivered by cesarean section. The physician may elect to assist the delivery with the use of forceps, vacuum extraction, or rupture of membranes. The physician may also elect to do an episiotomy, which is an incision in the perineum to widen the external opening. Episiotomy and laceration repair are included as well. This procedure covers both antepartum and postpartum care. Antepartum or prenatal care includes the initial and subsequent histories, physical examinations, recording of weight, blood pressures, fetal heart tones, and routine chemical urinalysis. It includes monthly visits up to 28 weeks gestation, biweekly visits to 36 weeks gestation, and weekly visits until delivery (approximately 12-15 visits). Because of the previous cesarean delivery, the physician monitors the patient during labor and delivery. Postpartum care includes hospital and office visits following delivery.

Coding Tips

Code 59610 includes total OB care; if services provided do not match the code description of vaginal delivery, including antepartum and postpartum care, following a previous cesarean delivery, use the appropriate stand-alone code. If care rendered was less than the listed service (i.e., the one that most closely describes the service performed), append modifier 52 and reduce the cost of the service. See notes in CPT for directions on the use of maternity care and delivery codes. For vaginal delivery only, after previous cesarean, without antepartum or postpartum care, see 59612. For vaginal delivery including postpartum care, after previous cesarean, see 59614.

ICD-9-CM Procedural

72.0	Low forceps operation
72.1	Low forceps operation with episiotomy
72.21	Mid forceps operation with episiotomy
72.29	Other mid forceps operation
72.31	High forceps operation with episiotomy
72.39	Other high forceps operation
72.4	Forceps rotation of fetal head
72.51	Partial breech extraction with forceps to aftercoming head
72.52	Other partial breech extraction
72.53	Total breech extraction with forceps to aftercoming head
72.54	Other total breech extraction
72.6	Forceps application to aftercoming head
72.71	Vacuum extraction with episiotomy
72.79	Other vacuum extraction
72.8	Other specified instrumental delivery
72.9	Unspecified instrumental delivery
73.01	Induction of labor by artificial rupture of membranes
73.09	Other artificial rupture of membranes
73.4	Medical induction of labor
73.59	Other manually assisted delivery
73.6	Episiotomy

Anesthesia

59610 01967

ICD-9-CM Diagnostic

The application of this code is too broad to adequately present ICD-9-CM diagnostic code links here. Refer to your ICD-9-CM book.

Terms To Know

elderly primigravida. Woman in her first pregnancy at an age beyond the norm, usually considered 35 years or older.

episiotomy. Deliberate incision in the perineal tissue to facilitate delivery of the fetus and avoid traumatic tearing. In a midline or median episiotomy, the incision is made from the vagina straight down toward the anus. In a mediolateral episiotomy, the incision slants to one side.

multigravida. Female who has had two or more pregnancies. Women in this category are considered to be at high risk during pregnancy.

multiparity. Condition of having had two or more pregnancies that resulted in viable fetuses; producing more than one fetus or offspring in the same gestation.

placenta previa. Implantation of the placenta in the lower segment of the uterus, over or near the internal cervical os. In total previa, the cervical os is completely covered by the placenta; in partial previa, only a portion is covered.

preeclampsia. Complication of pregnancy manifesting in the development of borderline hypertension, protein in the urine, and unresponsive swelling between the 20th week of pregnancy and the end of the first week following birth in mild to moderate cases. Severe preeclampsia presents with hypertension, associated with marked swelling, proteinuria, abdominal pain, and/or visual changes.

CCI Version 18.3

01958, 01960, 01967, 0213T, 0216T, 0230T, 12001-12007, 12011-12057, 13100-13153, 36000, 36410, 37202, 51701-51702, 59050-59051, 59300, 59414, 59430, 59510-59515, 59525, 59612-59618❖, 62311-62319, 64415-64417, 64430-64435, 64450, 64483, 64490, 64493, 69990, 81000, 81002, 96360, 96365, 96372, 96374-96376, 99201-99239, 99304-99310, 99315-99318, 99324-99328, 99334-99337, 99341-99350

Note: These CCI edits are used for Medicare. Other payers may reimburse on codes listed above.

Medicare Edits

	Fac RVU	Non-Fac RVU	FUD	Status
59610	65.46	65.46	N/A	A

	MUE		Modifiers		
59610	1	51	N/A	N/A	80*

* with documentation

Medicare References: 100-2,15,20.1; 100-2,15,180

59612-59614

59612 Vaginal delivery only, after previous cesarean delivery (with or without episiotomy and/or forceps);

59614 including postpartum care

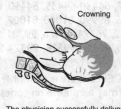

Crowning

The physician successfully delivers the infant through the vagina, after a previous cesarean delivery

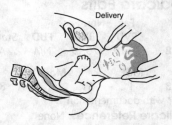

Delivery

59612 includes only delivery; 59614 includes delivery and postpartum care

Explanation

The physician delivers an infant and placenta through the vagina. The patient has previously delivered by cesarean section. The physician may elect to assist the delivery with the use of forceps. The physician may also elect to do an episiotomy, which is an incision in the perineum to widen the external opening. Episiotomy and laceration repair are included. Because of the previous cesarean delivery, the physician monitors the patient during labor and delivery. Code 59614 includes postpartum care, hospital office visits following delivery.

Coding Tips

If services provided do not match the code description of vaginal delivery only after previous cesarean (59612) or vaginal delivery including postpartum care, following a previous cesarean delivery (59614), use the appropriate stand-alone code. If care rendered was less than the listed service (i.e., the one that most closely describes the service performed), append modifier 52 and reduce the cost of the service. See notes in CPT for directions on the use of maternity care and delivery codes. For vaginal delivery, after previous cesarean delivery, with antepartum and postpartum care, see 59610.

ICD-9-CM Procedural

72.0 Low forceps operation

72.1 Low forceps operation with episiotomy

72.21 Mid forceps operation with episiotomy

72.29 Other mid forceps operation

72.31 High forceps operation with episiotomy

72.39 Other high forceps operation

72.4 Forceps rotation of fetal head

72.51 Partial breech extraction with forceps to aftercoming head

72.52 Other partial breech extraction

72.53 Total breech extraction with forceps to aftercoming head

72.54 Other total breech extraction

72.6 Forceps application to aftercoming head

72.71 Vacuum extraction with episiotomy

72.79 Other vacuum extraction

72.8 Other specified instrumental delivery

72.9 Unspecified instrumental delivery

73.01 Induction of labor by artificial rupture of membranes

73.09 Other artificial rupture of membranes

73.4 Medical induction of labor

73.59 Other manually assisted delivery

73.6 Episiotomy

Anesthesia

59612 01960
59614 01967

ICD-9-CM Diagnostic

The application of this code is too broad to adequately present ICD-9-CM diagnostic code links here. Refer to your ICD-9-CM book.

Terms To Know

delivery trauma. Perineal tears are classified by degree of tissue involvement, with or without an episiotomy: first-degree lacerations are superficial and involve vaginal mucosa and perineal skin in the fourchette; second-degree lacerations involve the pelvic floor and muscles; third-degree lacerations affect the anal sphincter; fourth-degree lacerations extend to the anal or rectal mucosa.

eclampsia. Tetany and toxemia producing seizure activity or coma in a pregnant patient who most often has presented with prior preeclampsia (i.e., hypertension, albuminuria, and edema).

elderly primigravida. Woman in her first pregnancy at an age beyond the norm, usually considered 35 years or older.

episiotomy. Deliberate incision in the perineal tissue to facilitate delivery of the fetus and avoid traumatic tearing. In a midline or median episiotomy, the incision is made from the vagina straight down toward the anus. In a mediolateral episiotomy, the incision slants to one side.

multiparity. Condition of having had two or more pregnancies that resulted in viable fetuses; producing more than one fetus or offspring in the same gestation.

oligohydramnios. Condition of less than the normal amount of amniotic fluid present, occurring most frequently in the last trimester.

polyhydramnios. Excess amniotic fluid surrounding the fetus, typically defined as a total fluid volume of greater than 24.0 cc.

CCI Version 18.3

01958, 01960, 01967, 0213T, 0216T, 0230T, 12001-12007, 12011-12057, 13100-13153, 36000, 36410, 37202, 51701-51702, 59050-59051, 59300, 59400-59410, 59414, 59525, 59618-59622❖, 62311-62319, 64415-64417, 64430-64435, 64450, 64483, 64490, 64493, 69990, 96360, 96365, 96372, 96374-96376

Also not with 59612: 59515

Also not with 59614: 59430, 59510-59515, 59612, 99201-99239, 99304-99310, 99315-99318, 99324-99328, 99334-99337, 99341-99350

Note: These CCI edits are used for Medicare. Other payers may reimburse on codes listed above.

Medicare Edits

	Fac RVU	Non-Fac RVU	FUD	Status
59612	27.57	27.57	N/A	A
59614	34.11	34.11	N/A	A

	MUE		Modifiers		
59612	-	51	N/A	N/A	80*
59614	1	51	N/A	N/A	80*

* with documentation

Medicare References: 100-2,15,20.1; 100-2,15,180

59618

59618 Routine obstetric care including antepartum care, cesarean delivery, and postpartum care, following attempted vaginal delivery after previous cesarean delivery

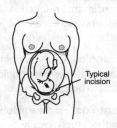

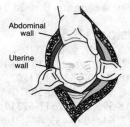

The physician delivers the infant through an abdominal incision, following attempted vaginal delivery after previous cesarean delivery

Explanation

After first attempting a vaginal delivery, the physician delivers an infant through a horizontal or vertical incision in the abdomen and uterus. The patient has previously delivered by cesarean section. Once the incisions are made, the infant is delivered and the placenta separated and removed. The uterine and abdominal incisions are closed with layered sutures. This procedure includes both antepartum and postpartum care. Antepartum or prenatal care includes the initial and subsequent histories, physical examinations, recording of weight, blood pressures, fetal heart tones, and routine chemical urinalysis. It includes monthly visits up to 28 weeks gestation, biweekly visits to 36 weeks gestation, and weekly visits until delivery (approximately 13-15 visits). Because of the previous cesarean delivery and the attempted vaginal delivery, the physician monitors the patient during labor and delivery. Postpartum care includes hospital and office visits following delivery.

Coding Tips

Code 59618 includes total OB care; if services provided do not match the code description of cesarean delivery, including antepartum and postpartum care, after attempted vaginal delivery, following a previous cesarean, use the appropriate stand-alone code. If care rendered was less than the listed service (i.e., the one that most closely describes the service performed), append modifier 52 and reduce the cost of the service. See notes in CPT for directions on the use of the maternity care and delivery codes. For cesarean delivery only, following attempted vaginal delivery after previous cesarean, see 59620. For cesarean delivery, following attempted vaginal delivery after previous cesarean, including postpartum care, see 59622.

ICD-9-CM Procedural

73.3	Failed forceps
74.0	Classical cesarean section
74.1	Low cervical cesarean section
74.4	Cesarean section of other specified type

Anesthesia

59618 01961

ICD-9-CM Diagnostic

The application of this code is too broad to adequately present ICD-9-CM diagnostic code links here. Refer to your ICD-9-CM book.

Terms To Know

eclampsia. Tetany and toxemia producing seizure activity or coma in a pregnant patient who most often has presented with prior preeclampsia (i.e., hypertension, albuminuria, and edema).

multigravida. Female who has had two or more pregnancies. Women in this category are considered to be at high risk during pregnancy.

multiparity. Condition of having had two or more pregnancies that resulted in viable fetuses; producing more than one fetus or offspring in the same gestation.

placenta previa. Implantation of the placenta in the lower segment of the uterus, over or near the internal cervical os. In total previa, the cervical os is completely covered by the placenta; in partial previa, only a portion is covered.

preeclampsia. Complication of pregnancy manifesting in the development of borderline hypertension, protein in the urine, and unresponsive swelling between the 20th week of pregnancy and the end of the first week following birth in mild to moderate cases. Severe preeclampsia presents with hypertension (blood pressure greater than 150/100), associated with marked swelling, proteinuria, abdominal pain, and/or visual changes.

CCI Version 18.3

01958, 01961, 01968, 0213T, 0216T, 0230T, 12001-12007, 12011-12057, 13100-13153, 36000, 36410, 37202, 44602-44605, 44820-44850, 49000-49010, 49255, 49570, 51701-51702, 59050-59051, 59300, 59400-59410, 59414, 59425-59430, 59510-59515, 59620-59622, 62311-62319, 64415-64417, 64430-64435, 64450, 64483, 64490, 64493, 69990, 81000, 81002, 96360, 96365, 96372, 96374-96376, 99201-99239, 99304-99310, 99315-99318, 99324-99328, 99334-99337, 99341-99350

Note: These CCI edits are used for Medicare. Other payers may reimburse on codes listed above.

Medicare Edits

	Fac RVU	Non-Fac RVU	FUD	Status
59618	70.19	70.19	N/A	A

	MUE		Modifiers	
59618	1	51	N/A N/A	80*

* with documentation

Medicare References: None

59620-59622

59620 Cesarean delivery only, following attempted vaginal delivery after previous cesarean delivery;

59622 including postpartum care

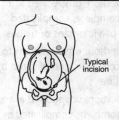

Typical incision

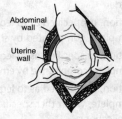

Abdominal wall

Uterine wall

The physician delivers the infant through an abdominal incision, following attempted vaginal delivery after previous cesarean delivery

59620 includes only delivery; 59622 includes delivery and postpartum care

Explanation

After first attempting a vaginal delivery, the physician delivers an infant through a horizontal or vertical incision in the abdomen and uterus. The patient has previously delivered by cesarean section. Once the incisions are made, the infant is delivered and the placenta separated and removed. The uterine and abdominal incisions are closed with layered sutures because of the previous cesarean delivery and the attempted vaginal delivery, the physician monitors the patient during labor and delivery. Only delivery is included in 59620. Postpartum care is included in 59622. Postpartum care includes hospital and office visits following delivery.

Coding Tips

Code 59620 represents a cesarean delivery following attempted vaginal delivery after previous cesarean delivery only and does not include postpartum care. Code 59622 represents a cesarean delivery including postpartum care, following attempted vaginal delivery, after previous cesarean delivery. See notes in CPT for directions on the use of the maternity care and delivery codes. For cesarean delivery including antepartum and postpartum care, following attempted vaginal delivery after previous cesarean delivery, see 59618.

ICD-9-CM Procedural

73.3	Failed forceps
74.0	Classical cesarean section
74.1	Low cervical cesarean section
74.4	Cesarean section of other specified type

Anesthesia
01961

ICD-9-CM Diagnostic

The application of this code is too broad to adequately present ICD-9-CM diagnostic code links here. Refer to your ICD-9-CM book.

Terms To Know

eclampsia. Tetany and toxemia producing seizure activity or coma in a pregnant patient who most often has presented with prior preeclampsia (i.e., hypertension, albuminuria, and edema).

elderly primigravida. Woman in her first pregnancy at an age beyond the norm, usually considered 35 years or older.

multiparity. Condition of having had two or more pregnancies that resulted in viable fetuses; producing more than one fetus or offspring in the same gestation.

placenta previa. Implantation of the placenta in the lower segment of the uterus, over or near the internal cervical os. In total previa, the cervical os is completely covered by the placenta; in partial previa, only a portion is covered.

preeclampsia. Complication of pregnancy manifesting in the development of borderline hypertension, protein in the urine, and unresponsive swelling between the 20th week of pregnancy and the end of the first week following birth in mild to moderate cases. Severe preeclampsia presents with hypertension (blood pressure greater than 150/100), associated with marked swelling, proteinuria, abdominal pain, and/or visual changes.

secundines. Placenta and membranes; the afterbirth.

CCI Version 18.3

01958, 01961, 01968, 0213T, 0216T, 0230T, 12001-12007, 12011-12057, 13100-13153, 36000, 36410, 37202, 44005, 44180, 44602-44605, 44820-44850, 49255, 49570, 51701-51702, 59050-59051, 59300, 59400-59410, 59414, 59510-59515, 59610❖, 62311-62319, 64415-64417, 64430-64435, 64450, 64483, 64490, 64493, 69990, 96360, 96365, 96372, 96374-96376

Also not with 59620: 49000-49002

Also not with 59622: 49000-49010, 59430, 59620, 99201-99239, 99304-99310, 99315-99318, 99324-99328, 99334-99337, 99341-99350

Note: These CCI edits are used for Medicare. Other payers may reimburse on codes listed above.

Medicare Edits

	Fac RVU	Non-Fac RVU	FUD	Status
59620	28.72	28.72	N/A	A
59622	38.9	38.9	N/A	A

	MUE		Modifiers		
59620	1	51	N/A	N/A	80
59622	1	51	N/A	N/A	80*

* with documentation

Medicare References: None

Coding Companion for Ob/Gyn

© 2012 OptumInsight, Inc.

59812

59812 Treatment of incomplete abortion, any trimester, completed surgically

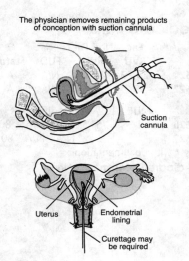

The physician removes remaining products of conception with suction cannula

Suction cannula

Uterus

Endometrial lining

Curettage may be required

Explanation

The physician removes the products of conception remaining after an incomplete spontaneous abortion in any trimester. To evacuate the uterus, the physician performs a dilation and suction curettage. The physician inserts a speculum into the vagina to view the cervix. A tenaculum is used to grasp the cervix, pull it down, and exert traction. If the cervix is not sufficiently dilated, a dilator is inserted into the endocervix and through the cervical canal to enlarge the opening. The physician places a cannula in the endocervical canal and passes it into the uterus. The suction machine is activated and the uterine contents are evacuated by rotation of the cannula. After suction curettage, a sharp curette may be used to gently scrape the uterus to ensure that it is empty.

Coding Tips

For medical treatment of a spontaneous complete abortion, any trimester, see 99201–99233. For treatment of a missed abortion completed surgically, see 59820–59821. For induced abortion, see 59840–59857.

ICD-9-CM Procedural

69.02   Dilation and curettage following delivery or abortion

Anesthesia

59812   01965

ICD-9-CM Diagnostic

634.01   Incomplete spontaneous abortion complicated by genital tract and pelvic infection

634.11   Incomplete spontaneous abortion complicated by delayed or excessive hemorrhage

634.21   Incomplete spontaneous abortion complicated by damage to pelvic organs or tissues

634.41   Incomplete spontaneous abortion complicated by metabolic disorder

634.51   Incomplete spontaneous abortion complicated by shock

634.61   Incomplete spontaneous abortion complicated by embolism

634.91   Incomplete spontaneous abortion without mention of complication

635.01   Incomplete legally induced abortion complicated by genital tract and pelvic infection

635.11   Incomplete legally induced abortion complicated by delayed or excessive hemorrhage

635.21   Legally induced abortion complicated by damage to pelvic organs or tissues, incomplete

635.41   Incomplete legally induced abortion complicated by metabolic disorder

635.51   Legally induced abortion, complicated by shock, incomplete

635.61   Incomplete legally induced abortion complicated by embolism

635.91   Incomplete legally induced abortion without mention of complication

636.01   Incomplete illegally induced abortion complicated by genital tract and pelvic infection

636.11   Incomplete illegally induced abortion complicated by delayed or excessive hemorrhage

636.21   Incomplete illegally induced abortion complicated by damage to pelvic organs or tissues

636.41   Incomplete illegally induced abortion complicated by metabolic disorder

636.51   Incomplete illegally induced abortion complicated by shock

636.61   Incomplete illegally induced abortion complicated by embolism

636.71   Incomplete illegally induced abortion with other specified complications

636.81   Incomplete illegally induced abortion with unspecified complication

636.91   Incomplete illegally induced abortion without mention of complication

637.01   Abortion, unspecified as to legality, incomplete, complicated by genital tract and pelvic infection

637.11   Abortion, unspecified as to legality, incomplete, complicated by delayed or excessive hemorrhage

637.21   Abortion, unspecified as to legality, incomplete, complicated by damage to pelvic organs or tissues

637.31   Abortion, unspecified as to legality, incomplete, complicated by renal failure

637.41   Abortion, unspecified as to legality, incomplete, complicated by metabolic disorder

637.51   Abortion, unspecified as to legality, incomplete, complicated by shock

637.61   Abortion, unspecified as to legality, incomplete, complicated by embolism

637.71   Abortion, unspecified as to legality, incomplete, with other specified complications

637.91   Abortion, unspecified as to legality, incomplete, without mention of complication

Terms To Know

legally induced abortion. Elective or therapeutic termination of pregnancy performed within legal parameters by a licensed physician or other qualified medical professionals.

CCI Version 18.3

01965-01966, 0213T, 0216T, 0228T, 0230T, 12001-12007, 12011-12057, 13100-13153, 36000, 36400-36410, 36420-36430, 36440, 36600, 36640, 37202, 43752, 51701-51703, 57410, 59855-59866❖, 62310-62319, 64400-64435, 64445-64450, 64479, 64483, 64490, 64493, 64505-64530, 69990, 93000-93010, 93040-93042, 93318, 94002, 94200, 94250, 94680-94690, 94770, 95812-95816, 95819, 95822, 95829, 95955, 96360, 96365, 96372, 96374-96376, 99148-99149, 99150, J0670, J2001

Note: These CCI edits are used for Medicare. Other payers may reimburse on codes listed above.

Medicare Edits

	Fac RVU	Non-Fac RVU	FUD	Status
59812	8.86	9.52	90	A

	MUE		Modifiers		
59812	1	51	N/A	N/A	N/A

* with documentation

Medicare References: 100-2,15,20.1

Coding Companion for Ob/Gyn

Maternity Care

59820-59821

59820 Treatment of missed abortion, completed surgically; first trimester
59821 second trimester

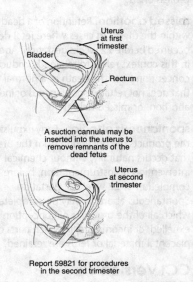

Uterus at first trimester
Bladder
Rectum

A suction cannula may be inserted into the uterus to remove remnants of the dead fetus

Uterus at second trimester

Report 59821 for procedures in the second trimester

Explanation

The physician treats a missed abortion in the first trimester by suction curettage. In missed abortion, the fetus remains in the uterus four to eight weeks following its death. Ultrasonography may be needed to determine the size of the fetus prior to the procedure. The physician inserts a speculum into the vagina to view the cervix. A tenaculum is used to grasp the cervix, pull it down, and exert traction. A dilator is then inserted into the endocervix and up through the cervical canal to enlarge the opening. The physician places a cannula in the endocervical canal and passes it into the uterus. The suction machine is then activated and the uterine contents are evacuated by rotation of the cannula. After suction curettage, a sharp curette may be used to gently scrape the uterus to ensure that it is empty.

Coding Tips

For medical treatment of a spontaneous complete abortion, any trimester, see 99201–99233. For induced abortion, see 59840–59857.

ICD-9-CM Procedural

69.02 Dilation and curettage following delivery or abortion

Anesthesia

01965

ICD-9-CM Diagnostic

631.8 Other abnormal products of conception
632 Missed abortion — (Use additional code from category 639 to identify any associated complications)
656.41 Intrauterine death affecting management of mother, delivered
656.43 Intrauterine death affecting management of mother, antepartum

Terms To Know

abortion. Premature expulsion or extraction of the products of conception.

curettage. Removal of tissue by scraping.

curette. Spoon-shaped instrument used to scrape out abnormal tissue from a cavity or bone.

D&C. Dilation and curettage.

dilation. Artificial increase in the diameter of an opening or lumen made by medication or by instrumentation.

missed abortion. Retention of a dead fetus within the uterus in cases where fetal demise occurred before 22 weeks gestation. Abortion in this context refers to retained products of conception from the death of a normal fetus that does not result in spontaneous or induced abortion, or missed delivery.

secundines. Placenta and membranes; the afterbirth.

speculum. Tool used to enlarge the opening of any canal or cavity.

suction. Vacuum evacuation of fluid or tissue.

CCI Version 18.3

01965-01966, 0213T, 0216T, 0228T, 0230T, 12001-12007, 12011-12057, 13100-13153, 36000, 36400-36410, 36420-36430, 36440, 36600, 36640, 37202, 43752, 51701-51703, 57410, 62310-62319, 64400-64435, 64445-64450, 64479, 64483, 64490, 64493, 64505-64530, 69990, 93000-93010, 93040-93042, 93318, 94002, 94200, 94250, 94680-94690, 94770, 95812-95816, 95819, 95822, 95829, 95955, 96360, 96365, 96372, 96374-96376, 99148-99149, 99150, J0670, J2001

Also not with 59820: 59821❖, 59855-59866❖

Also not with 59821: 59855-59857❖

Note: These CCI edits are used for Medicare. Other payers may reimburse on codes listed above.

Medicare Edits

	Fac RVU	Non-Fac RVU	FUD	Status
59820	10.7	11.4	90	A
59821	10.74	11.49	90	A

	MUE		Modifiers		
59820	1	51	N/A	N/A	N/A
59821	1	51	N/A	N/A	80*

* with documentation

Medicare References: 100-2,15,20.1

59830

59830 Treatment of septic abortion, completed surgically

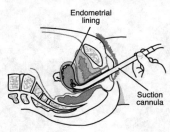

The physician removes remaining matter using a suction cannula; intravenous antibiotics and fluids may be required

Endometrial lining

Suction cannula

Explanation

The physician treats a septic abortion with prompt evacuation of the uterus and vigorous medical treatment of the patient. A septic abortion is one complicated by generalized fever and infection. There is also inflammation and infection of the endometrium and in the cellular tissue around the uterus. The physician treats the infection with intravenous antibiotics and blood transfusions as necessary. To evacuate the uterus, the physician inserts a speculum into the vagina to view the cervix. A tenaculum is used to grasp the cervix, pull it down, and exert traction. A dilator is inserted into the endocervix and through the cervical canal to enlarge the opening. The physician places a cannula in the endocervical canal and passes it into the uterus. The suction machine is activated and the uterine contents are evacuated by rotation of the cannula. After suction curettage, a sharp curette may be used to gently scrape the uterus to ensure that it is empty.

Coding Tips

To report surgical treatment of an incomplete abortion, any trimester, see 59812. For medical treatment of a spontaneous complete abortion, any trimester, see 99201–99233. For treatment of a missed abortion, completed surgically, see 59820–59821. For induced abortion, see 59840–59857.

ICD-9-CM Procedural

69.02 Dilation and curettage following delivery or abortion

Anesthesia

59830 01965

ICD-9-CM Diagnostic

634.01 Incomplete spontaneous abortion complicated by genital tract and pelvic infection

634.71 Incomplete spontaneous abortion with other specified complications

634.81 Incomplete spontaneous abortion with unspecified complication

634.91 Incomplete spontaneous abortion without mention of complication

635.01 Incomplete legally induced abortion complicated by genital tract and pelvic infection

635.81 Incomplete legally induced abortion with unspecified complication

635.91 Incomplete legally induced abortion without mention of complication

636.01 Incomplete illegally induced abortion complicated by genital tract and pelvic infection

636.71 Incomplete illegally induced abortion with other specified complications

636.81 Incomplete illegally induced abortion with unspecified complication

636.91 Incomplete illegally induced abortion without mention of complication

637.01 Abortion, unspecified as to legality, incomplete, complicated by genital tract and pelvic infection

637.71 Abortion, unspecified as to legality, incomplete, with other specified complications

637.81 Abortion, unspecified as to legality, incomplete, with unspecified complication

638.0 Failed attempted abortion complicated by genital tract and pelvic infection

638.7 Failed attempted abortion with other specified complication

656.41 Intrauterine death affecting management of mother, delivered

656.43 Intrauterine death affecting management of mother, antepartum

Terms To Know

legally induced abortion. Elective or therapeutic termination of pregnancy performed within legal parameters by a licensed physician or other qualified medical professionals.

missed abortion. Retention of a dead fetus within the uterus in cases where fetal demise occurred before 22 weeks gestation. Abortion in this context refers to retained products of conception from the death of a normal fetus that does not result in spontaneous or induced abortion, or missed delivery.

spontaneous abortion. Early expulsion of the products of conception from the uterus that occurs naturally, without chemical intervention or instrumentation, before completion of 22 weeks of gestation. Spontaneous abortion may be complete, in which all of the products of conception are expelled; or incomplete, in which parts of the placental material or fetus are retained.

CCI Version 18.3

01965-01966, 0213T, 0216T, 0228T, 0230T, 12001-12007, 12011-12057, 13100-13153, 36000, 36400-36410, 36420-36430, 36440, 36600, 36640, 37202, 43752, 51701-51703, 57410, 59856-59857❖, 62310-62319, 64400-64435, 64445-64450, 64479, 64483, 64490, 64493, 64505-64530, 69990, 93000-93010, 93040-93042, 93318, 94002, 94200, 94250, 94680-94690, 94770, 95812-95816, 95819, 95822, 95829, 95955, 96360, 96365, 96372, 96374-96376, 99148-99149, 99150

Note: These CCI edits are used for Medicare. Other payers may reimburse on codes listed above.

Medicare Edits

	Fac RVU	Non-Fac RVU	FUD	Status
59830	13.13	13.13	90	A

	MUE		Modifiers		
59830	1	51	N/A	N/A	80*

* with documentation

Medicare References: None

Coding Companion for Ob/Gyn

59840

59840 Induced abortion, by dilation and curettage

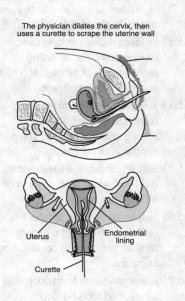

The physician dilates the cervix, then uses a curette to scrape the uterine wall

Explanation

The physician terminates a pregnancy by dilation and curettage. The physician inserts a speculum into the vagina to view the cervix. A tenaculum is used to grasp the cervix, pull it down, and exert traction. A dilator is inserted into the endocervix and through the cervical canal to enlarge the opening. The physician places a curette in the endocervical canal and passes it into the uterus. The uterine contents are removed by rotating the curette and gently scraping the uterus until all the products of conception are removed.

Coding Tips

To report induced abortion by dilation and evacuation, see 59841. For other induced abortion, see 59850–59857. For medical treatment of a spontaneous complete abortion, any trimester, see 99201–99233. For surgical treatment of an incomplete abortion, any trimester, see 59812. For treatment of a missed abortion, completed surgically, see 59820–59821. Because this procedure may not be done out of medical necessity, the patient may be responsible for charges. Verify with the insurance carrier for coverage.

ICD-9-CM Procedural

69.01 Dilation and curettage for termination of pregnancy

69.99 Other operations on cervix and uterus

Anesthesia

59840 01966

ICD-9-CM Diagnostic

635.00 Unspecified legally induced abortion complicated by genital tract and pelvic infection

635.01 Incomplete legally induced abortion complicated by genital tract and pelvic infection

635.02 Complete legally induced abortion complicated by genital tract and pelvic infection

635.10 Unspecified legally induced abortion complicated by delayed or excessive hemorrhage

635.11 Incomplete legally induced abortion complicated by delayed or excessive hemorrhage

635.12 Complete legally induced abortion complicated by delayed or excessive hemorrhage

635.20 Unspecified legally induced abortion complicated by damage to pelvic organs or tissues

635.21 Legally induced abortion complicated by damage to pelvic organs or tissues, incomplete

635.22 Complete legally induced abortion complicated by damage to pelvic organs or tissues

635.40 Unspecified legally induced abortion complicated by metabolic disorder

635.41 Incomplete legally induced abortion complicated by metabolic disorder

635.42 Complete legally induced abortion complicated by metabolic disorder

635.50 Unspecified legally induced abortion complicated by shock

635.51 Legally induced abortion, complicated by shock, incomplete

635.52 Complete legally induced abortion complicated by shock

635.60 Unspecified legally induced abortion complicated by embolism

635.61 Incomplete legally induced abortion complicated by embolism

635.62 Complete legally induced abortion complicated by embolism

646.03 Papyraceous fetus, antepartum — (Use additional code to further specify complication)

655.03 Central nervous system malformation in fetus, antepartum

655.13 Chromosomal abnormality in fetus, affecting management of mother, antepartum

655.33 Suspected damage to fetus from viral disease in mother, affecting management of mother, antepartum condition or complication

655.43 Suspected damage to fetus from other disease in mother, affecting management of mother, antepartum condition or complication

655.53 Suspected damage to fetus from drugs, affecting management of mother, antepartum

655.83 Other known or suspected fetal abnormality, not elsewhere classified, affecting management of mother, antepartum condition or complication

656.23 Isoimmunization from other and unspecified blood-group incompatibility, affecting management of mother, antepartum

656.43 Intrauterine death affecting management of mother, antepartum

CCI Version 18.3

01965-01966, 0213T, 0216T, 0228T, 0230T, 12001-12007, 12011-12057, 13100-13153, 36000, 36400-36410, 36420-36430, 36440, 36600, 36640, 37202, 43752, 51701-51703, 57410, 59855-59866❖, 62310-62319, 64400-64435, 64445-64450, 64479, 64483, 64490, 64493, 64505-64530, 69990, 93000-93010, 93040-93042, 93318, 94002, 94200, 94250, 94680-94690, 94770, 95812-95816, 95819, 95822, 95829, 95955, 96360, 96365, 96372, 96374-96376, 99148-99149, 99150

Note: These CCI edits are used for Medicare. Other payers may reimburse on codes listed above.

Medicare Edits

	Fac RVU	Non-Fac RVU	FUD	Status
59840	6.21	6.46	10	R

	MUE		Modifiers		
59840	1	51	N/A	N/A	80*

* with documentation

Medicare References: 100-2,1,90; 100-3,140.1; 100-4,3,100.1

59841

59841 Induced abortion, by dilation and evacuation

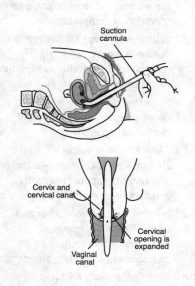

Suction cannula

Cervix and cervical canal

Vaginal canal

Cervical opening is expanded

Explanation

The physician terminates a pregnancy by dilation and evacuation (D&E). Because D&E requires wider cervical dilation than curettage, the physician may dilate the cervix with a laminaria several hours to several days before the procedure. At the time of the procedure, the physician inserts a speculum into the vagina to view the cervix. A tenaculum is used to grasp the cervix, pull it down, and exert traction. The physician places a cannula in the dilated endocervical canal and passes it into the uterus. The suction machine is activated and the uterine contents are evacuated by rotation of the cannula. For pregnancies through 16 weeks, the cannula will usually evacuate the pregnancy. For later pregnancies, the cannula is used to drain amniotic fluid and to draw tissue into the lower uterus for extraction by forceps. In either case, a sharp curette may be used to gently scrape the uterus to ensure that it is empty.

Coding Tips

To report induced abortion by dilation and curettage, see 59840. For other induced abortion, see 59850–59857. For medical treatment of a spontaneous complete abortion, any trimester, see 99201–99233. For surgical treatment of an incomplete abortion, any trimester, see 59812. For treatment of a missed abortion, completed surgically, see 59820–59821. Because this procedure may not be done out of medical necessity, the patient may be responsible for

charges. Verify with the insurance carrier for coverage.

ICD-9-CM Procedural

69.01	Dilation and curettage for termination of pregnancy
69.51	Aspiration curettage of uterus for termination of pregnancy
69.99	Other operations on cervix and uterus

Anesthesia

59841 01966

ICD-9-CM Diagnostic

631.8	Other abnormal products of conception
635.01	Incomplete legally induced abortion complicated by genital tract and pelvic infection
635.02	Complete legally induced abortion complicated by genital tract and pelvic infection
635.11	Incomplete legally induced abortion complicated by delayed or excessive hemorrhage
635.12	Complete legally induced abortion complicated by delayed or excessive hemorrhage
635.21	Legally induced abortion complicated by damage to pelvic organs or tissues, incomplete
635.22	Complete legally induced abortion complicated by damage to pelvic organs or tissues
635.31	Incomplete legally induced abortion complicated by renal failure
635.32	Complete legally induced abortion complicated by renal failure
635.41	Incomplete legally induced abortion complicated by metabolic disorder
635.42	Complete legally induced abortion complicated by metabolic disorder
635.51	Legally induced abortion, complicated by shock, incomplete
635.52	Complete legally induced abortion complicated by shock
635.61	Incomplete legally induced abortion complicated by embolism
635.62	Complete legally induced abortion complicated by embolism
646.03	Papyraceous fetus, antepartum — (Use additional code to further specify complication)
655.03	Central nervous system malformation in fetus, antepartum
655.13	Chromosomal abnormality in fetus, affecting management of mother, antepartum
655.20	Hereditary disease in family possibly affecting fetus, affecting management of mother, unspecified as to episode of care in pregnancy
655.33	Suspected damage to fetus from viral disease in mother, affecting management of mother, antepartum condition or complication
655.43	Suspected damage to fetus from other disease in mother, affecting management of mother, antepartum condition or complication
655.53	Suspected damage to fetus from drugs, affecting management of mother, antepartum
655.63	Suspected damage to fetus from radiation, affecting management of mother, antepartum condition or complication
656.23	Isoimmunization from other and unspecified blood-group incompatibility, affecting management of mother, antepartum
656.43	Intrauterine death affecting management of mother, antepartum
V61.7	Other unwanted pregnancy

CCI Version 18.3

01965-01966, 0213T, 0216T, 0228T, 0230T, 12001-12007, 12011-12057, 13100-13153, 36000, 36400-36410, 36420-36430, 36440, 36600, 36640, 37202, 43752, 51701-51703, 57410, 59855-59857❖, 62310-62319, 64400-64435, 64445-64450, 64479, 64483, 64490, 64493, 64505-64530, 69990, 93000-93010, 93040-93042, 93318, 94002, 94200, 94250, 94680-94690, 94770, 95812-95816, 95819, 95822, 95829, 95955, 96360, 96365, 96372, 96374-96376, 99148-99149, 99150, J0670, J2001

Note: These CCI edits are used for Medicare. Other payers may reimburse on codes listed above.

Medicare Edits

	Fac RVU	Non-Fac RVU	FUD	Status
59841	10.84	11.48	10	R

	MUE		Modifiers	
59841	1	51	N/A N/A	80*

* with documentation

Medicare References: 100-2,1,90; 100-3,140.1; 100-4,3,100.1

Maternity Care

59850

59850 Induced abortion, by 1 or more intra-amniotic injections (amniocentesis-injections), including hospital admission and visits, delivery of fetus and secundines;

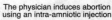
The physician induces abortion using an intra-amniotic injection

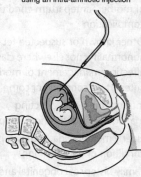

Explanation

The physician terminates a pregnancy by inducing labor with amniocentesis and intra-amniotic injections. This method is usually used after the first trimester (13 weeks or more). The physician inserts an amniocentesis needle into the abdomen to obtain a free flow of clear amniotic fluid. A hypertonic solution is administered by gravity drip. The hypertonic solution results in fetal death and labor usually results. The fetus and placenta are delivered through the vagina.

Coding Tips

For induced abortion by one or more intra-amniotic injections, with dilation and curettage and/or evacuation, see 59851; with hysterotomy, see 59852; by other methods, see 59855–59857. For medical treatment of a spontaneous complete abortion, any trimester, see 99201–99233. For surgical treatment of an incomplete abortion, any trimester, see 59812.

ICD-9-CM Procedural

75.0   Intra-amniotic injection for abortion

Anesthesia

59850   00940, 01966

ICD-9-CM Diagnostic

631.8   Other abnormal products of conception

635.01   Incomplete legally induced abortion complicated by genital tract and pelvic infection

635.02   Complete legally induced abortion complicated by genital tract and pelvic infection

635.11   Incomplete legally induced abortion complicated by delayed or excessive hemorrhage

635.12   Complete legally induced abortion complicated by delayed or excessive hemorrhage

635.21   Legally induced abortion complicated by damage to pelvic organs or tissues, incomplete

635.22   Complete legally induced abortion complicated by damage to pelvic organs or tissues

635.31   Incomplete legally induced abortion complicated by renal failure

635.32   Complete legally induced abortion complicated by renal failure

635.41   Incomplete legally induced abortion complicated by metabolic disorder

635.42   Complete legally induced abortion complicated by metabolic disorder

635.51   Legally induced abortion, complicated by shock, incomplete

635.52   Complete legally induced abortion complicated by shock

635.61   Incomplete legally induced abortion complicated by embolism

635.62   Complete legally induced abortion complicated by embolism

635.71   Incomplete legally induced abortion with other specified complications

635.72   Complete legally induced abortion with other specified complications

635.90   Unspecified legally induced abortion without mention of complication

635.91   Incomplete legally induced abortion without mention of complication

635.92   Complete legally induced abortion without mention of complication

638.0   Failed attempted abortion complicated by genital tract and pelvic infection

638.1   Failed attempted abortion complicated by delayed or excessive hemorrhage

638.2   Failed attempted abortion complicated by damage to pelvic organs or tissues

638.4   Failed attempted abortion complicated by metabolic disorder

638.5   Failed attempted abortion complicated by shock

638.6   Failed attempted abortion complicated by embolism

646.03   Papyraceous fetus, antepartum — (Use additional code to further specify complication)

655.03   Central nervous system malformation in fetus, antepartum

655.13   Chromosomal abnormality in fetus, affecting management of mother, antepartum

655.23   Hereditary disease in family possibly affecting fetus, affecting management of mother, antepartum condition or complication

655.83   Other known or suspected fetal abnormality, not elsewhere classified, affecting management of mother, antepartum condition or complication

656.43   Intrauterine death affecting management of mother, antepartum

659.63   Elderly multigravida, with antepartum condition or complication

V19.5   Family history of congenital anomalies

CCI Version 18.3

01965-01966, 0213T, 0216T, 0228T, 0230T, 12001-12007, 12011-12057, 13100-13153, 36000, 36400-36410, 36420-36430, 36440, 36600, 36640, 37202, 43752, 51701-51703, 57410, 59200, 59856-59857❖, 62310-62319, 64400-64435, 64445-64450, 64479, 64483, 64490, 64493, 64505-64530, 69990, 93000-93010, 93040-93042, 93318, 94002, 94200, 94250, 94680-94690, 94770, 95812-95816, 95819, 95822, 95829, 95955, 96360, 96365, 96372, 96374-96376, 99148-99149, 99150

Note: These CCI edits are used for Medicare. Other payers may reimburse on codes listed above.

Medicare Edits

	Fac RVU	Non-Fac RVU	FUD	Status
59850	10.19	10.19	90	R

	MUE		Modifiers		
59850	1	51	N/A	N/A	80*

* with documentation

Medicare References: 100-2,1,90; 100-3,140.1; 100-3,230.3; 100-4,3,100.1

59851

59851 Induced abortion, by 1 or more intra-amniotic injections (amniocentesis-injections), including hospital admission and visits, delivery of fetus and secundines; with dilation and curettage and/or evacuation

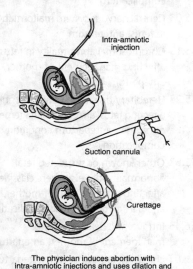

Intra-amniotic injection

Suction cannula

Curettage

The physician induces abortion with intra-amniotic injections and uses dilation and curettage and/or evacuation when all products of conception are not expelled

Explanation

The physician begins the termination of a pregnancy by inducing labor with amniocentesis and intra-amniotic injections. This method is usually used after the first trimester (13 weeks or more). The physician inserts an amniocentesis needle into the abdomen to obtain a free flow of clear amniotic fluid. A hypertonic solution is then administered by gravity drip. The hypertonic solution results in fetal death and labor usually results. Code 59851 is used when this method fails to expel all products of conception, and a dilation and curettage and/or evacuation is used to remove the remaining tissue.

Coding Tips

For induced abortion, by one or more intra-amniotic injections, see 59850; with hysterotomy, see 59852; by other methods, see 59855–59857. For medical treatment of a spontaneous complete abortion, any trimester, see 99201–99233. For surgical treatment of an incomplete abortion, any trimester, see 59812.

ICD-9-CM Procedural

69.01 Dilation and curettage for termination of pregnancy

69.51 Aspiration curettage of uterus for termination of pregnancy

75.0 Intra-amniotic injection for abortion

Anesthesia
59851 00940, 01965, 01966

ICD-9-CM Diagnostic

631.8 Other abnormal products of conception

635.01 Incomplete legally induced abortion complicated by genital tract and pelvic infection

635.02 Complete legally induced abortion complicated by genital tract and pelvic infection

635.11 Incomplete legally induced abortion complicated by delayed or excessive hemorrhage

635.12 Complete legally induced abortion complicated by delayed or excessive hemorrhage

635.21 Legally induced abortion complicated by damage to pelvic organs or tissues, incomplete

635.22 Complete legally induced abortion complicated by damage to pelvic organs or tissues

635.31 Incomplete legally induced abortion complicated by renal failure

635.32 Complete legally induced abortion complicated by renal failure

635.41 Incomplete legally induced abortion complicated by metabolic disorder

635.42 Complete legally induced abortion complicated by metabolic disorder

635.51 Legally induced abortion, complicated by shock, incomplete

635.52 Complete legally induced abortion complicated by shock

635.61 Incomplete legally induced abortion complicated by embolism

635.62 Complete legally induced abortion complicated by embolism

638.0 Failed attempted abortion complicated by genital tract and pelvic infection

638.1 Failed attempted abortion complicated by delayed or excessive hemorrhage

638.2 Failed attempted abortion complicated by damage to pelvic organs or tissues

638.4 Failed attempted abortion complicated by metabolic disorder

638.5 Failed attempted abortion complicated by shock

638.6 Failed attempted abortion complicated by embolism

646.03 Papyraceous fetus, antepartum — (Use additional code to further specify complication)

655.03 Central nervous system malformation in fetus, antepartum

655.13 Chromosomal abnormality in fetus, affecting management of mother, antepartum

655.23 Hereditary disease in family possibly affecting fetus, affecting management of mother, antepartum condition or complication

655.83 Other known or suspected fetal abnormality, not elsewhere classified, affecting management of mother, antepartum condition or complication

656.43 Intrauterine death affecting management of mother, antepartum

659.63 Elderly multigravida, with antepartum condition or complication

V19.5 Family history of congenital anomalies

V61.7 Other unwanted pregnancy

CCI Version 18.3
01965-01966, 0213T, 0216T, 0228T, 0230T, 12001-12007, 12011-12057, 13100-13153, 36000, 36400-36410, 36420-36430, 36440, 36600, 36640, 37202, 43752, 51701-51703, 57410, 59200, 59850, 59856❖, 62310-62319, 64400-64435, 64445-64450, 64479, 64483, 64490, 64493, 64505-64530, 69990, 93000-93010, 93040-93042, 93318, 94002, 94200, 94250, 94680-94690, 94770, 95812-95816, 95819, 95822, 95829, 95955, 96360, 96365, 96372, 96374-96376, 99148-99149, 99150

Note: These CCI edits are used for Medicare. Other payers may reimburse on codes listed above.

Medicare Edits

	Fac RVU	Non-Fac RVU	FUD	Status
59851	12.01	12.01	90	R

	MUE		Modifiers		
59851	1	51	N/A	N/A	80*

* with documentation

Medicare References: 100-2,1,90; 100-3,140.1; 100-4,3,100.1

Maternity Care

59852

59852 Induced abortion, by 1 or more intra-amniotic injections (amniocentesis-injections), including hospital admission and visits, delivery of fetus and secundines; with hysterotomy (failed intra-amniotic injection)

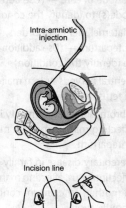

Intra-amniotic injection

Incision line

The physician induces abortion with intra-amniotic injections and when all products of conception are not expelled, performs a hysterotomy

Explanation

The physician begins the termination of a pregnancy by inducing labor with amniocentesis and intra-amniotic injections. This method is usually used after the first trimester (13 weeks or more). The physician inserts an amniocentesis needle into the abdomen to obtain a free flow of clear amniotic fluid. A hypertonic solution is administered by gravity drip. The hypertonic solution results in fetal death and labor usually results. Code 59852 is used when this method fails to expel all products of conception, and a hysterotomy, through an incision in the abdominal wall and uterus, is used to remove the remaining tissue. Following removal, the incision is closed with sutures.

Coding Tips

For induced abortion, by one or more intra-amniotic injections, see 59850; with dilation and curettage and/or evacuation, see 59851; by other methods, see 59855–59857. For medical treatment of a spontaneous complete abortion, any trimester, see 99201–99233. For surgical treatment of an incomplete abortion, any trimester, see 59812.

ICD-9-CM Procedural

74.91 Hysterotomy to terminate pregnancy
75.0 Intra-amniotic injection for abortion

Anesthesia
59852 00840, 01966

ICD-9-CM Diagnostic

635.01 Incomplete legally induced abortion complicated by genital tract and pelvic infection
635.02 Complete legally induced abortion complicated by genital tract and pelvic infection
635.11 Incomplete legally induced abortion complicated by delayed or excessive hemorrhage
635.12 Complete legally induced abortion complicated by delayed or excessive hemorrhage
635.21 Legally induced abortion complicated by damage to pelvic organs or tissues, incomplete
635.22 Complete legally induced abortion complicated by damage to pelvic organs or tissues
635.41 Incomplete legally induced abortion complicated by metabolic disorder
635.42 Complete legally induced abortion complicated by metabolic disorder
635.51 Legally induced abortion, complicated by shock, incomplete
635.52 Complete legally induced abortion complicated by shock
635.61 Incomplete legally induced abortion complicated by embolism
635.62 Complete legally induced abortion complicated by embolism
635.71 Incomplete legally induced abortion with other specified complications
635.72 Complete legally induced abortion with other specified complications
635.92 Complete legally induced abortion without mention of complication
638.0 Failed attempted abortion complicated by genital tract and pelvic infection
638.1 Failed attempted abortion complicated by delayed or excessive hemorrhage
638.2 Failed attempted abortion complicated by damage to pelvic organs or tissues
638.4 Failed attempted abortion complicated by metabolic disorder
638.5 Failed attempted abortion complicated by shock
638.6 Failed attempted abortion complicated by embolism

646.03 Papyraceous fetus, antepartum — (Use additional code to further specify complication)
648.40 Maternal mental disorders, complicating pregnancy, childbirth, or the puerperium, unspecified as to episode of care — (Use additional code(s) to identify the condition)
655.03 Central nervous system malformation in fetus, antepartum
655.13 Chromosomal abnormality in fetus, affecting management of mother, antepartum
655.20 Hereditary disease in family possibly affecting fetus, affecting management of mother, unspecified as to episode of care in pregnancy
655.23 Hereditary disease in family possibly affecting fetus, affecting management of mother, antepartum condition or complication
655.83 Other known or suspected fetal abnormality, not elsewhere classified, affecting management of mother, antepartum condition or complication
656.43 Intrauterine death affecting management of mother, antepartum
659.63 Elderly multigravida, with antepartum condition or complication

CCI Version 18.3

01965-01966, 0213T, 0216T, 0228T, 0230T, 12001-12007, 12011-12057, 13100-13153, 36000, 36400-36410, 36420-36430, 36440, 36600, 36640, 37202, 43752, 44602-44605, 49000-49002, 49320, 51701-51703, 57410, 59200, 59850, 59857❖, 62310-62319, 64400-64435, 64445-64450, 64479, 64483, 64490, 64493, 64505-64530, 69990, 93000-93010, 93040-93042, 93318, 94002, 94200, 94250, 94680-94690, 94770, 95812-95816, 95819, 95822, 95829, 95955, 96360, 96365, 96372, 96374-96376, 99148-99149, 99150

Note: These CCI edits are used for Medicare. Other payers may reimburse on codes listed above.

Medicare Edits

	Fac RVU	Non-Fac RVU	FUD	Status
59852	14.76	14.76	90	R

	MUE		Modifiers		
59852	1	51	N/A	N/A	80*

* with documentation

Medicare References: 100-2,1,90; 100-3,140.1; 100-3,230.3; 100-4,3,100.1

59855

59855 Induced abortion, by 1 or more vaginal suppositories (eg, prostaglandin) with or without cervical dilation (eg, laminaria), including hospital admission and visits, delivery of fetus and secundines;

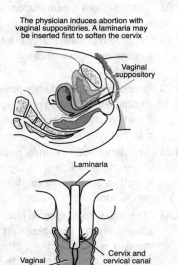

The physician induces abortion with vaginal suppositories. A laminaria may be inserted first to soften the cervix

Vaginal suppository

Laminaria

Vaginal canal

Cervix and cervical canal

Explanation

The physician terminates a pregnancy by inducing labor with vaginal suppositories. Before using the suppositories, a laminaria, which is an applicator made of kelp or synthetic material, may be inserted in the cervix to soften and expand the cervical canal. Once the cervix is ready, the physician inserts the vaginal suppositories and labor usually results. The fetus and placenta are delivered through the vagina.

Coding Tips

To report with dilation and curettage and/or evacuation, see 59856. If performed with a hysterotomy, see 59857. For medical treatment of a spontaneous complete abortion, any trimester, see 99201–99233. For insertion of a cervical dilator only, see 59200.

ICD-9-CM Procedural

69.93   Insertion of laminaria
96.49   Other genitourinary instillation

Anesthesia

59855   00940, 01966

ICD-9-CM Diagnostic

635.01   Incomplete legally induced abortion complicated by genital tract and pelvic infection
635.02   Complete legally induced abortion complicated by genital tract and pelvic infection
635.11   Incomplete legally induced abortion complicated by delayed or excessive hemorrhage
635.12   Complete legally induced abortion complicated by delayed or excessive hemorrhage
635.21   Legally induced abortion complicated by damage to pelvic organs or tissues, incomplete
635.22   Complete legally induced abortion complicated by damage to pelvic organs or tissues
635.31   Incomplete legally induced abortion complicated by renal failure
635.32   Complete legally induced abortion complicated by renal failure
635.41   Incomplete legally induced abortion complicated by metabolic disorder
635.42   Complete legally induced abortion complicated by metabolic disorder
635.51   Legally induced abortion, complicated by shock, incomplete
635.52   Complete legally induced abortion complicated by shock
635.61   Incomplete legally induced abortion complicated by embolism
635.62   Complete legally induced abortion complicated by embolism
635.71   Incomplete legally induced abortion with other specified complications
635.72   Complete legally induced abortion with other specified complications
635.81   Incomplete legally induced abortion with unspecified complication
635.82   Complete legally induced abortion with unspecified complication
638.0   Failed attempted abortion complicated by genital tract and pelvic infection
638.1   Failed attempted abortion complicated by delayed or excessive hemorrhage
638.2   Failed attempted abortion complicated by damage to pelvic organs or tissues
638.4   Failed attempted abortion complicated by metabolic disorder
638.5   Failed attempted abortion complicated by shock

638.6   Failed attempted abortion complicated by embolism
646.03   Papyraceous fetus, antepartum — (Use additional code to further specify complication)
648.40   Maternal mental disorders, complicating pregnancy, childbirth, or the puerperium, unspecified as to episode of care — (Use additional code(s) to identify the condition)
648.43   Maternal mental disorders, antepartum — (Use additional code(s) to identify the condition)
655.03   Central nervous system malformation in fetus, antepartum
655.13   Chromosomal abnormality in fetus, affecting management of mother, antepartum
655.23   Hereditary disease in family possibly affecting fetus, affecting management of mother, antepartum condition or complication
655.83   Other known or suspected fetal abnormality, not elsewhere classified, affecting management of mother, antepartum condition or complication
659.63   Elderly multigravida, with antepartum condition or complication
V19.5   Family history of congenital anomalies
V61.7   Other unwanted pregnancy

CCI Version 18.3

01965-01966, 0213T, 0216T, 0228T, 0230T, 12001-12007, 12011-12057, 13100-13153, 36000, 36400-36410, 36420-36430, 36440, 36600, 36640, 37202, 43752, 51701-51703, 57410, 59100❖, 59120-59121❖, 59130-59200, 59510-59515❖, 59525❖, 59610-59622❖, 59830❖, 59850-59852❖, 62310-62319, 64400-64435, 64445-64450, 64479, 64483, 64490, 64493, 64505-64530, 69990, 93000-93010, 93040-93042, 93318, 94002, 94200, 94250, 94680-94690, 94770, 95812-95816, 95819, 95822, 95829, 95955, 96360, 96365, 96372, 96374-96376, 99148-99149, 99150

Note: These CCI edits are used for Medicare. Other payers may reimburse on codes listed above.

Medicare Edits

	Fac RVU	Non-Fac RVU	FUD	Status
59855	12.49	12.49	90	R

	MUE		Modifiers		
59855	1	51	N/A	N/A	80*

* with documentation

Medicare References: 100-2,1,90; 100-3,140.1; 100-4,3,100.1

Coding Companion for Ob/Gyn

Maternity Care

59856

59856 Induced abortion, by 1 or more vaginal suppositories (eg, prostaglandin) with or without cervical dilation (eg, laminaria), including hospital admission and visits, delivery of fetus and secundines; with dilation and curettage and/or evacuation

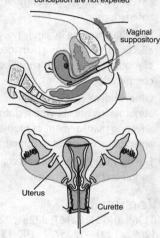

The physician induces abortion with vaginal suppositories and uses dilation and curettage and/or evacuation when all products of conception are not expelled

Vaginal suppository

Uterus

Curette

Explanation

The physician begins the termination of a pregnancy by inducing labor with vaginal suppositories. Before using the suppositories, a laminaria, which is an applicator made of kelp or synthetic material, may be inserted in the cervix to soften and expand the cervical canal. Once the cervix is ready, the physician inserts the vaginal suppositories and labor usually results. 59856 is used when this method fails to expel all products of conception, and a dilation and curettage and/or evacuation is used to remove the remaining tissue.

Coding Tips

If performed with a hysterotomy, see 59857. For medical treatment of a spontaneous complete abortion, any trimester, see 99201–99233. For insertion of a cervical dilator only, see 59200.

ICD-9-CM Procedural

69.01 Dilation and curettage for termination of pregnancy

69.51 Aspiration curettage of uterus for termination of pregnancy

69.93 Insertion of laminaria

96.49 Other genitourinary instillation

Anesthesia

59856 00940, 01966

ICD-9-CM Diagnostic

635.01 Incomplete legally induced abortion complicated by genital tract and pelvic infection

635.02 Complete legally induced abortion complicated by genital tract and pelvic infection

635.11 Incomplete legally induced abortion complicated by delayed or excessive hemorrhage

635.12 Complete legally induced abortion complicated by delayed or excessive hemorrhage

635.21 Legally induced abortion complicated by damage to pelvic organs or tissues, incomplete

635.22 Complete legally induced abortion complicated by damage to pelvic organs or tissues

635.31 Incomplete legally induced abortion complicated by renal failure

635.32 Complete legally induced abortion complicated by renal failure

635.41 Incomplete legally induced abortion complicated by metabolic disorder

635.42 Complete legally induced abortion complicated by metabolic disorder

635.51 Legally induced abortion, complicated by shock, incomplete

635.52 Complete legally induced abortion complicated by shock

635.61 Incomplete legally induced abortion complicated by embolism

635.62 Complete legally induced abortion complicated by embolism

635.71 Incomplete legally induced abortion with other specified complications

635.72 Complete legally induced abortion with other specified complications

635.81 Incomplete legally induced abortion with unspecified complication

635.82 Complete legally induced abortion with unspecified complication

638.0 Failed attempted abortion complicated by genital tract and pelvic infection

638.1 Failed attempted abortion complicated by delayed or excessive hemorrhage

638.2 Failed attempted abortion complicated by damage to pelvic organs or tissues

638.4 Failed attempted abortion complicated by metabolic disorder

638.5 Failed attempted abortion complicated by shock

638.6 Failed attempted abortion complicated by embolism

646.03 Papyraceous fetus, antepartum — (Use additional code to further specify complication)

648.43 Maternal mental disorders, antepartum — (Use additional code(s) to identify the condition)

655.03 Central nervous system malformation in fetus, antepartum

655.13 Chromosomal abnormality in fetus, affecting management of mother, antepartum

655.20 Hereditary disease in family possibly affecting fetus, affecting management of mother, unspecified as to episode of care in pregnancy

655.23 Hereditary disease in family possibly affecting fetus, affecting management of mother, antepartum condition or complication

659.63 Elderly multigravida, with antepartum condition or complication

V61.7 Other unwanted pregnancy

CCI Version 18.3

01965-01966, 0213T, 0216T, 0228T, 0230T, 12001-12007, 12011-12057, 13100-13153, 36000, 36400-36410, 36420-36430, 36440, 36600, 36640, 37202, 43752, 51701-51703, 57410, 59130-59136❖, 59151❖, 59200, 59510-59515❖, 59525❖, 59610-59622❖, 59852❖, 62310-62319, 64400-64435, 64445-64450, 64479, 64483, 64490, 64493, 64505-64530, 69990, 93000-93010, 93040-93042, 93318, 94002, 94200, 94250, 94680-94690, 94770, 95812-95816, 95819, 95822, 95829, 95955, 96360, 96365, 96372, 96374-96376, 99148-99149, 99150

Note: These CCI edits are used for Medicare. Other payers may reimburse on codes listed above.

Medicare Edits

	Fac RVU	Non-Fac RVU	FUD	Status
59856	14.68	14.68	90	R

	MUE		Modifiers			
59856	1	51	N/A	N/A	80*

* with documentation

Medicare References: 100-2,1,90; 100-3,140.1; 100-4,3,100.1

Coding Companion for Ob/Gyn

59857

59857 Induced abortion, by 1 or more vaginal suppositories (eg, prostaglandin) with or without cervical dilation (eg, laminaria), including hospital admission and visits, delivery of fetus and secundines; with hysterotomy (failed medical evacuation)

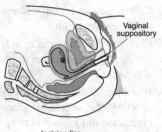

The physician induces abortion with vaginal suppositories and when all products of conception are not expelled, performs a hysterotomy

Vaginal suppository

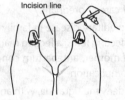

Incision line

Explanation
The physician begins the termination of a pregnancy by inducing labor with vaginal suppositories. Before using the suppositories, a laminaria, which is an applicator made of kelp or synthetic material, may be inserted in the cervix to soften and expand the cervical canal. Once the cervix is ready, the physician inserts the vaginal suppositories and labor usually results. 59857 is used when this method fails to expel all products of conception, and a hysterotomy, through an incision in the abdominal wall and uterus, is used to remove the remaining tissue. Following removal, the incision is closed with sutures.

Coding Tips
To report with dilation and curettage and/or evacuation, see 59856. For medical treatment of a spontaneous complete abortion, any trimester, see 99201–99233. For insertion of a cervical dilator only, see 59200.

ICD-9-CM Procedural
69.01 Dilation and curettage for termination of pregnancy
69.51 Aspiration curettage of uterus for termination of pregnancy
69.93 Insertion of laminaria

74.91 Hysterotomy to terminate pregnancy
96.49 Other genitourinary instillation

Anesthesia
59857 00840, 01966

ICD-9-CM Diagnostic
635.01 Incomplete legally induced abortion complicated by genital tract and pelvic infection
635.02 Complete legally induced abortion complicated by genital tract and pelvic infection
635.11 Incomplete legally induced abortion complicated by delayed or excessive hemorrhage
635.12 Complete legally induced abortion complicated by delayed or excessive hemorrhage
635.21 Legally induced abortion complicated by damage to pelvic organs or tissues, incomplete
635.22 Complete legally induced abortion complicated by damage to pelvic organs or tissues
635.31 Incomplete legally induced abortion complicated by renal failure
635.32 Complete legally induced abortion complicated by renal failure
635.41 Incomplete legally induced abortion complicated by metabolic disorder
635.42 Complete legally induced abortion complicated by metabolic disorder
635.51 Legally induced abortion, complicated by shock, incomplete
635.52 Complete legally induced abortion complicated by shock
635.61 Incomplete legally induced abortion complicated by embolism
635.62 Complete legally induced abortion complicated by embolism
635.71 Incomplete legally induced abortion with other specified complications
638.0 Failed attempted abortion complicated by genital tract and pelvic infection
638.1 Failed attempted abortion complicated by delayed or excessive hemorrhage
638.2 Failed attempted abortion complicated by damage to pelvic organs or tissues
638.4 Failed attempted abortion complicated by metabolic disorder
638.5 Failed attempted abortion complicated by shock

638.6 Failed attempted abortion complicated by embolism
646.03 Papyraceous fetus, antepartum — (Use additional code to further specify complication)
648.43 Maternal mental disorders, antepartum — (Use additional code(s) to identify the condition)
655.03 Central nervous system malformation in fetus, antepartum
655.13 Chromosomal abnormality in fetus, affecting management of mother, antepartum
655.23 Hereditary disease in family possibly affecting fetus, affecting management of mother, antepartum condition or complication
655.83 Other known or suspected fetal abnormality, not elsewhere classified, affecting management of mother, antepartum condition or complication
659.63 Elderly multigravida, with antepartum condition or complication

CCI Version 18.3
01965-01966, 0213T, 0216T, 0228T, 0230T, 12001-12007, 12011-12057, 13100-13153, 36000, 36400-36410, 36420-36430, 36440, 36600, 36640, 37202, 43752, 44005, 44180, 44602-44605, 44820-44850, 49000-49010, 49255, 49320, 51701-51703, 57410, 59135❖, 59200, 59510-59515❖, 59610-59622❖, 59851, 59855, 62310-62319, 64400-64435, 64445-64450, 64479, 64483, 64490, 64493, 64505-64530, 69990, 93000-93010, 93040-93042, 93318, 94002, 94200, 94250, 94680-94690, 94770, 95812-95816, 95819, 95822, 95829, 95955, 96360, 96365, 96372, 96374-96376, 99148-99149, 99150

Note: These CCI edits are used for Medicare. Other payers may reimburse on codes listed above.

Medicare Edits

	Fac RVU	Non-Fac RVU	FUD	Status
59857	15.16	15.16	90	R

	MUE		Modifiers		
59857	1	51	N/A	N/A	80*

* with documentation

Medicare References: 100-2,1,90; 100-3,140.1; 100-4,3,100.1

Maternity Care

59866

59866 Multifetal pregnancy reduction(s) (MPR)

Typically, under ultrasound guidance, a potassium chloride solution is injected into the fetal thorax

The number of a multiple pregnancy is reduced to improve the viability of the remaining fetus or fetuses

Explanation

Selective reduction is performed to eliminate one or more fetuses of a multiple pregnancy in an attempt to increase the viability of the remaining fetuses. Fetuses are usually eliminated in this procedure until only a twin or triplet pregnancy remains. Physicians most often use ultrasound guided intracardiac injection of potassium chloride to reduce the number of fetuses, although injection of potassium chloride in any part of the fetal body accomplishes the same result. When an intracardiac injection is performed, a 22 gauge spinal needle is advanced through the abdominal and uterine walls toward a cardiac echo using high-resolution ultrasound as a guide. With the needle position in the heart, a solution of potassium chloride is injected at intervals until prolonged cardiac standstill is observed. The physician withdraws the needle and redirects it into another gestational sac, as needed. The embryo(s) or fetus(es) that have been injected shrivel and decompose, leaving the remaining fetuses in utero an increased chance of surviving to term. Any sacs that remain intact are removed during delivery of the surviving fetus(es).

Coding Tips

For induced abortion, see 59840–59857. For medical treatment of a spontaneous complete abortion, any trimester, see 99201–99233.

ICD-9-CM Procedural

75.0   Intra-amniotic injection for abortion

75.99 Other obstetric operations

Anesthesia

59866   00840

ICD-9-CM Diagnostic

651.13 Triplet pregnancy, antepartum

651.23 Quadruplet pregnancy, antepartum

651.73 Multiple gestation following (elective) fetal reduction, antepartum condition or complication

651.83 Other specified multiple gestation, antepartum

651.93 Unspecified multiple gestation, antepartum

V23.0   Pregnancy with history of infertility

V23.41 Supervision of pregnancy with history of pre-term labor

V23.49 Supervision of pregnancy with other poor obstetric history

V23.5   Pregnancy with other poor reproductive history

V23.81 Supervision of high-risk pregnancy of elderly primigravida

V23.82 Supervision of high-risk pregnancy of elderly multigravida

V23.83 Supervision of high-risk pregnancy of young primigravida

V23.84 Supervision of high-risk pregnancy of young multigravida

V23.89 Supervision of other high-risk pregnancy

Terms To Know

elderly primigravida. Woman in her first pregnancy at an age beyond the norm, usually considered 35 years or older.

multigravida. Female who has had two or more pregnancies. Women in this category are considered to be at high risk during pregnancy.

CCI Version 18.3

01965-01966, 0213T, 0216T, 0228T, 0230T, 12001-12007, 12011-12057, 13100-13153, 36000, 36400-36410, 36420-36430, 36440, 36600, 36640, 37202, 43752, 51701-51703, 57410, 59160, 59821-59830❖, 59841-59857❖, 62310-62319, 64400-64435, 64445-64450, 64479, 64483, 64490, 64493, 64505-64530, 69990, 93000-93010, 93040-93042, 93318, 94002, 94200, 94250, 94680-94690, 94770, 95812-95816, 95819, 95822, 95829, 95955, 96360, 96365, 96372, 96374-96376, 99148-99149, 99150, J2001

Note: These CCI edits are used for Medicare. Other payers may reimburse on codes listed above.

Medicare Edits

	Fac RVU	Non-Fac RVU	FUD	Status
59866	6.32	6.32	0	R

	MUE		Modifiers	
59866	1	51	N/A	62*	80

* with documentation

Medicare References: 100-2,1,90; 100-3,140.1; 100-4,3,100.1

CPT only © 2012 American Medical Association. All Rights Reserved.

Coding Companion for Ob/Gyn

© 2012 OptumInsight, Inc.

59870

59870 Uterine evacuation and curettage for hydatidiform mole

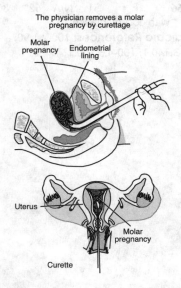

The physician removes a molar pregnancy by curettage

Molar pregnancy
Endometrial lining

Uterus

Molar pregnancy

Curette

Explanation

The physician treats a hydatidiform mole (molar pregnancy) by evacuation and curettage of the uterus. The physician inserts a speculum into the vagina to view the cervix. A tenaculum is used to grasp the cervix, pull it down, and exert traction. A dilator is inserted into the endocervix and through the cervical canal to enlarge the opening. The physician places a cannula in the endocervical canal and passes it into the uterus. The suction machine is activated and the hydatidiform mole is evacuated by rotation of the cannula. After suction curettage, a sharp curette may be used to scrape the uterus and confirm that it is empty.

Coding Tips

For treatment of a hydatidiform mole by hysterotomy, see 59100. For insertion of a cervical dilator, see 59200. For induced abortion, see 59840–59857.

ICD-9-CM Procedural

69.01 Dilation and curettage for termination of pregnancy

69.02 Dilation and curettage following delivery or abortion

69.59 Other aspiration curettage of uterus

Anesthesia

59870 00940

ICD-9-CM Diagnostic

630 Hydatidiform mole — (Use additional code from category 639 to identify any associated complications)

Terms To Know

curettage. Removal of tissue by scraping.

dilation. Artificial increase in the diameter of an opening or lumen made by medication or by instrumentation.

evacuation. Removal or purging of waste material.

hydatidiform mole. Trophoblastic neoplasm that mimics pregnancy by proliferating from a pathologic ovum and resulting only in a mass of cysts resembling grapes, 80 percent of which are benign, but require surgical removal. Hydatidiform moles can be complete, in which there is no fetal tissue, or partial, in which fetal tissue is frequently present.

speculum. Tool used to enlarge the opening of any canal or cavity.

suction. Vacuum evacuation of fluid or tissue.

CCI Version 18.3

01965-01966, 0213T, 0216T, 0228T, 0230T, 12001-12007, 12011-12057, 13100-13153, 36000, 36400-36410, 36420-36430, 36440, 36600, 36640, 37202, 43752, 51701-51703, 57410, 59855-59866, 62310-62319, 64400-64435, 64445-64450, 64479, 64483, 64490, 64493, 64505-64530, 69990, 93000-93010, 93040-93042, 93318, 94002, 94200, 94250, 94680-94690, 94770, 95812-95816, 95819, 95822, 95829, 95955, 96360, 96365, 96372, 96374-96376, 99148-99149, 99150

Note: These CCI edits are used for Medicare. Other payers may reimburse on codes listed above.

Medicare Edits

	Fac RVU	Non-Fac RVU	FUD	Status
59870	14.22	14.22	90	A

	MUE			Modifiers	
59870	1	51	N/A	N/A	80

* with documentation

Medicare References: None

Coding Companion for Ob/Gyn

Maternity Care

59871

59871 Removal of cerclage suture under anesthesia (other than local)

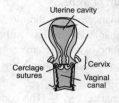

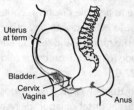

Cerclage sutures encircle the cervical opening, keeping it from premature dilation. When a fetus reaches term, the sutures are removed. Cerclage may also be employed for other circumstances as well

Code 59871 reports the removal of cerclage sutures in a session that requires the patient to be under anesthesia

Explanation

The physician removes a cervical cerclage, a suture that had been placed to hold the cervix closed. A cerclage is most often placed when a cervix dilates too early during pregnancy and risks a miscarriage. The physician severs the sutures and removes them. This code includes anesthesia other than local.

Coding Tips

For cerclage of cervix, during pregnancy, vaginal, see 59320; abdominal, see 59325. For non-obstetric cerclage, see 57700.

ICD-9-CM Procedural

69.96   Removal of cerclage material from cervix

Anesthesia

59871   00940

ICD-9-CM Diagnostic

622.3   Old laceration of cervix

654.53   Cervical incompetence, antepartum condition or complication — (Code first any associated obstructed labor, 660.2)

654.63   Other congenital or acquired abnormality of cervix, antepartum condition or complication — (Code first any associated obstructed labor, 660.2)

654.93   Other and unspecified abnormality of organs and soft tissues of pelvis, antepartum condition or complication — (Code first any associated obstructed labor, 660.2)

V23.2   Pregnancy with history of abortion

V23.81   Supervision of high-risk pregnancy of elderly primigravida

V23.82   Supervision of high-risk pregnancy of elderly multigravida

V23.83   Supervision of high-risk pregnancy of young primigravida

V23.84   Supervision of high-risk pregnancy of young multigravida

V23.89   Supervision of other high-risk pregnancy

Terms To Know

cerclage. Looping or encircling an organ or tissue with wire or ligature for positional support.

elderly primigravida. Woman in her first pregnancy at an age beyond the norm, usually considered 35 years or older.

McDonald operation. Surgical procedure in which the opening of the cervix is decreased via pursestring sutures around the bottom of the cervix.

multigravida. Female who has had two or more pregnancies. Women in this category are considered to be at high risk during pregnancy.

obstetric cerclage. Surgical procedure that encircles an incompetent cervix with suture material for support in an attempt to retain a pregnancy, usually performed between 12 and 14 weeks' gestation and often employed in patients with a history of spontaneous abortion in otherwise normal pregnancies.

CCI Version 18.3

0213T, 0216T, 0228T, 0230T, 12001-12007, 12011-12057, 13100-13153, 15851, 36000, 36400-36410, 36420-36430, 36440, 36600, 36640, 37202, 43752, 51701-51703, 57410, 62310-62319, 64400-64435, 64445-64450, 64479, 64483, 64490, 64493, 64505-64530, 69990, 93000-93010, 93040-93042, 93318, 94002, 94200, 94250, 94680-94690, 94770, 95812-95816, 95819, 95822, 95829, 95955, 96360, 96365, 96372, 96374-96376, 99148-99149, 99150, J0670, J2001

Note: These CCI edits are used for Medicare. Other payers may reimburse on codes listed above.

Medicare Edits

	Fac RVU	Non-Fac RVU	FUD	Status
59871	4.04	4.04	0	A

	MUE		Modifiers		
59871	1	51	N/A	N/A	80*

* with documentation

Medicare References: None

Coding Companion for Ob/Gyn

64430-64435

64430 Injection, anesthetic agent; pudendal nerve
64435 paracervical (uterine) nerve

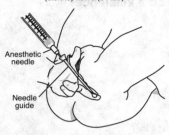

An anesthetic agent is injected to block the pudendal nerve (64430) or the paracervical (uterine) nerve (64435)

Anesthetic needle

Needle guide

A needle guide may be used to direct the injection using anatomical landmarks

The pudendal nerve (64430) and the para-cervical or uterine nerve (64435) are typically blocked by a transvaginal injection to both sides

The nerve may also be blocked by an extra-vaginal injection. A common use of these blocks is to prepare for a vaginal delivery

Explanation

The physician anesthetizes the pudendal nerve for anesthesia of the perineum, rectum, and parts of the bladder and genitals. In 64430, the pudendal nerve is blocked, typically for perineal pain control, for example, during vaginal delivery. Code 64435 is a female-only procedure in which the area around the cervix is injected with a local anesthetic to supply pain control for the first stage of labor.

Coding Tips

For anesthetic injection into the superior hypogastric plexus, see 64517. Surgical trays, A4550, are not separately reimbursed by Medicare; however, other third-party payers may cover them. Check with the specific payer to determine coverage.

ICD-9-CM Procedural

04.81 Injection of anesthetic into peripheral nerve for analgesia

Anesthesia

N/A

ICD-9-CM Diagnostic

218.0 Submucous leiomyoma of uterus
218.1 Intramural leiomyoma of uterus
218.2 Subserous leiomyoma of uterus
219.0 Benign neoplasm of cervix uteri
219.1 Benign neoplasm of corpus uteri
219.8 Benign neoplasm of other specified parts of uterus

221.0 Benign neoplasm of fallopian tube and uterine ligaments
239.5 Neoplasm of unspecified nature of other genitourinary organs
616.0 Cervicitis and endocervicitis — (Use additional code to identify organism: 041.00-041.09, 041.10-041.19)
616.2 Cyst of Bartholin's gland — (Use additional code to identify organism: 041.00-041.09, 041.10-041.19)
622.11 Mild dysplasia of cervix
622.12 Moderate dysplasia of cervix
622.7 Mucous polyp of cervix
625.3 Dysmenorrhea
626.2 Excessive or frequent menstruation
626.8 Other disorder of menstruation and other abnormal bleeding from female genital tract
632 Missed abortion — (Use additional code from category 639 to identify any associated complications)
635.01 Incomplete legally induced abortion complicated by genital tract and pelvic infection
635.11 Incomplete legally induced abortion complicated by delayed or excessive hemorrhage
635.21 Legally induced abortion complicated by damage to pelvic organs or tissues, incomplete
635.31 Incomplete legally induced abortion complicated by renal failure
635.41 Incomplete legally induced abortion complicated by metabolic disorder
635.51 Legally induced abortion, complicated by shock, incomplete
635.61 Incomplete legally induced abortion complicated by embolism
635.71 Incomplete legally induced abortion with other specified complications
635.72 Complete legally induced abortion with other specified complications
637.20 Abortion, unspecified as to completion or legality, complicated by damage to pelvic organs or tissues
637.21 Abortion, unspecified as to legality, incomplete, complicated by damage to pelvic organs or tissues
637.60 Abortion, unspecified as to completion or legality, complicated by embolism
637.71 Abortion, unspecified as to legality, incomplete, with other specified complications
638.0 Failed attempted abortion complicated by genital tract and pelvic infection

638.1 Failed attempted abortion complicated by delayed or excessive hemorrhage
638.2 Failed attempted abortion complicated by damage to pelvic organs or tissues
646.31 Pregnancy complication, recurrent pregnancy loss, with or without mention of antepartum condition — (Use additional code to further specify complication)
650 Normal delivery — (This code is for use as a single diagnosis code and is not to be used with any other code in the range 630-676. Use additional code to indicate outcome of delivery: V27.0.)
660.01 Obstruction caused by malposition of fetus at onset of labor, delivered — (Use additional code from 652.0-652.9 to identify condition)
664.01 First-degree perineal laceration, with delivery

CCI Version 18.3

0178T-0179T, 0180T, 01991-01992, 36000, 36400-36410, 36420-36430, 36440, 36600, 51701-51703, 69990, 76000-76001, 76998, 77001-77002, 90862, 92585, 93000-93010, 93040-93042, 93318, 94002, 94200, 94250, 94680-94690, 94770, 95812-95816, 95819, 95822, 95829, 95860-95861, 95867-95868, 95870, 95900, 95904, 95920, 95925-95934, 95936-95939, 95955, 96360, 96365, 96372, 96374-96376, 99148-99149, 99150, J0670, J2001

Also not with 64430: 20550-20553

Note: These CCI edits are used for Medicare. Other payers may reimburse on codes listed above.

Medicare Edits

	Fac RVU	Non-Fac RVU	FUD	Status
64430	2.43	4.13	0	A
64435	2.47	4.13	0	A

	MUE		Modifiers		
64430	1	51	50	N/A	N/A
64435	1	51	50	N/A	N/A

* with documentation

Medicare References: None

Nervous

64517

64517 Injection, anesthetic agent; superior hypogastric plexus

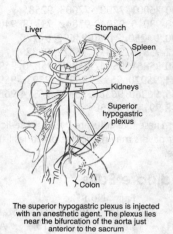

The superior hypogastric plexus is injected with an anesthetic agent. The plexus lies near the bifurcation of the aorta just anterior to the sacrum

Explanation

The physician performs a nerve block on the superior hypogastric plexus by injecting an anesthetic agent through a needle inserted in the L5/S1 interspace. The superior hypogastric plexus, also called the presacral nerve, is located in front of the upper part of the sacrum and is formed by lower lumbar nerves responsible for pain sensation in the pelvic area. This nerve block is done in such cases as severe, intractable menstrual pain and pain due to pelvic area metastases from cancer such as prostatic malignancy. The patient is placed in the prone position and prepped. A 6-inch needle is guided under radiological imaging, such as fluoroscopy (reported separately), into the ventral lateral spine and through the L5/S1 interspace. Needle position is checked by injecting contrast material and aspirating for the return of any blood, urine, or cerebral spinal fluid. With negative aspiration results and imaging verifying that the needle position is in the prevertebral space and not within a blood vessel, a ureter, or spinal nerves, local anesthetic is injected on both sides.

Coding Tips

Local anesthesia is included in this service. Fluoroscopic guidance is reported separately. Surgical trays, A4550, are not separately reimbursed by Medicare; however, other third-party payers may cover them. Check with the specific payer to determine coverage.

ICD-9-CM Procedural

05.31 Injection of anesthetic into sympathetic nerve for analgesia

Anesthesia

64517 N/A

ICD-9-CM Diagnostic

617.0	Endometriosis of uterus
617.1	Endometriosis of ovary
617.2	Endometriosis of fallopian tube
617.3	Endometriosis of pelvic peritoneum
617.4	Endometriosis of rectovaginal septum and vagina
617.5	Endometriosis of intestine
617.8	Endometriosis of other specified sites
617.9	Endometriosis, site unspecified
625.0	Dyspareunia
625.2	Mittelschmerz
625.3	Dysmenorrhea
625.9	Unspecified symptom associated with female genital organs
719.45	Pain in joint, pelvic region and thigh

Terms To Know

dysmenorrhea. Painful menstruation that may be primary, or essential, due to prostaglandin production and the onset of menstruation; secondary due to uterine, tubal, or ovarian abnormality or disease; spasmodic arising uterine contractions; or obstructive due to some mechanical blockage or interference with the menstrual flow.

endometriosis. Aberrant uterine mucosal tissue appearing in areas of the pelvic cavity outside of its normal location, lining the uterus and inflaming surrounding tissues, and can result in infertility and spontaneous abortion.

fluoroscopy. Radiology technique that allows visual examination of part of the body or a function of an organ using a device that projects an x-ray image on a fluorescent screen.

injection. Forcing a liquid substance into a body part such as a joint or muscle.

nerve block. Regional anesthesia/analgesia administered by injection that prevents sensory nerve impulses from reaching the central nervous system.

plexus. Bundle of nerves that serve a particular region of the body that lies relatively deep in the body as opposed to superficial nerves, which are close to the surface of the skin.

prone. Lying face downward.

sacrum. Lower portion of the spine composed of five fused vertebrae designated as S1-S5.

CCI Version 18.3

0178T-0179T, 0180T, 01991-01992, 0282T-0285T, 36000, 36400-36410, 36420-36430, 36440, 36600, 51701-51703, 69990, 76000-76001, 76800, 76998, 77001, 90862, 92585, 93000-93010, 93040-93042, 93318, 94002, 94200, 94250, 94680-94690, 94770, 95812-95816, 95819, 95822, 95829, 95860-95861, 95867-95868, 95870, 95900, 95904, 95920, 95925-95934, 95936-95939, 95955, 96360, 96365, 96372, 96374-96376, 99148-99149, 99150, J0670, J2001

Note: These CCI edits are used for Medicare. Other payers may reimburse on codes listed above.

Medicare Edits

	Fac RVU	Non-Fac RVU	FUD	Status
64517	3.69	5.42	0	A

	MUE		Modifiers		
64517	1	51	N/A	N/A	N/A

* with documentation

Medicare References: None

Coding Companion for Ob/Gyn

64681

64681 Destruction by neurolytic agent, with or without radiologic monitoring; superior hypogastric plexus

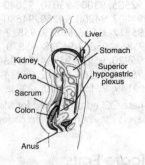

The sympathetic nerve system of the abdominal viscera is distributed largely via the celiac plexus, a network of ganglia on either side of the abdominal aorta just under the diaphragm and extending into the superior hypogastric plexus. The nerve is injected with a neurolytic agent. This plexus lies near the bifurcation of the aorta just anterior to the sacrum

Explanation

The physician performs a neurolysis on the superior hypogastric plexus by injecting a chemical, thermal, or electrical agent through a needle inserted in the L5/S1 interspace. The superior hypogastric plexus, also called the presacral nerve, is located in front of the upper part of the sacrum and is formed by lower lumbar nerves responsible for pain sensation in the pelvic area. Nerve destruction is done in such cases as severe, intractable menstrual pain and pain due to pelvic area metastases from cancer such as prostatic malignancy when an anesthetic nerve block does not offer sufficient relief. The patient is placed in the prone position and prepped. A 6-inch needle is guided under radiological imaging, such as fluoroscopy (reported separately), into the ventral lateral spine and through the L5/S1 interspace. Needle position is checked by injecting contrast material and aspirating for the return of any blood, urine, or cerebral spinal fluid. With negative aspiration results and imaging verifying that the needle position is in the prevertebral space and not within a blood vessel, a ureter, or spinal nerves, the neurolytic agent is injected, or delivered, to both sides.

Coding Tips

Code 64681 includes the injection of other therapeutic agents (e.g., corticosteroids). For destruction by neurolytic agent, with or without radiologic monitoring, celiac plexus, see 64680.

ICD-9-CM Procedural

05.32 Injection of neurolytic agent into sympathetic nerve

Anesthesia

64681 N/A

ICD-9-CM Diagnostic

617.0 Endometriosis of uterus
617.1 Endometriosis of ovary
617.2 Endometriosis of fallopian tube
617.3 Endometriosis of pelvic peritoneum
617.4 Endometriosis of rectovaginal septum and vagina
617.5 Endometriosis of intestine
617.8 Endometriosis of other specified sites
617.9 Endometriosis, site unspecified
625.0 Dyspareunia
625.2 Mittelschmerz
625.3 Dysmenorrhea
625.9 Unspecified symptom associated with female genital organs

Terms To Know

dysmenorrhea. Painful menstruation that may be primary, or essential, due to prostaglandin production and the onset of menstruation; secondary due to uterine, tubal, or ovarian abnormality or disease; spasmodic arising uterine contractions; or obstructive due to some mechanical blockage or interference with the menstrual flow.

endometriosis. Aberrant uterine mucosal tissue appearing in areas of the pelvic cavity outside of its normal location, lining the uterus and inflaming surrounding tissues, and can result in infertility and spontaneous abortion.

fluoroscopy. Radiology technique that allows visual examination of part of the body or a function of an organ using a device that projects an x-ray image on a fluorescent screen.

neurolytic. Destruction of nerve tissue.

plexus. Bundle of nerves that serve a particular region of the body that lies relatively deep in the body as opposed to superficial nerves, which are close to the surface of the skin.

prone. Lying face downward.

sacrum. Lower portion of the spine composed of five fused vertebrae designated as S1-S5.

CCI Version 18.3

0216T, 0228T, 0230T, 12001-12007, 12011-12057, 13100-13153, 20550-20553, 36000, 36400-36410, 36420-36430, 36440, 36600, 36640, 37202, 43752, 51701-51703, 62310-62319, 64400-64435, 64445-64450, 64479, 64483, 64493, 64505-64530, 69990, 76000-76001, 77001-77003, 92585, 93000-93010, 93040-93042, 93318, 94002, 94200, 94250, 94680-94690, 94770, 95812-95816, 95819, 95822, 95829, 95860-95861, 95867-95868, 95870, 95900, 95904, 95920, 95925-95934, 95936-95939, 95955, 96360, 96365, 96372, 96374-96376, 99148-99149, 99150

Note: These CCI edits are used for Medicare. Other payers may reimburse on codes listed above.

Medicare Edits

	Fac RVU	Non-Fac RVU	FUD	Status
64681	5.86	11.17	10	A

	MUE		Modifiers		
64681	1	51	N/A	N/A	N/A

* with documentation

Medicare References: None

Nervous

69990

69990 Microsurgical techniques, requiring use of operating microscope (List separately in addition to code for primary procedure)

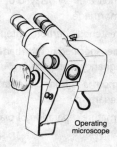

Operating microscope

Explanation

The physician uses a surgical microscope when the services are performed using the techniques of microsurgery, except when the microscopy is part of the procedure (such as in 15756). This code is reported in addition to the primary procedure.

Coding Tips

This reports surgical services performed using techniques of microsurgery. It should not be used for visualization with magnifying loupes or corrected vision. It should not be reported with procedures where use of an operating microscope is an inclusive component. As an "add-on" code, 69990 is not subject to multiple procedure rules. No reimbursement reduction or modifier 51 is applied. "Add-on" codes describe additional intraservice work associated with the primary procedure. They are performed by the same physician on the same date of service as the primary service/procedure, and must never be reported as a stand-alone code.

ICD-9-CM Procedural

The ICD-9-CM procedural code(s) would be the same as the actual procedure performed because these are in-addition-to codes.

Anesthesia

69990 N/A

ICD-9-CM Diagnostic

This is an add-on code. Refer to the corresponding primary procedure code for ICD-9-CM diagnosis code links.

Terms To Know

microsurgery. Surgical procedures performed under magnification using a surgical microscope.

operating microscope. Compound microscope with two or more lens systems or several grouped lenses in one unit that provides magnifying power to the surgeon up to 40X.

CCI Version 18.3

No CCI Edits apply to this code.

Medicare Edits

	Fac RVU	Non-Fac RVU	FUD	Status
69990	6.44	6.44	N/A	R

	MUE		Modifiers		
69990	1	N/A	N/A	N/A	80

* with documentation

Medicare References: None

Coding Companion for Ob/Gyn

Operating Microscope

76801-76802

76801 Ultrasound, pregnant uterus, real time with image documentation, fetal and maternal evaluation, first trimester (< 14 weeks 0 days), transabdominal approach; single or first gestation

76802 each additional gestation (List separately in addition to code for primary procedure)

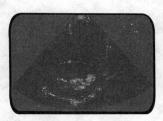

A real time ultrasound is taken of a pregnant uterus in the first trimester. Report 76801 for the first gestation and 76802 for each additional gestation

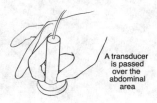

A transducer is passed over the abdominal area

Explanation

Diagnostic ultrasound is an imaging technique bouncing sound waves far above the level of human perception through interior body structures. The sound waves pass through different densities of tissue and reflect back to a receiving unit at varying speeds. The unit converts the waves to electrical pulses that are immediately displayed in picture form on screen. Real time scanning displays both two-dimensional structure images and movement with time. Use 76801 to report real time ultrasound, transabdominal, with image documentation on a pregnant uterus for fetal and maternal evaluation in the first trimester of a single or first gestation. This includes determining the number of fetuses and gestational sacs and taking their measurements, surveying the visible fetal and placental structure, assessing amniotic fluid volume and sac shape, and examining the maternal uterus and adnexa. Report 76802 for each additional gestation evaluation.

Coding Tips

As an "add-on" code, 76802 is not subject to multiple procedure rules. No reimbursement reduction or modifier 51 is applied. "Add-on" codes describe additional intra-service work associated with the primary procedure. They are performed by the same physician on the same date of service as the primary service/procedure, and must never be reported as a stand-alone code. These codes include the determination of the number of gestational sacs and fetuses along with gestational measurements for the first trimester (gestational age less than 14 weeks, 0 days). Results must be documented in the report for each of the following elements, including the reason that nonvisualization occurred: the visible fetal and placental structure, a qualitative assessment of the volume of amniotic fluid, and the shape of the gestational sac, as well as an examination of the maternal uterus and adnexa. It is appropriate to code an obstetrical ultrasound for a patient who has an established diagnosis of pregnancy, who presents with indications necessitating the exam that may be pregnancy related, even when the outcome shows that the patient is no longer currently pregnant.

ICD-9-CM Procedural

88.78 Diagnostic ultrasound of gravid uterus

Anesthesia
N/A

ICD-9-CM Diagnostic

630 Hydatidiform mole — (Use additional code from category 639 to identify any associated complications)

631.0 Inappropriate change in quantitative human chorionic gonadotropin (hCG) in early pregnancy

631.8 Other abnormal products of conception

632 Missed abortion — (Use additional code from category 639 to identify any associated complications)

633.01 Abdominal pregnancy with intrauterine pregnancy — (Use additional code from category 639 to identify any associated complications)

633.11 Tubal pregnancy with intrauterine pregnancy — (Use additional code from category 639 to identify any associated complications)

633.21 Ovarian pregnancy with intrauterine pregnancy — (Use additional code from category 639 to identify any associated complications)

633.81 Other ectopic pregnancy with intrauterine pregnancy — (Use additional code from category 639 to identify any associated complications)

633.91 Unspecified ectopic pregnancy with intrauterine pregnancy — (Use additional code from category 639 to identify any associated complications)

634.00 Unspecified spontaneous abortion complicated by genital tract and pelvic infection

634.01 Incomplete spontaneous abortion complicated by genital tract and pelvic infection

634.02 Complete spontaneous abortion complicated by genital tract and pelvic infection

634.11 Incomplete spontaneous abortion complicated by delayed or excessive hemorrhage

640.03 Threatened abortion, antepartum

640.83 Other specified hemorrhage in early pregnancy, antepartum

641.13 Hemorrhage from placenta previa, antepartum

641.23 Premature separation of placenta, antepartum

642.43 Mild or unspecified pre-eclampsia, antepartum

642.53 Severe pre-eclampsia, antepartum

646.33 Pregnancy complication, recurrent pregnancy loss, antepartum condition or complication — (Use additional code to further specify complication)

651.03 Twin pregnancy, antepartum

651.33 Twin pregnancy with fetal loss and retention of one fetus, antepartum

655.13 Chromosomal abnormality in fetus, affecting management of mother, antepartum

655.23 Hereditary disease in family possibly affecting fetus, affecting management of mother, antepartum condition or complication

V23.89 Supervision of other high-risk pregnancy

CCI Version 18.3
76998

Also not with 76801: 76805-76810, 76812, 76815-76816, 76830❖

Note: These CCI edits are used for Medicare. Other payers may reimburse on codes listed above.

Medicare Edits

	Fac RVU	Non-Fac RVU	FUD	Status
76801	3.87	3.87	N/A	A
76802	2.04	2.04	N/A	A

	MUE			Modifiers		
76801	1	N/A	N/A	N/A	80*
76802	3	N/A	N/A	N/A	80*

* with documentation

Medicare References: None

Radiology

76805-76810

76805 Ultrasound, pregnant uterus, real time with image documentation, fetal and maternal evaluation, after first trimester (> or = 14 weeks 0 days), transabdominal approach; single or first gestation

76810 each additional gestation (List separately in addition to code for primary procedure)

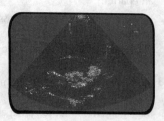

A real time ultrasound is taken of a pregnant uterus after the first trimester. Report 76805 for studies on the first or a single gestation and 76810 for each additional gestation

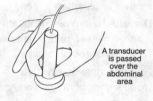

A transducer is passed over the abdominal area

Explanation

Diagnostic ultrasound is an imaging technique bouncing sound waves far above the level of human perception through interior body structures. The sound waves pass through different densities of tissue and reflect back to a receiving unit at varying speeds. The unit converts the waves to electrical pulses that are immediately displayed in picture form on screen. Real time scanning displays both two-dimensional structure images and movement with time. Use 76805 to report real time ultrasound, transabdominal, with image documentation on a pregnant uterus for fetal and maternal evaluation after the first trimester of a single or first gestation. This includes determining the number of fetuses and amniotic/chorionic sacs, taking measurements appropriate for gestational age, surveying intracranial, spinal, abdominal, and heart chamber anatomy as well as the insertion site of the umbilical cord and the location of the placenta, and assessing amniotic fluid and maternal adnexa. Report 76810 for each additional gestation evaluation.

Coding Tips

As an "add-on" code, 76810 is not subject to multiple procedure rules. No reimbursement reduction or modifier 51 is applied. "Add-on" codes describe additional intra-service work associated with the primary procedure. They are performed by the same physician on the same date of service as the primary service/procedure, and must never be reported as a stand-alone code. These codes include the determination of the number of chorionic sacs and fetuses along with gestational measurements after the first trimester (gestational age greater than or equal to 14 weeks, 0 days). Results must be documented in the report for each of the following elements, including the reason that nonvisualization occurred: surveying the structure of the fetus' intracranial, spinal, and abdominal anatomy, its four-chambered heart, the insertion site of the umbilical cord, location of the placenta, and an assessment of the amniotic fluid, as well as an examination of the maternal adnexa. It is appropriate to code an obstetrical ultrasound for a patient who has an established diagnosis of pregnancy, who presents with indications necessitating the exam that may be pregnancy related, even when the outcome shows that the patient is no longer currently pregnant.

ICD-9-CM Procedural

88.78 Diagnostic ultrasound of gravid uterus

Anesthesia

N/A

ICD-9-CM Diagnostic

630 Hydatidiform mole — (Use additional code from category 639 to identify any associated complications)

631.0 Inappropriate change in quantitative human chorionic gonadotropin (hCG) in early pregnancy

631.8 Other abnormal products of conception

634.11 Incomplete spontaneous abortion complicated by delayed or excessive hemorrhage

640.03 Threatened abortion, antepartum

640.83 Other specified hemorrhage in early pregnancy, antepartum

640.93 Unspecified hemorrhage in early pregnancy, antepartum

641.03 Placenta previa without hemorrhage, antepartum

641.13 Hemorrhage from placenta previa, antepartum

641.23 Premature separation of placenta, antepartum

641.33 Antepartum hemorrhage associated with coagulation defect, antepartum

642.43 Mild or unspecified pre-eclampsia, antepartum

642.53 Severe pre-eclampsia, antepartum

646.33 Pregnancy complication, recurrent pregnancy loss, antepartum condition or complication — (Use additional code to further specify complication)

651.03 Twin pregnancy, antepartum

651.33 Twin pregnancy with fetal loss and retention of one fetus, antepartum

652.03 Unstable lie of fetus, antepartum — (Code first any associated obstructed labor, 660.0)

653.53 Unusually large fetus causing disproportion, antepartum — (Code first any associated obstructed labor, 660.1)

655.13 Chromosomal abnormality in fetus, affecting management of mother, antepartum

655.23 Hereditary disease in family possibly affecting fetus, affecting management of mother, antepartum condition or complication

V23.89 Supervision of other high-risk pregnancy

CCI Version 18.3

51701-51702, 76998

Also not with 76805: 76802, 76812, 76815-76816, 76830-76831❖, 76856-76857❖

Also not with 76810: 76815

Note: These CCI edits are used for Medicare. Other payers may reimburse on codes listed above.

Medicare Edits

	Fac RVU	Non-Fac RVU	FUD	Status
76805	4.48	4.48	N/A	A
76810	2.93	2.93	N/A	A

	MUE		Modifiers		
76805	1	N/A	N/A	N/A	80*
76810	3	N/A	N/A	N/A	80*

* with documentation

Medicare References: None

76811-76812

76811 Ultrasound, pregnant uterus, real time with image documentation, fetal and maternal evaluation plus detailed fetal anatomic examination, transabdominal approach; single or first gestation

76812 each additional gestation (List separately in addition to code for primary procedure)

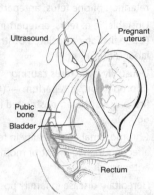

Ultrasound is performed on a pregnant uterus, real time with documentation. The fetus is examed for length of limb bones, cranial development, as well as other landmarks. A full evaluation of the mother is performed as well. Report 76811 for single or first gestation and 76812 for each additional gestation

Explanation

Diagnostic ultrasound is an imaging technique bouncing sound waves far above the level of human perception through interior body structures. The sound waves pass through different densities of tissue and reflect back to a receiving unit at varying speeds. The unit converts the waves to electrical pulses that are immediately displayed in picture form on screen. Real time scanning displays both two-dimensional structure images and movement with time. Use 76811 to report real time ultrasound, transabdominal, with image documentation on a pregnant uterus for fetal and maternal evaluation plus detailed fetal anatomic examination of a single or first gestation. This includes determining the number of fetuses and amniotic/chorionic sacs, taking measurements appropriate for gestational age, and surveying intracranial, spinal, abdominal, and heart chamber anatomy plus a detailed evaluation of the brain and ventricles, face, heart and outflow tracts, chest, abdominal organs, and number, length, and structure of the limbs. Assessing amniotic fluid, maternal adnexa, and any other fetal anatomy is also done with a detailed evaluation of the umbilical cord and the placenta. Report 76812 for each additional gestation evaluation.

Coding Tips

As an "add-on" code, 76812 is not subject to multiple procedure rules. No reimbursement reduction or modifier 51 is applied. "Add-on" codes describe additional intra-service work associated with the primary procedure. They are performed by the same physician on the same date of service as the primary service/procedure, and must never be reported as a stand-alone code. Results must be documented in the report for each of the following elements, including the reason that nonvisualization occurred: surveying the structure of the fetus' spinal, abdominal, and intracranial anatomy with a detailed evaluation of the brain and ventricles and specifics of the fetus' abdominal structures, surveying the four-chambered heart and its outflow tracts along with chest anatomy, an assessment of the limbs and face, a detailed evaluation of the umbilical cord along with its insertion site, location and details of the placenta, and an assessment of the amniotic fluid, as well as an examination of the maternal adnexa. It is appropriate to code an obstetrical ultrasound for a patient who has an established diagnosis of pregnancy, who presents with indications necessitating the exam that may be pregnancy related, even when the outcome shows that the patient is no longer currently pregnant.

ICD-9-CM Procedural

88.78 Diagnostic ultrasound of gravid uterus

Anesthesia

N/A

ICD-9-CM Diagnostic

651.03 Twin pregnancy, antepartum

651.33 Twin pregnancy with fetal loss and retention of one fetus, antepartum

652.03 Unstable lie of fetus, antepartum — (Code first any associated obstructed labor, 660.0)

652.53 High fetal head at term, antepartum — (Code first any associated obstructed labor, 660.0)

652.73 Prolapsed arm of fetus, antepartum condition or complication — (Code first any associated obstructed labor, 660.0)

653.43 Fetopelvic disproportion, antepartum — (Code first any associated obstructed labor, 660.1)

653.53 Unusually large fetus causing disproportion, antepartum — (Code first any associated obstructed labor, 660.1)

653.63 Hydrocephalic fetus causing disproportion, antepartum — (Code

first any associated obstructed labor, 660.1)

653.73 Other fetal abnormality causing disproportion, antepartum — (Code first any associated obstructed labor, 660.1)

653.83 Fetal disproportion of other origin, antepartum — (Code first any associated obstructed labor, 660.1)

655.13 Chromosomal abnormality in fetus, affecting management of mother, antepartum

655.23 Hereditary disease in family possibly affecting fetus, affecting management of mother, antepartum condition or complication

655.33 Suspected damage to fetus from viral disease in mother, affecting management of mother, antepartum condition or complication

655.53 Suspected damage to fetus from drugs, affecting management of mother, antepartum

655.73 Decreased fetal movements, affecting management of mother, antepartum condition or complication

656.53 Poor fetal growth, affecting management of mother, antepartum condition or complication

656.63 Excessive fetal growth affecting management of mother, antepartum

V28.3 Encounter for routine screening for malformation using ultrasonics

V28.4 Antenatal screening for fetal growth retardation using ultrasonics

CCI Version 18.3

51701-51702, 76998

Also not with 76811: 76801, 76805, 76815-76816, 76830-76831✛, 76856-76857✛, 76941

Note: These CCI edits are used for Medicare. Other payers may reimburse on codes listed above.

Medicare Edits

	Fac RVU	Non-Fac RVU	FUD	Status
76811	5.68	5.68	N/A	A
76812	6.26	6.26	N/A	A

	MUE		Modifiers		
76811	1	N/A	N/A	N/A	80*
76812	3	N/A	N/A	N/A	80*

* with documentation

Medicare References: None

76813-76814

76813 Ultrasound, pregnant uterus, real time with image documentation, first trimester fetal nuchal translucency measurement, transabdominal or transvaginal approach; single or first gestation

76814 each additional gestation (List separately in addition to code for primary procedure)

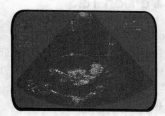

A real time ultrasound is taken of a pregnant uterus to exam nuchal translucency measurement via transabdominal or transvaginal approach.

Report 76813 for single gestation and 76814 for each additional gestation

Explanation

Fetal nuchal translucency provides a noninvasive method to screen for chromosomal abnormalities or heart defects in the first trimester. Nuchal pertains to the back of the neck. Until the lymphatic system of the fetus develops, the back of the neck is a good predictor of fetal health, because the fetus will lie on its back and edema will form in the neck if circulatory problems are present. In a fetal nuchal translucency test, ultrasound transducers on the maternal abdomen or vagina focus on the fetal neck, and the depth of tissue there is measured. The examination includes a calculation of fetal length, and the two measurements are correlated. Fetal nuchal edema does not provide a definitive diagnosis, but would warrant further testing (e.g., chorionic villus sampling). Report 76813 for fetal nuchal translucency testing of one fetus and 76814 for each additional fetus.

Coding Tips

As an "add-on" code, 76814 is not subject to multiple procedure rules. No reimbursement reduction or modifier 51 is applied. "Add-on" codes describe additional intra-service work associated with the primary procedure. They are performed by the same physician on the same date of service as the primary service/procedure, and must never be reported as a stand-alone code. Use 76814 in conjunction with 76813. If fetal and maternal evaluation with detailed fetal anatomic examination is performed, see codes 76811–76812.

ICD-9-CM Procedural

88.78   Diagnostic ultrasound of gravid uterus

Anesthesia

N/A

ICD-9-CM Diagnostic

630   Hydatidiform mole — (Use additional code from category 639 to identify any associated complications)

631.0   Inappropriate change in quantitative human chorionic gonadotropin (hCG) in early pregnancy

631.8   Other abnormal products of conception

633.11   Tubal pregnancy with intrauterine pregnancy — (Use additional code from category 639 to identify any associated complications)

633.21   Ovarian pregnancy with intrauterine pregnancy — (Use additional code from category 639 to identify any associated complications)

633.81   Other ectopic pregnancy with intrauterine pregnancy — (Use additional code from category 639 to identify any associated complications)

633.91   Unspecified ectopic pregnancy with intrauterine pregnancy — (Use additional code from category 639 to identify any associated complications)

640.83   Other specified hemorrhage in early pregnancy, antepartum

641.03   Placenta previa without hemorrhage, antepartum

641.13   Hemorrhage from placenta previa, antepartum

641.23   Premature separation of placenta, antepartum

641.83   Other antepartum hemorrhage, antepartum

644.03   Threatened premature labor, antepartum

646.33   Pregnancy complication, recurrent pregnancy loss, antepartum condition or complication — (Use additional code to further specify complication)

655.03   Central nervous system malformation in fetus, antepartum

655.13   Chromosomal abnormality in fetus, affecting management of mother, antepartum

655.23   Hereditary disease in family possibly affecting fetus, affecting management of mother, antepartum condition or complication

655.93   Unspecified fetal abnormality affecting management of mother, antepartum condition or complication

V23.3   Pregnancy with grand multiparity

V23.5   Pregnancy with other poor reproductive history

V23.81   Supervision of high-risk pregnancy of elderly primigravida

V23.82   Supervision of high-risk pregnancy of elderly multigravida

V23.83   Supervision of high-risk pregnancy of young primigravida

V23.84   Supervision of high-risk pregnancy of young multigravida

V23.89   Supervision of other high-risk pregnancy

V23.9   Unspecified high-risk pregnancy

V28.3   Encounter for routine screening for malformation using ultrasonics

V28.4   Antenatal screening for fetal growth retardation using ultrasonics

Terms To Know

ultrasound. Imaging using ultra-high sound frequency bounced off body structures.

CCI Version 18.3

Also not with 76813: 51701-51702, 76830❖, 76857❖, 76998

Note: These CCI edits are used for Medicare. Other payers may reimburse on codes listed above.

Medicare Edits

	Fac RVU	Non-Fac RVU	FUD	Status
76813	3.76	3.76	N/A	A
76814	2.42	2.42	N/A	A

	MUE		Modifiers		
76813	1	N/A	N/A	N/A	80*
76814	3	N/A	N/A	N/A	80*

* with documentation

Medicare References: None

Coding Companion for Ob/Gyn

© 2012 OptumInsight, Inc.

Radiology

76815-76816

76815 Ultrasound, pregnant uterus, real time with image documentation, limited (eg, fetal heart beat, placental location, fetal position and/or qualitative amniotic fluid volume), 1 or more fetuses

76816 Ultrasound, pregnant uterus, real time with image documentation, follow-up (eg, re-evaluation of fetal size by measuring standard growth parameters and amniotic fluid volume, re-evaluation of organ system(s) suspected or confirmed to be abnormal on a previous scan), transabdominal approach, per fetus

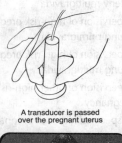

A transducer is passed over the pregnant uterus

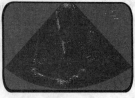

The fetus is visualized on-screen and recordings taken for later analysis

Explanation

Diagnostic ultrasound is an imaging technique bouncing sound waves far above the level of human perception through interior body structures. The sound waves pass through different densities of tissue and reflect back to a receiving unit at varying speeds. The unit converts the waves to electrical pulses that are immediately displayed in picture form on screen. Real time scanning displays both two-dimensional structure images and movement with time. Use 76815 to report real time ultrasound with image documentation on a pregnant uterus for a limited evaluation focused on the assessment of one or more of the following: fetal heartbeat, placental location, fetal position, and/or qualitative amniotic fluid volume for one or more fetuses.

Coding Tips

Code 76815 is an exam focused only on evaluating one or more of the elements listed in the code descriptor based on certain clinical

indications that necessitate a quick look assessment by ultrasound. Report 76816 for a reassessment of fetal size and growth or when re-evaluation of specific abnormalities already demonstrated on ultrasound is done. If multiple fetuses are evaluated, report 76816 for each fetus after the first and append modifier 59. It is appropriate to code an obstetrical ultrasound for a patient who has an established diagnosis of pregnancy, who presents with indications necessitating the exam that may be pregnancy related, even when the outcome shows that the patient is no longer currently pregnant.

ICD-9-CM Procedural

88.78   Diagnostic ultrasound of gravid uterus

Anesthesia

76815   N/A
76816   01922

ICD-9-CM Diagnostic

644.03   Threatened premature labor, antepartum

645.13   Post term pregnancy, antepartum condition or complication

651.33   Twin pregnancy with fetal loss and retention of one fetus, antepartum

652.03   Unstable lie of fetus, antepartum — (Code first any associated obstructed labor, 660.0)

652.43   Fetal face or brow presentation, antepartum — (Code first any associated obstructed labor, 660.0)

652.53   High fetal head at term, antepartum — (Code first any associated obstructed labor, 660.0)

656.53   Poor fetal growth, affecting management of mother, antepartum condition or complication

656.63   Excessive fetal growth affecting management of mother, antepartum

657.03   Polyhydramnios, antepartum complication

658.03   Oligohydramnios, antepartum

659.73   Abnormality in fetal heart rate or rhythm, antepartum condition or complication

Terms To Know

placenta. Temporary organ within the uterus during pregnancy, joining the mother and fetus. It is attached to the fetus via the umbilical cord and provides oxygen and nutrients and helps to eliminate carbon dioxide and waste through the selective exchange of soluble substances carried via the blood. The placenta is expelled from the uterus after the baby is delivered, and is then termed the afterbirth.

real-time. Immediate imaging, with movement as it happens.

CCI Version 18.3

51701-51702, 76857❖, 76998

Also not with 76816: 76810❖, 76815❖

Note: These CCI edits are used for Medicare. Other payers may reimburse on codes listed above.

Medicare Edits

	Fac RVU	Non-Fac RVU	FUD	Status
76815	2.74	2.74	N/A	A
76816	3.58	3.58	N/A	A

	MUE		Modifiers		
76815	1	N/A	N/A	N/A	80*
76816	-	N/A	N/A	N/A	80*

* with documentation

Medicare References: None

76817

76817 Ultrasound, pregnant uterus, real time with image documentation, transvaginal

Pregnant uterus
Pubic bone
Bladder
Ultrasonic lead in vaginal canal
Rectum

Ultrasound is performed in real time with image documentation by a transvaginal approach

Explanation

Diagnostic ultrasound is an imaging technique bouncing sound waves far above the level of human perception through interior body structures. The sound waves pass through different densities of tissue and reflect back to a receiving unit at varying speeds. The unit converts the waves to electrical pulses that are immediately displayed in picture form on screen. Real time scanning displays both two-dimensional structure images and movement with time. Use 76817 to report real time ultrasound on a pregnant uterus done transvaginally, with image documentation.

Coding Tips

A transvaginal ultrasound may be performed separately or in addition to a transabdominal ultrasound. When this procedure is done in addition to a transabdominal obstetrical ultrasound examination, report this code and the appropriate transabdominal exam code. See 76830 for a non-obstetrical transvaginal ultrasound. It is appropriate to code an obstetrical ultrasound for a patient who has an established diagnosis of pregnancy, who presents with indications necessitating the exam that may be pregnancy related, even when the outcome shows that the patient is no longer currently pregnant.

ICD-9-CM Procedural

88.78   Diagnostic ultrasound of gravid uterus

Anesthesia

76817   N/A

ICD-9-CM Diagnostic

630   Hydatidiform mole — (Use additional code from category 639 to identify any associated complications)

634.11   Incomplete spontaneous abortion complicated by delayed or excessive hemorrhage

640.03   Threatened abortion, antepartum

640.83   Other specified hemorrhage in early pregnancy, antepartum

642.53   Severe pre-eclampsia, antepartum

642.63   Eclampsia, antepartum

643.13   Hyperemesis gravidarum with metabolic disturbance, antepartum

643.23   Late vomiting of pregnancy, antepartum

645.13   Post term pregnancy, antepartum condition or complication

646.33   Pregnancy complication, recurrent pregnancy loss, antepartum condition or complication — (Use additional code to further specify complication)

648.03   Maternal diabetes mellitus, antepartum — (Use additional code(s) to identify the condition)

648.63   Other maternal cardiovascular diseases, antepartum — (Use additional code(s) to identify the condition)

651.03   Twin pregnancy, antepartum

651.33   Twin pregnancy with fetal loss and retention of one fetus, antepartum

652.03   Unstable lie of fetus, antepartum — (Code first any associated obstructed labor, 660.0)

652.53   High fetal head at term, antepartum — (Code first any associated obstructed labor, 660.0)

653.43   Fetopelvic disproportion, antepartum — (Code first any associated obstructed labor, 660.1)

653.53   Unusually large fetus causing disproportion, antepartum — (Code first any associated obstructed labor, 660.1)

654.33   Retroverted and incarcerated gravid uterus, antepartum — (Code first any associated obstructed labor, 660.2)

655.13   Chromosomal abnormality in fetus, affecting management of mother, antepartum

655.53   Suspected damage to fetus from drugs, affecting management of mother, antepartum

655.73   Decreased fetal movements, affecting management of mother, antepartum condition or complication

656.43   Intrauterine death affecting management of mother, antepartum

656.53   Poor fetal growth, affecting management of mother, antepartum condition or complication

656.63   Excessive fetal growth affecting management of mother, antepartum

659.63   Elderly multigravida, with antepartum condition or complication

V23.89   Supervision of other high-risk pregnancy

V28.3   Encounter for routine screening for malformation using ultrasonics

V28.4   Antenatal screening for fetal growth retardation using ultrasonics

Terms To Know

habitual aborter. Spontaneous abortions or miscarriages in three or more successive pregnancies.

ultrasound. Imaging using ultra-high sound frequency bounced off body structures.

CCI Version 18.3

51701-51702, 76830-76831❖, 76856-76857❖, 76941❖, 76998

Note: These CCI edits are used for Medicare. Other payers may reimburse on codes listed above.

Medicare Edits

	Fac RVU	Non-Fac RVU	FUD	Status
76817	3.09	3.09	N/A	A

	MUE		Modifiers		
76817	1	N/A	N/A	N/A	80*

* with documentation

Medicare References: None

Radiology

76818-76819

76818 Fetal biophysical profile; with non-stress testing
76819 without non-stress testing

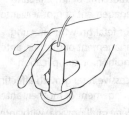

A transducer is passed over the pregnant uterus

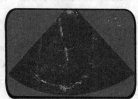

A non-stress test is taken to monitor the fetus' heart rate

Explanation

The health of a term or near-term fetus is assessed using ultrasound to monitor the fetus' movements, tone, and breathing, as well as to check amniotic fluid volume. The fetal heart rate is also monitored electronically in a biophysical profile. The physician conducts a non-stress test which monitors the baby's heart rate over a period of 20 minutes or more to look for accelerations with the baby's movement. Report 76819 if the fetal profile is done without non-stress testing.

Coding Tips

If biophysical profile assessments are done on multiple fetuses, report 76818 or 76819 separately, as appropriate, for each fetus after the first and append modifier 59. For qualitative amniotic fluid volume assessment, use 76815.

ICD-9-CM Procedural

75.34 Other fetal monitoring
88.78 Diagnostic ultrasound of gravid uterus

Anesthesia

N/A

ICD-9-CM Diagnostic

641.83 Other antepartum hemorrhage, antepartum
642.33 Transient hypertension of pregnancy, antepartum

642.63 Eclampsia, antepartum
644.03 Threatened premature labor, antepartum
645.13 Post term pregnancy, antepartum condition or complication
651.03 Twin pregnancy, antepartum
651.13 Triplet pregnancy, antepartum
652.03 Unstable lie of fetus, antepartum — (Code first any associated obstructed labor, 660.0)
652.23 Breech presentation without mention of version, antepartum — (Code first any associated obstructed labor, 660.0)
652.33 Transverse or oblique fetal presentation, antepartum — (Code first any associated obstructed labor, 660.0)
652.53 High fetal head at term, antepartum — (Code first any associated obstructed labor, 660.0)
652.63 Multiple gestation with malpresentation of one fetus or more, antepartum — (Code first any associated obstructed labor, 660.0)
653.43 Fetopelvic disproportion, antepartum — (Code first any associated obstructed labor, 660.1)
653.53 Unusually large fetus causing disproportion, antepartum — (Code first any associated obstructed labor, 660.1)
653.63 Hydrocephalic fetus causing disproportion, antepartum — (Code first any associated obstructed labor, 660.1)
655.13 Chromosomal abnormality in fetus, affecting management of mother, antepartum
655.43 Suspected damage to fetus from other disease in mother, affecting management of mother, antepartum condition or complication
655.73 Decreased fetal movements, affecting management of mother, antepartum condition or complication
656.03 Fetal-maternal hemorrhage, antepartum condition or complication
656.53 Poor fetal growth, affecting management of mother, antepartum condition or complication
657.03 Polyhydramnios, antepartum complication
658.03 Oligohydramnios, antepartum
659.73 Abnormality in fetal heart rate or rhythm, antepartum condition or complication

761.7 Fetus or newborn affected by malpresentation before labor — (Use additional code(s) to further specify condition)
V23.49 Supervision of pregnancy with other poor obstetric history
V23.89 Supervision of other high-risk pregnancy

Terms To Know

fetus. Unborn offspring past the embryonic stage that has developed major structures. It is the period defined from nine weeks after fertilization until birth.

ultrasound. Imaging using ultra-high sound frequency bounced off body structures.

CCI Version 18.3

51701-51702, 76376-76377, 76998
Also not with 76818: 59025, 76819
Also not with 76819: 59020-59025

Note: These CCI edits are used for Medicare. Other payers may reimburse on codes listed above.

Medicare Edits

	Fac RVU	Non-Fac RVU	FUD	Status
76818	3.69	3.69	N/A	A
76819	2.73	2.73	N/A	A

	MUE			Modifiers
76818	-	N/A	N/A	N/A	80*
76819	-	N/A	N/A	N/A	80*

* with documentation
Medicare References: None

76820-76821

76820 Doppler velocimetry, fetal; umbilical artery
76821 middle cerebral artery

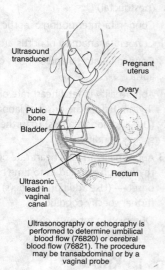

Ultrasound transducer
Pregnant uterus
Ovary
Pubic bone
Bladder
Rectum
Ultrasonic lead in vaginal canal

Ultrasonography or echography is performed to determine umbilical blood flow (76820) or cerebral blood flow (76821). The procedure may be transabdominal or by a vaginal probe

Explanation

Doppler ultrasonography, or echography, is performed for fetal surveillance to determine the velocity of blood flow through the umbilical artery (76820) or the middle cerebral artery (76821). Doppler works off the principle that when emitted sound waves reflect back off a moving object, the frequency of the reflected waves will vary in relation to the speed of the moving object. The frequency of sound waves bouncing back off moving blood cells is converted to the velocity of blood flow through the vessel and is seen on screen as a wave with peak, systole, and diastole. Velocity waveforms through the umbilical artery of a normally growing fetus are different from those of a growth-retarded fetus. The peak systolic velocity through the middle cerebral artery is inversely related to the amount of hematocrit in fetal blood. These tests help determine the timing of labor induction and when fetal anemia is severe enough to require a transfusion. The ultrasound is carried out either transabdominally or endovaginally.

Coding Tips

For fetal dopplar echocardiography, see 76827–76828.

ICD-9-CM Procedural

75.35   Other diagnostic procedures on fetus and amnion

Anesthesia

N/A

ICD-9-CM Diagnostic

655.70   Decreased fetal movements, unspecified as to episode of care

760.3   Fetus or newborn affected by other chronic maternal circulatory and respiratory diseases — (Use additional code(s) to further specify condition)

764.90   Unspecified fetal growth retardation, unspecified (weight) — (Use additional code(s) to further specify condition)

764.91   Unspecified fetal growth retardation, less than 500 grams — (Use additional code(s) to further specify condition)

764.92   Unspecified fetal growth retardation, 500-749 grams — (Use additional code(s) to further specify condition)

764.93   Unspecified fetal growth retardation, 750-999 grams — (Use additional code(s) to further specify condition)

764.94   Unspecified fetal growth retardation, 1,000-1,249 grams — (Use additional code(s) to further specify condition)

764.95   Unspecified fetal growth retardation, 1,250-1,499 grams — (Use additional code(s) to further specify condition)

764.96   Unspecified fetal growth retardation, 1,500-1,749 grams — (Use additional code(s) to further specify condition)

764.97   Unspecified fetal growth retardation, 1,750-1,999 grams — (Use additional code(s) to further specify condition)

764.98   Unspecified fetal growth retardation, 2,000-2,499 grams — (Use additional code(s) to further specify condition)

764.99   Unspecified fetal growth retardation, 2,500 or more grams — (Use additional code(s) to further specify condition)

Terms To Know

echography. Radiographic imaging that uses sound waves reflected off the different densities of anatomic structures to create images.

fetus. Unborn offspring past the embryonic stage that has developed major structures. It is the period defined from nine weeks after fertilization until birth.

ultrasound. Imaging using ultra-high sound frequency bounced off body structures.

CCI Version 18.3

76828❖

Also not with 76821: 76376-76377

Note: These CCI edits are used for Medicare. Other payers may reimburse on codes listed above.

Medicare Edits

	Fac RVU	Non-Fac RVU	FUD	Status
76820	1.3	1.3	N/A	A
76821	2.92	2.92	N/A	A

	MUE		Modifiers		
76820	-	N/A	N/A	N/A	80*
76821	-	N/A	N/A	N/A	80*

* with documentation

Medicare References: None

76825-76826

76825 Echocardiography, fetal, cardiovascular system, real time with image documentation (2D), with or without M-mode recording;

76826 follow-up or repeat study

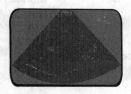

An echocardiogram study is performed on a fetus. Report code 76826 for a follow-up or repeat study

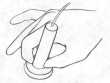

A transducer is passed over the patient's pregnant abdominal area

Explanation

Diagnostic ultrasound is an imaging technique bouncing sound waves far above the level of human perception through interior body structures. The sound waves pass through different densities of tissue and reflect back to a receiving unit at varying speeds. The unit then converts the waves to electrical pulses that are immediately displayed in picture form on screen. These codes report fetal echocardiography, real time, with or without M-mode recording. Real time scanning displays both two-dimensional structure images and movement with time. M-mode is a single dimension method of recording amplitude and velocity of a moving structure producing the echoes being studied. Report 76825 for a complete evaluation of a fetal cardiovascular system and 76826 for a follow-up or repeat study.

Coding Tips

Procedures 76825 and 76826 have both a technical and professional component. To claim only the professional component, append modifier 26. To claim only the technical component, append modifier TC. To claim the complete procedure (i.e., both the professional and technical components), submit without a modifier. When 76825 or 76826 is performed with another separately identifiable procedure, the highest dollar value

code is listed as the primary procedure and subsequent procedures are appended with modifier 51. For fetal Doppler echocardiography, see 76827–76828.

ICD-9-CM Procedural

88.78 Diagnostic ultrasound of gravid uterus

Anesthesia

N/A

ICD-9-CM Diagnostic

655.13 Chromosomal abnormality in fetus, affecting management of mother, antepartum

655.23 Hereditary disease in family possibly affecting fetus, affecting management of mother, antepartum condition or complication

655.53 Suspected damage to fetus from drugs, affecting management of mother, antepartum

745.10 Complete transposition of great vessels

745.11 Transposition of great vessels, double outlet right ventricle

745.19 Other transposition of great vessels

745.2 Tetralogy of Fallot

745.3 Bulbus cordis anomalies and anomalies of cardiac septal closure, common ventricle

745.4 Ventricular septal defect

745.5 Ostium secundum type atrial septal defect

745.61 Ostium primum defect

745.7 Cor biloculare

745.8 Other bulbus cordis anomalies and anomalies of cardiac septal closure

746.01 Congenital atresia of pulmonary valve

746.1 Congenital tricuspid atresia and stenosis

746.2 Ebstein's anomaly

746.3 Congenital stenosis of aortic valve

746.4 Congenital insufficiency of aortic valve

746.5 Congenital mitral stenosis

746.6 Congenital mitral insufficiency

746.7 Hypoplastic left heart syndrome

746.81 Congenital subaortic stenosis

746.82 Cor triatriatum

746.83 Congenital infundibular pulmonic stenosis

746.84 Congenital obstructive anomalies of heart, not elsewhere classified — (Use additional code for associated anomalies: 746.5, 746.81, 747.10)

746.85 Congenital coronary artery anomaly

746.86 Congenital heart block

746.87 Congenital malposition of heart and cardiac apex

747.0 Patent ductus arteriosus

747.10 Coarctation of aorta (preductal) (postductal)

747.11 Congenital interruption of aortic arch

747.21 Congenital anomaly of aortic arch

747.22 Congenital atresia and stenosis of aorta

763.81 Abnormality in fetal heart rate or rhythm before the onset of labor — (Use additional code(s) to further specify condition)

763.83 Abnormality in fetal heart rate or rhythm, unspecified as to time of onset — (Use additional code(s) to further specify condition)

V71.7 Observation for suspected cardiovascular disease

Terms To Know

antepartum. Period of pregnancy between conception and the onset of labor.

imaging. Radiologic means of producing pictures for clinical study of the internal structures and functions of the body, such as x-ray, ultrasound, magnetic resonance, or positron emission tomography.

real-time. Immediate imaging, with movement as it happens.

CCI Version 18.3

51701-51702, 76998

Also not with 76826: 76825

Note: These CCI edits are used for Medicare. Other payers may reimburse on codes listed above.

Medicare Edits

	Fac RVU	Non-Fac RVU	FUD	Status
76825	6.58	6.58	N/A	A
76826	3.87	3.87	N/A	A

	MUE		Modifiers		
76825	-	N/A	N/A	N/A	80*
76826	-	N/A	N/A	N/A	80*

* with documentation

Medicare References: None

Radiology

76827-76828

76827 Doppler echocardiography, fetal, pulsed wave and/or continuous wave with spectral display; complete

76828 follow-up or repeat study

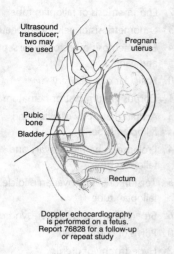

Doppler echocardiography is performed on a fetus. Report 76828 for a follow-up or repeat study.

Explanation

Diagnostic ultrasound is an imaging technique bouncing sound waves far above the level of human perception through interior body structures. The sound waves pass through different densities of tissue and reflect back to a receiving unit at varying speeds. The unit converts the waves to electrical pulses that are immediately displayed in picture form on screen. These codes report fetal doppler echocardiography by pulsed or continuous sound wave. Fetal echocardiography is done to study the unborn baby's heart in much greater detail than is possible with a routine pregnancy ultrasound when the mother is at risk for giving birth to a baby with heart defects. Doppler echography uses the frequency shifts of the emitted waves against their echoes to measure velocity, such as for blood flow through the heart. Pulsed wave transmits and records from a single source to determine a precise site of signal origin but not high velocity. Continuous wave uses two transducers: one to continually transmit and the other to record. This scan determines high velocities. Report 76827 for a complete fetal echocardiographic evaluation and 76828 for a follow-up or repeat study.

Coding Tips

Procedures 76827 and 76828 have both a technical and professional component. To claim only the professional component, append modifier 26. To claim only the technical component, append modifier TC. To claim the complete procedure (i.e., both the professional and technical components), submit without a modifier. When 76827 or 76828 is performed with another separately identifiable procedure, the highest dollar value code is listed as the primary procedure and subsequent procedures are appended with modifier 51. For color flow velocity mapping for Doppler echocardiography, use 93325.

ICD-9-CM Procedural

88.78 Diagnostic ultrasound of gravid uterus

Anesthesia

N/A

ICD-9-CM Diagnostic

659.73 Abnormality in fetal heart rate or rhythm, antepartum condition or complication

745.0 Bulbus cordis anomalies and anomalies of cardiac septal closure, common truncus

745.10 Complete transposition of great vessels

745.11 Transposition of great vessels, double outlet right ventricle

745.2 Tetralogy of Fallot

745.3 Bulbus cordis anomalies and anomalies of cardiac septal closure, common ventricle

745.4 Ventricular septal defect

745.5 Ostium secundum type atrial septal defect

745.61 Ostium primum defect

745.7 Cor biloculare

746.01 Congenital atresia of pulmonary valve

746.02 Congenital stenosis of pulmonary valve

746.1 Congenital tricuspid atresia and stenosis

746.2 Ebstein's anomaly

746.3 Congenital stenosis of aortic valve

746.4 Congenital insufficiency of aortic valve

746.5 Congenital mitral stenosis

746.6 Congenital mitral insufficiency

746.7 Hypoplastic left heart syndrome

746.81 Congenital subaortic stenosis

746.82 Cor triatriatum

746.83 Congenital infundibular pulmonic stenosis

746.85 Congenital coronary artery anomaly

746.86 Congenital heart block

746.87 Congenital malposition of heart and cardiac apex

747.0 Patent ductus arteriosus

747.10 Coarctation of aorta (preductal) (postductal)

747.21 Congenital anomaly of aortic arch

747.22 Congenital atresia and stenosis of aorta

747.31 Pulmonary artery coarctation and atresia

747.32 Pulmonary arteriovenous malformation

747.39 Other anomalies of pulmonary artery and pulmonary circulation

747.41 Total congenital anomalous pulmonary venous connection

747.42 Partial congenital anomalous pulmonary venous connection

CCI Version 18.3

51701-51702, 76376-76377, 76998

Also not with 76828: 76827❖

Note: These CCI edits are used for Medicare. Other payers may reimburse on codes listed above.

Medicare Edits

	Fac RVU	Non-Fac RVU	FUD	Status
76827	1.91	1.91	N/A	A
76828	1.39	1.39	N/A	A

	MUE		Modifiers		
76827	-	N/A	N/A	N/A	80*
76828	-	N/A	N/A	N/A	80*

* with documentation

Medicare References: None

Coding Companion for Ob/Gyn

76830

76830 Ultrasound, transvaginal

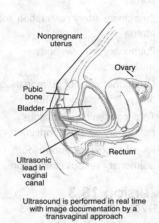

Nonpregnant uterus

Ovary

Pubic bone

Bladder

Rectum

Ultrasonic lead in vaginal canal

Ultrasound is performed in real time with image documentation by a transvaginal approach

Explanation

Diagnostic ultrasound is an imaging technique bouncing sound waves far above the level of human perception through interior body structures. The sound waves pass through different densities of tissue and reflect back to a receiving unit at varying speeds. The unit converts the waves to electrical pulses that are immediately displayed in picture form on screen. This code reports transvaginal ultrasonography.

Coding Tips

When 76830 is performed with another separately identifiable procedure, the highest dollar value code is listed as the primary procedure and subsequent procedures are appended with modifier 51. If transvaginal ultrasound (nonobstetric) is done in addition to a transabdominal ultrasound exam, report 76830 in addition to the appropriate code for the transabdominal ultrasound. For transvaginal ultrasound on a gravid uterus, see 76817.

ICD-9-CM Procedural

88.79   Other diagnostic ultrasound

Anesthesia

76830   01922

ICD-9-CM Diagnostic

180.0   Malignant neoplasm of endocervix
180.1   Malignant neoplasm of exocervix
180.8   Malignant neoplasm of other specified sites of cervix
182.0   Malignant neoplasm of corpus uteri, except isthmus
182.1   Malignant neoplasm of isthmus
182.8   Malignant neoplasm of other specified sites of body of uterus
183.0   Malignant neoplasm of ovary — (Use additional code to identify any functional activity)
183.2   Malignant neoplasm of fallopian tube
183.3   Malignant neoplasm of broad ligament of uterus
183.5   Malignant neoplasm of round ligament of uterus
184.0   Malignant neoplasm of vagina
195.3   Malignant neoplasm of pelvis
198.1   Secondary malignant neoplasm of other urinary organs
218.0   Submucous leiomyoma of uterus
218.1   Intramural leiomyoma of uterus
218.2   Subserous leiomyoma of uterus
219.0   Benign neoplasm of cervix uteri
219.1   Benign neoplasm of corpus uteri
220   Benign neoplasm of ovary — (Use additional code to identify any functional activity: 256.0-256.1)
221.0   Benign neoplasm of fallopian tube and uterine ligaments
221.1   Benign neoplasm of vagina
223.3   Benign neoplasm of bladder
233.1   Carcinoma in situ of cervix uteri
256.4   Polycystic ovaries
614.0   Acute salpingitis and oophoritis — (Use additional code to identify organism: 041.00-041.09, 041.10-041.19)
614.1   Chronic salpingitis and oophoritis — (Use additional code to identify organism: 041.00-041.09, 041.10-041.19)
614.2   Salpingitis and oophoritis not specified as acute, subacute, or chronic — (Use additional code to identify organism: 041.00-041.09, 041.10-041.19)
614.3   Acute parametritis and pelvic cellulitis — (Use additional code to identify organism: 041.00-041.09, 041.10-041.19)
614.4   Chronic or unspecified parametritis and pelvic cellulitis — (Use additional code to identify organism: 041.00-041.09, 041.10-041.19)
615.0   Acute inflammatory disease of uterus, except cervix — (Use additional code

to identify organism: 041.00-041.09, 041.10-041.19)
615.1   Chronic inflammatory disease of uterus, except cervix — (Use additional code to identify organism: 041.00-041.09, 041.10-041.19)
617.0   Endometriosis of uterus
617.1   Endometriosis of ovary
617.2   Endometriosis of fallopian tube
617.3   Endometriosis of pelvic peritoneum
617.4   Endometriosis of rectovaginal septum and vagina
620.0   Follicular cyst of ovary
620.1   Corpus luteum cyst or hematoma
620.3   Acquired atrophy of ovary and fallopian tube
620.4   Prolapse or hernia of ovary and fallopian tube
620.5   Torsion of ovary, ovarian pedicle, or fallopian tube
620.6   Broad ligament laceration syndrome
621.0   Polyp of corpus uteri
621.2   Hypertrophy of uterus
621.30   Endometrial hyperplasia, unspecified
621.5   Intrauterine synechiae
625.3   Dysmenorrhea
626.0   Absence of menstruation
626.2   Excessive or frequent menstruation
626.4   Irregular menstrual cycle
626.5   Ovulation bleeding
627.1   Postmenopausal bleeding
752.49   Other congenital anomaly of cervix, vagina, and external female genitalia

Terms To Know

exocervix. Region of the cervix uteri that protrudes into the vagina.

ultrasound. Imaging using ultra-high sound frequency bounced off body structures.

CCI Version 18.3

51701-51702, 76815-76816❖, 76998

Note: These CCI edits are used for Medicare. Other payers may reimburse on codes listed above.

Medicare Edits

	Fac RVU	Non-Fac RVU	FUD	Status
76830	3.79	3.79	N/A	A

	MUE		Modifiers		
76830	1	N/A	N/A	N/A	80*

* with documentation

Medicare References: None

Radiology

76831

76831 Saline infusion sonohysterography (SIS), including color flow Doppler, when performed

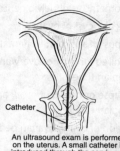

Catheter

An ultrasound exam is performed on the uterus. A small catheter is introduced through the cervix and radiographic contrast material is introduced

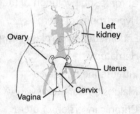

Ovary
Left kidney
Uterus
Cervix
Vagina

Explanation

Diagnostic ultrasound is an imaging technique bouncing sound waves far above the level of human perception through interior body structures. The sound waves pass through different densities of tissue and reflect back to a receiving unit at varying speeds. The unit converts the waves to electrical pulses that are immediately displayed in picture form on screen. This code reports saline infusion sonohysterography, with or without color flow Doppler. The addition of color flow Doppler monitors the behavior of a moving structure, such as flowing blood. The color image that is produced depicts the various levels of fluid concentration within a given area. In the case of saline infusion sonohysterography, a thin catheter, the size of uncooked spaghetti, is introduced into the cervical opening and into the uterus and one to two teaspoons of saline solution is injected into the uterine cavity. Fluid enhanced endovaginal ultrasound is done with the saline solution acting as a contrast medium to view any abnormal anatomic findings in the uterus that needs to be further evaluated. This code reports only the radiological supervision and interpretation.

Coding Tips

When 76831 is performed with another separately identifiable procedure, the highest dollar value code is listed as the primary procedure and subsequent procedures are appended with modifier 51. For the catheterization and introduction of saline or

contrast material for the hysterosonography, see 58340.

ICD-9-CM Procedural

88.79   Other diagnostic ultrasound

Anesthesia

76831   01922

ICD-9-CM Diagnostic

180.0   Malignant neoplasm of endocervix
180.1   Malignant neoplasm of exocervix
182.0   Malignant neoplasm of corpus uteri, except isthmus
182.1   Malignant neoplasm of isthmus
183.0   Malignant neoplasm of ovary — (Use additional code to identify any functional activity)
183.2   Malignant neoplasm of fallopian tube
183.3   Malignant neoplasm of broad ligament of uterus
183.4   Malignant neoplasm of parametrium of uterus
183.5   Malignant neoplasm of round ligament of uterus
218.0   Submucous leiomyoma of uterus
218.1   Intramural leiomyoma of uterus
218.2   Subserous leiomyoma of uterus
219.0   Benign neoplasm of cervix uteri
219.1   Benign neoplasm of corpus uteri
233.1   Carcinoma in situ of cervix uteri
256.31   Premature menopause — (Use additional code for states associated with natural menopause: 627.2)
614.0   Acute salpingitis and oophoritis — (Use additional code to identify organism: 041.00-041.09, 041.10-041.19)
614.1   Chronic salpingitis and oophoritis — (Use additional code to identify organism: 041.00-041.09, 041.10-041.19)
614.3   Acute parametritis and pelvic cellulitis — (Use additional code to identify organism: 041.00-041.09, 041.10-041.19)
614.5   Acute or unspecified pelvic peritonitis, female — (Use additional code to identify organism: 041.00-041.09, 041.10-041.19)
615.0   Acute inflammatory disease of uterus, except cervix — (Use additional code to identify organism: 041.00-041.09, 041.10-041.19)
615.1   Chronic inflammatory disease of uterus, except cervix — (Use

additional code to identify organism: 041.00-041.09, 041.10-041.19)
617.0   Endometriosis of uterus
617.1   Endometriosis of ovary
617.2   Endometriosis of fallopian tube
617.3   Endometriosis of pelvic peritoneum
620.0   Follicular cyst of ovary
620.1   Corpus luteum cyst or hematoma
620.4   Prolapse or hernia of ovary and fallopian tube
620.5   Torsion of ovary, ovarian pedicle, or fallopian tube
621.0   Polyp of corpus uteri
621.1   Chronic subinvolution of uterus
621.2   Hypertrophy of uterus
621.30   Endometrial hyperplasia, unspecified
621.5   Intrauterine synechiae
621.6   Malposition of uterus
626.0   Absence of menstruation
626.2   Excessive or frequent menstruation
626.3   Puberty bleeding
626.5   Ovulation bleeding
628.3   Female infertility of uterine origin — (Use additional code for any associated tuberculous endometriosis: 016.7)
752.2   Congenital doubling of uterus
752.32   Hypoplasia of uterus
752.33   Unicornuate uterus
752.34   Bicornuate uterus
752.35   Septate uterus
752.36   Arcuate uterus

Terms To Know

infusion. Introduction of a therapeutic fluid, other than blood, into the bloodstream.

CCI Version 18.3

51701-51702, 76801❖, 76813❖, 76815-76816❖, 76830, 76998

Note: These CCI edits are used for Medicare. Other payers may reimburse on codes listed above.

Medicare Edits

	Fac RVU	Non-Fac RVU	FUD	Status
76831	3.83	3.83	N/A	A

	MUE			Modifiers	
76831	1	51	N/A	N/A	80*

* with documentation

Medicare References: None

Radiology

76856-76857

76856 Ultrasound, pelvic (nonobstetric), real time with image documentation; complete
76857 limited or follow-up (eg, for follicles)

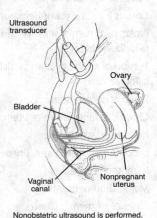

Nonobstetric ultrasound is performed. Report 76857 for follow-up or limited study, such as a study for follicles on an ovary

Explanation

Diagnostic ultrasound is an imaging technique bouncing sound waves far above the level of human perception through interior body structures. The sound waves pass through different densities of tissue and reflect back to a receiving unit at varying speeds. The unit converts the waves to electrical pulses that are immediately displayed in picture form on screen. Real time scanning displays both structure images and movement with time. Report 76856 for a complete pelvic evaluation in a patient who is not pregnant and 76857 for a limited or follow-up pelvic evaluation, for example, to monitor real time follicle development on the ovary to evaluate gonadotrophin therapy.

Coding Tips

It is appropriate to code a nonobstetrical pelvic ultrasound in cases where a patient, without an established diagnosis of pregnancy, has gynecological signs and symptoms that would necessitate an ultrasound even when the outcome results in a diagnosis of pregnancy or a complication of a pregnancy.

ICD-9-CM Procedural

88.79   Other diagnostic ultrasound

Anesthesia

01922

ICD-9-CM Diagnostic

182.0   Malignant neoplasm of corpus uteri, except isthmus
183.0   Malignant neoplasm of ovary — (Use additional code to identify any functional activity)
183.2   Malignant neoplasm of fallopian tube
183.3   Malignant neoplasm of broad ligament of uterus
183.4   Malignant neoplasm of parametrium of uterus
183.5   Malignant neoplasm of round ligament of uterus
218.0   Submucous leiomyoma of uterus
218.1   Intramural leiomyoma of uterus
218.2   Subserous leiomyoma of uterus
219.1   Benign neoplasm of corpus uteri
220   Benign neoplasm of ovary — (Use additional code to identify any functional activity: 256.0-256.1)
221.0   Benign neoplasm of fallopian tube and uterine ligaments
256.2   Postablative ovarian failure — (Use additional code for states associated with artificial menopause: 627.4)
256.31   Premature menopause — (Use additional code for states associated with natural menopause: 627.2)
256.4   Polycystic ovaries
614.0   Acute salpingitis and oophoritis — (Use additional code to identify organism: 041.00-041.09, 041.10-041.19)
614.1   Chronic salpingitis and oophoritis — (Use additional code to identify organism: 041.00-041.09, 041.10-041.19)
614.2   Salpingitis and oophoritis not specified as acute, subacute, or chronic — (Use additional code to identify organism: 041.00-041.09, 041.10-041.19)
614.3   Acute parametritis and pelvic cellulitis — (Use additional code to identify organism: 041.00-041.09, 041.10-041.19)
614.6   Pelvic peritoneal adhesions, female (postoperative) (postinfection) — (Use additional code to identify organism: 041.00-041.09, 041.10-041.19) (Use additional code to identify any associated infertility: 628.2)
615.0   Acute inflammatory disease of uterus, except cervix — (Use additional code to identify organism: 041.00-041.09, 041.10-041.19)

615.1   Chronic inflammatory disease of uterus, except cervix — (Use additional code to identify organism: 041.00-041.09, 041.10-041.19)
617.1   Endometriosis of ovary
617.2   Endometriosis of fallopian tube
617.3   Endometriosis of pelvic peritoneum
620.0   Follicular cyst of ovary
620.1   Corpus luteum cyst or hematoma
620.3   Acquired atrophy of ovary and fallopian tube
620.4   Prolapse or hernia of ovary and fallopian tube
620.5   Torsion of ovary, ovarian pedicle, or fallopian tube
620.7   Hematoma of broad ligament
621.1   Chronic subinvolution of uterus
621.2   Hypertrophy of uterus
621.30   Endometrial hyperplasia, unspecified
621.4   Hematometra
621.5   Intrauterine synechiae
621.6   Malposition of uterus
621.7   Chronic inversion of uterus
625.5   Pelvic congestion syndrome
752.0   Congenital anomalies of ovaries
752.11   Embryonic cyst of fallopian tubes and broad ligaments
752.2   Congenital doubling of uterus

CCI Version 18.3

51701-51702, 51798, 76801❖, 76941❖, 76998

Also not with 76856: 76813❖, 76815-76816❖, 76857, 93976❖, 93980❖

Also not with 76857: 76810❖, 93975-93981❖

Note: These CCI edits are used for Medicare. Other payers may reimburse on codes listed above.

Medicare Edits

	Fac RVU	Non-Fac RVU	FUD	Status
76856	3.75	3.75	N/A	A
76857	2.97	2.97	N/A	A

	MUE		Modifiers		
76856	1	51	N/A	N/A	80*
76857	1	51	N/A	N/A	80*

* with documentation

Medicare References: None

90384-90386

90384 Rho(D) immune globulin (RhIg), human, full-dose, for intramuscular use

90385 Rho(D) immune globulin (RhIg), human, mini-dose, for intramuscular use

90386 Rho(D) immune globulin (RhIgIV), human, for intravenous use

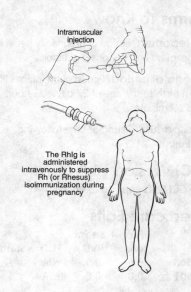

Intramuscular injection

The RhIg is administered intravenously to suppress Rh (or Rhesus) isoimmunization during pregnancy

Explanation

Code 90384 identifies the human Rho(D) immune globulin (RhIg) for intramuscular use, full-dose; 90385 is for a mini-dose. Code 90386 identifies the human Rho(D) immune globulin (RhIgIV) for intravenous use. This immune globulin is a passive immunization agent that gives protection against reactions between blood that is negative for the presence of Rh antigens on the surface of red blood cells to blood that is positive for the presence of Rh antigens on the RBC. Report these codes with the appropriate administration code.

Coding Tips

Modifier 51 should not be reported with the immune globulin codes when performed with another procedure. Report with the appropriate administration code. Assign the appropriate E/M service code when a significant and separately identifiable service is performed in addition to the administration of the vaccine/toxoid. Supplies used when providing this procedure may be reported with the appropriate HCPCS Level II code. Check with the specific payer to determine coverage.

ICD-9-CM Procedural

99.11 Injection of Rh immune globulin

Anesthesia

N/A

ICD-9-CM Diagnostic

656.10 Rhesus isoimmunization unspecified as to episode of care in pregnancy

656.11 Rhesus isoimmunization affecting management of mother, delivered

656.13 Rhesus isoimmunization affecting management of mother, antepartum condition

V07.2 Need for prophylactic immunotherapy

Terms To Know

intramuscular. Within a muscle.

intravenous. Within a vein or veins.

CCI Version 18.3

No CCI Edits apply to this code.

Medicare Edits

	Fac RVU	Non-Fac RVU	FUD	Status
90384	0.0	0.0	N/A	I
90385	0.0	0.0	N/A	E
90386	0.0	0.0	N/A	I

	MUE	Modifiers			
90384	-	N/A	N/A	N/A	N/A
90385	1	N/A	N/A	N/A	N/A
90386	-	N/A	N/A	N/A	N/A

* with documentation

Medicare References: None

Coding Companion for Ob/Gyn

Medicine

99500-99501

99500 Home visit for prenatal monitoring and assessment to include fetal heart rate, non-stress test, uterine monitoring, and gestational diabetes monitoring

99501 Home visit for postnatal assessment and follow-up care

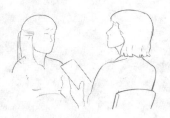

Code 99500 reports a home visit for prenatal monitoring and assessment. Code 99501 reports a home visit for postnatal assessment and follow-up care

Explanation

The home health provider may visit patients with prenatal complications from the first month until the birth of the baby in 99500. The home nurse may obtain vaginal-anorectal/cervical cultures, perform a non-stress test and uterine and fetal heart rate monitoring, draw blood for serology (including offering of AFP/HIV testing), and other tests such as glucose screening to check for gestational diabetes. In 99501, the home visit for postnatal assessment may include a review of plans for future health maintenance and care, including routine infant immunizations, identification of illness and periodic health evaluations, and linking the family with other sources of support such as social services, parenting classes, and lactation consultants as necessary.

Coding Tips

A home visit constitutes the patient's place of residence and may include assisted living residences, group homes, non-traditional private homes, and custodial care facilities. These codes are reported by non-physician health care professionals. Home visits performed by a physician should be reported with the appropriate E/M home visit codes (99341–99350) in conjunction with any appropriate codes other than those in the 99500–99602 range for any additional procedures or services provided by the physician in the patient's home. Health care professionals who are allowed to report E/M home visit codes (99341–99350) may report these codes in addition when both services are performed.

ICD-9-CM Procedural

89.04 Other interview and evaluation
89.26 Gynecological examination

Anesthesia

N/A

ICD-9-CM Diagnostic

641.03 Placenta previa without hemorrhage, antepartum
642.03 Benign essential hypertension antepartum
642.13 Hypertension secondary to renal disease, antepartum
642.23 Other pre-existing hypertension, antepartum
642.43 Mild or unspecified pre-eclampsia, antepartum
643.03 Mild hyperemesis gravidarum, antepartum
643.13 Hyperemesis gravidarum with metabolic disturbance, antepartum
643.23 Late vomiting of pregnancy, antepartum
644.03 Threatened premature labor, antepartum
644.13 Other threatened labor, antepartum
648.03 Maternal diabetes mellitus, antepartum — (Use additional code(s) to identify the condition)
648.04 Maternal diabetes mellitus, complicating pregnancy, childbirth, or the puerperium, postpartum condition or complication — (Use additional code(s) to identify the condition)
648.83 Abnormal maternal glucose tolerance, antepartum — (Use additional code(s) to identify the condition. Use additional code, if applicable, for associated long-term (current) insulin use: V58.67)
648.84 Abnormal maternal glucose tolerance complicating pregnancy, childbirth, or the puerperium, postpartum condition or complication — (Use additional code(s) to identify the condition. Use additional code, if applicable, for associated long-term (current) insulin use: V58.67)

V22.0 Supervision of normal first pregnancy
V22.1 Supervision of other normal pregnancy
V24.0 Postpartum care and examination immediately after delivery
V24.1 Postpartum care and examination of lactating mother
V24.2 Routine postpartum follow-up

Terms To Know

antepartum. Period of pregnancy between conception and the onset of labor.

neonatal period. Period of an infant's life from birth to the age of 27 days, 23 hours, and 59 minutes.

postpartum. Period of time following childbirth.

CCI Version 18.3

No CCI Edits apply to this code.

Medicare Edits

	Fac RVU	Non-Fac RVU	FUD	Status
99500	0.0	0.0	N/A	I
99501	0.0	0.0	N/A	I

	MUE	Modifiers			
99500	-	N/A	N/A	N/A	N/A
99501	-	N/A	N/A	N/A	N/A

* with documentation

Medicare References: None

Medicine

71010

71010 Radiologic examination, chest; single view, frontal

Explanation

A radiograph is taken of the patient's chest from front to back (AP). Typically, this is done when the patient is too ill to stand or be turned to the prone position. The key element of this code is that it reports a single, frontal view.

71020

71020 Radiologic examination, chest, 2 views, frontal and lateral;

Explanation

Films are taken of the patient's chest to include a frontal and side to side (lateral) view. This code specifically reports these two views.

72170

72170 Radiologic examination, pelvis; 1 or 2 views

Explanation

One or two views are taken of the pelvis. The most common view is from front to back (AP) with the patient lying supine with feet inverted 15 degrees to overcome the anteversion (or rotation) of the femoral necks. The pelvic girdle, femoral head, neck, trochanters, and upper femurs are also shown.

72190

72190 Radiologic examination, pelvis; complete, minimum of 3 views

Explanation

A minimum of three films are taken of the pelvis, typically front to back (AP) with the patient lying supine. The patient's legs are placed in what is termed a "frogleg" lateral position, wherein the patient's feet are drawn up toward the buttocks, at which point the knees are allowed to drop down to the table with feet together. A third film may be taken with the patient lying on his or her side for a lateral view of the pelvis, as well as unilateral views of the hips, if necessary.

72191

72191 Computed tomographic angiography, pelvis, with contrast material(s), including noncontrast images, if performed, and image postprocessing

Explanation

Computed tomographic angiography (CTA) of the pelvis is performed with contrast materials and image postprocessing. CTA produces images of vessels to detect aneurysms, blood clots, and other vascular irregularities. Contrast medium is rapidly infused intravenously, at intervals, usually with an automatic injector, and the patient is scanned with thin section axial or spiral mode x-ray beams. The images are acquired with narrower collimation and reconstructed at shorter intervals than standard CT images. Three-dimensional images are generated and postprocessing reconstruction is done at a workstation on the scanner. CTA also provides information unavailable with conventional angiography, such as vessel wall thickness (mural thrombus) and the venous anatomy of a target organ and/or associated organs within the scan range. Noncontrast images, if performed, are also included in this procedure.

72192-72194

72192 Computed tomography, pelvis; without contrast material
72193 with contrast material(s)
72194 without contrast material, followed by contrast material(s) and further sections

Explanation

Computed tomography directs multiple narrow beams of x-rays around the body structure being studied and uses computer imaging to produce thin cross-sectional views of various layers (or slices) of the body. It is useful for the evaluation of trauma, tumor, and foreign bodies as CT is able to visualize soft tissue as well as bones. Patients are required to remain motionless during the study and sedation may need to be administered as well as a contrast medium for image enhancement. These codes report an exam of the pelvis. Report 72192 if no contrast is used. Report 72193 if performed with contrast and 72194 if performed first without contrast and again following the injection of contrast.

72195-72197

72195 Magnetic resonance (eg, proton) imaging, pelvis; without contrast material(s)
72196 with contrast material(s)
72197 without contrast material(s), followed by contrast material(s) and further sequences

Explanation

Magnetic resonance imaging (MRI) is a radiation-free, noninvasive, technique to produce high quality sectional images of the inside of the body in multiple planes. MRI uses the natural magnetic properties of the hydrogen atoms in our bodies that emit radiofrequency signals when exposed to radio waves within a strong electro-magnetic field. These signals are processed and converted by the computer into high-resolution, three-dimensional, tomographic images. Patients with metallic or electronic implants or foreign bodies cannot be exposed to MRI. The patient must remain still while lying on a motorized table within the large, circular MRI tunnel. A sedative may be administered as well as contrast material for image enhancement. These codes report an exam of the pelvis. Report 72195 if no contrast is used. Report 72196 if performed with contrast and 72197 if performed first without contrast and again following the injection of contrast.

72198

72198 Magnetic resonance angiography, pelvis, with or without contrast material(s)

Explanation

Magnetic resonance angiography (MRA) is magnetic resonance imaging (MRI) that specifically visualizes blood vessels and blood flow to evaluate vascular disorders within the structure being studied. Unlike CT, it does not rely on the absorption of x-ray energy. Magnetic resonance imaging uses the natural magnetic properties of the hydrogen atoms in our bodies that emit radiofrequency signals when exposed to radio waves within a strong electro-magnetic field. These signals are processed and converted by the computer into high-resolution, three-dimensional tomographic images. Patients with metallic or electronic implants or foreign bodies cannot be exposed to MRI. The patient must remain still while lying on a motorized table within the large, circular MRI tunnel. A sedative may be administered as well as contrast material for image enhancement. This code reports an exam of the pelvis.

72220

72220 Radiologic examination, sacrum and coccyx, minimum of 2 views

Explanation

Films are taken (minimum of two views) of the sacrum and the coccyx. The sacrum is a triangular bone located between the fifth lumbar vertebra and the coccyx. It is formed by five connected vertebrae and is wedged between the two innominate bones. The coccyx is the small bone at the very base of the spinal column, and is formed by the fusion of four vertebrae. The sacrum and the coccyx form the posterior (back) boundary of the pelvis. While anteroposterior (AP; front to back) and lateral (side) views are the most common views taken, this procedure is used for any two or more views reported.

74000

74000 Radiologic examination, abdomen; single anteroposterior view

Explanation

Films are taken of the abdominal cavity in one view from front to back. Because an abdominal x-ray usually precedes another diagnostic imaging procedure, it is not coded separately unless performed as a separately identifiable examination.

74010

74010 Radiologic examination, abdomen; anteroposterior and additional oblique and cone views

Explanation

Films are taken of the abdominal cavity from front to back, with an oblique view and a focused (coned down or spot) view. Because an abdominal x-ray usually precedes another diagnostic imaging procedure, it is not coded separately unless performed as a separately identifiable examination.

74020

74020 Radiologic examination, abdomen; complete, including decubitus and/or erect views

Explanation

Films are taken of the abdominal cavity from front to back, back to front, or front to back with the patient lying on the side and/or standing. Because an abdominal x-ray usually precedes another diagnostic imaging procedure, it is not coded separately unless performed as a separately identifiable examination.

74022

74022 Radiologic examination, abdomen; complete acute abdomen series, including supine, erect, and/or decubitus views, single view chest

Explanation

Films are taken of the abdominal cavity with the patient lying flat, standing, and/or lying on the side. This procedure includes a single view chest x-ray. Because an abdominal x-ray usually precedes another diagnostic imaging procedure, it is not coded separately unless performed as a separately identifiable examination.

74150-74170

74150 Computed tomography, abdomen; without contrast material
74160 with contrast material(s)
74170 without contrast material, followed by contrast material(s) and further sections

Explanation

Computed tomography directs multiple thin beams of x-rays at the body structure being studied and uses computer imaging to produce thin cross-sectional views of various layers (or slices) of the body. It is useful for the evaluation of trauma, tumor, and foreign bodies as CT is able to visualize soft tissue as well as bones. Patients are required to remain motionless during the study and sedation may need to be administered as well as a contrast medium for image enhancement. These codes report an exam of the abdomen. Report 74150 if no contrast is used. Report 74160 if performed with contrast and 74170 if performed first without contrast and again following the injection of contrast.

74174

74174 Computed tomographic angiography, abdomen and pelvis, with contrast material(s), including noncontrast images, if performed, and image postprocessing

Explanation

Computed tomographic angiography (CTA) of the abdomen and pelvis is performed with contrast material and image postprocessing. CTA is a procedure used for the imaging of vessels. CTA of the abdomen and pelvis may detect aneurysms, thrombosis, and ischemia in the arteries supplying blood to the digestive system, as well as locate gastrointestinal bleeding. Contrast medium is rapidly infused at intervals, usually with an automatic injector, and the patient is scanned with thin section axial or spiral mode x-ray beams. The images obtained are acquired with narrower collimation and reconstructed at shorter intervals than standard CT images. Three-dimensional images are generated and postprocessing reconstruction is done at a workstation on the scanner. Noncontrast images, if performed, are also included in this procedure.

74175

74175 Computed tomographic angiography, abdomen, with contrast material(s), including noncontrast images, if performed, and image postprocessing

Explanation

Computed tomographic angiography (CTA) of the abdomen is performed with contrast material and image postprocessing. CTA is a procedure used for the imaging of vessels. CTA of the abdomen may detect aneurysms, thrombosis, and ischemia in the arteries supplying blood to the digestive system, as well as locate gastrointestinal bleeding. Contrast medium is rapidly infused at intervals, usually with an automatic injector, and the patient is scanned with thin section axial or spiral mode x-ray beams. The images obtained are acquired with narrower collimation and reconstructed at shorter intervals than standard CT images. Three-dimensional images are generated and postprocessing reconstruction is done at a workstation on the scanner. Noncontrast images, if performed, are also included in this procedure.

74176-74178

74176 Computed tomography, abdomen and pelvis; without contrast material
74177 with contrast material(s)
74178 without contrast material in 1 or both body regions, followed by contrast material(s) and further sections in 1 or both body regions

Explanation

Computed tomography directs multiple thin beams of x-rays at the body structure being studied and uses computer imaging to produce thin, cross-sectional views of various layers (or slices) of the body. It is useful for the evaluation of trauma, tumor, and foreign bodies as CT is able to visualize soft tissue as well as bones. Patients are required to remain motionless during the study and sedation may need to be administered, as well as a contrast medium for image enhancement. These codes report an exam of the abdomen and pelvis. Report 74176 if no contrast is used; 74177 if performed with contrast; and 74178 if performed first without contrast in one or both body regions followed by the injection of contrast and further sections in one or both body regions.

74181-74183

74181 Magnetic resonance (eg, proton) imaging, abdomen; without contrast material(s)
74182 with contrast material(s)
74183 without contrast material(s), followed by with contrast material(s) and further sequences

Explanation

Magnetic resonance imaging (MRI) is a radiation-free, noninvasive, technique to produce high quality sectional images of the inside of the body in multiple planes. MRI uses the natural magnetic properties of the hydrogen atoms in our bodies that emit radiofrequency signals when exposed to radio waves within a strong electro-magnetic field. These signals are processed and converted by the computer into high-resolution, three-dimensional, tomographic images. Patients with metallic or electronic implants or foreign bodies cannot be exposed to MRI. The patient must remain still while lying on a motorized table within the large, circular MRI tunnel. A sedative may be administered as well as contrast material for image enhancement. These codes report an exam of the abdomen. Report 74181 if no contrast is used; 74182 if performed with contrast; and 74183 if performed first without contrast and again following the injection of contrast.

74185

74185 Magnetic resonance angiography, abdomen, with or without contrast material(s)

Explanation

Magnetic resonance angiography (MRA) is magnetic resonance imaging (MRI) that specifically visualizes blood vessels and blood flow to evaluate vascular disorders within the structure being studied. Unlike CT, it does not rely on the absorption of x-ray energy. Magnetic resonance imaging uses the natural magnetic properties of the hydrogen atoms in our bodies that emit radiofrequency signals when exposed to radio waves within a strong electro-magnetic field. These signals are processed and converted by the computer into high-resolution, three-dimensional tomographic images. Patients with metallic or electronic implants or foreign bodies cannot be exposed to MRI. The patient must remain still while lying on a motorized table within the large, circular MRI tunnel. A sedative may be administered as well as contrast material for image enhancement. This code reports an exam of the abdomen.

74190

74190 Peritoneogram (eg, after injection of air or contrast), radiological supervision and interpretation

Explanation

A radiographic exam is done on the peritoneal cavity to define the pattern of air in the cavity after injection of air or contrast. The physician inserts a needle or catheter in to the peritoneal cavity and injects air or contrast as a diagnostic procedure. X-rays are then taken. The needle or catheter is removed. This code reports the radiological supervision and interpretation for a peritoneogram. Use a separately reportable code for the procedure.

74710

74710 Pelvimetry, with or without placental localization

Explanation

Although most abnormalities of the pelvis can be suspected by using clinical measurements, x-ray pelvimetry is the most accurate means of determining adequacy of the pelvic bony structures for a normal vaginal delivery. With pelvimetry, comparison is made with the capacity of the pelvis to the size of the infant's head, in order to discover any disproportion. However, radiographic pelvimetry is not used often in modern obstetrics because of the risks associated with radiation. This code is reported with or without locating the placenta.

74740

74740 Hysterosalpingography, radiological supervision and interpretation

Explanation

In hysterosalpingography, the uterine cavity and fallopian tubes are visualized radiographically after the injection of contrast material through the cervix. Uterine tumors, intrauterine adhesions, and developmental anomalies can be seen. Tubal obstruction caused by internal scarring, tumor, or kinking can also be detected. This code reports only the radiological supervision and interpretation. The injection portion of this study is reported separately.

74742

74742 Transcervical catheterization of fallopian tube, radiological supervision and interpretation

Explanation

The physician introduces a catheter into the cervix and takes it into the uterus and through the fallopian tube to diagnose any blockages or to re-establish patency. The physician may elect to inject liquid radiographic contrast material into the endometrial cavity with mild pressure to force the material into the tubes (hysterosalpingogram). The shadow of this material on x-ray film permits examination of the uterus and tubes for any abnormalities or blockages. This code reports only the radiological supervision and interpretation. The introduction of the catheter into the fallopian tube is reported separately.

74775

74775 Perineogram (eg, vaginogram, for sex determination or extent of anomalies)

Explanation

The perineum, which is the area between the vulva and the anus in the female, is viewed to determine the sex of the patient. It is used mainly in cases where an infant is born with ambiguous genitalia. The procedure also may be used to check for an abnormal opening (fistula) between the vagina and bladder or the vagina and rectum. When locating a fistula, the use of contrast material is included.

75984

75984 Change of percutaneous tube or drainage catheter with contrast monitoring (eg, genitourinary system, abscess), radiological supervision and interpretation

Explanation

An existing percutaneous drainage tube or catheter (e.g., genitourinary system or abscess) is replaced with contrast monitoring. A guidewire is usually inserted into the existing catheter to guide the new one. The old catheter is removed and the replacement catheter is threaded back over the guidewire. Contrast injection allows for correct positioning to be visualized with fluoroscopic images displayed on a screen. This code reports the radiological supervision and interpretation only.

75989

75989 Radiological guidance (ie, fluoroscopy, ultrasound, or computed tomography), for percutaneous drainage (eg, abscess, specimen collection), with placement of catheter, radiological supervision and interpretation

Explanation

Fluoroscopic, ultrasonic, or CT guidance may be used for percutaneous drainage of an abscess or to obtain a specimen and place a tube or catheter. Once the abscess is located, the skin is punctured with a needle to begin draining. A catheter may be advanced over a guidewire inserted through the

needle and into the abscess cavity. The tract to the outside is dilated to facilitate placing a percutaneous drainage tube. The cavity is aspirated and the drainage tube placed at the lowest point to ensure complete drainage. The drainage tube is then secured to suction drainage. This code reports the radiological supervision and interpretation only for this procedure.

76001

76001 Fluoroscopy, physician or other qualified health care professional time more than 1 hour, assisting a nonradiologic physician or other qualified health care professional (eg, nephrostolithotomy, ERCP, bronchoscopy, transbronchial biopsy)

Explanation

A radiologist, or other qualified health care provider, supplies fluoroscopic monitoring of the body for more than one hour while assisting a nonradiologic physician (e.g., nephrologist, pulmonologist) or other nonradiologic qualified provider. This code describes the professional work component entailed in providing fluoroscopic monitoring during procedures such as nephrostolithotomy and bronchoscopy. If formal contrast x-ray studies are done and included as a part of the procedure to produce films with written interpretation and report, fluoroscopy is already included and cannot be separately reported.

Coding Tips

This code has been revised for 2013 in the official CPT description.

76604

76604 Ultrasound, chest (includes mediastinum), real time with image documentation

Explanation

Diagnostic ultrasound is an imaging technique bouncing sound waves far above the level of human perception through interior body structures. The sound waves pass through different densities of tissue and reflect back to a receiving unit at varying speeds. The unit converts the waves to electrical pulses that are immediately displayed in picture form on screen. Real time scanning displays structure images and movement with time. This code reports ultrasound and real time for the chest, including the mediastinum.

76645

76645 Ultrasound, breast(s) (unilateral or bilateral), real time with image documentation

Explanation

Diagnostic ultrasound is an imaging technique bouncing sound waves far above the level of human perception through interior body structures. The sound waves pass through different densities of tissue and reflect back to a receiving unit at varying speeds. The unit converts the waves to electrical pulses that are immediately displayed in picture form on screen. Real time scanning displays structure images and movement with time. This code reports ultrasound and real time for one or both breasts.

76700-76705

76700 Ultrasound, abdominal, real time with image documentation; complete
76705 limited (eg, single organ, quadrant, follow-up)

Explanation
Diagnostic ultrasound is an imaging technique bouncing sound waves far above the level of human perception through interior body structures. The sound waves pass through different densities of tissue and reflect back to a receiving unit at varying speeds. The unit converts the waves to electrical pulses that are immediately displayed in picture form on screen. Real time scanning displays structure images and movement with time. Report 76700 for ultrasound and real time of the entire abdomen and 76705 for a single quadrant or organ of the abdomen.

76941

76941 Ultrasonic guidance for intrauterine fetal transfusion or cordocentesis, imaging supervision and interpretation

Explanation
The physician performs a blood transfusion to a fetus or inserts an amniocentesis needle through the abdominal wall into the umbilical vessels of the pregnant uterus and obtains fetal blood guided by ultrasound. Ultrasound is an imaging technique bouncing sound waves far above the level of human perception through interior body structures. The sound waves pass through different densities of tissue and reflect back to a receiving unit, which converts the waves to electrical pulses that are immediately displayed in picture form on screen. For fetal blood transfusion, the physician locates the umbilical vein. A needle is directed through the abdominal wall into the amniotic cavity. The umbilical vein is pierced and fetal blood is exchanged with transfused blood. This code reports the imaging supervision and interpretation only for this procedure.

76942

76942 Ultrasonic guidance for needle placement (eg, biopsy, aspiration, injection, localization device), imaging supervision and interpretation

Explanation
Ultrasonic guidance is used for guiding needle placement required for procedures such as breast biopsies, needle aspirations, injections, or placing

localizing devices. Ultrasound is the process of bouncing sound waves far above the level of human perception through interior body structures. The sound waves pass through different densities of tissue and reflect back to a receiving unit at varying speeds. The unit converts the waves to electrical pulses that are immediately displayed in picture form on screen. Once the exact needle entry site is determined along with the depth of the lesion, the optimal route from the skin to the lesion is decided. The needle is inserted and advanced to the lesion under ultrasonic guidance. This code reports the imaging supervision and interpretation only for this procedure.

76945

76945 Ultrasonic guidance for chorionic villus sampling, imaging supervision and interpretation

Explanation
The physician aspirates cells from the chorionic villus (early stage of the placenta) under ultrasonic guidance. Ultrasound is an imaging technique bouncing sound waves far above the level of human perception through interior body structures. The sound waves pass through different densities of tissue and reflect back to a receiving unit, which converts the waves to electrical pulses that are immediately displayed in picture form on screen. In the transcervical method, a catheter is inserted through the cervix and into the uterine cavity toward the chorionic villus or early placenta. Aspirated cells are obtained for abnormal chromosome analysis. The procedure may also be done transvaginally or transabdominally. The transabdominal approach can be done throughout pregnancy while the other approaches are usually done between 9 and 12 weeks gestation. This code reports the imaging supervision and interpretation only for this procedure.

76946

76946 Ultrasonic guidance for amniocentesis, imaging supervision and interpretation

Explanation
The physician withdraws fluid from the amniotic sac under ultrasonic guidance. Ultrasound is an imaging technique bouncing sound waves far above the level of human perception through interior body structures. The sound waves pass through different densities of tissue and reflect back to a receiving unit, which converts the waves to electrical pulses that are immediately displayed in picture form on screen. Following preparation of the skin and administration of a local anesthetic, a small gauge needle is introduced into the amniotic sac and fluid aspirated. This code reports the imaging supervision and interpretation only for this procedure.

76948

76948 Ultrasonic guidance for aspiration of ova, imaging supervision and interpretation

Explanation
The physician aspirates ova under ultrasonic guidance. Ultrasound is an imaging technique bouncing sound waves far above the level of human perception through interior body structures. The sound waves pass through different densities of tissue and reflect back to a receiving unit, which converts the waves to electrical pulses that are immediately displayed in picture form on screen. Following preparation of the skin and administration of a local anesthetic, a small gauge needle is introduced into the ovary and the ova are aspirated. This code reports the imaging supervision and interpretation only for this procedure.

76950

76950 Ultrasonic guidance for placement of radiation therapy fields

Explanation
Ultrasound is used for placing radiation therapy fields. Ultrasound is an imaging technique bouncing sound waves far above the level of human perception through interior body structures. The sound waves pass through different densities of tissue and reflect back to a receiving unit, which converts the waves to electrical pulses that are immediately displayed in picture form on screen. Images of both normal and abnormal tissue structures are obtained and the treatment field area volume is determined. The normal tissues surrounding the treatment area are also defined. Acquiring this data is an important step in planning the patient's radiation treatment.

76965

76965 Ultrasonic guidance for interstitial radioelement application

Explanation
Ultrasonic guidance is used for the accurate guiding and placement of an interstitial radioactive implant into a tumor during the course of brachytherapy for malignant neoplasms, such as in the prostate. Ultrasound is an imaging technique bouncing sound waves far above the level of human perception through interior body structures. The sound waves pass through different densities of tissue and reflect back to a receiving unit, which converts the waves to electrical pulses that are immediately displayed in picture form on screen. Radioactive implants may be enclosed in various apparatus modes such as tubes, needles, wires, or seeds. Common materials used are radium, cobalt-60, cesium-137, gold-198, and iridium-192.

76970

76970 Ultrasound study follow-up (specify)

Explanation

A follow-up study is performed after a previous ultrasonic study has been completed. The follow-up study may include a repeat A-scan, B-scan, or both. A-scan utilizes sound waves introduced in a straight line to display a single dimension image of vertical peaks and B-scan utilizes sound waves in a two-dimensional scanning procedure to display a two-dimensional image.

76998

76998 Ultrasonic guidance, intraoperative

Explanation

Ultrasonography is used during a procedure to guide the physician in successfully accomplishing the surgery. Ultrasonic guidance may be used by the physician intraoperatively during many different types of operations on various areas of the body. Examples of intraoperative ultrasonic guidance include evaluating tissue removal in anatomical structures such as the breast, brain, abdominal organs, etc. This procedure may also be used to determine the location and depth of incisions to be made. This code is not to be used for ultrasound guidance for open or laparoscopic radiofrequency tissue ablation.

77002

77002 Fluoroscopic guidance for needle placement (eg, biopsy, aspiration, injection, localization device)

Explanation

Needle biopsy or fine needle aspiration is guided by fluoroscopic visualization. A cutting biopsy or fine needle is inserted into the target area and the position reaffirmed by fluoroscopy. This is done for an internal mass or lesion that has been positively identified by other diagnostic imaging performed earlier.

77012

77012 Computed tomography guidance for needle placement (eg, biopsy, aspiration, injection, localization device), radiological supervision and interpretation

Explanation

Computed tomography (CT) is used for guiding needle biopsies. CT scanning directs multiple narrow beams of x-rays around the body structure(s) being studied and uses computer imaging to produce thin cross-sectional views of various layers (or slices) of the body. It is able to visualize soft tissue as well as bones. Patients are required to remain motionless during the study. Once the exact needle entry site is determined along with the depth of the lesion, the optimal route from the skin to the lesion is decided. The needle is inserted and advanced to the lesion and another CT scan image is done to confirm placement for the biopsy. This code reports

the radiological supervision and interpretation only for this procedure.

77013

77013 Computed tomography guidance for, and monitoring of, parenchymal tissue ablation

Explanation

Computed tomographic guidance is used for the ablation of parenchymal (vital organ) tissue. The patient receives intravenous pain medication and sedation. Grounding pads are placed on the patient's thigh. A needle-electrode with an insulated shaft and a noninsulated distal tip is inserted through the skin and directly into the tissue to be ablated. Computed tomography (CT) is used to guide the needle to the correct spot and to monitor treatment. Each treatment session has about 10 to 15 minutes of active ablation. The energy at the needle tip causes ionic agitation and frictional heat in the surrounding tissue, which leads to cell death and coagulative necrosis. This results in a 3 to 5 cm sphere of dead tissue per treatment session. In large tumors, the physician may create more than one sphere next to each other to try to turn the tumor edges in three dimensions. A small margin of normal tissue next to tumors is also burned. The dead tumor cells are not removed, but are gradually replaced by fibrosis and scar tissue. This code reports the CT guidance and monitoring of the ablation procedure.

77022

77022 Magnetic resonance guidance for, and monitoring of, parenchymal tissue ablation

Explanation

A needle-electrode with an insulated shaft and a noninsulated distal tip is inserted through the skin and directly into the tissue to be ablated. Magnetic resonance imaging (MRI) is used to guide the needle to the correct spot and to monitor treatment. Each treatment session has about 10 to 15 minutes of active ablation of parenchymal (vital organ) tissue. The energy at the needle tip causes ionic agitation and frictional heat in the surrounding tissue, which leads to cell death and coagulative necrosis. This results in a 3 to 5 cm sphere of dead tissue per treatment session. In large tumors, the physician may create more than one sphere next to each other to try to turn the tumor edges in three dimensions. A small margin of normal tissue next to tumors is also burned. The dead tumor cells are not removed, but are gradually replaced by fibrosis and scar tissue. This code reports the magnetic resonance guidance and monitoring of the ablation procedure.

77031

77031 Stereotactic localization guidance for breast biopsy or needle placement (eg, for wire localization or for injection), each lesion, radiological supervision and interpretation

Explanation

A lesion in the breast is localized for biopsy. In the localization process, a movable arm holding the needle works together with the mammography unit that images the lesion from different angles at different fixed points. The mammogram information tells a computer where the coordinates are to correctly align the biopsy needle. Needle position is confirmed with more views taken and a stab incision made in the skin. The needle is advanced to the lesion and additional stereotactic views confirm needle placement. This code reports the radiological supervision and interpretation only for this procedure.

77032

77032 Mammographic guidance for needle placement, breast (eg, for wire localization or for injection), each lesion, radiological supervision and interpretation

Explanation

A needle localization wire is inserted into a breast lesion preoperatively under radiologic visualization in preparation for biopsy or removal. The skin is marked over the area of the lesion and mammograms performed. A needle with a hooked wire is inserted into the lesion from a perpendicular angle and advanced deep enough to remain within the lesion when the patient moves. X-rays are again taken to confirm needle placement within the lesion. Adjustments may need to be made. The needle is withdrawn while the hooked wire remains anchored. A short length of wire extends beyond the skin surface of the breast, which is taped and covered. This code reports the radiological supervision and interpretation only for this procedure.

77051-77052

77051 Computer-aided detection (computer algorithm analysis of digital image data for lesion detection) with further review for interpretation, with or without digitization of film radiographic images; diagnostic mammography (List separately in addition to code for primary procedure)

77052 screening mammography (List separately in addition to code for primary procedure)

Explanation

Computer-aided detection of lesions obtained in the mammogram is performed, with further physician or other qualified provider's interpretive review of those films. Computer-aided detection (CAD) utilizes the x-ray taken of the breast, scans the analog mammography film with a laser beam, and analyzes the video display for suspicious areas, most often converting it into digital data for the computer first. The patient does not need to be present for the CAD process. Report 77051 when the test is diagnostic and 77052 when the test is a screening mammography.

Coding Tips
These codes have been revised for 2013 in the official CPT description.

77053-77054
77053 Mammary ductogram or galactogram, single duct, radiological supervision and interpretation

77054 Mammary ductogram or galactogram, multiple ducts, radiological supervision and interpretation

Explanation
The physician performs an injection procedure for mammary ductogram or galactogram. A needle and cannula are inserted into the duct of the breast. Contrast medium is introduced into the breast duct for the radiographic visualization. A dissecting microscope may be used to aid in placing the cannula. The needle and cannula are removed when the study is completed. Report code 77053 for a single duct studied and code 77054 for multiple ducts. These codes report the radiological supervision and interpretation only for this procedure.

77055-77057
77055 Mammography; unilateral

77056 bilateral

77057 Screening mammography, bilateral (2-view film study of each breast)

Explanation
Mammography is a radiographic technique used to diagnose breast cysts or tumors in women with symptoms of breast disease or to detect them before they are palpable in women who are asymptomatic. Mammography is done using a different type of x-ray than is used for routine exams that do not penetrate tissue as easily. The breast is compressed firmly between two planes and pictures are taken. This spreads the tissue and allows for a lower x-ray dose. Use 77055 for a single breast and 77056 for both breasts. Report 77057 for both breasts done in an asymptomatic screening with two views taken of each breast.

77058-77059
77058 Magnetic resonance imaging, breast, without and/or with contrast material(s); unilateral

77059 bilateral

Explanation
Magnetic resonance imaging (MRI) is a radiation-free, noninvasive technique to produce high-quality sectional images of the inside of the body in multiple planes. MRI uses the natural magnetic properties of the hydrogen atoms in our bodies that emit radiofrequency signals when exposed to radio waves within a strong electromagnetic field. These signals are processed and converted by the computer into high-resolution, three-dimensional, tomographic images. Patients with metallic or electronic implants or foreign bodies cannot be exposed to MRI. The patient must remain still while lying on a motorized table within the large, circular MRI tunnel. A sedative may be administered, as well as an IV injected contrast material for image enhancement. Report 77058 for magnetic resonance imaging of the left or right breast and 77059 for both breasts.

77761-77763
77761 Intracavitary radiation source application; simple

77762 intermediate

77763 complex

Explanation
Brachytherapy is the application of radioactive isotopes for internal radiation. Radioactive material is encapsulated for intracavitary or interstitial implantation or prepared in solutions for instillation or oral administration. For intracavitary application, the physician inserts encapsulated radioactive elements (e.g., metal seeds, wires, tubes, or needles) into the affected body cavity using appropriate applicators, surgically inserted under ultrasound or fluoroscopic guidance. The physician may suture the applicator into or near the tumor. A radioactive isotope, usually Cesium, Iridium, or Cobalt, is placed in the applicator. The isotopes are left in place for two to three days, but may be left longer. This method provides radiation to a limited body area while minimizing exposure to normal tissue. Report 77761 for simple intracavitary application of 1 to 4 sources/ribbons; 77762 for intermediate intracavitary application of 5 to 10 sources/ribbons; and 77763 for complex intracavitary application of more than 10 sources/ribbons.

77776-77778
77776 Interstitial radiation source application; simple

77777 intermediate

77778 complex

Explanation
Brachytherapy is the application of radioactive isotopes for internal radiation. Radioactive material is encapsulated for intracavitary or interstitial implantation or prepared in solutions for instillation or oral administration. For interstitial application, the physician inserts encapsulated radioactive elements (e.g., metal seeds, wires, tubes, or needles) directly into the affected tissue using appropriate applicators, surgically inserted under ultrasound or fluoroscopic guidance. The physician may suture the applicator into or near the tumor. A radioactive isotope, usually Cesium, Iridium, or Cobalt, is placed in the applicator. The isotopes are left in place for two to three days, but may be left longer. Tiny seeds of radioactive material may be inserted directly into the tumor area and left there permanently. This method provides radiation to a limited body area while minimizing exposure to normal tissue. Report 77776 for simple interstitial application of 1 to 4 sources/ribbons; 77777 for intermediate interstitial application of 5 to 10 sources/ribbons; and 77778 for complex interstitial application of more than 10 sources/ribbons.

80050
80050 General health panel

Explanation
A general health panel includes the following tests: albumin (82040), total bilirubin (82247), calcium (82310), carbon dioxide (bicarbonate) (82374), chloride (82435), creatinine (82565), glucose (82947), alkaline phosphatase (84075), potassium (84132), total protein (84155), sodium (84295), alanine amino transferase (ALT) (SGPT) (84460), aspartate amino transferase (AST) (SGOT) (84450), urea nitrogen (BUN) (84520), and thyroid stimulating hormone (84443). In addition, this panel includes a hemogram with automated differential (85025 or 85027 and 85004) or hemogram (85027) with manual differential (85007 or 85009). Blood specimen is obtained by venipuncture. See specific codes for additional information about the listed tests.

80051
80051 Electrolyte panel

Explanation
An electrolyte panel includes the following tests: carbon dioxide (82374), chloride (82435), potassium (84132), and sodium (84295). Blood specimen is obtained by venipuncture. See specific codes for additional information about the listed tests.

80055
80055 Obstetric panel

Explanation
An obstetric panel includes the following tests: hepatitis B surface antigen (HBsAg) (87340), rubella antibody (86762), qualitative non-treponemal antibody syphilis test (VDRL, RPR, ART) (86592), RBC antibody screen (86850), ABO blood typing (86900), and Rh (D) blood typing (86901). In addition, this panel includes either an automated complete blood count (CBC) and automated differential white blood count (WBC) as described by 85025 or 85027 and 85004 OR automated CBC (85027) and appropriate manual differential WBC count (85007 or 85009). Blood specimen is obtained by venipuncture. See specific codes for additional information about the listed tests.

80061
80061 Lipid panel

Appendix

Explanation

A lipid panel includes the following tests: total serum cholesterol (82465), high-density cholesterol (HDL cholesterol) by direct measurement (83718), and triglycerides (84478). Blood specimen is obtained by venipuncture. See specific codes for additional information about the listed tests.

80100 (80104)

80100 Drug screen, qualitative; multiple drug classes chromatographic method, each procedure

80104 Drug screen, qualitative; multiple drug classes other than chromatographic method, each procedure

Explanation

These tests may be requested as drug screens for multiple drug classes. In 80100, the screening test must be performed by a chromatographic technique that has good sensitivity, although it may not be as specific as a confirmatory test. Thin-layer chromatography is a common chromatographic technique for drug screening tests. It is performed by applying a thin layer adsorbent to a rectangular plate in the stationary phase. The specimen is applied to the plate and the end of the plate is placed in a solvent. As the solvent rises along the adsorbent on the plate, the different components of the specimen are carried along at varying rates and deposited along the plate. The different components can be separately visualized and analyzed. In 80104, a number of different methods are available to screen for qualitative, non-chromatographic, multiple drug class assays, including multiplexed screening kits, urine cups, test cards, or test strips. Positive tests are always confirmed with a second method. Specimen type varies.

Coding Tips

Code 80104 is a resequenced code and will not display in numeric order.

80101

80101 Drug screen, qualitative; single drug class method (eg, immunoassay, enzyme assay), each drug class

Explanation

This test may be requested as a drug screen for a single drug class. The screening test should be performed by a technique that has good sensitivity, although it may not be as specific as a confirmatory test. A number of different methods are available to screen for single drugs or drug classes, including simple drug screening kits that rely on immunoassay for detection of a single specific drug or drug class. For example, Placidyl (aka ethchlorvynol) can be screened in urine with a very simple colorimetric test where equal parts of urine and a single reagent are mixed and observed for a visual color change.

This would be reported with 80101. Positive tests are always confirmed with a second method.

80102

80102 Drug confirmation, each procedure

Explanation

This test may be requested as drug screen confirmation. It is performed when the initial drug screen (80100-80101) is positive. Confirmatory tests must be both sensitive and specific and involve a different technique than the initial screen. For example, if the initial screen is performed by thin layer chromatography identifying a spot on the chromatogram that is the right color and in the right place to be consistent with a particular drug, it is confirmed with a more specific method, like high performance liquid chromatography (HPLC), gas chromatography-mass spectrometry (GC-MS), or immunoassay. If the drug suspected is a barbiturate, for example, a confirmatory HPLC method might be done to prove that the compound had the correct retention time, etc., and to identify it exactly as a particular barbiturate. This would be reported with 80102.

80103

80103 Tissue preparation for drug analysis

Explanation

Tissue is sometimes tested for the presence of drugs. This code reports the tissue preparation only.

80150

80150 Amikacin

Explanation

Amikacin is a type of antibiotic. Test specimens are frequently collected at peak and trough periods, which is shortly after administration of amikacin and again just before the next administration when serum concentration is at its lowest. This is an effective approach to determine a therapeutic level of drug. Method is radioimmunoassay (RIA) or high performance liquid chromatography (HPLC).

80170

80170 Gentamicin

Explanation

This drug is classified as an aminoglycoside, an antibiotic. In its injectable form, the drug may be prescribed for gram-negative infections, septicemia, and other serious infections, as well as unknown causative organisms. Common trade names include Garamycin and Gentacidin. A typical course will run seven to 10 days. Monitoring may be initiated to measure drug clearance via the kidneys. Patients with impaired renal function may accumulate the drug. Peak serum concentrations can be expected about 30 to 60 minutes following an intramuscular injection though concentrations occur just before

the next dose. Dosage is highly dependent on the severity of infection. Methodology varies.

80200

80200 Tobramycin

Explanation

This drug is also known as Nebcin. This drug has bactericidal properties and is usually injected. Specimen collection is at peak and trough. Peak will occur about one hour after an intramuscular injection and trough will occur about 12 hours after that. Method will often be by radioimmunoassay (RIA), microbiological assay, or high performance liquid chromatography (HPLC).

80202

80202 Vancomycin

Explanation

This drug may also be known as Vancocin. Specimen collection may be drawn during the trough period. This occurs around 30 minutes prior to the next dose. It is sometimes also drawn at peak. Toxic and therapeutic dosages for vancomycin can be difficult to determine due to the way the drug is metabolized. Methods include radioimmunoassay (RIA), high performance liquid chromatography (HPLC), and microbiological assay.

80414

80414 Chorionic gonadotropin stimulation panel; testosterone response

Explanation

This test may be ordered as a HCG "Stim" or human chorionic gonadotropin panel. Blood specimens may be drawn on two separate mornings before HCG is administered, usually by intramuscular injection. Injections may be repeated on two following days. Blood collection times may vary following HCG administration. The test is useful in diagnosis of certain cases of hypogonadotrophism as well as certain steroid deficiencies.

80415

80415 Chorionic gonadotropin stimulation panel; estradiol response

Explanation

This test may be ordered as a HCG "Stim" or human chorionic gonadotropin panel. Blood specimens may be drawn on two separate mornings before HCG is administered, usually by intramuscular injection and sometimes in several sessions. Timing of blood draws may vary, but just prior to the first administration of HCG and four hours after is common for women. Estradiol is among the more active endogenous estrogens. The panel is useful in the diagnosis of certain menstrual disorders, fertility problems, and estrogen-producing tumors.

Appendix

80418

80418   Combined rapid anterior pituitary evaluation panel This panel must include the following: Adrenocorticotropic hormone (ACTH) (82024 x 4) Luteinizing hormone (LH) (83002 x 4) Follicle stimulating hormone (FSH) (83001 x 4) Prolactin (84146 x 4) Human growth hormone (HGH) (83003 x 4) Cortisol (82533 x 4) Thyroid stimulating hormone (TSH) (84443 x 4)

Explanation

This series of tests may also be ordered as a pituitary panel and many large facilities will have an internal code name for this panel. This is a complex panel with numerous tests. Facilities with proper capabilities can offer a rapid, combined series where stimulation agents (i.e., insulin, thyrotropin-releasing hormone, and luteinizing hormone-releasing hormone) are administered simultaneously on a single day. This panel may be used most often for a suspected pituitary tumor. See individual code listings for specifics about portions of the panel.

80426

80426   Gonadotropin releasing hormone stimulation panel This panel must include the following: Follicle stimulating hormone (FSH) (83001 x 4) Luteinizing hormone (LH) (83002 x 4)

Explanation

This panel may be ordered as a GnRH "Stim." The panel tests for a variety of disorders, including pituitary disorders and premature sexual development in children. Baseline blood work is usually drawn. The gonadotropin-releasing hormone (GnRH) is typically administered by intravenous bolus. The peak response for follicle stimulating hormone (FSH) will be somewhat different than for luteinizing hormone (LH). Blood is often drawn at 30 minutes, 60 minutes, and 120 minutes.

80434

80434   Insulin tolerance panel; for ACTH insufficiency This panel must include the following: Cortisol (82533 x 5) Glucose (82947 x 5)

Explanation

The insulin tolerance panel for ACTH insufficiency typically involves baseline blood work before testing. The insulin is administered following a fasting period, typically by an indwelling needle. The panel is specifically for adrenocorticosteroid hormone (ACTH). The cortisol test is an indirect but accurate measure of ACTH. The panel is useful to assess hypothalamic/pituitary/adrenal interaction.

81000

81000   Urinalysis, by dip stick or tablet reagent for bilirubin, glucose, hemoglobin, ketones, leukocytes, nitrite, pH, protein, specific gravity, urobilinogen, any number of these constituents; non-automated, with microscopy

Explanation

This type of test may be ordered by the brand name product and the analytes tested. Although screens are considered to show the presence of an analyte (qualitative), some newer products are semi-quantitative. Many are plastic strips that contain sites impregnated with chemicals that react with urine when the strip is dipped into a specimen. The result is a color change that is compared against a standardized chart. Most strips will test for numerous analytes, as well as for pH and specific gravity. Tablets work in a similar fashion. A drop of urine is placed on the tablet and a chemical reaction causes a color change that is compared to a standard chart. Usually only a single analyte is under consideration, per tablet. Code 81000 involves a manual (nonautomated) test and includes a microscopic examination. Microscopy involves examination of the urine sediments or solids. The urine is first centrifuged in a graduated tube to concentrate the sediments. Samples (either wet or dry) are examined, usually under both high and low power, and abnormal constituents are noted. These may include a wide range of biological abnormalities, such as blood cells, casts, and bacteria, as well as chemical anomalies, such as crystals.

81001

81001   Urinalysis, by dip stick or tablet reagent for bilirubin, glucose, hemoglobin, ketones, leukocytes, nitrite, pH, protein, specific gravity, urobilinogen, any number of these constituents; automated, with microscopy

Explanation

This type of test may be ordered by the type of processor used and the analytes tested. The testing methodology is similar to the manual strips, except that the color change caused by the chemical reaction with urine is processed and read mechanically. The strip is exposed to the urine sample and is mechanically fed through a processor that reads the colors emitted by the reaction. The unit will be calibrated according to international standards and readings have a high degree of accuracy. The result may be displayed on a monitor, but is always printed or recorded in some form. Code 81001 also includes a microscopy. Microscopy involves examination of the urine sediments or solids. The urine is first centrifuged in a graduated tube to concentrate the sediments. Samples (either wet or dry) are examined, usually under both high and low power, and abnormal constituents are

noted. These may include a wide range of biological abnormalities, such as blood cells, casts, and bacteria, as well as chemical anomalies, such as crystals.

81002

81002   Urinalysis, by dip stick or tablet reagent for bilirubin, glucose, hemoglobin, ketones, leukocytes, nitrite, pH, protein, specific gravity, urobilinogen, any number of these constituents; non-automated, without microscopy

Explanation

This type of test may be ordered by the brand name product and the analytes tested. Although usually considered screens to show the presence of an analyte (qualitative), some newer products are semi-quantitative. Many are plastic strips that contain sites impregnated with chemicals that react with urine when the strip is dipped into a specimen. The result is a color change that is compared against a standardized chart. Most strips will test for numerous analytes, as well as for pH and specific gravity. Tablets work in a similar fashion. A drop of urine is placed on the tablet and a chemical reaction causes a color change that is compared to a standard chart. Usually only a single analyte is under consideration per tablet, however. Code 81002 does not include a microscopic examination of the urine sample or its components.

81003

81003   Urinalysis, by dip stick or tablet reagent for bilirubin, glucose, hemoglobin, ketones, leukocytes, nitrite, pH, protein, specific gravity, urobilinogen, any number of these constituents; automated, without microscopy

Explanation

This type of test may be ordered by the type of processor used and the analytes tested. The testing methodology is similar to the manual strips, except that the color change caused by the chemical reaction with urine is processed and read mechanically. The strip is exposed to the urine sample and is mechanically fed through a processor that reads the colors emitted by the reaction. The unit will be calibrated according to international standards and readings have a high degree of accuracy. The result may be displayed on a monitor, but is always printed or recorded in some form. Code 81003 does not include a microscopic examination of the urine sample or its components.

81005

81005   Urinalysis; qualitative or semiquantitative, except immunoassays

Appendix

Explanation

This test may be ordered by the type of processor used and the analytes under examination. The method will be any type of automated analyzer, usually colorimetry. The results of a semi-quantitative test indicate the presence or absence of an analyte and may be expressed as simply positive or negative. A qualitative result may be indicated as trace, 1+, 2+, etc.

81007

81007 Urinalysis; bacteriuria screen, except by culture or dipstick

Explanation

This type of test may be ordered by the brand name of the commercial kit used and the bacteria that the kit screens for. Human urine is normally almost entirely free of bacteria. However, bacteria can easily be introduced upon voiding. In addition, specimens containing any amount of pathological bacteria can have the organisms rapidly multiply after collection. For this reason, specimens are often examined shortly after collection. Method includes any method except culture or dipstick. The test is often performed by commercial kit. The type of kit used should be specified in the report.

81015

81015 Urinalysis; microscopic only

Explanation

This test may be ordered as a microscopic analysis. Human urine is normally free of bacteria. However, bacteria can easily be introduced upon voiding. In addition, specimens containing any amount of pathological bacteria can have the organisms rapidly multiply after collection. For this reason, specimens are often examined shortly after collection. The sample may first be centrifuged into a graduated tube to concentrate the sediments, or solid matter, held in suspension. The concentration of bacteria as well as cell types, crystals, and other elements seen is reported.

81020

81020 Urinalysis; 2 or 3 glass test

Explanation

This test may be ordered as a two-glass or three-glass test, a MacConkey-blood agar test, an MC-blood agar test, or any of the previous with a gram-positive plate. This is a culture for bacteria and will typically involve a culture plate of 5 percent sheep's blood agar and a MacConkey plate (a medium containing differentiate for lactose and nonlactose fermenters). A third plate of gram-positive media may offer further discrimination of bacteria cultured. The test is useful in determining the types and prevalence of bacteria in the urine.

81025

81025 Urine pregnancy test, by visual color comparison methods

Explanation

This test may be ordered by any of the brand name kits available. The tests typically involve a dipstick impregnated with reagents that chemically react upon contact with urine. A change in color indicates positive or negative for the presence of hormones found in the urine of women in early pregnancy.

81050

81050 Volume measurement for timed collection, each

Explanation

This test may be ordered as simply a volume measurement, a flow study, uroflowmetry, or urodynamic study. Timed collections are typically collected over a given period (24 hours is common). This test may be performed as a preliminary study to determine the volume of urine voided per second. A flowmeter device may be used or a simple timing of the flow into a graduated container may be employed. The test is sometimes also administered as a baseline or otherwise in conjunction with urinary tract procedures that might affect flow.

81200

81200 ASPA (aspartoacylase) (eg, Canavan disease) gene analysis, common variants (eg, E285A, Y231X)

Explanation

This test may be requested as ASPA genetic analysis, CANW, or Canavan disease mutation analysis. Specimen is whole blood. Methodology is multiplex PCR amplification. This is a blood test that screens for the missing enzyme aspartoacylase or for mutations in the gene that controls aspartoacylase. A mutation of the gene for the enzyme aspartoacylase results in Canavan disease, a common gene-linked birth disorder manifesting as cerebral degeneration during infancy. Canavan disease occurs in any ethnic group, however, it is more prevalent among Ashkenazi Jews from eastern Poland, Lithuania, and western Russia, and Saudi Arabians. Both parents must be carriers of the Canavan gene mutation, and there is a one in four (25 percent) chance with each pregnancy that the child will be affected.

81201-81203

81201 APC (adenomatous polyposis coli) (eg, familial adenomatosis polyposis [FAP], attenuated FAP) gene analysis; full gene sequence
81202 known familial variants
81203 duplication/deletion variants

Explanation

This test may be requested as APC (adenomatous polyposis coli), familial adenomatosis polyposis (FAP), or attenuated FAP analysis. Specimen is peripheral blood leukocytes. Methodology is bi-directional sequence analysis and/or multiplex ligation-dependent probe amplification (MLPA). A normal APC gene produces a protein that prevents polyps and tumors from forming. When this gene is mutated, the protein no longer is effective and polyps develop. This test screens for mutations in the APC gene that cause polyposis conditions such as FAP, colon cancer predisposition, Gardner syndrome, and Turcot syndrome. Report 81201 when the full gene sequence is analyzed. Report 81202 for the analysis of known familial variants only. Report 81203 if only the duplication/deletion variants are analyzed.

Coding Tips

These codes are new for 2013.

81205

81205 BCKDHB (branched-chain keto acid dehydrogenase E1, beta polypeptide) (eg, Maple syrup urine disease) gene analysis, common variants (eg, R183P, G278S, E422X)

Explanation

This test may be ordered as BCKDHB analysis, MSUD gene analysis, or maple syrup disease analysis. Specimen is whole blood. Methodology is multiplex PCR amplification. Maple syrup urine disease is an inherited disease in which some amino acids are not processed by the body. A symptom of the disease is a distinct sweet odor of the urine of affected infants, thus the name of the disease.

81209

81209 BLM (Bloom syndrome, RecQ helicase-like) (eg, Bloom syndrome) gene analysis, 2281del6ins7 variant

Explanation

This test may be ordered as a Bloom syndrome analysis. Specimen is whole blood, chorionic villi, or amniotic fluid. Methodology is multiplex PCR amplification. Bloom syndrome causes growth problems, immune deficiencies, and places the patient at high risk for all types of cancer. It is the result of mutations of the BLM gene.

81211-81213

81211 BRCA1, BRCA2 (breast cancer 1 and 2) (eg, hereditary breast and ovarian cancer) gene analysis; full sequence analysis and common duplication/deletion variants in BRCA1 (ie, exon 13 del 3.835kb, exon 13 dup 6kb, exon 14-20 del 26kb, exon 22 del 510bp, exon 8-9 del 7.1kb)

81212 185delAG, 5385insC, 6174delT variants

81213 uncommon duplication/deletion variants

Explanation

BRCA1 and BRCA2 genes are a class of genes that are known as tumor suppressors. Mutations to the BRCA1 and BRCA2 gene have been linked to hereditary breast and ovarian cancers. Specimen is blood. These tests are performed to determine what, if any, mutations have affected the BRCA1 and BRCA2 genes. Code selection is dependent on the type of mutation being tested for.

81214-81215

81214 BRCA1 (breast cancer 1) (eg, hereditary breast and ovarian cancer) gene analysis; full sequence analysis and common duplication/deletion variants (ie, exon 13 del 3.835kb, exon 13 dup 6kb, exon 14-20 del 26kb, exon 22 del 510bp, exon 8-9 del 7.1kb)

81215 known familial variant

Explanation

BRCA1 is a gene within a class of genes that are known as tumor suppressors. Mutations to the BRCA1 gene have been linked to hereditary breast and ovarian cancers. Specimen is blood. This test is performed to determine what, if any, mutations have affected the BRCA1 gene. Code selection is dependent on the type of mutation being tested for.

81216-81217

81216 BRCA2 (breast cancer 2) (eg, hereditary breast and ovarian cancer) gene analysis; full sequence analysis

81217 known familial variant

Explanation

BRCA2 is a gene within a class of genes that are known as tumor suppressors. Mutations to the BRCA2 gene have been linked to hereditary breast and ovarian cancers. Specimen is blood. This test is performed to determine what, if any, mutations have affected the BRCA2 gene. Code selection is dependent on the type of mutation being tested for.

81220-81221

81220 CFTR (cystic fibrosis transmembrane conductance regulator) (eg, cystic fibrosis) gene analysis; common variants (eg, ACMG/ACOG guidelines)

81221 known familial variants

Explanation

Specimen may be blood, amniotic fluid, or chorionic villus sample. Methodology is PCR sequencing or multiplex ligation dependent probe amplification (MLPA). Testing is performed to identify the specific gene mutation when a diagnosis of cystic fibrosis has been made. Code 81220 is used to report analysis for the more common variants of the CFTR gene mutations. Report 81221 for the familial mutation(s) only, which does not rule out the presence of other mutations within the CFTR gene. Report 81222 or 81223 for identification of mutations in individuals with atypical presentations of cystic fibrosis or when detection rates by targeted mutation analysis are low or unknown.

81222-81223

81222 CFTR (cystic fibrosis transmembrane conductance regulator) (eg, cystic fibrosis) gene analysis; duplication/deletion variants

81223 full gene sequence

Explanation

Specimen is whole blood. Methodology is PCR sequencing or multiplex ligation dependent probe amplification (MLPA). Mutations to the CFTR gene found on chromosome 7 are numerous and therefore there is a wide variability in clinical manifestation of cystic fibrosis. Report 81222 when analysis is performed for the identification of mutations in individuals with atypical presentations of cystic fibrosis or 81223 when full gene sequence analysis is performed. Full gene sequence analysis is usually performed when detection rates by targeted mutation analysis are low or unknown.

81225-81227

81225 CYP2C19 (cytochrome P450, family 2, subfamily C, polypeptide 19) (eg, drug metabolism), gene analysis, common variants (eg, *2, *3, *4, *8, *17)

81226 CYP2D6 (cytochrome P450, family 2, subfamily D, polypeptide 6) (eg, drug metabolism), gene analysis, common variants (eg, *2, *3, *4, *5, *6, *9, *10, *17, *19, *29, *35, *41, *1XN, *2XN, *4XN)

81227 CYP2C9 (cytochrome P450, family 2, subfamily C, polypeptide 9) (eg, drug metabolism), gene analysis, common variants (eg, *2, *3, *5, *6)

Explanation

Specimen is whole blood. Methodology is PCR amplification followed by DNA sequence analysis and mutation detection with hybridization probes. These tests identify patients who are poor metabolizers or extensive metabolizers of drugs because of mutations to certain genes. This allows physicians to adjust drug levels, including non-conventional doses, or to select drugs that are not affected by the mutation. Report 81225 for CYP2C19, 81226 for CYP2D6, and 81227 for CYP2C9 gene analysis.

81228-81229

81228 Cytogenomic constitutional (genome-wide) microarray analysis; interrogation of genomic regions for copy number variants (eg, Bacterial Artificial Chromosome [BAC] or oligo-based comparative genomic hybridization [CGH] microarray analysis)

81229 interrogation of genomic regions for copy number and single nucleotide polymorphism (SNP) variants for chromosomal abnormalities

Explanation

These tests may be ordered as aCGH, CGH, or CMA. Specimen is whole blood. Methodology is array comparative genomic hybridization. These tests are useful in identifying chromosomal abnormalities in patients with mental retardation, developmental delay, autism, dysmorphic features, or multiple congenital anomalies, particularly those patients with normal chromosome or FISH studies. The most common type of genetic variation occurs at the SNPs (pronounced "snips"). While most SNPs have no effect on a person's health or normal development, some may help to predict a patient's response to certain drugs and risk factors for developing certain diseases such as cancer, diabetes, and heart disease. Report 81229 when single nucleotide polymorphisms (SNP) are also interrogated.

81242

81242 FANCC (Fanconi anemia, complementation group C) (eg, Fanconi anemia, type C) gene analysis, common variant (eg, IVS4+4A>T)

Explanation

Specimen is whole blood. Methodology is PCR-based assay using Luminex. Mutations that have been associated with Fanconi anemia have been found in several genes; however, the IVS4(+4)A->T mutation is common in the Ashkenazi Jewish population. Fanconi anemia, an aplastic anemia, causes bone marrow failure and myelodysplasia or acute myelogenous leukemia.

81243-81244

81243 FMR1 (Fragile X mental retardation 1) (eg, fragile X mental retardation) gene analysis; evaluation to detect abnormal (eg, expanded) alleles

81244 characterization of alleles (eg, expanded size and methylation status)

Explanation

Sample can be blood, amniotic fluid, or chorionic villus. Prenatal sampling must be accompanied by maternal blood specimen. Methodology for 81243 is direct mutation analysis. Report 81244 when methylation-specific PCR, which assesses the methylation status, is performed. These tests are useful for determining carrier status, as well as confirmation of fragile X syndrome.

81250

81250 G6PC (glucose-6-phosphatase, catalytic subunit) (eg, Glycogen storage disease, Type 1a, von Gierke disease) gene analysis, common variants (eg, R83C, Q347X)

Explanation

Specimen type varies. Methodology is PCR-assay. The G6PC gene family contains three members designated G6PC, G6PC2, and G6PC3. The tissue-specific expression patterns of these genes differ, and mutations in all three genes have been linked to distinct diseases in humans. This test is useful for genetic screening, as well as definitive diagnosis.

81251-81255

81251 GBA (glucosidase, beta, acid) (eg, Gaucher disease) gene analysis, common variants (eg, N370S, 84GG, L444P, IVS2+1G>A)

81255 HEXA (hexosaminidase A [alpha polypeptide]) (eg, Tay-Sachs disease) gene analysis, common variants (eg, 1278insTATC, 1421+1G>C, G269S)

Explanation

Sample can be blood, amniotic fluid, or chorionic villus. Prenatal sampling must be accompanied by maternal blood specimen. Methodology is PCR-based assay. These tests are used for prenatal diagnosis in high-risk pregnancies, for genetic screening, or as confirmation of a clinical diagnosis. Report 81251 for analysis of the GBA gene (Gaucher disease) or 81255 for analysis of the HEXA gene (Tay-Sachs disease).

81252-81253

81252 GJB2 (gap junction protein, beta 2, 26kDa, connexin 26) (eg, nonsyndromic hearing loss) gene analysis; full gene sequence

81253 GJB2 (gap junction protein, beta 2, 26kDa; connexin 26) (eg, nonsyndromic hearing loss) gene analysis; known familial variants

Explanation

This test may be requested as GJB2 (gap junction protein, beta 2, 26kDa, connexin 26) or nonsyndromic hearing loss gene analysis. Specimen is whole blood. Methodology is bidirectional sequence analysis and/or PCR amplification. This test screens for a genetic mutation of GJB2, which is accountable for a high frequency of nonsyndromic autosomal recessive deafness (DFNA3). Report 81252 for the analysis of the full gene sequence. Report 81253 if only the known familial variants are analyzed.

Coding Tips

These codes are new for 2013.

81254

81254 GJB6 (gap junction protein, beta 6, 30kDa, connexin 30) (eg, nonsyndromic hearing loss) gene analysis, common variants (eg, 309kb [del(GJB6-D13S1830)] and 232kb [del(GJB6-D13S1854)])

Explanation

This test may be requested as GJB6 (gap junction protein, beta 6, 30kDa, connexin 30) or nonsyndromic hearing loss gene analysis. Specimen is whole blood. Methodology is bidirectional sequence analysis and/or PCR amplification. This test screens for a genetic mutation of GJB6, which is accountable for a high frequency of recessively inherited deafness (DFNB1).

Coding Tips

This code is new for 2013.

81256

81256 HFE (hemochromatosis) (eg, hereditary hemochromatosis) gene analysis, common variants (eg, C282Y, H63D)

Explanation

Sample is whole blood. Methodology is PCR-based assay. This study is useful in establishing or confirming the clinical diagnosis of hereditary hemochromatosis. It is not recommended for general patient genetic screening; however, it is appropriate for predictive testing of patients who have a family history of hereditary hemochromatosis.

81257

81257 HBA1/HBA2 (alpha globin 1 and alpha globin 2) (eg, alpha thalassemia, Hb Bart hydrops fetalis syndrome, HbH disease), gene analysis, for common deletions or variant (eg, Southeast Asian, Thai, Filipino, Mediterranean, alpha3.7, alpha4.2, alpha20.5, and Constant Spring)

Explanation

Specimen is whole blood or amniotic fluid. Prenatal screening of amniotic fluid must be accompanied by maternal blood sample. Methodology is PCR amplification followed by bidirectional sequencing. Alpha thalassemia is one of the most common inherited disorders of hemoglobin worldwide. There are two main forms of this condition: Hb Bart hydrops fetalis syndrome where there is loss of all four alpha globin genes and Hemoglobin H disease where there is loss of three alpha globin gene function. Carrier states include the loss of two alpha globin genes (trait carrier status) and the loss of a single alpha globin gene (silent carrier status).

81260

81260 IKBKAP (inhibitor of kappa light polypeptide gene enhancer in B-cells, kinase complex-associated protein) (eg, familial dysautonomia) gene analysis, common variants (eg, 2507+6T>C, R696P)

Explanation

Sample is whole blood, amniotic fluid, or chorionic villus sampling. Prenatal testing should be accompanied by maternal whole blood sample. Methodology is PCR-based assay and fluorescent hybridization probes. This study is useful in carrier screening, prenatal diagnosis, and clinical diagnosis confirmation. Mutations in the IKBKAP gene result in the manifestations of familial dysautonomia. There are two common mutations prevalent in the Ashkenazi Jewish population: IVS20(+6)T->C and R696P, and the carrier rate is one in 31.

81265-81266

81265 Comparative analysis using Short Tandem Repeat (STR) markers; patient and comparative specimen (eg, pre-transplant recipient and donor germline testing, post-transplant non-hematopoietic recipient germline [eg, buccal swab or other germline tissue sample] and donor testing, twin zygosity testing, or maternal cell contamination of fetal cells)

81266 each additional specimen (eg, additional cord blood donor, additional fetal samples from different cultures, or additional zygosity in multiple birth pregnancies) (List separately in addition to code for primary procedure)

Explanation

Short tandem repeat (STR) sequences are used as identity markers. This test is useful in fraternal and identical twin determination, donor matches, and maternal cell contamination (MCC). The potential presence of MCC in chorionic villus or amniotic fluid samples poses a serious risk for prenatal misdiagnosis. Report 81265 for the first specimen and 81266 for each additional specimen.

Coding Companion for Ob/Gyn

81290

81290   MCOLN1 (mucolipin 1) (eg, Mucolipidosis, type IV) gene analysis, common variants (eg, IVS3-2A>G, del6.4kb)

Explanation

Specimen is blood, amniotic fluid, or chorionic villus. Prenatal samples should include a maternal blood specimen. Methodology is PCR-based assay. This test is useful for carrier status testing in individuals of Ashkenazi Jewish ancestry, prenatal screening for at-risk pregnancies, and confirmation of clinical diagnosis of mucolipidosis IV. Mucolipidosis IV is a lysosomal storage disease that results in mental retardation, hypotonia, corneal clouding, and retinal degeneration.

81291

81291   MTHFR (5,10-methylenetetrahydrofolate reductase) (eg, hereditary hypercoagulability) gene analysis, common variants (eg, 677T, 1298C)

Explanation

Specimen is whole blood. Methodology is direct mutation analysis based on the amplification of fluorescent signal released by cleavage of sequence specific alleles. Several MTHFR mutations have been associated with homocystinuria. Homocystinuria presents with a wide range of clinical manifestations, including developmental delay, mental retardation, and premature vascular disease.

81302-81304

81302   MECP2 (methyl CpG binding protein 2) (eg, Rett syndrome) gene analysis; full sequence analysis
81303   known familial variant
81304   duplication/deletion variants

Explanation

Specimen is blood. Methodology is PCR-analysis. Genetic mutations in MECP2 can be associated with variable phenotypes in females, including classic Rett syndrome, variant or atypical Rett syndrome, mild mental retardation, and asymptomatic carriers. Males with MECP2 mutations can present with variable phenotypes as well. These tests can be useful in the screening and diagnosis of Rett syndrome. Report 81302 for full gene sequence analysis, 81303 when analysis is for known familial gene variations, and 81304 when duplication/deletion variants are determined.

81321-81323

81321   *PTEN (phosphatase and tensin homolog)* (eg, Cowden syndrome, PTEN hamartoma tumor syndrome) gene analysis; full sequence analysis
81322   PTEN (phosphatase and tensin homolog) (eg, Cowden syndrome, PTEN hamartoma tumor syndrome) gene analysis; known familial variant
81323   duplication/deletion variant

Explanation

This test may be requested as PTEN (phosphatase and tensin homolog), Cowden syndrome, or PTEN hamartoma tumor syndrome gene analysis. Specimen is whole blood or saliva. Methodology is bidirectional sequence analysis and FISH (fluorescent in situ hybridization) testing. This test screens for mutations of the PTEN gene, which causes defects in or omission of the PTEN enzyme, a tumor suppressor. A mutation of this gene results in diseases such as Cowden syndrome, which presents a high risk for benign and malignant tumors of the thyroid, breast, and endometrium, and hamartoma tumor syndrome. Report 81321 for analysis of the full gene sequence. Report 81322 if only the known familial variants are analyzed. Report 81323 when only the duplication/deletion variants are analyzed.

Coding Tips

These codes are new for 2013.

81324-81326

81324   PMP22 (peripheral myelin protein 22) (eg, Charcot-Marie-Tooth, hereditary neuropathy with liability to pressure palsies) gene analysis; duplication/deletion analysis
81325   full sequence analysis
81326   known familial variant

Explanation

This test screens for mutations in the peripheral myelin protein 22 gene, which is responsible for development and maintenance of myelin in the nervous system. Specimen is whole blood. Methodology is multiplex ligation-dependent probe amplification (MLPA). Mutations of this gene, most commonly duplication, result in Charcot-Marie-Tooth syndrome type 1A. Deletion of this gene causes demyelinization, resulting in hereditary neuropathy with liability to pressure palsies. Report 81324 if only the duplication/deletion variants are analyzed. Report 81325 when the full gene sequence is analyzed. Report 81326 if only the known familial variants are analyzed.

Coding Tips

These codes are new for 2013.

81330

81330   SMPD1(sphingomyelin phosphodiesterase 1, acid lysosomal) (eg, Niemann-Pick disease, Type A) gene analysis, common variants (eg, R496L, L302P, fsP330)

Explanation

Specimen is whole blood. Methodology is PCR-assay. There are three types of Niemann-Pick disease: A, B, and C. Niemann-Pick disease type A is a lysosomal storage disease resulting from three common gene mutations (R4961, K302P, and fsP330). These mutations cause a deficiency of the enzyme acid sphingomyelinase resulting in jaundice, the progressive loss of motor skills, difficulties with feeding, enlargement of the liver and spleen, and learning disabilities. This test is useful for carrier screening. The mutation is more common in patients of the Ashkenazi Jewish heritage.

81331

81331   SNRPN/UBE3A (small nuclear ribonucleoprotein polypeptide N and ubiquitin protein ligase E3A) (eg, Prader-Willi syndrome and/or Angelman syndrome), methylation analysis

Explanation

This test is useful for the confirmation of Prader-Willi or Angelman syndromes. These syndromes result in global developmental delay, as well as other symptoms, and are thought to be the result of mutations to chromosome 15. Specimen is blood or amniotic fluid. Amniotic fluid must be accompanied by maternal blood. Methodology is methylation-sensitive multiple ligation-dependent probe amplification (MLPA).

81350

81350   UGT1A1 (UDP glucuronosyltransferase 1 family, polypeptide A1) (eg, irinotecan metabolism), gene analysis, common variants (eg, *28, *36, *37)

Explanation

This test is used to identify the UGT1A1 mutation and carrier status. Specimen is whole blood. Methodology is PCR-assay. Mutations to the UGT1A1 gene result in hyperbilirubinemia.

81355

81355   VKORC1 (vitamin K epoxide reductase complex, subunit 1) (eg, warfarin metabolism), gene analysis, common variants (eg, -1639/3673)

Explanation

This test may also be ordered as Coumadin genotype or warfarin genotype. Specimen is whole blood. Methodology is PCR-assay. This test is used to identify patients who are poor metabolizers or

Appendix

extensive metabolizers of warfarin because of mutations to the VKORC1 gene. This allows physicians to adjust drug levels, including non-conventional doses, or to select drugs that are not affected by the mutation.

81370-81371

81370 HLA Class I and II typing, low resolution (eg, antigen equivalents); HLA-A, -B, -C, -DRB1/3/4/5, and -DQB1

81371 HLA-A, -B, and -DRB1/3/4/5 (eg, verification typing)

Explanation

These tests are commonly used to determine the histocompatibility between a patient and a donor to predict and prevent graft versus host disease (GVHD). Variations may also be used to detect susceptibility to certain genetic autoimmune diseases. Human leukocyte antigens (HLA) are a group of genes found on chromosome 6. There are two types of HLA: class I and class II. Low resolution (or generic) HLA typing can be performed via serology, cellular, or molecular technique, the molecular technique being the most common. In this technique, whole blood must be obtained and DNA extracted. The genes of interest are amplified and identification of HLA type is made via detection of the DNA sequence polymorphism. High resolution typing involves identifying groups of alleles and approximating the specific HLA characteristics. Report 81370 for low resolution typing of HLA-A-, -B, -C, -DRB1/3/4/5, and -DQB1. Report 81371 for low resolution typing of HLA-A, -B, and DRB1/3/4/5.

81372-81374

81372 HLA Class I typing, low resolution (eg, antigen equivalents); complete (ie, HLA-A, -B, and -C)

81373 1 locus (eg, HLA-A, -B, or -C), each

81374 1 antigen equivalent (eg, B*27), each

Explanation

These tests are commonly used to determine the histocompatibility between a patient and a donor to predict and prevent graft versus host disease (GVHD). Variations may also be used to detect susceptibility to certain genetic autoimmune diseases. Human leukocyte antigens (HLA) are a group of genes found on chromosome 6. There are two types of HLA: class I and class II. Low resolution (or generic) HLA typing can be performed via serology, cellular, or molecular technique, the molecular technique being the most common. In this technique, whole blood must be obtained and DNA extracted. The genes of interest are amplified and identification of HLA type is made via detection of the DNA sequence polymorphism. High resolution typing involves identifying groups of alleles and approximating the specific HLA characteristics. Report 81372 for complete low resolution HLA class I typing, including HLA-A, -B, and -C. Report 81373 for HLA low resolution typing

of each individual class I loci (HLA-A, -B, or -C) when complete class I typing is not performed. Report 81374 for low resolution class I typing of each serological HLA equivalent or subtype (e.g., HLA-B*27).

81375-81377

81375 HLA Class II typing, low resolution (eg, antigen equivalents); HLA-DRB1/3/4/5 and -DQB1

81376 1 locus (eg, HLA-DRB1/3/4/5, -DQB1, -DQA1, -DPB1, or -DPA1), each

81377 1 antigen equivalent, each

Explanation

These tests are commonly used to determine the histocompatibility between a patient and a donor to predict and prevent graft versus host disease (GVHD). Variations may also be used to detect susceptibility to certain genetic autoimmune diseases. Human leukocyte antigens (HLA) are a group of genes found on chromosome 6. There are two types of HLA: class I and class II. Low resolution (or generic) HLA typing can be performed via serology, cellular, or molecular technique, the molecular technique being the most common. In this technique, whole blood must be obtained and DNA extracted. The genes of interest are amplified and identification of HLA type is made via detection of the DNA sequence polymorphism. High resolution typing involves identifying groups of alleles and approximating the specific HLA characteristics. Report 81375 for complete low resolution HLA class II typing, including HLA-DRB1/3/4/5 and HLA-DQB1. Report 81376 for HLA low resolution typing of each individual class II loci (HLA-DRB1/3/4/5, -DQB1, -DQA1, -DPB1, or -DPA1) when complete class II typing is not performed. Report 81377 for low resolution class II typing of each serological HLA equivalent or subtype.

81378

81378 HLA Class I and II typing, high resolution (ie, alleles or allele groups), HLA-A, -B, -C, and -DRB1

Explanation

This test is commonly used to determine the histocompatibility between a patient and a donor to predict and prevent graft versus host disease (GVHD). Variations may be used to detect susceptibility to certain genetic autoimmune diseases. Human leukocyte antigens (HLA) are a group of genes found on chromosome 6. There are two types of HLA: class I and class II. Low resolution (or generic) HLA typing can be performed via serology, cellular, or molecular technique, the molecular technique being the most common. In this technique, whole blood must be obtained and DNA extracted. The genes of interest are amplified and identification of HLA type is made via detection of the DNA sequence polymorphism. High resolution typing involves identifying alleles or allele

groups by examining and determining the specific HLA characteristics. Code 81378 is reported for high resolution typing of both HLA class I and II (HLA-A, -B, -C, and -DRB1).

81379-81381

81379 HLA Class I typing, high resolution (ie, alleles or allele groups); complete (ie, HLA-A, -B, and -C)

81380 1 locus (eg, HLA-A, -B, or -C), each

81381 1 allele or allele group (eg, B*57:01P), each

Explanation

These tests are commonly used to determine the histocompatibility between a patient and a donor to predict and prevent graft versus host disease (GVHD). Variations may also be used to detect susceptibility to certain genetic autoimmune diseases. Human leukocyte antigens (HLA) are a group of genes found on chromosome 6. There are two types of HLA: class I and class II. Low resolution (or generic) HLA typing can be performed via serology, cellular, or molecular technique, the molecular technique being the most common. In this technique, whole blood must be obtained and DNA extracted. The genes of interest are amplified and identification of HLA type is made via detection of the DNA sequence polymorphism. High resolution typing involves identifying alleles or allele groups by examining and determining the specific HLA characteristics. Report 81379 for complete high resolution HLA class I typing, including HLA-A, -B, and -C. Report 81380 for HLA high resolution typing of each individual class I loci (HLA-A, -B, or -C) when complete class I typing is not performed. Report 81381 for high resolution typing of each class I allele or allele group (e.g., B*57:01P).

81382-81383

81382 HLA Class II typing, high resolution (ie, alleles or allele groups); one locus (eg, HLA-DRB1, -DRB3, -DRB4, -DRB5, -DQB1, -DQA1, -DPB1, or -DPA1), each

81383 1 allele or allele group (eg, HLA-DQB1*06:02P), each

Explanation

These tests are commonly used to determine the histocompatibility between a patient and a donor to predict and prevent graft versus host disease (GVHD). Variations may also be used to detect susceptibility to certain genetic autoimmune diseases. Human leukocyte antigens (HLA) are a group of genes found on chromosome 6. There are two types of HLA: class I and class II. Low resolution (or generic) HLA typing can be performed via serology, cellular, or molecular technique, the molecular technique being the most common. In this technique, whole blood must be obtained and DNA extracted. The genes of interest are amplified and identification of HLA type is made via detection of the DNA sequence polymorphism. High

Appendix

resolution typing involves identifying alleles or allele groups by examining and determining the specific HLA characteristics. Report 81382 for high resolution typing of an individual HLA class II locus, including HLA-DRB1/3/4/5, -DQA1, -DPB1, or -DPA1. Report 81383 for high resolution typing of each individual class II allele or allele group (e.g., HLA-DQB1*06:02P).

81500-81503

81500 Oncology (ovarian), biochemical assays of two proteins (CA-125 and HE4), utilizing serum, with menopausal status, algorithm reported as a risk score

81503 Oncology (ovarian), biochemical assays of five proteins (CA-125, apolipoprotein A1, beta-2 microglobulin, transferrin and pre-albumin), utilizing serum, algorithm reported as a risk score

Explanation

Multianalyte Assays with Algorithmic Analyses (MAAA) are procedures that are typically performed by a single clinical laboratory or manufacturer. These analyses utilize results obtained from assays of various types, including molecular pathology, fluorescent in situ hybridization, and non-nucleic acid based assays, to perform proprietary analysis using the results, as well as other patient information, to assess risk. This risk factor is reported typically as a numeric score(s) or as a probability. Report 81500 for the Risk of Ovarian Malignancy Algorithm analysis, also known as ROMA, which utilizes the results of CA-125 and HE4 tests in the algorithm. Report 81503 when the OVA1 analysis, utilizing CA-125, apolipoprotein A1, beta-2 microglobulin, transferrin, and pre-albumin tests in the algorithm, is performed.

Coding Tips

These codes are new for 2013.

81508-81512

81508 Fetal congenital abnormalities, biochemical assays of two proteins (PAPP-A, hCG [any form]), utilizing maternal serum, algorithm reported as a risk score

81509 Fetal congenital abnormalities, biochemical assays of three proteins (PAPP-A, hCG [any form], DIA), utilizing maternal serum, algorithm reported as a risk score

81510 Fetal congenital abnormalities, biochemical assays of three analytes (AFP, uE3, hCG [any form]), utilizing maternal serum, algorithm reported as a risk score

81511 Fetal congenital abnormalities, biochemical assays of four analytes (AFP, uE3, hCG [any form], DIA) utilizing maternal serum, algorithm reported as a risk score (may include additional results from previous biochemical testing)

81512 Fetal congenital abnormalities, biochemical assays of five analytes (AFP, uE3, total hCG, hyperglycosylated hCG, DIA) utilizing maternal serum, algorithm reported as a risk score

Explanation

These analyses utilize results obtained from assays of various types, including molecular pathology, fluorescent in situ hybridization, and non-nucleic acid based assays. Analysis, using the results as well as other patient information, is then performed and reported typically as a numeric score(s) or as a probability. Report 81508 or 81509 for analyses utilizing proteins in the algorithm. Code 81508 represents two proteins (PAPP-A and any form of hCG). Code 81509 includes three proteins (PAPP-A, DIA, and any form of hCG). Report 81510, 81511, or 81512 when the analyses use analytes in the algorithm. Code 81510 is reported for three analytes (AFP, uE3, and any form of hCG); 81511 is reported for four analytes (AFP, uE3, any form of hCG and DIA), and 81512 is reported for five analytes (AFP, uE3, total hCG, DIA, and hyperglycosylated hCG).

Coding Tips

These codes are new for 2013.

82013

82013 Acetylcholinesterase

Explanation

This test is also referred to as red blood cell (RBC) acetylcholinesterase, erythrocytic cholinesterase, or true cholinesterase. Method is colorimetric or spectrophotometric rate of hydrolysis determination. This test may be performed to determine certain RBC disorders such as thalassemias, spherocytosis, and other anemias. It may also be used to determine toxicity or exposure to certain insecticides. For amniotic fluid specimen, a separately reportable amniocentesis is performed. The presence of acetylcholinesterase activity and increased alpha-fetoprotein in amniotic fluid are presumptive evidence of an open neural tube defect in the fetus.

82016-82017

82016 Acylcarnitines; qualitative, each specimen
82017 quantitative, each specimen

Explanation

These tests may be requested as qualitative acylcarnitine (carnitine esters) and quantitative acylcarnitine (carnitine esters). Acylcarnitine is a condensation product formed from carboxylic acid and carnitine. It has a variety of metabolic roles and may be an indicator of inborn errors of metabolism, chronic disease, or acute and critical illness. Methods include enzymatic, chromatography, and mass-spectrometry. Qualitative analysis (82016) tests for the presence of acylcarnitine while quantitative analysis (82017) measures the amount of acylcarnitine.

82040

82040 Albumin; serum, plasma or whole blood

Explanation

This test measures the concentration of albumin in serum, plasma, or whole blood. It is often used to determine nutritional status, renal disease, and other chronic diseases, particularly those involving the kidneys or liver. A blood sample is typically drawn from a vein in the hand or forearm. The skin over the vein is cleaned with an antiseptic, and a tourniquet is wrapped around the upper arm to enlarge the lower arm veins by restricting the blood flow. A thin needle is inserted into the vein, the tourniquet is removed, and blood flows from the vein through the needle and is collected into a vial or syringe. The needle is withdrawn and the puncture site covered to prevent bleeding. The blood sample is sent to the laboratory for testing.

82042

82042 Albumin; urine or other source, quantitative, each specimen

Explanation

This code reports quantitative analysis for albumin on urine, CSF, or amniotic fluid. Urine tests are usually performed on a 24-hour urine specimen to measure protein loss of patients with hypoalbuminemia. Patients typically perform specimen collection over a 24-hour period. Method is colorimetry. CSF analysis requires separately reportable spinal puncture and the test is performed using nephelometry. Amniotic fluid analysis requires separately reportable ultrasound guidance and amniocentesis and test is usually performed by autoanalyzer.

82043-82044

82043 Albumin; urine, microalbumin, quantitative
82044   urine, microalbumin, semiquantitative (eg, reagent strip assay)

Explanation

"Microalbuminuria" is defined as albuminuria of 30 to 300 mg/24 hours and is requested to determine early increase of proteinuria, usually in diabetes and in pre-eclampsia before protein becomes evident by conventional urinalysis. Patients commonly perform specimen collection over a 24-hour period. Methods include radioimmunoassay (RIA) or enzyme-linked immunosorbent assay (ELISA). Report 82043 for quantitative microalbumin and 82044 for semi-quantitative or reagent strip microalbumin.

82088

82088 Aldosterone

Explanation

For serum aldosterone, blood is obtained by post-fasting venipuncture. Extreme care must be taken in preparing the patient before specimen collection and handling the specimen in order to obtain an accurate measurement. Blood specimens are usually taken early in the morning and a notation is made as to whether the patient was sitting or supine. A second test may be performed approximately four hours later. A radioimmunoassay (RIA) is typically employed for analysis of the specimen. This test is most commonly used in the diagnosis of specific types of adrenal adenomas, or secondary aldosteronism caused by cirrhosis, congestive heart failure, nephrosis, potassium loading, toxemia of pregnancy, and other states of contraction of plasma volume. Urine aldosterone requires a 24-hour non-fasting urine specimen. The patient flushes the first urine of the day. All voided urine for the next 24 hours is collected. Method is radioimmunoassay.

82105

82105 Alpha-fetoprotein (AFP); serum

Explanation

This test may be abbreviated as AFP. It may also be referred to as fetal alpha globulin. While this test is most often associated with pregnancy, it is also used to diagnose a variety of other conditions. During pregnancy, the test is normally performed between the 16th and 18th week of gestation. If levels are abnormal, it may be repeated approximately one week after the first test. Analysis is normally performed by radioimmunoassay (RIA).

82106

82106 Alpha-fetoprotein (AFP); amniotic fluid

Explanation

The test may be abbreviated as AFP. The test is normally performed on pregnant women initially between the 16th and 18th week of gestation. An amniotic AFP may be performed when serum AFP (82105) results are abnormal to confirm a diagnosis. An ultrasound is performed to determine the exact location of the fetus. AFP levels are measured, generally by radioimmunoassay (RIA).

82107

82107 Alpha-fetoprotein (AFP); AFP-L3 fraction isoform and total AFP (including ratio)

Explanation

This test may also be ordered as an AFP-L3. The test is a measure of the L3 form of alpha fetoprotein in a patient with chronic liver disease. The specimen is blood. Using a special fluorescent reagent, the L3 form of AFP is separated from other forms of alpha fetoprotein and tagged with a special fluorescent reagent. L3 is then measured as a percentage of total AFP. The calculations occur within an instrument developed for this test. The test is primarily used in the clinical evaluation of patient risk, as elevated levels of AFP-L3 in a patient with chronic liver disease are associated with hepatocellular carcinoma.

82143

82143 Amniotic fluid scan (spectrophotometric)

Explanation

This prenatal procedure may be requested as an amniotic fluid spectral analysis, Lily test, and amniotic fluid OD 450 spectral analysis. Amniotic fluid is collected by amniocentesis and the specimen is protected from exposure to light. A separately reported ultrasound is performed to determine the exact location of the fetus prior to the amniocentesis. Method of testing is spectrophotometry. This test measures the amount of free bilirubin in the amniotic fluid.

82150

82150 Amylase

Explanation

Serum amylase is elevated in acute pancreatitis and is, therefore, a common test when abdominal pain, epigastric tenderness, nausea, and vomiting are present. There are multiple methods of testing for amylase.

82154

82154 Androstanediol glucuronide

Explanation

This test may be requested as 3-Alpha-diol G. Androstanediol glucuronide is an androgen formed in the peripheral tissues. Elevated levels are frequently seen in females with hirsutism (excessive body hair). When androstanediol glucuronide is elevated, treatment of hirsutism is directed at the peripheral tissue sites rather than at other sites that are sometimes responsible for overproduction of androgens (adrenal cortex, ovary). Method is radioimmunoassay (RIA).

82157

82157 Androstenedione

Explanation

An androgenic steroid secreted by the testes, adrenal cortex, and ovaries. This test is used primarily to evaluate androgen production in females with hirsutism. Blood is obtained by venipuncture. Method is radioimmunoassay (RIA).

82160

82160 Androsterone

Explanation

Androsterone is a steroid hormone metabolite in the androgen series that is measured for evaluation of syndromes of androgen excess such as hirsutism and polycystic ovary syndrome. It has been measured typically by methods involving extraction and chromatography, followed by detection and quantification by colorimetric or immunometric techniques. Measurement of this compound has largely been replaced by determination of other specific plasma androgens (e.g., testosterone) by modern, sensitive assays.

82180

82180 Ascorbic acid (Vitamin C), blood

Explanation

This test is used to evaluate vitamin C deficiency. It may be performed with or without vitamin C saturation. When performed as a saturation test, megadoses of vitamin C are given over a three-to-four day period. The amount of vitamin C is measured (quantified).

82190

82190 Atomic absorption spectroscopy, each analyte

Explanation

AAS is a method for detecting the absorption of specific wavelengths of light by analyte that have been vaporized in a flame. The analysis is performed using a specialized instrument known as an atomic absorption spectrometer. Analytes are typically pure elements, since each element has a specific absorption spectrum.

82247-82248

82247 Bilirubin; total
82248   direct

Explanation

Bilirubin is a bile pigment formed by the breakdown of hemoglobin during both normal and abnormal erythrocyte destruction. Direct (conjugated) bilirubin is that portion of the bilirubin that has been taken up by the liver cells to form bilirubin diglucuronide. Indirect (unconjugated) bilirubin is that portion of the bilirubin that has not been taken up by the liver cells. Total bilirubin is the sum of direct and indirect bilirubin present in the specimen. Method is diazotization. Spectrophotometry may be used in neonates six weeks or younger. Report 82247 for total bilirubin. Report 82248 for direct bilirubin.

82306

82306 Vitamin D; 25 hydroxy, includes fraction(s), if performed

Explanation

This test may be requested as 25-OHD3, 25(OH) Calciferol, Vitamin D 25-Hydroxy, Vitamin D3 25-OH, or Calciferol 25-Hydroxy. Specimen is serum or plasma and method is high performance liquid chromatography (HPLC), competitive protein binding (CPB), or radioimmunoassay (RIA). This code includes fractions, if performed.

(82652)

82652 Vitamin D; 1, 25 dihydroxy, includes fraction(s), if performed

Explanation

This test may be requested as 1,25 (OH) Vitamin D, 1,25-Dihydroxy Vitamin D, 1,25-Dihydroxycholecalciferal, and Vitamin D, 1,25-Dihydroxy. This is the most active form of Vitamin D. It is formed by the renal cells and is essential for calcium absorption. Specimen is serum or plasma, and method is radioimmunoassay (RIA) or column chromatography. This code includes fractions, if performed.

Coding Tips

Code 82652 is a resequenced code and will not display in numeric order.

82308

82308 Calcitonin

Explanation

This test may be requested as thyrocalcitonin. This test may be used to screen for specific malignant neoplasms. A fasting blood specimen should be taken. The specimen is collected in a chilled tube and the test performed within 10 minutes of collection. Serum (plasma) is separated in a refrigerated centrifuge and frozen. The test is performed by assay or radioimmunoassay (RIA).

82310

82310 Calcium; total

Explanation

This test may be abbreviated Ca. Blood is obtained by venipuncture or heel stick. Specimen is obtained in the morning and a fasting sample is preferable. Postural changes and venous stasis may provide misleading results. Accurate diagnosis may require obtaining additional specimens on subsequent days. Method is spectrophotometry or atomic absorption spectroscopy (AAS). The test may be used to assess thyroid and parathyroid function.

82330

82330 Calcium; ionized

Explanation

This test may also be referred to as free calcium. It may be abbreviated iCa, Ca++ or Ca+2. Ionized or free calcium refers to calcium that is not bound to proteins in the blood. It is the metabolically active portion of the calcium in the blood. Blood is obtained by venipuncture and collected anaerobically. Method is by ion-selective electrode (ISE). The test may be used to assess thyroid and parathyroid function.

82331

82331 Calcium; after calcium infusion test

Explanation

The calcium infusion test is a provocative test for evaluation of medullary thyroid carcinoma (MTC). Calcitonin levels are measured following an IV infusion of calcium solution, and sometimes calcium levels are also measured to evaluate calcium incorporation or monitor hypercalcemia.

82340

82340 Calcium; urine quantitative, timed specimen

Explanation

This test may be abbreviated Ca urine, Ca++ or Ca+2. A 24-hour urine specimen is generally required. The patient flushes the first urine of the day and discards it. All voided urine for the next 24 hours is collected and refrigerated. Method is spectrophotometry or atomic absorption spectrometry (AAS).

82374

82374 Carbon dioxide (bicarbonate)

Explanation

This test may be requested as CO2, HCO3, or bicarbonate. Bicarbonate (carbon dioxide) is an indicator of electrolyte and acid-base status (alkalosis, acidosis). It is elevated in metabolic alkalosis, compensated respiratory acidosis, and hypokalemia. It is decreased in metabolic acidosis, compensated respiratory alkalosis, and in diabetic ketoacidosis. Blood specimen is normally obtained by arterial puncture, but venipuncture may also be used. Bicarbonate is usually calculated using the Henderson-Hasselbalch equation (HCO3 = Total CO2 – H2CO3). However, it can also be determined by titration.

82378

82378 Carcinoembryonic antigen (CEA)

Explanation

This test may be abbreviated as CEA. While CEA occurs normally in the gastrointestinal tract, it may be elevated for certain benign and malignant neoplasms and other diseases. CEA is used primarily to monitor patients with colorectal cancer and to a lesser extent advanced breast cancer. Method is immunofluorescence, enzyme immunoassay (EIA), and radioimmunoassay (RIA).

82380

82380 Carotene

Explanation

This test may also be requested as beta-carotene. Carotene is an isomeric pigment found in a number of vegetables and fruits. In the liver, carotene is converted to Vitamin A, which, in turn, is converted to retinal, the major molecule that enables vision. Method is high performance liquid chromatography (HPLC), colorimetry.

82387

82387 Cathepsin-D

Explanation

Cathepsin D is an indicator of metastatic breast cancer. Neoplastic tissue must be dissected free of fat and normal breast tissue, sliced into small pieces, placed in a tube, and quick frozen in liquid nitrogen. The tissue is analyzed by means of enzymatic immunoassay (EIA) or immunoradiometric assay (IRMA).

82397

82397 Chemiluminescent assay

Explanation

Chemiluminescent assay refers to a detection method, whereby a chemiluminogenic substrate is converted to a chemiluminescent (light emitting) product.

82415

82415 Chloramphenicol

Explanation

This test may be requested as a chloramphenicol, Chloromycetin, or Mychel-S level. Chloramphenicol is a broad spectrum antibiotic. This test is used to monitor therapeutic and toxic levels. Several methods may be used, including high performance liquid chromatography (HPLC), gas-liquid chromatography (GLC), microbiological assay (MB), colorimetry, or enzymatic immunoassay (EIA).

82435

82435 Chloride; blood

Explanation

This test may be requested as Cl, blood. Chloride is a salt of hydrochloric acid and is important in maintaining electrolyte balance. Methods include colorimetry, coulometry, and ion-selective electrode (ISE).

82436

82436 Chloride; urine

Explanation

This test may be requested as Cl, urine. Chloride is important in maintaining proper electrolyte balance. A 24-hour urine test is preferred, but shorter timed collections and random specimens may also be used. If a timed specimen is used, the patient flushes the first urine of the day and discards it. All voided urine for the next 24 hours (or shorter time increment) is collected and refrigerated. Methods include colorimetry, coulometry, and ion-selective electrode (ISE).

82465

82465 Cholesterol, serum or whole blood, total

Explanation

Cholesterol level is a risk indicator for atherosclerosis and myocardial infarction. Blood specimen is obtained by venipuncture. Method is enzymatic. This test reports total cholesterol in serum or whole blood.

82486

82486 Chromatography, qualitative; column (eg, gas liquid or HPLC), analyte not elsewhere specified

Explanation

This code reports a specific chromatography technique for analyzing substances that are not specifically listed elsewhere in the chemistry section. Chromatography, itself, uses a number of different techniques to separate and analyze the specimen components. Code 82486 reports column chromatography, which uses a sorbent packed in a column. The specimen is dissolved in a solvent and poured into the column. Some of the specimen components bind to the sorbent and are retained in the column, while others escape. Subsequent washings with the same or different solvents cause more strongly bound components to escape. These components can then be individually analyzed. This code tests for the presence (qualitative analysis) of a single analyte.

82487-82488

82487 Chromatography, qualitative; paper, 1-dimensional, analyte not elsewhere specified

82488 paper, 2-dimensional, analyte not elsewhere specified

Explanation

These codes report specific chromatography techniques for analyzing substances that are not specifically listed elsewhere in the chemistry section. Chromatography uses a number of different techniques to separate and analyze the specimen components. Codes 82487 and 82488 report paper chromatography, which uses a special-grade filter paper in the stationary phase. The specimen is applied to the paper and the end of the paper is placed in a solvent. The solvent rises along the paper, carrying and depositing the different components of the specimen along the filter paper. The different components can be separately visualized and analyzed. These codes test for the presence (qualitative analysis) of a single analyte. Report 82487 for 1-dimensional and 82488 for 2-dimensional.

82489

82489 Chromatography, qualitative; thin layer, analyte not elsewhere specified

Explanation

This code reports a specific chromatography technique for analyzing substances that are not specifically listed elsewhere in the chemistry section. Chromatography uses a number of different techniques to separate and analyze the specimen components. Code 82489 reports thin-layer chromatography, which uses a thin layer adsorbent applied to a rectangular plate in the stationary phase. The specimen is applied to the plate and the end of the plate is placed in a solvent. As the solvent rises along the adsorbent on the plate, the different components of the specimen are carried along at varying rates and deposited along the plate. The different components can then be separately visualized and analyzed. This code tests for the presence (qualitative analysis) of a single analyte.

82491-82492

82491 Chromatography, quantitative, column (eg, gas liquid or HPLC); single analyte not elsewhere specified, single stationary and mobile phase

82492 multiple analytes, single stationary and mobile phase

Explanation

These codes report specific chromatography techniques for analyzing substances that are not specifically listed elsewhere in the chemistry section. Chromatography uses a number of different

techniques to separate and analyze the specimen components. Codes 82491-82492 report column chromatography, which uses a sorbent packed in a column. The specimen is dissolved in a solvent and poured into the column. Some of the specimen components bind to the sorbent and are retained in the column, while others escape. Subsequent washings with the same or different solvents cause more strongly bound components to escape. These components can be individually analyzed. Code 82491 measures (quantifies) the amount of a single analyte, while 82492 measures (quantifies) the amount of multiple analytes.

82495

82495 Chromium

Explanation

Chromium is an essential nutrient that is toxic in large doses. The test monitors for environmental or occupational chromium toxicity that is associated with skin respiratory and other diseases such as lung cancer. Blood, urine or hair may be tested. Methods used include atomic absorption spectrometry (AAS) and neutron activation analysis (NAA).

82530

82530 Cortisol; free

Explanation

Cortisol is a naturally occurring glucocorticoid responsible for metabolism of glucose, protein, and fats and is important in immune system function. Urinary free cortisol is used in initial screening for Cushing's syndrome. Amniotic fluid levels of free cortisol are useful in evaluating fetal lung maturation. To obtain an amniotic fluid specimen, an ultrasound is performed to determine the exact location of the fetus. Methods include high performance liquid chromatography (HPLC) for urine and radioimmunoassay (RIA) for amniotic fluid. This test measures free (unbound) cortisol only.

82533

82533 Cortisol; total

Explanation

Cortisol is a naturally occurring glucocorticoid responsible for metabolism of glucose, protein, and fats and is important in immune system function. To obtain an amniotic fluid specimen, an ultrasound is performed to determine the exact location of the fetus. The fluid is sent to the lab for analysis. Method is radioimmunoassay (RIA), competitive protein binding (CPB), or fluorescent assay. This test measures total cortisol (both free and bound) in various specimen types.

82541-82542

82541 Column chromatography/mass spectrometry (eg, GC/MS, or HPLC/MS), analyte not elsewhere specified; qualitative, single stationary and mobile phase

82542 quantitative, single stationary and mobile phase

Explanation

These codes report specific chromatography techniques combined with mass spectrometry for analyzing substances that are not specifically listed elsewhere in the chemistry section. Chromatography uses different techniques to separate and analyze the specimen components. Codes 82541-82542 report column chromatography combined with mass spectrometry. Column chromatography uses a sorbent packed in a column. The specimen is dissolved in a solvent and poured into the column. Some of the specimen components bind to the sorbent and are retained in the column, while others escape. Subsequent washings with the same or different solvents cause more strongly bound components to escape. These components can be individually analyzed. Mass spectrometry represents one of the most powerful new tools available for studying complex substances. Mass spectrometry isolates specific substances by sorting a stream of electrified particles (ions) based on their mass. Code 82541 screens for the presence (qualitative analysis) of an analyte using a single stationary and mobile phase, while 82542 measures (quantifies) the amount of an analyte using a single stationary and mobile phase.

82543-82544

82543 Column chromatography/mass spectrometry (eg, GC/MS, or HPLC/MS), analyte not elsewhere specified; stable isotope dilution, single analyte, quantitative, single stationary and mobile phase

82544 stable isotope dilution, multiple analytes, quantitative, single stationary and mobile phase

Explanation

These codes report specific chromatography techniques combined with mass spectrometry for analyzing substances that are not specifically listed elsewhere in the chemistry section. Chromatography uses different techniques to separate and analyze the specimen components. Codes 82543-82544 report column chromatography combined with mass spectrometry. Column chromatography uses a sorbent packed in a column. The specimen is dissolved in a solvent and poured into the column. Some of the specimen components bind to the sorbent and are retained in the column, while others escape. Subsequent washings with the same or different solvents cause more strongly bound components to escape. These components can be

individually analyzed. Mass spectrometry represents one of the most powerful new tools available for studying complex substances. Mass spectrometry isolates specific substances by sorting a stream of electrified particles (ions) based on their mass. These two tests are also performed with a stable isotope dilution. Code 82543 measures (quantifies) a single analyte using a single stationary and mobile phase, while 82544 measures (quantifies) the amount of multiple analytes using a single stationary and mobile phase.

82565

82565 Creatinine; blood

Explanation

Serum creatinine is the most common laboratory test for evaluating renal function. Method is enzymatic or colorimetry.

82570

82570 Creatinine; other source

Explanation

Urine creatinine levels are not normally used to evaluate disease processes except as part of a creatinine clearance test, but they are a good indicator of the adequacy of timed urine specimens. Amniotic fluid creatinine is used to evaluate fetal maturity. For amniotic fluid specimen, a separately reportable amniocentesis is performed. Method is enzymatic, Jaffe reaction, or manual.

82575

82575 Creatinine; clearance

Explanation

This test may be requested as urea clearance or urea nitrogen clearance. Both blood and urine specimens are required. Blood specimen is obtained by venipuncture. A 24-hour urine specimen is preferred, but timed shorter increments may also be acceptable. Method is enzymatic or Jaffe reaction, or alkaline picrate. Creatinine clearance is a calculation of urine and serum creatinine content adjusted by urine volume and body size. The test is a general indicator of glomerular filtration function of the kidneys.

82610

82610 Cystatin C

Explanation

Code 82610 reports the quantitative determination of Cystatin C, which is used to diagnose impaired kidney function. Serum Cystatin C is a useful indicator of glomerular filtration rate (GFR), particularly in elderly, very obese, and malnourished patients whose serum creatinine can be misleading. It is also used in renal function assessment in patients suspected of having renal disease, and for monitoring the response to treatment in those with

kidney disease. The method of testing varies by laboratory.

82626

82626 Dehydroepiandrosterone (DHEA)

Explanation

This test may be requested as unconjugated DHEA. Serum DHEA levels may be used to evaluate delayed puberty and hirsutism. Elevations may be indicative of ovarian disorders, neoplasm of the adrenal gland, Cushing's disease, or ectopic ACTH-producing neoplasm. Decreased levels in amniotic fluid may be indicative of congenital adrenal hypoplasia. For amniotic fluid specimen, a separately reportable amniocentesis is performed. Method is radioimmunoassay (RIA) or gas-liquid chromatography (GLC).

82627

82627 Dehydroepiandrosterone-sulfate (DHEA-S)

Explanation

This test may be requested as DHEA-S or DHEAS. Serum DHEA-S levels may be used to evaluate hirsutism. Elevations may be indicative of ovarian or adrenal disorders, neoplasm of the adrenal cortex, Cushing's disease, or ectopic ACTH-producing neoplasm. Decreased levels in amniotic fluid may be indicative of anencephaly. Blood specimen is obtained by venipuncture. For amniotic fluid specimen, an amniocentesis is performed. Method is typically radioimmunoassay (RIA).

82633

82633 Desoxycorticosterone, 11-

Explanation

This test may be requested as DOC. Deoxycorticosterone is a hormone produced in small quantities by the adrenal cortex. A normal circadian rise and fall in levels is noted. Method is radioimmunoassay (RIA). The test may be ordered during pregnancy for a variety of reasons, including preeclampsia.

82657-82658

82657 Enzyme activity in blood cells, cultured cells, or tissue, not elsewhere specified; nonradioactive substrate, each specimen

82658 radioactive substrate, each specimen

Explanation

These codes report enzyme assays using a variety of different methods, some established and some relatively new. Code 82657 reports enzyme assay with nonradioactive substrate (substance upon which an enzyme acts), while 82658 reports enzyme assay with radioactive substrate.

82664

82664 Electrophoretic technique, not elsewhere specified

Explanation

This code reports various electrophoretic techniques. Electrophoresis is a test method that uses an electrical field to move particles toward electrical poles. It separates ionic substances based on differences in their rates of migration toward the poles. Some types of electrophoresis include disc, gel, isoenzyme, and thin layer.

82666

82666 Epiandrosterone

Explanation

Epiandrosterone is a steroid hormone metabolite in the androgen series that is measured for evaluation of syndromes of androgen excess such as hirsutism and polycystic ovary syndrome. It has been measured typically by methods involving extraction and chromatography, followed by detection and quantification by colorimetric or immunometric techniques. Measurement of this compound has largely been replaced by determination of other specific plasma androgens (e.g., testosterone) by modern, sensitive assays.

82670

82670 Estradiol

Explanation

This test may be requested as unconjugated estradiol (E2). Estradiol is derived from ovaries, testes, and the placenta and is the most active endogenous estrogen. Method is radioimmunoassay (RIA).

82671

82671 Estrogens; fractionated

Explanation

This test may be requested as fractionated estrogens. Estrogens are the female sex hormones and include estradiol, estrone, and estriol. Blood specimen is obtained by venipuncture. Method is radioimmunoassay. Fractionation involves separating total estrogen into its components.

82672

82672 Estrogens; total

Explanation

This test may be requested as total estrogen, serum or urine. Because the serum assay does not measure estriol levels, urine assay is perhaps more commonly ordered. Estrogens are the female sex hormones and include estradiol, estrone, and estriol. Method is spectroscopy or fluorometry.

82677

82677 Estriol

Explanation

This test may be requested as estriol (E3). Estriol is a relatively weak estrogen, present in high concentrations during pregnancy. Low levels may be indicative of maternal complications (e.g., diabetes, preeclampsia), fetal growth retardation, or fetal anomaly (e.g., anencephaly). For amniotic fluid specimen, a separately reportable amniocentesis is performed. Method is radioimmunoassay (RIA) for serum or urine and gas-liquid chromatography (GLC) for amniotic fluid.

82679

82679 Estrone

Explanation

This test may be requested as estrone (E1). Estrone is a moderately potent estrogen, derived primarily from oxidation of estradiol, but also secreted by the ovaries. For amniotic fluid specimen, a separately reportable amniocentesis is performed. Method is radioimmunoassay (RIA) for serum or urine and gas-liquid chromatography-mass spectrometry (GLC-MC) for amniotic fluid.

82696

82696 Etiocholanolone

Explanation

Etiocholanolone is a steroid hormone metabolite in the androgen series that is measured for evaluation of syndromes of androgen excess such as hirsutism and polycystic ovary syndrome. It has been measured typically by methods involving extraction and chromatography, followed by detection and quantification by colorimetric or immunometric techniques. Measurement of this compound has largely been replaced by determination of other specific plasma androgens (e.g., testosterone) by modern, sensitive assays.

82728

82728 Ferritin

Explanation

Serum ferritin level measures available iron stores and is a reliable indicator of normal, as well as deficient, levels. Blood specimen is obtained by venipuncture. Method is radioimmunoassay (RIA), immunoradiometric assay (IRMA), enzyme immunoassay (EIA), or enzyme linked immunosorbent assay (ELISA).

82731

82731 Fetal fibronectin, cervicovaginal secretions, semi-quantitative

Explanation

Fibronectin is an adhesive glycoprotein. The presence of fetal fibronectin in cervicovaginal secretions is an indicator that a pregnant woman will soon go into labor, and it is tested for the purpose of predicting premature labor. Rapid enzyme-linked immunosorbent assay (ELISA) tests are available to perform the assay on cervical swab specimens. The test is a semi-quantitative (positive or negative) test.

82746

82746 Folic acid; serum

Explanation

This test may be requested as serum folate. This test is used to detect folic acid deficiency. Folic acid is a B vitamin necessary for normal red blood cell production. It is stored in the body as folates. Folic acid deficiency results in a form of megaloblastic anemia. Blood specimen is obtained by venipuncture. Method is competitive binding protein (CPB) radioimmunoassay, chemiluminescence, or microbiological assay.

82747

82747 Folic acid; RBC

Explanation

This test may be requested as RBC folate or red cell folate. It is used to detect folic acid deficiency. Folic acid is a B vitamin necessary for normal red blood cell production. It is stored in the body as folates. Folic acid deficiency results in a form of megaloblastic anemia. Method is radioimmunoassay (RIA), competitive binding protein (CPB) radioimmunoassay, or chemiluminescence.

82784

82784 Gammaglobulin (immunoglobulin); IgA, IgD, IgG, IgM, each

Explanation

This test may be requested as immunoglobulin, IgA, IgD, IgG, or IgM. Immunoglobulins are in the group of proteins classified as antibodies. Immunoglobulins are produced in response to foreign proteins referred to antigens. IgG is the most abundant immunoglobulin. It is produced in response to secondary exposure to viral and bacterial antigens. IgA is found primarily in the respiratory, gastrointestinal, and genitourinary tracts, as well as in tears and saliva. It is responsible for protecting the mucous membranes from viral and bacterial antigens. Congenital IgA deficiency is also associated with autoimmune disease. IgM is produced following primary exposure to an antigen and is active against rheumatoid factors, gram-negative organisms, and the ABO blood group. IgD properties are not well understood but increases with chronic infection, connective tissue disorders, and some liver disease. Serum immunoglobulins may be tested for the four types (IgA, IgD, IgG, and

right
Appendix

IgM) reported with this code. Saliva may be tested for IgA. CSF may be tested for IgA, IgD, IgG, and IgM. CSF is obtained by spinal puncture, which is reported separately. Method is dependent on specimen source and specific immunoglobulins being tested. Serum is usually analyzed using radial immunodiffusion (RID), enzyme linked immunosorbent assay (ELISA), nephelometry, or turbidimetry. Urine uses electroimmunodiffusion (EID). Saliva uses radial immunodiffusion (RID). CSF is analyzed with radioimmunoassay (RIA).

82785

82785 Gammaglobulin (immunoglobulin); IgE

Explanation

This test may be requested as immunoglobulin, IgE. Immunoglobulins are in the group of proteins classified as antibodies. Immunoglobulins are produced in response to foreign proteins referred to as antigens. IgE is produced in response to allergic reactions and anaphylaxis. CSF is obtained by spinal puncture, which is reported separately. Method is radioimmunoassay (RIA). Paper radioimmunosorbent test may also be used for serum specimen only.

82787

82787 Gammaglobulin (immunoglobulin); immunoglobulin subclasses (eg, IgG1, 2, 3, or 4), each

Explanation

This test may be requested as immunoglobulin subclasses or IgG subclasses. There are four IgG subclasses, which are designated as IgG1, IgG2, IgG3, and IgG4. IgG is part of the body's defense system against infection. Deficiencies of single subclasses, particularly IgG1, can significantly impair this defense. Blood specimen is obtained by venipuncture. Method is radial immunodiffusion (RID), enzyme linked immunosorbent assay (ELISA), nephelometry, or turbidimetry.

82800

82800 Gases, blood, pH only

Explanation

This test may be requested as blood pH. Blood pH is tested to identify acidemia or alkalemia. Arterial puncture is preferred, but venipuncture may also be performed. Method is glass pH electrode or potentiometry.

82803-82805

82803 Gases, blood, any combination of pH, pCO2, pO2, CO2, HCO3 (including calculated O2 saturation);

82805 with O2 saturation, by direct measurement, except pulse oximetry

Explanation

These tests may be requested as arterial blood gases (ABGs). Blood gases are usually requested to evaluate disturbances of acid-base balance, which may be caused by respiratory or metabolic disorders. Blood specimen is obtained by arterial puncture. Code 82803 reports any combination of pH, pCO2, pO2, CO2, and HCO3, including calculated O2 saturation. Code 82805 reports any combination of the same gases, but O2 saturation is performed by direct measurement. Method is selective electrode, potentiometry, or spectrophotometry (O2 saturation).

82810

82810 Gases, blood, O2 saturation only, by direct measurement, except pulse oximetry

Explanation

This test may be requested as O2. Oxygen saturation is the percent of the oxygen in the blood that combines with hemoglobin. Blood specimen is obtained by arterial puncture. Method is spectrophotometry.

82820

82820 Hemoglobin-oxygen affinity (pO2 for 50% hemoglobin saturation with oxygen)

Explanation

This test may be requested as oxygen, P50 or as pO2, P50. This test is performed to measure the affinity of hemoglobin for oxygen, which allows evaluation of oxygen delivery to body tissues. Blood specimen is obtained by arterial puncture. Method is spectrophotometry or potentiometry.

82943

82943 Glucagon

Explanation

Glucagon is a hormone secreted by the pancreas. It stimulates the conversion of glycogen stored in the liver to glucose. Glucagon levels may be requested to evaluate suspected diabetes mellitus or glucagonoma. Method is radioimmunoassay (RIA).

82945

82945 Glucose, body fluid, other than blood

Explanation

Glucose is the end product of carbohydrate metabolism, providing energy for living organisms. It is found in body fluids including joint fluid and CSF. Both elevated and decreased levels of glucose may be indicative of disease processes. Joint fluid specimen is obtained by separately reportable arthrocentesis. CSF specimen is obtained by separately reportable spinal puncture. Method is enzymatic.

82946

82946 Glucagon tolerance test

Explanation

Glucagon is a hormone secreted by the pancreas. It stimulates the conversion of glycogen stored in the liver to glucose. Glucagon tolerance test may be requested to evaluate suspected diabetes mellitus or glucagonoma. A fasting glucagon level is obtained. A high carbohydrate meal or an oral dose of glucose is given. Glucagon levels are tested at 30, 60, and 120-minute intervals. Method is radioimmunoassay (RIA).

82947

82947 Glucose; quantitative, blood (except reagent strip)

Explanation

This test may be requested as a fasting blood sugar (FBS). This quantitative test is used to evaluate disorders of carbohydrate metabolism. The patient has ordinarily fasted for eight hours. Method is enzymatic.

82948

82948 Glucose; blood, reagent strip

Explanation

This test is used to monitor disorders of carbohydrate metabolism. Blood specimen is obtained by finger stick. A drop of blood is placed on the reagent strip for a specified amount of time. When the prescribed amount of time has elapsed, the strip is blotted and the reagent strip is compared to a color chart. Method is reagent strip with visual comparison.

82950

82950 Glucose; post glucose dose (includes glucose)

Explanation

This test may also be requested as glucose, postprandial (PP). This test is used to monitor disorders of carbohydrate metabolism. The patient consumes a high carbohydrate meal or an oral glucose solution. Blood glucose levels are checked two hours after the meal or glucose solution. A one-hour postprandial screen may be used to evaluate pregnant women for gestational diabetes mellitus. Method of testing varies.

82951-82952

82951 Glucose; tolerance test (GTT), 3 specimens (includes glucose)

82952 tolerance test, each additional beyond 3 specimens (List separately in addition to code for primary procedure)

Appendix

Explanation

This test may be requested as GTT, oral GTT, OGTT, intravenous GTT, or IVGTT. This test monitors disorders of carbohydrate metabolism. This test is normally performed using an oral dose of glucose, but may also be performed using intravenous glucose. A blood specimen is obtained prior to glucose administration and at intervals following glucose administration. Report 82951 for up to three specimens and 82952 for each additional specimen. Testing method varies.

82953

82953 Glucose; tolbutamide tolerance test

Explanation

This test may be requested as a tolbutamide tolerance test. It is used to evaluate pancreatic tumor and functional hypoglycemia. Baseline glucose and insulin levels are obtained. Tolbutamide is administered intravenously. Glucose and insulin levels are obtained at 3, 30, 60, 90, 120, and 180 minutes following the tolbutamide administration.

82955-82960

82955 Glucose-6-phosphate dehydrogenase (G6PD); quantitative
82960　　　screen

Explanation

These tests may be requested as G6PD quantitative or G6PD screen. This test is used to identify genetic G6PD deficiency, which causes hemolytic anemia after ingestion of certain drugs and foods and may also cause hemolytic disease of the newborn (HDN). Blood specimen is obtained by venipuncture. Method is methemoglobin reduction (Brewer's test), modified Bishop (ultraviolet), dye reduction, or ascorbic or fluorescent spot tests. Code 82955 is used to report measurement of amount (quantitation) of G6PD in erythrocytes, while 82960 reports screening (qualitative analysis) for the presence of G6PD only.

82962

82962 Glucose, blood by glucose monitoring device(s) cleared by the FDA specifically for home use

Explanation

This test is used to monitor disorders of carbohydrate metabolism. This test reports blood glucose monitoring by an FDA-approved device. While the code states that it is for home use, these devices may also be used in the physician office. Blood is obtained by finger stick. Method is enzymatic, electrochemical, or spectrophotometry by small portable device designed for home glucose testing.

83001

83001 Gonadotropin; follicle stimulating hormone (FSH)

Explanation

This test may be requested as FSH or follitropin. FSH is a gonadotropic hormone produced by the pituitary gland. It stimulates growth and maturation of the ovarian follicle in females and promotes spermatogenesis in males. This test may be requested in an infertility work-up. Method is immunoassay.

83002

83002 Gonadotropin; luteinizing hormone (LH)

Explanation

This test may be requested as LH, lutropin, or interstitial cell-stimulating hormone (ICSH). LH is a gonadotropic hormone secreted by the pituitary gland. LH required for ovulation in females and stimulates testosterone production in males. LH may be ordered as part of an infertility work-up. Method is immunoassay.

83003

83003 Growth hormone, human (HGH) (somatotropin)

Explanation

This test may be requested as GH, HGH, or somatotropin. This test may be used to evaluate pituitary gigantism or dwarfism, acromegaly, hypopituitarism, adrenocortical hyperfunction, fetal anencephaly (amniotic fluid analysis), as well as other conditions. Amniotic fluid sample is obtained by amniocentesis, which is reported separately. Method is radioimmunoassay.

83010

83010 Haptoglobin; quantitative

Explanation

This test may be requested as Hp, HPT, or hemoglobin-binding protein. Method is turbidimetry or nephelometry. This procedure measures (quantifies) the amount of haptoglobin present in serum. Haptoglobin is a plasma glycoprotein. Haptoglobin prevents loss of free hemoglobin in the urine by binding with it and removing it to the liver. This test may be indicated to evaluate anemia or other indicators of hemolysis, pregnancy induced hypertension, transfusion reactions, as well as other conditions.

83020

83020 Hemoglobin fractionation and quantitation; electrophoresis (eg, A2, S, C, and/or F)

Explanation

This test may be requested as Hb electrophoresis. This test uses electrophoresis to test for several hemoglobin variants. It is used to identify the different types of hemoglobin present in the blood and measure (quantify) the amounts of each. The normal types of hemoglobin are Hb A1, Hb A2, and Hb F (fetal). When Hb F exceeds five percent of total hemoglobin after age 6 months, it may be an indicator of thalassemia. Increased amounts of Hb A2 may also indicate thalassemia. Abnormal variants, which can be identified by electrophoresis, include Hb S and Hb C. Hb S is the most common hemoglobin variant and is indicative of sickle cell anemia. Hb C is indicative of hemolytic anemia.

83021

83021 Hemoglobin fractionation and quantitation; chromatography (eg, A2, S, C, and/or F)

Explanation

This test may be requested as Hb chromatography. This test uses chromatography to test for several hemoglobin variants. It is used to identify the different types of hemoglobin present in the blood and measure (quantify) the amounts of each. The normal types of hemoglobin are Hb A1, Hb A2, and Hb F (fetal). When Hb F exceeds five percent of total hemoglobin after age 6 months, it may be an indicator of thalassemia. Increased amounts of Hb A2 may also indicate thalassemia. Abnormal variants, which can be identified by electrophoresis, include Hb S and Hb C. Hb S is the most common hemoglobin variant and is indicative of sickle cell anemia. Hb C is indicative of hemolytic anemia.

83026

83026 Hemoglobin; by copper sulfate method, non-automated

Explanation

The copper sulfate method for measuring hemoglobin is performed by placing a drop of blood into each of a series of containers containing copper sulfate solutions of varying specific gravity. If the drop sinks, the blood has greater specific gravity than the copper sulfate solution. The specific gravity of whole blood strongly correlates to the hemoglobin concentration, so the hemoglobin concentration may be accurately estimated. Specimen collection is by venipuncture.

83030

83030 Hemoglobin; F (fetal), chemical

Explanation

This is also known as Hb F. Hemoglobin F is the normal hemoglobin of the fetus. Most Hb F is replaced by hemoglobin A in the first days after birth. Hb F has an increased capacity to carry oxygen and is present in increased amounts in some pathologic conditions, including sickle cell anemia,

Appendix

aplastic anemia, and leukemia. Small amounts are produced throughout life.

83033

83033 Hemoglobin; F (fetal), qualitative

Explanation

Hemoglobin F (Hb F) is the normal hemoglobin of the term fetus. Most Hb F is replaced by hemoglobin A in the first days after birth. Elevated levels after age 6 months may be indicative of a blood disorder. Hb F has an increased capacity to carry oxygen and the test is also useful in determining whether bleeding disorders may have occurred preterm. Method for blood specimen is electrophoresis. Method for stool specimen may be by alkali denaturation visual screening. Hemoglobin F is alkali resistant. The procedure is used to examine fresh "red" blood taken from a fresh stool sample.

83036

83036 Hemoglobin; glycosylated (A1C)

Explanation

These tests may also be known as HbA1C. A blood specimen is collected. Glycosylated hemoglobin levels reflect the average level of glucose in the blood over a three-month period. Methods may include high-performance liquid chromatography and ion exchange chromatography (83036) or FDA approved home monitoring device (83037).

83497

83497 Hydroxyindolacetic acid, 5-(HIAA)

Explanation

This test may be performed to measure the levels of 5-HIAA for detecting and following the clinical course of patients with carcinoid tumors. Specimen collection is urine, collected over a 24-hour period. Method is high performance liquid chromatography. These tumors contain enteroendocrine cells that secrete stomach gastrin, a secretory hormone released upon nerve impulse. Neurohormones, such as gastrin, are metabolized by the liver and excreted in the urine. Rising levels of 5-HIAA may indicate a tumor is progressing; falling levels of 5-HIAA may indicate that a tumor is responding to antineoplastic therapy. This test measures (quantifies) the level of 5-HIAA present in the specimen.

83498

83498 Hydroxyprogesterone, 17-d

Explanation

This test may also be known as 17-OHP. Methodology may involve radioimmunoassay. This test is performed to diagnose and manage certain metabolic diseases. Insufficient amounts of hydroxyprogesterone can block the synthesis of cortisol, resulting in conditions such as adrenal hyperplasia, hirsutism (excessive body and facial hair, especially in women), and infertility.

83499

83499 Hydroxyprogesterone, 20-

Explanation

20-hydroxyprogesterone is a weakly active metabolite of progesterone with progestational activity. Levels have been measured in evaluation of ovulation, and gestagenic activity during the menstrual cycle and pregnancy. Typical methodology is column separation (chromatography) with radioimmunoassay detection.

83516-83518

83516 Immunoassay for analyte other than infectious agent antibody or infectious agent antigen; qualitative or semiquantitative, multiple step method

83518 qualitative or semiquantitative, single step method (eg, reagent strip)

Explanation

Immunoassay uses highly specific antigen to antibody binding to identify specific chemical substances. This code reports a number of immunoassay techniques for identifying analytes (chemical substances) that are not specifically identified elsewhere, excluding infectious agent antibody or infectious agent antigen. More specific methods reported with these codes include enzyme immunoassay (EIA) and fluoroimmunoassay (FIA). This test identifies (qualitative analysis) the substance or roughly measures (semi-quantitative analysis) the amount of the substance. Code 83516 reports multiple step method, while 83518 reports single step method.

83519

83519 Immunoassay for analyte other than infectious agent antibody or infectious agent antigen; quantitative, by radioimmunoassay (eg, RIA)

Explanation

Immunoassay uses highly specific antigen to antibody binding to identify specific chemical substances. This code reports measurement (quantitative analysis) using radioimmunoassay (RIA) technique for identifying analytes (chemical substances) that are not specifically identified elsewhere, excluding infectious agent antibody or infectious agent antigen.

83520

83520 Immunoassay for analyte other than infectious agent antibody or infectious agent antigen; quantitative, not otherwise specified

Explanation

Immunoassay uses highly specific antigen to antibody binding to identify specific chemical substances. This code reports measurement (quantitative analysis) using a technique other than radioimmunoassay (RIA) for identifying analytes (chemical substances) that are not specifically identified elsewhere, excluding infectious agent antibody or infectious agent antigen.

83540

83540 Iron

Explanation

This test may be requested as Fe. Iron is an essential constituent of hemoglobin, which is present in foods and absorbed through the small bowel (duodenum and jejunum). Method is colorimetry or atomic absorption spectrophotometry. This test is often used in combination with other tests to evaluate anemia, acute leukemia, lead poisoning, acute hepatitis, and vitamin B6 deficiency. It is also used to evaluate iron poisoning caused by accidental overdose (children) or excessive use of supplements.

83550

83550 Iron binding capacity

Explanation

This test may be abbreviated as TIBC. Iron is an essential constituent of hemoglobin, which is present in foods and absorbed through the small bowel (duodenum and jejunum). Method is colorimetry or atomic absorption spectrophotometry. TIBC measures the total amount of iron capable of binding to the protein transferrin. This test is often used in combination with other tests to evaluate anemia, various neoplasms, acute hepatitis and other liver disease, hemochromatosis, thalassemia, and renal disease.

83605

83605 Lactate (lactic acid)

Explanation

This test is used to assess lactic blood levels to document the presence of tissue hypoxia, determine the degree of hypoxia, and monitor the effect of therapy in blood, plasma, or cerebrospinal fluid (CSF). Specimen collection is either CSF from a spinal puncture or arterial or venous blood. Hand clenching and the use of a tourniquet should be avoided to prevent the build-up of potassium and lactic acid. Method is enzymatic or gas chromatography (GS). This test may be used to determine lactic acidosis when unaccountable anion gap metabolic acidosis is detected.

83615

83615 Lactate dehydrogenase (LD), (LDH);

Explanation

This test may also be ordered as LD or LDH. The test is a measure of LD or LDH, which is found in many body tissues, particularly the heart, liver, red blood cells, and kidneys. Methods used are lactate to pyruvate or pyruvate to lactate. This test may be ordered for a wide variety of disorders, including renal diseases and congestive heart failure.

83625

83625 Lactate dehydrogenase (LD), (LDH); isoenzymes, separation and quantitation

Explanation

This test may be ordered as LDH isoenzymes or LD isoenzymes. Three serial blood specimens are collected at 6-8 hour intervals to detect changes in the LD isoenzymes. Shifts in the values of five clinically significant LD fractions monitored over time create diagnostic patterns that correlate with diseases such as myocardial infarction, renal infarction and hepatic congestion. This allows for the differential diagnosis of numerous conditions. Method is by electrophoresis or immunochemical methods, including immunoprecipitation. This test may be ordered for a wide variety of reasons, and results may point to numerous diagnoses.

83632

83632 Lactogen, human placental (HPL) human chorionic somatomammotropin

Explanation

This test may be called maternal serum hPL. Specimen collection is obtained by venipuncture. Method used is radioimmunoassay (RIA) or turbidimetric latex immunoassay. This test may be used to evaluate antepartum placental function and fetal health. It is also used as an indicator of intrauterine growth retardation in twin pregnancy, evaluation of placental function, and may be used to assess gestational age. Other uses are in detecting non-germ cell neoplasms.

83655

83655 Lead

Explanation

This test may be ordered using Pb, the chemical abbreviation for lead. A whole blood test may be used to identify more recent lead exposures; the urine test is used to determine lead body burden, rather than to diagnose lead poisoning. In some instances, serum, hair samples, or bronchoalveolar lavage fluids may be tested. Specimen collection for urine is usually a 24-hour collection. Method used is source dependent, but commonly electrothermal atomic absorption spectrometry (AAS). Bronchoalveolar lavage specimens may be tested by x-ray fluorescence spectrometry.

83661

83661 Fetal lung maturity assessment; lecithin sphingomyelin (L/S) ratio

Explanation

Specimen collection is by amniocentesis, but amniotic fluid may be collected vaginally after rupture of the amniotic membrane. This test determines fetal pulmonary maturation and may be an indicator for the possibility of development of respiratory distress syndrome (RDS). Method used is thin-layer chromatography (TLC) and a 1D or 2D approach may be specified.

83662

83662 Fetal lung maturity assessment; foam stability test

Explanation

This test may also be ordered as pulmonary surfactant or the "shake test." Specimen collection is by amniocentesis. Method involves diluting amniotic fluid with ethanol and shaking the specimen. This test indicates fetal pulmonary maturation and newborn risk for respiratory distress syndrome. The test may also be useful in managing other conditions in both mother and fetus during late stages of pregnancy.

83663

83663 Fetal lung maturity assessment; fluorescence polarization

Explanation

Specimen collection is by amniocentesis. The amniotic fluid is analyzed by fluorescent polarization (FPOL). A fluorescent phospholipid analogue is added to amniotic fluid and its fluorescence polarization is measured using a fluorescence polarimeter. The presence of increased amounts of surfactant indicating increased lung maturity result in lower polarization levels. Therefore, polarization values decrease during gestation in conjunction with maturation of the pulmonary surfactant system. This test indicates fetal pulmonary maturation and newborn risk for respiratory distress syndrome.

83664

83664 Fetal lung maturity assessment; lamellar body density

Explanation

Specimen collection is by amniocentesis. Lamellar body density is calculated by measuring the number of surfactant containing particles per microliter of amniotic fluid. Method is automated cell count. This test indicates fetal pulmonary maturation and newborn risk for respiratory distress syndrome.

83718

83718 Lipoprotein, direct measurement; high density cholesterol (HDL cholesterol)

Explanation

This test may be requested as HDL, HDLC, or HDL cholesterol. Lipoproteins are compounds composed of lipids bound to proteins, which are transported through the blood. High-density lipoprotein (HDL) is frequently referred to as "good cholesterol," or "friendly lipid," as it is responsible for decreasing plaque deposits in blood vessels. High levels of HDL decrease the risk of premature coronary artery disease. This code reports direct measurement only, normally performed using an enzymatic or precipitation method.

83719

83719 Lipoprotein, direct measurement; VLDL cholesterol

Explanation

This test measures VLDL, the lipoprotein that carries triglycerides in the blood. The test is useful to determine a patient's risk of arteriosclerotic occlusive disease, as well as other cholesterol-related disorders. The method used is electrophoresis and may first involve ultracentrifugation.

83721

83721 Lipoprotein, direct measurement; LDL cholesterol

Explanation

This test may also be referred to as LDL-C. It measures the amount of low-density lipoprotein (LDL), also known as "bad cholesterol." The test is useful to determine the patient's risk of coronary heart disease (CHD), among other disorders. Method may be by precipitation procedure with results derived by the Friedewald formula.

83727

83727 Luteinizing releasing factor (LRH)

Explanation

This test may also be referred to as the LH-RH test. Natural bursts of LH-RH govern the release of luteinizing hormone and follicular stimulating hormone, both essential to ovulation. The test is useful in diagnosing problems in LH-RH transport or production, as well as associated fertility problems. Methodology may entail administration of a stimulation agent with a baseline blood sample drawn before the injection and several after. Samples may be tested by immunoassay.

83735

83735 Magnesium

Explanation

Magnesium, abbreviated Mg, is an inorganic cation essential for many physiochemical processes. It is an enzyme activator found in body fluids and cells. Magnesium depletion is clinically associated with weakness and neuromuscular disorders including cardiac arrhythmias and seizures. IV therapy, malabsorption, dialysis, pregnancy, toxicity and conditions such as hyperparathyroidism and hyperaldosteronism deplete magnesium. Specimen types and methods of testing vary. Colorimetry or spectrophotometry are methods frequently used.

83788

83788 Mass spectrometry and tandem mass spectrometry (MS, MS/MS), analyte not elsewhere specified; qualitative, each specimen

Explanation

This test identifies the presence (qualitative) of specific analytes in protein. The specimen varies. Method is mass spectrometry. The test is used for identifying the chemical makeup and structure of a substance. Tandem MS (MS/MS) is a method using sequential analysis to provide structural information by establishing relationships between substances. This test assists in analyzing viruses, sequencing and analyzing peptides and proteins, and providing information on such life-threatening diseases as AIDS and various types of skin cancers.

83789

83789 Mass spectrometry and tandem mass spectrometry (MS, MS/MS), analyte not elsewhere specified; quantitative, each specimen

Explanation

This test is used for identifying the chemical makeup and structure of a substance. The specimen type varies. Method is mass spectometry (MS). This test is used to analyze viruses, sequence and analyze peptides and proteins, and to provide information on such life-threatening diseases as AIDS and various types of skin cancers. This test quantifies (measures) the amount of analyte in the specimen.

83857

83857 Methemalbumin

Explanation

This test measures methemalbumin. It is representative of intravascular hemolysis. The specimen is serum or amniotic fluid. Methods may include Schumm test, ether, ammonium sulfide, EP for serum, and spectrophotometry for serum or plasma.

83883

83883 Nephelometry, each analyte not elsewhere specified

Explanation

Nephelometry is a method to measure the concentration of a suspension using an instrument (nephelometer) for assessing turbidity of a solution. For example, this code can be used to measure the concentration of albumin in body fluid. Albumins make up about 60 percent of plasma proteins, and exert considerable pressure in maintaining water balance between blood and tissues. Report this nephelometry test when the analyte is not specifically cited elsewhere in this section.

84061

84061 Phosphatase, acid; forensic examination

Explanation

This test is performed to detect acid phosphatase, a constituent of semen, as part of evidence collection following a sex crime. The specimen is vaginal fluid. Some specimens may be placed in transport tubes; others may be submitted on slides as smears. This test does not detect the presence of spermatozoa. Levels of phosphatase may be elevated due to vaginal infection, which may confuse test results.

84075

84075 Phosphatase, alkaline;

Explanation

This test may be requested as ALP. ALP is an enzyme. It is an indicator of liver cell damage. Amniotic fluid ALP may be screened for cystic fibrosis in mothers who have had a child affected with the disease. Methods include a number of kinetic spectrophotometry and fluorescent techniques, as well as 4-nitrylphenophosphate (4-NPP) and diethanolamine (DEA).

84081

84081 Phosphatidylglycerol

Explanation

These tests together are frequently ordered as LS/PG. Testing is performed in conjunction with an L/S (lecithin/sphingomyelin) ratio for assessment of fetal maturity based on pulmonary surfactant. This test may be performed to determine fetal lung maturity and to establish the possibility of the development of respiratory distress syndrome in the fetus. The specimen is by amniocentesis, a separately reportable procedure Methods may include thin-layer chromatography (TLC) and immunologic and enzymatic assays.

84100

84100 Phosphorus inorganic (phosphate);

Explanation

This test may be ordered as PO4. Methods may include phosphomolybdate colorimetric and modified molybdate enzymatic, and colorimetric. The testing may be performed to measure high or low levels of phosphorus to determine a variety of differential diagnoses. Potassium supplements increase phosphate levels. Also, phosphate levels may increase during the last trimester of pregnancy.

84105

84105 Phosphorus inorganic (phosphate); urine

Explanation

This test is performed to identify the calcium/phosphorus balance. High values may be associated with primary hyperparathyroidism, vitamin D deficiency, and renal tubular acidosis; low values may be due to hypoparathyroidism, pseudohypoparathyroidism, and vitamin D toxicity. The test may also be used for nephrolithiasis assessment.

84112

84112 Placental alpha microglobulin-1 (PAMG-1), cervicovaginal secretion, qualitative

Explanation

This is a noninvasive test for the rupture of fetal membranes (ROM) in a pregnant patient. During pregnancy, large quantities of placental alpha microglobulin-1 (PAMG-1) are secreted into the amniotic fluid. If the fetal membranes are intact, a low background level of PAMG-1 is measured in cervicovaginal secretions, while high levels may be indicative of ROM. A swab is inserted two to three inches into the vagina and is withdrawn after one minute. The swab tip is placed into a vial and rinsed with solvent. A test strip is then placed into the vial with the solvent. Depending on the size of the amniotic fluid leak, results may be visible within five to 10 minutes.

84132

84132 Potassium; serum, plasma or whole blood

Explanation

This test may be requested as K or K+. Potassium is the major electrolyte found in intracellular fluids. Potassium influences skeletal and cardiac muscle activity. Very small fluctuations outside the normal range may cause significant health risk, including muscle weakness and cardiac arrhythmias. Blood specimen is serum, plasma, or whole blood. Methods include atomic absorption spectrometry (AAS), ion-selective electrode (ISE), and flame emission spectroscopy (FES).

84133

84133 Potassium; urine

Explanation

This test may be ordered as urine K+. The specimen is collected by the patient over a 24-hour period or is random urine sample. Methods may include flame emission photometry and ion-selective electrode (ISE). The test may be ordered to determine elevated levels for the differential diagnoses of chronic renal failure, renal tubular acidosis, and for diuretic therapy.

84135

84135 Pregnanediol

Explanation

This test measures pregnanediol to evaluate progesterone production by the ovaries and placenta. Methods may involve gas-liquid chromatography and radioimmunoassay. Progesterone initiates the phase in ovulation that prepares the endometrium for implantation of a fertilized ovum. The serum and urine level of the progesterone metabolite pregnanediol increases rapidly during this phase, making it a useful measure in documenting and charting ovulation.

84138

84138 Pregnanetriol

Explanation

This test is also known as 17-Hydroxyprogesterone or 17-OH-Progesterone. Methods may include extraction/gas-liquid chromatography (GLC) and spectrophotometry. This test may be performed to determine differential diagnoses of adrenogenital syndrome, tumors of ovary and adrenal cortices, Stein-Leventhal syndrome, and congenital adrenal hyperplasia, among others.

84140

84140 Pregnenolone

Explanation

This test is used for detecting and measuring the levels of pregnenolone, a steroid involved in the synthesis of numerous hormones. The specimen is blood (to include cord blood) or a 24 hour timed urine collection. Method is typically radioimmunoassay.

84143

84143 17-hydroxypregnenolone

Explanation

Serum or urine from a female patient may be examined using radioimmunoassay in this test for detecting and measuring the levels of 17-hydroxypregnenolone, a hormonal metabolite.

84144

84144 Progesterone

Explanation

This test is performed to determine corpus luteum function, confirm ovulation, and to diagnose incompetent luteal phase and insufficient progesterone production, which may be the cause of habitual abortions. The specimen is serum. Methods may include radioimmunoassay (RIA) and direct time-resolved fluorescence immunoassay.

84145

84145 Procalcitonin (PCT)

Explanation

Procalcitonin (PCT) is produced in the thyroid cells of healthy individuals as a precursor for the hormone calcitonin and is not normally found in human blood. However, bacterial infections may cause many of the body's organs to produce PCT, resulting in a rapid elevation of PCT blood levels. This increase is not caused by viral infections. PCT blood levels reflect the severity of bacterial infection, making it a useful biomarker in the diagnosis of bacterial infection and sepsis. Specimen is serum or plasma; test method is by various assays.

84146

84146 Prolactin

Explanation

Prolactin is a hormone secreted by the anterior pituitary gland. This test may be performed for the differential diagnoses of prolactinemia, galactorrhea (lactation disorder), pituitary adenomas, pituitary prolactinoma, and other pituitary tumors. The specimen is post-fasting serum. Methods may include immunoassay and radioimmunoassay (RIA).

84150

84150 Prostaglandin, each

Explanation

Method is enzyme immunoassay. Prostaglandin (PG) is a potent unsaturated fatty acid that can act against organs in exceedingly low concentrations, and in their pharmaceutical form may be used for terminating pregnancy or treating asthma. This test may also be known as PG.

84155-84157

84155	Protein, total, except by refractometry; serum, plasma or whole blood
84156	urine
84157	other source (eg, synovial fluid, cerebrospinal fluid)

Explanation

A total protein test may be performed to assess nutritional status. Serum, plasma, or whole blood is tested for protein in 84155. Synovial, cerebrospinal, or other fluid is obtained in 84157. A urine specimen is required for 84156. For amniotic fluid specimen (84157), a separately reportable amniocentesis is performed. Aspiration of other body fluids (CSF, bronchial fluid, exudates) may also require separately reportable procedures. The method is biuret for blood (serum) and amniotic fluid. The method is turbidimetry or nephelometry for urine and CSF. For other body fluids, the method is turbidimetry or biuret.

84163

84163 Pregnancy-associated plasma protein-A (PAPP-A)

Explanation

Pregnancy associated plasma protein-A (PAPP-A, PAPPA) is a large zinc binding protein that acts as an enzyme. The test is used as a marker for Down's syndrome in the fetus. It can also be used as a marker for acute coronary syndromes such as angina and acute myocardial infarction. Blood specimen is obtained by venipuncture. Testing for Down's syndrome requires a maternal blood sample. Purified human PAPP-A is used as the immunogen (antigen). Methods include enzyme linked immunosorbent assay (ELISA) and Western blot.

84202-84203

84202	Protoporphyrin, RBC; quantitative
84203	screen

Explanation

This test is performed to diagnose various anemias and lead toxicity. Code 84203 is a qualitative test used as a screen to determine if protoporphyrin is present in the specimen. Code 84202 measures (quantifies) the level of protoporphyrin present. The specimen is whole blood. Methods may include hematofluorometry methods and high performance liquid chromatography.

84233

84233 Receptor assay; estrogen

Explanation

This test may be ordered to assist in identifying a breast cancer patient's ability to respond to chemotherapy and endocrine therapy. The specimen is surgical tissue. The surgical procedure is separately billable. Methods may include biochemical measurement in cytosol fractions of tumor homogenate, dextranestradiol conjugate, immunoperoxidase using tissue sections, enzyme immunoassay (EIA), and in situ hybridization.

84234

84234 Receptor assay; progesterone

Explanation

This test assists in identifying a patient's ability to respond to treatment in breast and other cancers and may be ordered as a PgR assay. The specimen is surgical tissue. Methods may include sucrose density gradient, steroid binding assay, and enzyme immunoassay.

84235

84235 Receptor assay; endocrine, other than estrogen or progesterone (specify hormone)

Explanation

The test may be used to predict or monitor patient response to hormonal therapy. The specimen is whole blood or plasma; separately reportable biopsy or surgical excision for tumor tissue. Methods are radioimmunoassay (most commonly used technique), gas-liquid and liquid chromatography or electrophoresis.

84238

84238   Receptor assay; non-endocrine (specify receptor)

Explanation

This test may be used to predict or monitor patient response to therapy, including AChR. Methods include radioimmunoassay (most commonly used technique), gas-liquid and liquid chromatography, or electrophoresis. The test is performed to determine the concentration of the target substance.

84270

84270   Sex hormone binding globulin (SHBG)

Explanation

The test may be used to predict or monitor patient response to hormonal therapy and to assist in certain diagnoses, including hypothyroidism and hyperthyroidism. This test may also be ordered as SHBG. The specimen is serum which requires special handling or amniotic fluid. Methods include CMA or radioimmunoassay.

84295-84302

84295   Sodium; serum, plasma or whole blood
84300   urine
84302   other source

Explanation

Sodium is an electrolyte found in extracellular fluid. Blood specimen for serum, plasma, or whole blood sodium (Na) in 84295 is obtained by venipuncture. Methods include atomic absorption spectrometry (AAS), flame emission photometry, and ion-selective electrode (ISE). The specimen for urine Na in 84300 is collected over a 24-hour period or by random urine sample. Methods may include flame emission photometry and ISE. This test is used to identify increased (hypernatremia) and decreased (hyponatremia) levels of sodium due to various conditions or disease states. Report 84302 for a sodium level test done on another source of specimen other than blood serum or urine.

84305

84305   Somatomedin

Explanation

Somatomedin is a protein mainly produced in the liver. It is a peptide dependent on growth hormone for its actions. This test may be used to diagnose and evaluate response to therapy for a variety of growth disorders. The test may be performed to diagnose acromegaly, dwarfism, pituitary disease and disorders, nutritional deficiencies, and to monitor response to therapies. The specimen is plasma, which requires special handling. Methodology may use a process of dissociation from binding protein and chromatography, followed by radioimmunoassay (RIA).

84311

84311   Spectrophotometry, analyte not elsewhere specified

Explanation

Specimen types include blood, random urine, or a 24-hour timed urine collection. Method is typically spectrophotometry, which provides a quantitative measure of the amount of a material in a solution absorbing applied light. Report this test for an analyte not elsewhere specified. Measuring the absorption of visible, ultraviolet or infrared light makes quantitative measurements of concentrations of reagents. The specimen is by the bodily fluid chosen as a sample (e.g., gastric secretions). Method is by specific gravity, which measures the concentration or the weight of a substance as compared to an equal volume of water. For laboratory testing, specific gravity shows the density of a specific material.

84315

84315   Specific gravity (except urine)

Explanation

Specific gravity is a measure of concentration. It is the weight of a substance, as compared with that of an equal volume of water. Body fluids are typically collected by needle aspiration or lavage. The method of testing is refractometer.

84376-84379

84376   Sugars (mono-, di-, and oligosaccharides); single qualitative, each specimen
84377   multiple qualitative, each specimen
84378   single quantitative, each specimen
84379   multiple quantitative, each specimen

Explanation

These tests may be used for infants who are failing to thrive due to lactose, sucrose, or fructose imbalances. Methods include gas chromatography and mass spectrometry to test for sugars, mono-, di-, and oligosaccharides in body fluids.

84402-84403

84402   Testosterone; free
84403   total

Explanation

These tests may be used to evaluate testosterone levels. Testosterone is an androgenic hormone responsible for, among other biological activities, secondary male characteristics in women. Increased testosterone levels in women may be linked to a variety of conditions, including hirsutism. Code 84403 reports total testosterone, which includes both protein bound and free testosterone. Code 84402 reports testosterone as a free unbound protein. This test may be ordered to assist in diagnosis of hypogonadism, hypopituitarism, and Klinefelter's syndrome, among other disorders. The specimen is serum. Method may be by radioimmunoassay (RIA) and immunoassay (non-isotopic).

84432

84432   Thyroglobulin

Explanation

This test is also known as Tg. The specimen is serum. This test is performed to determine thyroglobulin levels to identify thyroid disorders and tumors.

84436

84436   Thyroxine; total

Explanation

This test may be ordered as a T4. The specimen is serum. Methods may include radioimmunoassay (RIA), enzyme-linked immunosorbent assay (ELISA), fluorescence polarization immunoassay (FPIA), and chemiluminescence assay (CIA). The test is performed to determine thyroid function screening test; total thyroxine makes up approximately 99 percent of the thyroid hormone.

84437

84437   Thyroxine; requiring elution (eg, neonatal)

Explanation

This test may be ordered as a neonatal T4. The specimen is whole blood. The specimen may be taken at the same time as a PKU (Phenylalanine) test. Method is typically radioimmunoassay (RIA). The test may be performed to determine hypothyroidism in newborns (performed in all 50 states) to prevent mental retardation and to monitor suppressive and replacement therapy.

84439

84439   Thyroxine; free

Explanation

This test may be ordered as a FT4, free T4, FTI or FT4 index. The specimen is serum, requiring special handling. Methods may include radioimmunoassay and equilibrium dialysis for reference method. Free thyroxine is a minimal amount of the total T4 level (approximately one percent). This test is not influenced by thyroid-binding abnormalities and perhaps correlates more closely with the true hormonal status. It may be effective in the diagnosis of hyperthyroidism and hypothyroidism.

84442

84442   Thyroxine binding globulin (TBG)

Explanation
Thyroxin binding globulin is a plasma protein that binds with thyroxine and transports it in the blood. Elevated levels may be associated with pregnancy and newborn states, hepatitis, and other disorders. Decreased levels may be associated with liver diseases and acromegaly, among other disorders. The specimen is serum. Methods may include chemiluminescent immunoassay, equilibrium dialysis, ultrafiltration, and solid phase enzyme immunoassay (EIA) technology.

84443
84443 Thyroid stimulating hormone (TSH)

Explanation
TSH is produced in the pituitary gland and stimulates the secretion of thyrotropin (T3) and thyroxine (T4); these secretory products monitor TSH. The specimen is serum, requiring special handling. Heel stick or umbilical cord sample is drawn from newborns and may be collected on a special paper. Methods may include radioimmunoassay (RIA), sandwich immunoradiometric assay (IRMA), fluorometric enzyme immunoassay with use of monoclonal antibodies, or microparticle enzyme immunoassay on IMx (MEIA). This test may be performed to determine thyroid function, to differentiate from various types of hypothyroidism (e.g., primary, and pituitary/hypothalamic), or to diagnose hyperthyroidism. The test may be ordered to evaluate therapy in patients receiving hypothyroid treatment, and to detect congenital hypothyroidism.

84445
84445 Thyroid stimulating immune globulins (TSI)

Explanation
This test may also be ordered as TSI. This serum test measures the amount of thyroid stimulating antibody, which stimulates the thyroid to produce excessive amounts of thyroid hormone. Methods may include vitro bioassay and radioimmunoassay. The test may be useful in diagnosis of Grave's disease (hyperthyroidism).

84446
84446 Tocopherol alpha (Vitamin E)

Explanation
This test may also be known as a-tocopherol. The specimen is serum or plasma, requiring special handling. Methods may include high performance liquid chromatography (HPLC), fluorometry after solvent extraction, and colorimetry. The test may be performed to determine vitamin E deficiency, to evaluate patients on long-term parenteral nutrition, and to evaluate numerous disorders.

84450
84450 Transferase; aspartate amino (AST) (SGOT)

Explanation
This test is usually referred to as aspartate aminotransferase (AST) or as serum glutamic oxaloacetic transaminase (SGOT). AST is an enzyme found primarily in heart muscle and the liver. Serum levels are low unless there is cellular damage, at which time large amounts are released into circulation. AST levels are increased following acute myocardial infarction (MI). Liver disease may also cause elevated levels of AST. Blood specimen is serum or plasma. Method is spectrophotometry, kinetic assay, and enzymatic.

84460
84460 Transferase; alanine amino (ALT) (SGPT)

Explanation
This test is usually referred to as alanine aminotransferase (ALT) or as serum glutamic pyruvic transaminase (SGPT). ALT is an enzyme found primarily in liver cells and elevations may be indicative of liver disease. Blood specimen is serum or plasma. Method is spectrophotometry or enzymatic.

84478
84478 Triglycerides

Explanation
This test may be requested as TG. Triglycerides are blood lipids that are transported through the circulatory system by lipoproteins. Triglycerides contribute to atherosclerosis and other arterial diseases. Blood specimen is serum or plasma. Method is enzymatic or colorimetry.

84479
84479 Thyroid hormone (T3 or T4) uptake or thyroid hormone binding ratio (THBR)

Explanation
This test may be requested as T3 uptake and T4 uptake or THBR. The specimen is serum. Method is chemiluminescent immunoassay.

84480
84480 Triiodothyronine T3; total (TT-3)

Explanation
This test may be ordered as a T3 (RIA) or total T3. The specimen is serum. Methods may include radioimmunoassay (RIA), immunochemiluminometric assay, and fluorometric immunoassay. Abnormal results may be diseases and disorders related to the thyroid.

84481
84481 Triiodothyronine T3; free

Explanation
This test may also be known as FT3, or free T3. The specimen is serum. Method may involve equilibrium dialysis (tracer). This test may be used to identify thyroid dysfunction, such as hyperthyroidism and hypothyroidism.

84482
84482 Triiodothyronine T3; reverse

Explanation
Reverse T3 (rT3) is an inactive form of the thyroid hormone T3, and is found in the blood of normal people. The specimen is serum. Measurement of rT3 has been suggested in differentiating euthyroid sick syndrome from true hypothyroidism, and in identifying factitious hyperthyroidism. RT3 is typically measured by radioimmunoassay.

84510
84510 Tyrosine

Explanation
This test may also be known by the abbreviation Tyr. Measurement of tyrosine is useful in the evaluation of certain amino-acidopathies or inborn errors of metabolism, and to determine possible thyroid disorders and various other diseases Tyrosine has been measured by chromatographic techniques such as HPLC or gas chromatography combined with a variety of detection/evaluation technologies, including mass-spectrometry. Specimen types vary.

84520
84520 Urea nitrogen; quantitative

Explanation
This test may be requested as blood urea nitrogen (BUN). Urea is an end product of protein metabolism. BUN may be requested to evaluate dehydration or renal function. Blood specimen is serum or plasma. Method is colorimetry, enzymatic, or rate conductivity. This test measures (quantitates) the amount of urea in the blood.

84525
84525 Urea nitrogen; semiquantitative (eg, reagent strip test)

Explanation
This test may also be ordered as a BUN. This test may provide useful information regarding carbohydrate metabolism (diabetes), kidney function, and acid-base balance. The specimen is by random urine sample. Method is reagent strip.

84540
84540 Urea nitrogen, urine

Explanation
This test may provide useful information regarding carbohydrate metabolism (diabetes), kidney function, and acid-base balance, in addition to dietary protein. Urea is a measure of protein breakdown in the body. Urine urea excretion can

be measured to obtain a ratio between the plasma (blood) urea and the urine urea; this ratio is an indicator of kidney function. Urine collection over a 24-hour period. Methods may include enzymatic assay, colorimetry, and conductometric.

84545

84545 Urea nitrogen, clearance

Explanation

This test is also known as BUN-blood urea nitrogen. The specimen is taken over a 24-hour period. Urea nitrogen is formed in the liver as an end product of protein metabolism. Increased or decreased levels of urea nitrogen can indicate renal disease, dehydration, congestive heart failure, and gastrointestinal bleeding, starvation, shock or urinary tract obstruction (by tumor or prostate gland).

84590

84590 Vitamin A

Explanation

This vitamin is also known as retinol. The specimen is serum, and requires special handling. Methods are electrochemical, high performance liquid chromatography (HPLC), and fluorescence or UV/VIS spectroscopy. Levels of vitamin A can be increased in specific diseases and toxic states, and decreased levels are seen in other conditions, such as, nutritional deficiency.

84591

84591 Vitamin, not otherwise specified

Explanation

This test is used to analyze vitamin levels that are not specified elsewhere such as biotin and niacin. Methods are dependent on the specific vitamin level being analyzed and on the type of specimen, but include microbiological assay (urine biotin levels), high performance liquid chromatography (HPLC) (urine niacin levels) solid phase (cellulose) binding assay (plasma biotin levels), chemoluminescence (serum biotin levels).

84597

84597 Vitamin K

Explanation

This test is used to analyze vitamin K, a fat-soluble vitamin that plays an important role in blood clotting. The specimen is serum which requires special handling. Method is high-performance liquid chromatography A. A deficiency in vitamin K is characterized by the increased tendency to bleed, including internal bleeding. Such bleeding episodes may be severe in newborn infants.

84702

84702 Gonadotropin, chorionic (hCG); quantitative

Explanation

This test may be ordered as hCG or as a serum pregnancy test. The specimen is serum. Method may be radioimmunoassay (RIA), two-site immunoradiometric assay (IRMA), two-site enzyme-linked immunosorbent assay (ELISA), and radioreceptor assay (RRA). This test is quantitative and measures the amount of hCG present, a determinate of pregnancy and certain tumors.

84703

84703 Gonadotropin, chorionic (hCG); qualitative

Explanation

This test is also known as a beta-subunit human chorionic gonadotropin. The specimen is serum or random urine sample. Methods may include radioimmunoassay (RIA), immunoradiometric (IRMA), and enzyme immunoassay. The test may be ordered to determine pregnancy, ectopic pregnancy, and hCG tumors, and as a screening prior to select medical care (e.g., sterilization).

84704

84704 Gonadotropin, chorionic (hCG); free beta chain

Explanation

Free beta human chorionic gonadotropin (hCG) is a biochemical marker used in early (first trimester) screening to detect such abnormalities as Down syndrome, Trisomy 18, and neural tube defects. Maternal serum levels of free beta hCG are elevated in Down syndrome pregnancies and markedly reduced in Trisomy 18. This test is quantitative and identifies the free beta chain of human chorionic gonadotropin using an enzyme immunoassay methodology.

84830

84830 Ovulation tests, by visual color comparison methods for human luteinizing hormone

Explanation

This test is used for the qualitative detection of the luteinizing hormone (LH) in urine. The specimen is urine. Method is rapid chromatographic immunoassay. LH is always present in the blood and urine, though its levels are higher in urine during ovulation. The LH surge and actual release of the egg is considered as the most fertile time of the cycle, and the most likely time for becoming pregnant.

85002

85002 Bleeding time

Explanation

This test may be ordered as a bleeding time or as an Ivy bleeding time. A small, superficial wound is nicked in the patient's forearm. Essentially, the amount of time it takes for the wound to stop bleeding is recorded at bedside. The Ivy bleeding

time test is one standardized method. All methods are manual or point of care. A bleeding time is a rough measure of platelet (thrombocyte) function. The test is often performed on a preoperative patient.

85004

85004 Blood count; automated differential WBC count

Explanation

This test may be ordered as a blood count with automated differential. The specimen is whole blood. Method is automated cell counter. The blood count typically includes a measurement of normal cell constituents including white blood cells or leukocytes, red blood cells, and platelets. In addition, this test includes a differential count of the white blood cells or "diff" in which the following leukocytes are differentiated and counted automatically: neutrophils or granulocytes, lymphocytes, monocytes, eosinophils, and basophils.

85007-85008

85007 Blood count; blood smear, microscopic examination with manual differential WBC count
85008 blood smear, microscopic examination without manual differential WBC count

Explanation

This test may be ordered as a manual blood smear examination, RBC smear, peripheral blood smear, or RBC morphology without differential parameters in 85008 and with manual WBC differential in 85007. The specimen is whole blood. The method is manual testing. A blood smear is prepared and microscopically examined for the presence of normal cell constituents, including white blood cells, red blood cells, and platelets. In 85008, the white blood cell and platelet or thrombocyte counts are estimated and red cell morphology is commented on if abnormal. In 85007, a manual differential of white blood cells is included in which the following leukocytes are differentiated: neutrophils or granulocytes, lymphocytes, monocytes, eosinophils, and basophils.

85009

85009 Blood count; manual differential WBC count, buffy coat

Explanation

This test may be ordered as a buffy coat differential or as a differential WBC count, buffy coat. Blood is whole blood. Other collection types (e.g., finger stick or heel stick) do not yield the volume of blood required for this test. Method is manual testing. The whole blood is centrifuged to concentrate the white blood cells, and a manual WBC differential is performed in which the following leukocytes are differentiated: neutrophils or granulocytes, lymphocytes, monocytes, eosinophils, and basophils. This test is usually performed when the number of WBCs or leukocytes is abnormally low and the presence of abnormal white cells (e.g., blasts or cancer cells) is suspected clinically.

85013
85013 Blood count; spun microhematocrit

Explanation
This test may be ordered as a microhematocrit, a spun microhematocrit, or a "spun crit." The specimen (whole blood) is by finger stick or heel stick in infants. The sample is placed in a tube and into a microcentrifuge device. The vials can be read manually against a chart for the volume of packed red cells or a digital reader in the centrifuge device. A spun microhematocrit only reports the volume of packed red cells. It is typically performed at sites where limited testing is available, the patient is a very difficult blood draw, or on infants.

85014
85014 Blood count; hematocrit (Hct)

Explanation
This test may be ordered as a hematocrit, Hmt, or Hct. The specimen is whole blood. Method is automated cell counter. The hematocrit or volume of packed red cells (VPRC) in the blood sample is calculated by multiplying the red blood cell count or RBC times the mean corpuscular volume or MCV.

85018
85018 Blood count; hemoglobin (Hgb)

Explanation
This test may be ordered as hemoglobin, Hgb, or hemoglobin concentration. The specimen is whole blood. Method is usually automated cell counter but a manual method is seen in labs with a limited test menu and blood bank drawing stations. Hemoglobin is an index of the oxygen-carrying capacity of the blood.

85025-85027
85025 Blood count; complete (CBC), automated (Hgb, Hct, RBC, WBC and platelet count) and automated differential WBC count
85027 complete (CBC), automated (Hgb, Hct, RBC, WBC and platelet count)

Explanation
This test may be ordered as a complete automated blood count (CBC). The specimen is whole blood. Method is automated cell counter. This code includes the measurement of erythrocytes (red blood cells or RBC), leukocytes (white blood cells or WBC), hemoglobin, hematocrit (volume of packed red blood cells or VPRC), platelet or thrombocyte count, and indices (mean corpuscular hemoglobin or MCH, mean corpuscular hemoglobin concentration or MCHC, mean corpuscular volume

or MCV, and red cell distribution width or RDW). Code 85025 includes an automated differential of the white blood cells or "diff" in which the following leukocytes are differentiated: neutrophils or granulocytes, lymphocytes, monocytes, eosinophils, and basophils. Report 85027 if the complete CBC, or automated blood count, is done without the differential WBC count.

85032
85032 Blood count; manual cell count (erythrocyte, leukocyte, or platelet) each

Explanation
This code reports a manual cell count done for red blood cells (erythrocytes), white blood cells (leukocytes), or platelets (thrombocytes), each. The specimen is whole blood. The method is manual examination and counting.

85041
85041 Blood count; red blood cell (RBC), automated

Explanation
This test may be ordered as red blood cell count or RBC. The specimen is by whole blood Method is automated cell counter.

85044
85044 Blood count; reticulocyte, manual

Explanation
This test may be ordered as a manual reticulocyte count or as a manual "retic." The specimen is whole blood. Method is manual. A blood smear is prepared and stained with a dye that highlights the reticulum in the immature red blood cells, or the reticulocytes. The reticulocytes reported as a percentage of total red blood cells.

85045
85045 Blood count; reticulocyte, automated

Explanation
This test may be ordered as an automated reticulocyte count, an "auto retic," or a reticulocyte by flow cytometry. The specimen is whole blood. Method is automated cell counter or flow cytometer. Reticulocytes are immature red blood cells that still contain mitochondria and ribosomes. The reticulocytes are reported as a percentage of total red blood cells.

85046
85046 Blood count; reticulocytes, automated, including 1 or more cellular parameters (eg, reticulocyte hemoglobin content [CHr], immature reticulocyte fraction [IRF], reticulocyte volume [MRV], RNA content), direct measurement

Explanation
This test may be ordered as a reticulocyte count and hemoglobin concentration, "retics" and Hgb, or as an "auto retic" and hemoglobin. The specimen is whole blood. Method is automated cell counter. The blood is stained with a dye that marks the reticulum in immature red blood cells, or reticulocytes. The reticulocytes are reported as a percentage of total red blood cells. The automated reticulocyte blood count also includes one or more cellular parameters, such as the hemoglobin content of the reticulocytes (CHr), the fraction of immature reticulocytes (IRF), the RNA content, or the volume of reticulocytes.

85048-85049
85048 Blood count; leukocyte (WBC), automated
85049 platelet, automated

Explanation
This test may be ordered as an automated white blood cell or WBC count, white cell count, or leukocyte count for 85048 and as an automated platelet count in 85049. The specimen is whole blood. Method is automated cell counter. In 85048, the population of white blood cells, or WBCs in the blood sample, is counted by machine. Only the number of white blood cells or leukocytes is reported. In 85049, the population of platelets or thrombocytes in the blood sample is counted by machine. Only the number of platelets is reported.

85060
85060 Blood smear, peripheral, interpretation by physician with written report

Explanation
This test may be ordered as a peripheral blood smear with interpretation by a physician, with a written report. It would usually be ordered following a hemogram with WBC differential where the technologist noted the presence of significant abnormalities and requested a pathology review. Although lacking specificity, peripheral smears also provide a quick and cost-effective screening for the presence of bacteremia. The specimen is whole blood. The method is manual. A blood smear is prepared and reviewed by a physician/pathologist, who submits a written interpretation of the findings.

85415
85415 Fibrinolytic factors and inhibitors; plasminogen activator

Explanation
This test may be ordered as plasminogen activator, plasminogen activator inhibitor (PAI). The specimen is plasma. The method is chromogenic substrate or enzyme linked immunosorbent assay. Increased plasminogen activator levels are present during fibrinolytic or clot dissolving activity.

85420

85420 Fibrinolytic factors and inhibitors; plasminogen, except antigenic assay

Explanation

This test may be ordered as plasminogen level, functional plasminogen, or plasminogen activity. The specimen is plasma. The method is chromogenic substrate. Increased plasminogen levels are present during fibrinolytic or clot dissolving activity, intrauterine death, and some metastatic cancers.

85421

85421 Fibrinolytic factors and inhibitors; plasminogen, antigenic assay

Explanation

This test may be ordered as plasminogen antigen level. The specimen is plasma. The method is radial immunodiffusion. Increased plasminogen antigen levels may be present during fibrinolytic or clot dissolving activity, intrauterine death, and some metastatic cancers.

85460

85460 Hemoglobin or RBCs, fetal, for fetomaternal hemorrhage; differential lysis (Kleihauer-Betke)

Explanation

This test may be ordered as a Kleihauer-Betke stain or K-B stain, a Kleihauer-Betke stain for fetal hemoglobin, a Kleihauer-Betke stain for fetomaternal hemorrhage, acid-resistant fetal cells, or a differential lysis stain. The specimen is whole blood or finger stick. This test is not performed on infants. The method is semi-quantitative stain following acid elution. The blood smear is stained and examined microscopically. The number of red cells containing fetal hemoglobin or acid-resistant hemoglobin red cells are counted and reported as a percentage of the normal adult hemoglobin-containing red cells. This test is usually performed on post-partum mothers to determine if the newborn bled during delivery. The number of acid-resistant, or fetal cells, present is useful in developing postpartum treatment plans, especially with Rh-negative mothers.

85461

85461 Hemoglobin or RBCs, fetal, for fetomaternal hemorrhage; rosette

Explanation

This test may be ordered as a fetal hemoglobin screening test, a fetal red cell rosette, a FetalDex screen, or a fetal screen. The specimen is whole blood or finger stick. This test is not appropriate for infants. The blood is treated with a chemical (anti-D) that causes fetal cells to form a rosette, or circle, of cells. This test is a screen usually performed on Rh-negative post-partum mothers to determine if the newborn bled during delivery.

85520

85520 Heparin assay

Explanation

This test may be ordered as a heparin assay, a quantitative heparin analysis, or as a heparin level. The specimen is plasma. The method is chromogenic assay. This test measures the amount of heparin in a patient's blood and is usually ordered when the patient is on low-dose heparin therapy.

85525

85525 Heparin neutralization

Explanation

This test may be ordered as a heparin neutralization test, a heparin-thrombin coagulation time test, or as protamine neutralization test. The specimen plasma. The method is manual. This test is used to determine the dose of protamine needed to neutralize heparin-induced bleeding.

85530

85530 Heparin-protamine tolerance test

Explanation

This test may be ordered as a heparin-protamine tolerance test. Protamine is given as an antidote to heparin overdose. However, some patients develop hypersensitivity to protamine and may go into anaphylactic shock if they receive a dosage. Method is point of care testing. This test is used to assess hypersensitivity to protamine and measures the amount of protamine that can be safely administered.

85576

85576 Platelet, aggregation (in vitro), each agent

Explanation

This test may be ordered as a platelet aggregation study, or as an in vitro platelet aggregation study. Specimen is plasma. The method may be platelet aggregometer. Platelet function is measured by observing the amount of platelet clumping that occurs when certain chemicals are added to a solution of platelets. The test is an in vitro enactment of the platelet aggregation that occurs naturally at the site of vascular injury. The test may be used to detect von Willebrand's disease or other inherited platelet disjunction diseases.

85610

85610 Prothrombin time;

Explanation

This test may be ordered as a prothrombin time (PT), a prothrombin, or as simply PT. The specimen is plasma. Method is one-stage using an automated device. The prothrombin time is prolonged when deficiencies of coagulation factors II, V, VII, or X are present. More commonly, this test monitors the effectiveness of the anticoagulant drug Coumadin or warfarin, prescribed to patients who have had blood clots or myocardial infarction.

85611

85611 Prothrombin time; substitution, plasma fractions, each

Explanation

This test may be ordered as a diluted prothrombin time (PT), a prothrombin 1:1, or as plasma diluted PT. The specimen is plasma. Addition or dilution with normal plasma differentiates between a clotting factor deficiency and a circulating anticoagulant. Prolonged prothrombin times due to a clotting factor deficiency will shorten to normal with the addition of normal plasma while a prolonged prothrombin time due to a circulating anticoagulant may increase with the addition of normal plasma.

85651

85651 Sedimentation rate, erythrocyte; non-automated

Explanation

This test may be ordered as an erythrocyte sedimentation rate (ESR), a Westergren sedimentation rate, Wintrobe sedimentation rate, or simply as a "sed rate." The specimen is whole blood. This test is a non-specific screening test for a number of diseases including anemia, disorders of protein production such as multiple myeloma, other conditions that alter the size and/or shape of red cells or erythrocytes, and to screen diseases that cause an increase or decrease in the amount of protein in the plasma. Further studies are often launched by ESR results. The method is manual. A variety of procedures have been used over time to study sedimentation rate. A common one performed manually is the Westergren tube.

85652

85652 Sedimentation rate, erythrocyte; automated

Explanation

This test may be ordered as a Zeta sedimentation rate or as a Zeta sed rate. Specimen is whole blood. Method is centrifugation; this is an automated test. This test is a non-specific screening test for a number of diseases including anemia, disorders of protein production such as multiple myeloma, and other conditions that alter the size and/or shape of red cells or erythrocytes. This test may also be used to screen diseases that cause an increase or decrease in the amount of protein in the plasma or liquid portion of the blood.

85730

85730 Thromboplastin time, partial (PTT); plasma or whole blood

Explanation

This test may be ordered as a partial thromboplastin time or PTT, or as an activated partial thromboplastin time or APTT. The specimen is plasma. The method is automated coagulation instrument. The partial thromboplastin time is prolonged when deficiencies of coagulation factors VIII, IX, XI, and XII are present. This test is used to monitor the effectiveness of the anticoagulant drug heparin, which is prescribed for patients who have had blood clots or heart attacks.

85732

85732 Thromboplastin time, partial (PTT); substitution, plasma fractions, each

Explanation

This test may be ordered as a diluted partial thromboplastin time, a PTT or APTT 1:1, or as a plasma diluted PTT or APTT. The specimen is plasma. The method is automated coagulation instrument. Addition of or dilution with normal plasma differentiates between a clotting factor deficiency and a circulating anticoagulant. Prolonged partial thromboplastin times due to a clotting factor deficiency will shorten to normal with the addition of normal plasma while a prolonged PTT due to a circulating anticoagulant may increase with the addition of normal plasma.

85810

85810 Viscosity

Explanation

This test may be ordered as a serum viscosity test or as a viscosity. The specimen is serum. Finger stick or heel stick is not acceptable. The method is viscometer. This test measures the viscosity or thickness of serum as compared to saline. Increased viscosity may be found in disorders such as Waldenstrvm macroglobulinemia.

86021

86021 Antibody identification; leukocyte antibodies

Explanation

This test may also be ordered as alloantibody identification, or alloagglutinin identification (the term "isoantibodies" is archaic). The term autoantibody may also be used. Leukocyte antibodies correlate closely to human leukocyte antigens, a complex genetic code for the immune system. The leukocyte antibody side of the equation may be referred to as alloagglutinins. This type of test is usually ordered to predict for one of several disorders: severe immune reactions from fetomaternal leukocyte incompatibility and/or neonatal incompatibilities, post-blood transfusion reactions, and poor blood component viability following transfusion. Alloantibodies arising from previous pregnancies and transfusions may be evident years after antigen exposure. Autoantibodies

are usually identified with autoimmune disorders and infectious diseases. Methods may include agglutination and flow cytometry.

86147

86147 Cardiolipin (phospholipid) antibody, each Ig class

Explanation

This test may also be ordered as antiphospholipid antibody or anticardiolipin antibodies (ACA). The specimen is serum. Method is enzyme-linked immunoassay (ELISA). The test may be used to classify patients with recurrent venous or arterial thrombosis, thrombocytopenia (low platelet count), recurrent fetal loss, and acquired valvular heart disease, and systemic lupus erythematosus (SLE).

86171

86171 Complement fixation tests, each antigen

Explanation

This test may be ordered as a complement assay. The complementary system involves enzymes and regulatory proteins synthesized in the liver. Activation of the system triggers a cascading, or sequential, response that may lead to histamine release, inflammation, and other normal activities of the immune system. Blood specimen is serum. Complement fixation is widely used test that relies on these principles. The test may be used for a wide variety of suspected illnesses, including viral infections.

86255-86256

86255 Fluorescent noninfectious agent antibody; screen, each antibody
86256   titer, each antibody

Explanation

These codes report detection of noninfectious agents using fluorescent agent antibody technique. A number of noninfectious agents are reported with codes 86255 and 86256. Some antibodies reported with these codes include: acetylcholine receptor antibody (anti-AChR); adrenal cortex antibodies; anti D. S., DNA, IFA using C. Luciliae; mitochondrial antibody, liver; smooth muscle antibody; antineutrophil antibody; endomysial antibody; parietal cell antibody; and myositis-specific auto antibody. Code 86255 is a screen and reports the presence of the antibody only. Code 86256 is a titer and reports the level of antibody present.

86294

86294 Immunoassay for tumor antigen, qualitative or semiquantitative (eg, bladder tumor antigen)

Explanation

This code may be requested as single step qualitative or semi-quantitative immunoassay to

identify the presence of a specific tumor antigen. The specimen is serum. Method is immunoassay.

86300

86300 Immunoassay for tumor antigen, quantitative; CA 15-3 (27.29)

Explanation

This test may also be requested as CEA carbohydrate antigen 15-3. Method is immunoassay or ICMA. Quantitative analysis for CA 15-3 is used primarily to monitor patients for recurrence of breast cancer after diagnosis and initial treatment or to evaluate response to therapy. Elevated levels are often indicative of a recurrence or a failed treatment.

86301

86301 Immunoassay for tumor antigen, quantitative; CA 19-9

Explanation

This test may also be requested as carbohydrate antigen 19-9. The specimen is serum. Method is immunoassay. Quantitative analysis for CA 19-9 is used primarily as a marker for pancreatic cancer. It identifies recurrence and monitors patients. It is also used to monitor gastrointestinal, head/neck, and gynecological cancer. It may identify recurrence of stomach, colorectal, liver, gallbladder, and urothelial malignancies.

86304

86304 Immunoassay for tumor antigen, quantitative; CA 125

Explanation

This test may also be requested as cancer antigen 125. The specimen is serum. Method is immunoassay. CA 125 is found in ovarian cancers, and some endometrium and fallopian tube cancers. Testing for CA 125 is performed primarily to detect residual tumor in women who have been previously diagnosed with ovarian malignancy.

86316

86316 Immunoassay for tumor antigen, other antigen, quantitative (eg, CA 50, 72-4, 549), each

Explanation

This test is an immunoassay for tumor antigen and may be requested by the specific antigen. Some of the more common tumor antigens include carbohydrate antigen 549 (CA 549), carbohydrate antigen 72-4 (CA 72-4, TAG 72), and carbohydrate antigen 50 (CA 50). Each of these antigens is specific for certain types of cancer. CA 549 is found in Stage IV metastatic breast cancer and is used primarily to evaluate response to therapy.

© 2012 OptumInsight, Inc.

Appendix

86317

86317 Immunoassay for infectious agent antibody, quantitative, not otherwise specified

Explanation
This code may be requested to measure the amount of specific infectious disease antibodies in the blood that are not otherwise specified. It would normally be obtained subsequent to qualitative or semi-quantitative immunoassays (86318, 86602-86804), which identify the presence of specific antibodies but do not measure the amount of antibody present. Method is immunoassay.

86318

86318 Immunoassay for infectious agent antibody, qualitative or semiquantitative, single step method (eg, reagent strip)

Explanation
This code may be requested as single step qualitative or semi-quantitative immunoassay to identify the presence of a specific infectious agent antibodies. Specimen is serum. Method is immunoassay. Single step methods frequently use a reagent strip for the specific antibody.

86320

86320 Immunoelectrophoresis; serum

Explanation
This code may be abbreviated as serum IEP. Blood specimen is serum. This code is used to report a technique most often used to identify monoclonal gammopathy or lymphoproliferative processes, specifically myelomas. It combines electrophoresis and immunodiffusion. This test is qualitative only.

86325

86325 Immunoelectrophoresis; other fluids (eg, urine, cerebrospinal fluid) with concentration

Explanation
This code may be abbreviated as IEP. A random urine specimen is obtained. CSF is obtained by separately reportable spinal puncture. This code is used to report a technique most often used to identify monoclonal gammopathy or lymphoproliferative processes, specifically myelomas. It combines electrophoresis and immunodiffusion. This test is qualitative only.

86327

86327 Immunoelectrophoresis; crossed (2-dimensional assay)

Explanation
Two-dimensional or crossed immunoelectrophoresis (IEP) is similar to standard IEP as described in 86320 and 86325; however, following immunodiffusion, electrophoresis is performed a second time at right angles to the original separation.

86329-86331

86329 Immunodiffusion; not elsewhere specified
86331 gel diffusion, qualitative (Ouchterlony), each antigen or antibody

Explanation
These tests may be abbreviated as ID. Immunodiffusion (86329) involves an antibody-antigen reaction that causes a visible precipitate to form. It is a technique used in identifying immunoglobulin. Ouchterlony gel diffusion (86331) involves evaluation of the precipitin reaction in a clear gel. Immune complex assays were once thought to be a promising diagnostic technique. However, they have generally been replaced with tests that are more specific, more standardized, and less expensive. Blood specimen is serum which requires special handling. Method is a complement binding (CP) technique.

86592

86592 Syphilis test, non-treponemal antibody; qualitative (eg, VDRL, RPR, ART)

Explanation
This nontreponemal (screening) antibody test is commonly ordered as RPR (rapid plasma reagin), STS (serologic test for syphilis), VDRL (venereal disease research laboratory), or ART (automated reagin test). It may also be ordered as standard test for syphilis. The specimen is serum. The test is commonly used to provide a diagnosis (screening test) for syphilis. The method is by nontreponemal rapid plasma reagin (RPR)-particle agglutination test. More recently, it is being performed by automated methodology, such as enzyme-linked immunosorbent assay (ELISA).

86593

86593 Syphilis test, non-treponemal antibody; quantitative

Explanation
This nontreponemal (screening) test is commonly ordered as quantitative RPR (rapid plasma reagin), STS (serologic test for syphilis), VDRL (venereal disease research laboratory), or ART (automated reagin test). This test may also be ordered as a standard test for syphilis. The specimen is serum. It is most commonly used to provide a monitor for treatment, or to establish a diagnosis of reinfection with syphilis. The method is nontreponemal rapid plasma reagin-particle agglutination test or anticardiolipin antibodies. More recently, it is being performed by automated methodology, such as by enzyme-linked immunosorbent assay (ELISA).

86625

86625 Antibody; Campylobacter

Explanation
Campylobacter is a genus of bacteria, some of which are responsible for a wide variety of illnesses in humans. Enteritis is among the more common illnesses. Campylobacter is also implicated in Guillain-Barri syndrome, a type of arthritis. Blood specimen is obtained by venipuncture. The literature is unclear about methods and reasons to order such testing. Most clinical cases of Campylobacter infection resolve themselves spontaneously or following drug therapy.

86628

86628 Antibody; Candida

Explanation
Candida is a ubiquitous genus of fungi, some species of which are pathogenic to humans. The range of illnesses is quite large. This test is performed primarily to evaluate suspected systemic invasions by *Candida*. If confirmed, tests may be obtained at biweekly intervals to assess effectiveness of drug therapy. Blood specimen is serum. Methods include latex agglutination (LA), immunodiffusion (ID), crossed (2-dimensional) immunoelectrophoresis, and enzyme-linked immunosorbent assay (ELISA).

86631

86631 Antibody; Chlamydia

Explanation
This test may be ordered as chlamydia psittaci or LVG titer. The specimen is serum or finger stick in adults, or heel stick in infants. Methods are complement fixation (CF), enzyme-linked immunosorbent assay (ELISA), and immunofluorescent antibody (IFA). This test may be used to determine exposure to chlamydia, though the test should not be used as a specific type. *Chlamydomonas* is a genus of algae that can cause nongonococcal urethritis, among other infections.

86632

86632 Antibody; Chlamydia, IgM

Explanation
This test may be ordered as chlamydia IgM titer. The specimen is serum or finger stick in adults, or heel stick in infants. Complement fixation (CF), enzyme-linked immunosorbent assay (ELISA), and immunofluorescent antibody (IFA) are methods commonly used to determine previous exposure to chlamydia or a current infection. *Chlamydomonas* is a genus of algae that can cause nongonococcal urethritis, among other infections.

86687

86687 Antibody; HTLV-I

Explanation
This test is commonly ordered as HTLV-I antibody titer or Human T Cell Leukemia I Virus titer. The

specimen is by venipuncture or finger stick in adults, or heel stick in infants. Methods are Western blot, radioimmunoprecipitation, and screen enzyme immunoassay. This test may be performed to determine the presence of HTLV-I virus and to screen blood and blood products used for transfusions.

86688

86688   Antibody; HTLV-II

Explanation

This test is commonly ordered as HTLV-II antibody titer or human T cell leukemia II virus titer. The specimen is serum. Methods are Western blot, radioimmunoprecipitation, and screen enzyme immunoassay. This test may be performed to determine the presence of HTLV-II virus and to screen blood and blood products used for transfusions.

86689

86689   Antibody; HTLV or HIV antibody, confirmatory test (eg, Western Blot)

Explanation

This test is commonly ordered as HTLV or HIV by Western blot. The specimen is serum. This test may be performed as a confirmation of a positive test for human T cell leukemia II virus or human immunodeficiency virus (HIV), often by a previous enzyme-linked immunoassay (ELISA).

86692

86692   Antibody; hepatitis, delta agent

Explanation

This test may be ordered as hepatitis D antibody, hepatitis delta antibody, or superinfection antibody. Hepatitis D occurs concurrently with hepatitis B and may lead to more severe clinical symptoms than hepatitis B alone, a condition known as superinfection. Specimen is serum. Methodology may involve enzyme immunoassay (EIA).

86694-86696

86694   Antibody; herpes simplex, non-specific type test
86695   herpes simplex, type 1
86696   herpes simplex, type 2

Explanation

These tests may be ordered as HSV antibody titer, HSV titer, herpes simplex antibody titer, or HSV IgG/IGM. The specimen is serum or finger stick in adults, or heel stick in infants. A number of methodologies have been employed, such as complement fixation (CF), enzyme-linked immunosorbent assay (ELISA), indirect fluorescent antibody (IFA), enzyme immunoassay, and latex agglutination. This test has been used as a serologic method to detect previous or recent exposure to herpes simplex. To report non-specific type testing,

see 86694; testing for type 1, see 86695; testing for type 2, see 86696.

86701

86701   Antibody; HIV-1

Explanation

This test may be ordered as an HIV-1 serological test, an HIV-1 antibody, or by an internal code. HIV is a retrovirus and the causative agent of acquired immunodeficiency syndrome (AIDS). Specimen is serum. Numerous kits are now available that use a variety of viral proteins and serumsynthetic peptides as antigens. Methodology is enzyme immunoassay (EIA), enzyme-linked immunosorbent assay (ELISA), radioimmunoprecipitation assay (RIPA), or indirect fluorescent antibody (IFA). A negative test does not guarantee negative status and the test is often repeated several times.

86702

86702   Antibody; HIV-2

Explanation

This test may be ordered as an HIV-2 serological antibody. This is an antibody test for HIV-2, a retrovirus closely related to simian AIDS and found initially in West African nations and Portugal, but with cases also being reported in the United States since 1987. Blood specimen is serum. Specific kits are now available that use a variety of viral proteins and synthetic peptides as antigens to test for HIV-2. Methodology is enzyme immunoassay (EIA), enzyme-linked immunosorbent assay (ELISA), radioimmunoprecipitation assay (RIPA), or indirect fluorescent antibody (IFA). A negative test does not guarantee negative status and the test is often repeated several times.

86703

86703   Antibody; HIV-1 and HIV-2, single result

Explanation

This test may be ordered as a combined HIV-1 and -2 serological or a combined HIV-1 and -2 antibody. This is an antibody test that tests for both HIV-1 and HIV-2 with a single result. Both are retroviruses. HIV-1 is the causative agent of acquired immunodeficiency syndrome (AIDS), while HIV-2 is closely related to simian AIDS. Blood specimen is serum. Specific kits are now available that use a variety of viral proteins and synthetic peptides as antigens to test for both HIV-1 and HIV-2. Methodology is enzyme immunoassay (EIA), enzyme-linked immunosorbent assay (ELISA), radioimmunoprecipitation assay (RIPA), or indirect fluorescent antibody (IFA). A negative test does not guarantee negative status and the test is often repeated several times.

86704

86704   Hepatitis B core antibody (HBcAb); total

Explanation

This test may be ordered as hepatitis Bc Ab (HBcAb), total. It may also be ordered as HBcAb, anti-HBc, HBVc Ab, anti-HBVc. This test identifies Hepatitis B core total antibodies (IgG and IgM), which are markers available to identify individuals with acute, chronic, or past infection of hepatitis B. The presence of high-titered IgM specific HBcAb is always indicative of an acute infection. The presence of IgG may indicate acute or chronic infection. Blood specimen is serum. Methods include radioimmunoassay (RIA) and enzyme-linked immunosorbent assay (ELISA).

86705

86705   Hepatitis B core antibody (HBcAb); IgM antibody

Explanation

This test may be ordered as hepatitis Bc Ab (HBcAb), IgM. It may also be ordered as HBcAb, anti-HBc, HBVc Ab, anti-HBVc. This test identifies Hepatitis B core IgM antibodies, the presence of which always indicates an acute infection. Blood specimen is serum. Methods include radioimmunoassay (RIA) and enzyme-linked immunosorbent assay (ELISA).

86706

86706   Hepatitis B surface antibody (HBsAb)

Explanation

This test may be requested as Hepatitis B surface antibody (HBsAb), Hepatitis Bs Ab, HBV surface antibody, or anti-HBs. The presence of HBsAb is indicative of a previous resolved infection or vaccination against hepatitis B. Blood specimen is serum. Methods include radioimmunoassay (RIA), enzyme immunoassay (EIA), immunoradiometric assay (IRMA), and immunoenzymatic assay (IEMA).

86707

86707   Hepatitis Be antibody (HBeAb)

Explanation

This test may be ordered as hepatitis Be antibody (HBeAb) as Hepatitis Be Ab, HBVe, or anti-HBe. The presence of HBeAb usually indicates a high likelihood of a lesser infectivity and usually points to a benign outcome, although some individuals with HBeAb have chronic hepatitis. Blood specimen is serum. Methods include immunoradiometric assay (IRMA) and enzyme immunoassay (EIA).

86708

86708   Hepatitis A antibody (HAAb); total

Explanation

This test may be ordered as Hepatitis A Antibody (HAAb), HAV antibody, anti-Hep A or anti-HAV total (IgG and IgM). The presence of HAV IgG antibody may indicate acute infection or previous resolved infection, while IgM antibody always indicates acute infectious disease. Blood specimen is serum.

Appendix

Methods include radioimmunoassay (RIA), enzyme immunoassay (EIA), immunoradiometric assay (IRMA), immunoenzymatic assay (IEMA), and microparticle enzyme immunoassay (MEIA).

86709

86709 Hepatitis A antibody (HAAb); IgM antibody

Explanation

This test may be ordered as Hepatitis A Antibody (Haas), HAV IgM antibody, anti-Hep A IgM, or anti-HAV IgM. The presence of IgM antibody indicates acute infectious disease. Blood specimen is serum. Methods include radioimmunoassay (RIA), enzyme immunoassay (EIA), immunoradiometric assay (IRMA), immunoenzymatic assay (IEMA), and microparticle enzyme immunoassay (MEIA).

86762

86762 Antibody; rubella

Explanation

This test is ordered as rubella antibody titers. It may also be ordered as German measles antibody titers, and anti-rubella titers. The test is used primarily to evaluate immune status. The presence of rubella IgG and IgM antibodies may indicate previous exposure, vaccination, or current acute infection. Blood specimen is serum. Enzyme-linked immunosorbent assay (ELISA), enzyme immunoassay (EIA), and latex agglutination (LA) are among methods used in identifying antibody response, with ELISA being more common in larger, high volume laboratories.

86777

86777 Antibody; Toxoplasma

Explanation

This test is ordered as Toxoplasma IgG antibody titers. It may also be ordered as anti-Toxoplasma IgG titers, or toxo IgG titers. The presence of Toxoplasma IgG antibody may indicate current or past infection. Blood specimen is serum,. Amniotic fluid is collected by amniocentesis that is reported separately. Enzyme-linked immunosorbent assay (ELISA) or immunofluorescent assay (IFA) principles may be used for the identification of Toxoplasma antibody.

86778

86778 Antibody; Toxoplasma, IgM

Explanation

This test is ordered as Toxoplasma IgM antibody titers. It may also be ordered as anti-Toxoplasma IgM titers, or toxo IgM titers. The demonstration of Toxoplasma IgM antibodies may establish the diagnosis of a recent or current infection. Blood specimen is serum amniotic fluid collected by amniocentesis that is reported separately. Enzyme-linked immunosorbent assay (ELISA) or immunofluorescent assay (IFA) principles may be

used for the identification of toxoplasma IgM antibody.

86780

86780 Antibody; Treponema pallidum

Explanation

Treponema pallidum antibody tests are used to screen and confirm syphilis. This test may be ordered as a screening or confirmatory test for syphilis or as a screening or confirmatory test for a positive venereal disease research lab test (VDRL), rapid plasma reagent (RPR), or serologic test (STS) for syphilis. Blood specimen is serum. Fluorescent antibody (FA) or FTA principles are most commonly employed in identifying an antibody response to the specific syphilis. Agglutination or flocculation of cardiolipin principles may also be used for the identification of syphilis antibody.

86803

86803 Hepatitis C antibody;

Explanation

This test may be ordered as Hepatitis C antibody titers. It may also be ordered as anti-hepatitis C titers, HCV Ab titers, and anti-HCV titers. This test is normally used initially to screen for Hepatitis C. Positive or unequivocal tests are repeated using different techniques that are reported separately. Blood specimen is serum,. Methods may include enzyme-linked immunosorbent assay (ELISA) or enzyme immunoassay (EIA).

86804

86804 Hepatitis C antibody; confirmatory test (eg, immunoblot)

Explanation

These tests may be ordered as hepatitis C antibody titers, anti-hepatitis C titers, HCV Ab titers, or anti-HCV titers. The specimen is serum. Recombinant immunoblot assay (RIBA) principles may be employed in identifying an antibody response to the specific Hepatitis C virus. The presence of IgG antibody by RIBA is a confirmatory test.

86805-86806

86805 Lymphocytotoxicity assay, visual crossmatch; with titration
86806 without titration

Explanation

These tests may also be referred to as compatibility tests or major histocompatibility complex (MHC) tests. These tests pertain primarily to matching potential donor tissues to transplant patients, but uses may also include bench research. Methodology involves mixing purified donor lymphocytes with recipient sera or known antibodies. Cytotoxic reaction (cell death) is visually monitored, usually by incubation method. Indicator dyes may be used

to identify dead cells. Titration involves methodology to determine quantities. Report 86805 for testing with titration; 86806 for testing without titration.

86850

86850 Antibody screen, RBC, each serum technique

Explanation

This test may be ordered as an RBC antibody detection. The test is a screen for particular antibodies to red cell antigens that may present problems during a blood transfusion or childbirth. Blood specimen is whole blood. The test may be performed using tubes, microtiter plates, or gel cards. Another method is agglutination.

86860

86860 Antibody elution (RBC), each elution

Explanation

Elution is a technique for removing antibody from antibody/antigen complex on RBCs for identification purposes. Blood specimen is whole blood. The process is usually part of a workup to aid in diagnosis of certain autoimmune disorders such as autoimmune hemolytic anemia, and for resolution of incompatible crossmatches due to unidentified antibodies, and to identify the antibody causing hemolytic disease of a newborn (HDN).

86870

86870 Antibody identification, RBC antibodies, each panel for each serum technique

Explanation

This test is also known as an antibody panel. Blood specimen is whole blood. The test identifies an antibody isolated by techniques reported by 86850 and/or 86860 above. The test may be performed using tubes, microtiter plates, or gel cards. This code can be reported up to four times during the same session for differences in technique necessary for identification (i.e., regular panel, cold-panel, pre-warmed panel, and enzyme treated panel).

86880

86880 Antihuman globulin test (Coombs test); direct, each antiserum

Explanation

This test is also known as a direct Coombs or sometimes as a direct antiglobulin test (DAT). Blood specimen is whole blood. The test is used to detect coating of the RBCs by antibody or complement. It is useful in diagnosis of hemolytic disease of the newborn (HDN), detection of autoimmune hemolytic anemia, investigation of transfusion reactions, and detection of red cell sensitization reactions caused by medication. Method may be by gel test, flow cytometry, or enzyme-linked immunosorbent assay (ELISA) or hemagglutination.

86885

86885 Antihuman globulin test (Coombs test); indirect, qualitative, each reagent red cell

Explanation

This test is also known as an indirect Coombs, IAT, or sometimes as selective antibody screen. The indirect antiglobulin test indicates whether there is antibody in the serum, which will react to combine with antigen on the red cell. Uses for the IAT include determining if there are IgG antibodies (coating antibodies) in the patient's serum; investigating the ability to sensitize red blood cells; crossmatching, detection of Du (weak D) antigen; and investigation of transfusion reactions. The specimen is whole blood. Methodology includes agglutination, hemolysis of Type 0 test cells, flow cytometry, or enzyme-linked immunosorbent assay (ELISA). Report this code for each reagent red cell.

86900

86900 Blood typing; ABO

Explanation

This test may also be known as blood group. The test determines whether a patient is O, A, B, or AB by testing for the presence or absence of these antigens on the RBC surface. This typing of blood is the oldest and most widely recognized. Blood specimen is whole blood. The classic test method is by agglutination.

86901

86901 Blood typing; Rh (D)

Explanation

This test is known as Rh type. The test determines whether a patient is "positive" or "negative" by identifying the presence (Rh positive) or absence (Rh negative) of Rh antigens on the RBC surface. Blood specimen is whole blood. Method is enzyme-linked immunosorbent assay (ELISA), but may be performed by agglutination or gel test.

86906

86906 Blood typing; Rh phenotyping, complete

Explanation

Rh phenotyping may be required to assist in confirming the identity of an Rh antibody detected during screening, or when a family study is being undertaken for any number of reasons. Some donor centers maintain limited supplies of phenotyped blood to issue patients who have corresponding antibodies.

87015

87015 Concentration (any type), for infectious agents

Explanation

Concentration may also be referred to as thick smear preparation. The source samples are treated to concentrate the presence of suspect organisms, usually through sedimentation or flotation. There are two common methods of concentration for ova and parasite exams: formalin concentration and zinc sulfate flotation. The most common concentration methods for AFB stains or cultures are the N-acetyl-L cysteine method, cytocentrifuggation, and the Zephiran-trisodium phosphate method. Do not report 87015 in conjunction with 87177.

87040

87040 Culture, bacterial; blood, aerobic, with isolation and presumptive identification of isolates (includes anaerobic culture, if appropriate)

Explanation

Samples for bacterial blood culture are drawn by venipuncture and usually consist of a set of bottles, an aerobic and an anaerobic bottle. Drawing at least two sets of cultures increases the effectiveness of the test. This code includes anaerobic culture along with aerobic, if appropriate. Presumptive identification of aerobic pathogens or microorganisms in the blood sample is by means of identifying colony morphology. The test includes gram staining and subculturing to selective media for the detection of bacterial growth. There are several automated systems that detect the presence of bacteria using colorimetric, radiometric, or spectrophotometric means. The purpose of blood culture tests is to detect the presence of aerobic and anaerobic bacteria in blood and to identify the bacteria, but not to the specific level of genus or species requiring additional testing, such as slide cultures.

87045

87045 Culture, bacterial; stool, aerobic, with isolation and preliminary examination (eg, KIA, LIA), Salmonella and Shigella species

Explanation

This test may be called a stool culture, culture for *Salmonella* and *Shigella,* or routine culture when stool or rectal swab is the specimen. The testing method includes gram staining and subculturing to selective media for the detection of bacterial growth. This test cultures specifically for the initial identification of enteric pathogens *Salmonella* and *Shigella.*

87046

87046 Culture, bacterial; stool, aerobic, additional pathogens, isolation and presumptive identification of isolates, each plate

Explanation

This test may be requested by the name of the suspected pathogenic organism. Presumptive identification of aerobic pathogens or microorganisms in the stool sample is by means of identifying colony morphology. The test includes gram staining and subculturing to selective media for the detection of bacterial growth. There are several automated systems that detect the presence of bacteria using colorimetric, radiometric, or spectrophotometric means. The purpose of this stool culture test is to detect the presence of enteric pathogens in the form of aerobic bacteria and to identify the micro-organism(s), but not to the specific level of genus or species requiring additional testing, such as slide cultures. Report this code once for each plate prepared. Stool or rectal swab is the specimen.

87070-87071

87070 Culture, bacterial; any other source except urine, blood or stool, aerobic, with isolation and presumptive identification of isolates

87071 quantitative, aerobic with isolation and presumptive identification of isolates, any source except urine, blood or stool

Explanation

Common names for this test are numerous and may include routine culture, aerobic culture, or, using a body or source site, they may be referred to as vaginal culture, CSF culture, etc. The methodology is by bacterial culture and includes various identification procedures for the presumptive identification of any and multiple pathogens. The collection and transport of specimen is varied and specimen dependent.

87075

87075 Culture, bacterial; any source, except blood, anaerobic with isolation and presumptive identification of isolates

Explanation

The most common name for this procedure is anaerobic culture. Presumptive identification of anaerobic pathogens or microorganisms in the sample is by means of identifying colony morphology. The test includes gram staining and subculturing to selective media for the detection of bacterial growth. There are several automated systems that detect the presence of bacteria using colorimetric, radiometric, or spectrophotometric means. The purpose of this culture test is to detect the presence of any or multiple anaerobic bacteria from any body source or site, except blood, and to identify the micro-organism(s), but not to the specific level of genus or species requiring additional testing, such as slide cultures. Tissues, fluids, and aspirations, except blood samples, are collected in anaerobic vials or with anaerobic transport swabs and transported immediately. Anaerobic bacteria are sensitive to oxygen and cold.

Appendix

87076-87077

87076 Culture, bacterial; anaerobic isolate, additional methods required for definitive identification, each isolate

87077 aerobic isolate, additional methods required for definitive identification, each isolate

Explanation

This code reports definitive anaerobic (87076) or aerobic (87077) organism identification of an already-isolated anaerobic or aerobic bacterium. The pathogen has already been presumptively identified, but additional testing is required to identify the specific genus or species. The additional definitive testing methods include biochemical panels and slide cultures. Studies using chromatography, molecular probes, or specific immunological techniques may be employed for definitive testing, but are not included in this code and are reported separately.

87081-87084

87081 Culture, presumptive, pathogenic organisms, screening only;

87084 with colony estimation from density chart

Explanation

This is a presumptive screening culture for one or more pathogenic organisms. The methodology is by culture and the culture should be identified by type (e.g., anaerobic, aerobic) and specimen source (e.g., pleural, peritoneal, bronchial aspirates). If a specific organism is suspected, the person ordering the test will typically use common names, such as strep screen, staph screen, etc., to specify the organism for screening. Presumptive identification includes gram staining as well as up to three tests, such as a catalase, oxidase, or urease test. Screenings included in this code are nonmotile, catalase-positive, gram-positive rod bacteria. Report 87084 when an estimation of the number of organisms is also made, based on a density chart.

87086-87088

87086 Culture, bacterial; quantitative colony count, urine

87088 with isolation and presumptive identification of each isolate, urine

Explanation

These codes report the performance of a urine bacterial culture with a calibrated inoculating device so that a colony count accurately correlates with the number of organisms in the urine. In 87088, isolation and presumptive identification of bacteria recovered from the sample is done by means of identifying colony morphology, subculturing organisms to selective media and the performance of a gram stain or other simple test to identify bacteria to the genus level. There are several automated systems that detect the presence of bacteria using colorimetric, radiometric, or spectrophotometric means. In 87086, quantified colony count numbers within the urine sample are measured.

87101

87101 Culture, fungi (mold or yeast) isolation, with presumptive identification of isolates; skin, hair, or nail

Explanation

Dermatophyte culture and fungal culture are common names for this test. Fungi are divided into two broad categories, yeasts and molds. Skin, hair or nail scrapings from infected site are transferred to appropriate agar. Growth and confirmation by microscopic methods identify, or confirm, a presumptive identification of fungus isolated. Alternately, the scrapings are dropped onto dermatophyte test media (DMT) at the time of collection. The media changes color to indicate dermatophyte growth.

87102

87102 Culture, fungi (mold or yeast) isolation, with presumptive identification of isolates; other source (except blood)

Explanation

Fungal culture, yeast culture, and mold culture are common names for this procedure. Collection is as varied as the sources and the same specimen may be used for other tests. This test is to culture and isolate fungi (yeast or mold) with presumptive identification. Presumptive identification may include fungi (yeast or mold) present or a genus name with no species (e.g., Aspergillus).

87103

87103 Culture, fungi (mold or yeast) isolation, with presumptive identification of isolates; blood

Explanation

Fungal blood culture and blood culture for yeast are common names for this procedure. Blood is subcultured to fungal media. This test procedure is a culture to isolate fungi (yeast or mold) with presumptive identification. Presumptive identification may include fungi (yeast or mold) present or a genus name with no species (e.g., Aspergillus).

87106

87106 Culture, fungi, definitive identification, each organism; yeast

Explanation

This test is commonly known as a fungal yeast identification. Yeast isolates from fungal cultures are further tested for definitive identification. This code reports testing only for yeast pathogens. Various identification procedures, including growth patterns, and macroscopic and microscopic characteristics, are employed. Examples of fungal yeast pathogens that might require definitive identification include: Histoplasma, Coccidioides and Blastomyces.

87110

87110 Culture, chlamydia, any source

Explanation

This test is commonly known as a Chlamydia culture. A swab of the infected site is placed in a vial of sucrose transport media containing antibiotics and glass beads. The specimen is generally kept refrigerated. The test method is by cell culture, fluorescent stain. The cell culture technique is to isolate for Chlamydia.

87116

87116 Culture, tubercle or other acid-fast bacilli (eg, TB, AFB, mycobacteria) any source, with isolation and presumptive identification of isolates

Explanation

Common names include AFB culture, TB culture, mycobacterium culture, and acid-fast culture. Collection methods are source dependent. The methodology is by culture for the isolation and presumptive identification of mycobacterium. An acid-fast smear should be done at the time the specimen is cultured. Media for isolation should include both solid and liquid types.

87118

87118 Culture, mycobacterial, definitive identification, each isolate

Explanation

This procedure is a definitive identification of mycobacterial organisms isolated by procedure 87116. This procedure may be performed by a reference laboratory after isolation by a primary lab. Methodology is traditional biochemical tests for identification of mycobacterium.

87140

87140 Culture, typing; immunofluorescent method, each antiserum

Explanation

Specific antisera are combined with a fluorescent dye and used to stain slides of organisms. Stained slides are scanned with a fluorescent microscope to look for fluorescing organisms. Typing of organisms by immunofluorescent technique is usually to determine whether an organism is of a more pathogenic strain, to determine a treatment, or for epidemiological purposes.

87143

87143 Culture, typing; gas liquid chromatography (GLC) or high pressure liquid chromatography (HPLC) method

Explanation

This procedure is performed to provide more specific typing of cultured pathogenic organisms. The methodology is gas liquid chromatography (GLC) or high pressure liquid chromatography (HPLC) to analyze byproducts of rapidly growing organisms. GLC is an automated technique in which the culture specimen is dissolved in a solvent, vaporized, and transported by an inert gas through an adsorbent gas-liquid column containing detectors that analyze and graph the components of the specimen. HPLC is similar to GLC except that the liquid is forced under high pressure through a column packed with sorbent and separated by various methods including adsorption, gel filtration, ion-exchange, or partition. This procedure is performed on an isolated organism as in the definitive identification of mycobacterium.

87147

87147 Culture, typing; immunologic method, other than immunofluoresence (eg, agglutination grouping), per antiserum

Explanation

This test is used for more specifically identifying cultured specimens using an immunologic method other than immunofluorescence. For example, agglutination technique may be used to more specifically identify Salmonella usually to a group level since there are more than 2,000 serovar of Salmonella. The different species have been grouped by common antigens and are tested with polyvalent antisera and reported by group (e.g., Salmonella Group D).

87158

87158 Culture, typing; other methods

Explanation

Any methodology that would identify a microbial organism to the species level or a type level that does not involve the use of biochemical substrates (traditional bacteriology), antigen specific fluorescent stain, gas chromatography, phage testing, or agglutination or precipitation from antigen-antibody reactions. Lectin assays and bacteriocin typing are two tests that fit in this procedure description.

87164-87166

87164 Dark field examination, any source (eg, penile, vaginal, oral, skin); includes specimen collection

87166 without collection

Explanation

Names commonly used include dark field for syphilis and dark field exam. Dark field microscopic exams have generally been limited to the bacteria called spirochetes. *Treponema pallidum,* the agent of syphilis; *Borrelia burgdorferi,* the agent of Lyme disease; and *Leptospira* are among the better known spirochetes. Specimens for dark field exam are typically examined within 30 minutes of collection. Certain immunological tests have rendered this method to be somewhat outdated. The term "dark field" refers to the staining method. If the lab is responsible for specimen collection, report 87164. If the lab is not responsible for collection of the specimen, report 87166.

87181

87181 Susceptibility studies, antimicrobial agent; agar dilution method, per agent (eg, antibiotic gradient strip)

Explanation

A susceptibility study is performed to determine the susceptibility of a bacterium to an antibiotic. The methodology is agar diffusion (the E test is a method of agar diffusion). The specific antibiotics could be chosen and limited. The test is reported per antibiotic tested. The agar dilution is reported as minimum inhibitory concentration (MIC), which is a method of measuring the exact amount of antibiotic needed to inhibit an organism.

87184

87184 Susceptibility studies, antimicrobial agent; disk method, per plate (12 or fewer agents)

Explanation

This is commonly called a Kirby-Bauer or Bauer-Kirby sensitivity test. It is a sensitivity test to determine the susceptibility of a bacterium to an antibiotic. The methodology is disk diffusion and results are reported as sensitive, intermediate, or resistant. As many as 12 antibiotic disks may be used per plate and the procedure is billed per plate not per antibiotic disk.

87185

87185 Susceptibility studies, antimicrobial agent; enzyme detection (eg, beta lactamase), per enzyme

Explanation

Bacteria produce enzymes that can inactivate some types of antibiotics. This susceptibility test identifies those bacteria that will be resistant to certain types of antibiotics by detecting the presence of these enzymes.

87186

87186 Susceptibility studies, antimicrobial agent; microdilution or agar dilution (minimum inhibitory concentration [MIC] or breakpoint), each multi-antimicrobial, per plate

Explanation

This procedure may be called an MIC, or a sensitivity test. It is a sensitivity test to determine the susceptibility of a bacterium to an antibiotic. The methodology is microtiter dilution (several commercial panels use this method). Results are given as a minimum inhibitory concentration (MIC) with an interpretation of sensitive, intermediate, or resistant. The antibiotics on commercial plates are numerous, but predetermined. The procedure is charged by plate not by antibiotic.

87187

87187 Susceptibility studies, antimicrobial agent; microdilution or agar dilution, minimum lethal concentration (MLC), each plate (List separately in addition to code for primary procedure)

Explanation

This test may be called an MBC (minimum bactericidal concentration). MBC is the dilution of antibiotic needed to kill the bacteria. MICs are tube dilutions read visually. Tubes that may visually appear to have no growth are cultured to solid media to detect a concentration of antibiotic where no organisms grow (MBC).

87188

87188 Susceptibility studies, antimicrobial agent; macrobroth dilution method, each agent

Explanation

This test may be referred to as an MIC (minimum inhibitory concentration). It is a susceptibility test to determine the sensitivity of a bacterium to an antibiotic. The methodology is macrobroth dilution. Results are given as a minimum inhibitory concentration (MIC) with an interpretation of sensitive, intermediate, or resistant. The procedure is charged per antibiotic tested.

87190

87190 Susceptibility studies, antimicrobial agent; mycobacteria, proportion method, each agent

Explanation

Mycobacterium susceptibility test is a procedure done only on mycobacterium (e.g., M. tuberculosis, M. marinum, etc.). Proportion method is used and involves testing of a panel of antibiotics used only for the treatment of mycobacterium. Results are given as sensitive or resistant.

Coding Companion for Ob/Gyn

87205

87205 Smear, primary source with interpretation; Gram or Giemsa stain for bacteria, fungi, or cell types

Explanation

Any smear done on a primary source (e.g., sputum, CSF, etc.) to identify bacteria, fungi, and cell types. An interpretation of findings is provided. Bacteria, fungi, WBCs, and epithelial cells may be estimated in quantity with an interpretation as to the possibility of contamination by normal flora. A gram stain may be the most commonly performed smear of this type.

87206

87206 Smear, primary source with interpretation; fluorescent and/or acid fast stain for bacteria, fungi, parasites, viruses or cell types

Explanation

A fluorescent or acid-fast stain for bacteria, fungi, parasites, viruses, or cell types. These are stains usually for specific groups of organisms (e.g., mycobacterium and *Nocardia*). Identification of *Cryptosporidium* and related parasites are examples of parasites that can be identified by fluorescent or acid fast stain. An interpretation is included.

87207

87207 Smear, primary source with interpretation; special stain for inclusion bodies or parasites (eg, malaria, coccidia, microsporidia, trypanosomes, herpes viruses)

Explanation

This is a stain to look for inclusion bodies or parasites (e.g., malaria inside red cells). Its use to detect herpes has been outdated by amplification and immunological methods. An interpretation is included.

87210

87210 Smear, primary source with interpretation; wet mount for infectious agents (eg, saline, India ink, KOH preps)

Explanation

This test may be requested as a KOH prep. A wet mount is prepared from a primary source to detect bacteria, fungi, or ova and parasites. Motility of organisms is visible on wet mounts and the addition of a simple stain, such as iodine, India ink, or simple dyes, may aid detection of bacteria, fungi, and parasites. An interpretation of findings is included.

87220

87220 Tissue examination by KOH slide of samples from skin, hair, or nails for fungi or ectoparasite ova or mites (eg, scabies)

Explanation

Potassium hydroxide (KOH) prep and calcofluor stains are the most common methods of looking for hyphal elements and/ or yeast in tissue. The KOH causes a clearing of the specimen to make fungus more visible. The preparation is enhanced for microscopic observation by adding a drop of calcofluor, a type of fluorescent dye, to the slide and reading the preparation with a fluorescent microscope.

87270

87270 Infectious agent antigen detection by immunofluorescent technique; Chlamydia trachomatis

Explanation

This test may be requested as Chlamydia trachomatis or C. trachomatis by DFA or by immunofluorescence. C. trachomatis is a frequently occurring sexually transmitted disease. It may cause nonspecific urethritis or pelvic inflammatory disease (PID), although it is frequently asymptomatic in women. Another serotype also causes conjunctivitis. Infectious agent antigen detection by immunofluorescence includes direct and indirect fluorescent antibody technique and involves using monoclonal antibodies and immunofluorescence microscopy. Cellular material must be obtained from the site for immunofluorescence to be an effective diagnostic technique.

87271

87271 Infectious agent antigen detection by immunofluorescent technique; Cytomegalovirus, direct fluorescent antibody (DFA)

Explanation

A cytomegalovirus is detected by direct fluorescent antibody (DFA) staining technique. The presence of the infectious agent microorganism is detected indirectly when the fluorescent reaction of the dye is seen under a special microscope. The cytomegalovirus is isolated in cell culture for the test. Specimens include throat swabs, CSF, and blood samples. A cytomegalovirus is any virus in the Betaherpesvirinae subfamily.

87274

87274 Infectious agent antigen detection by immunofluorescent technique; Herpes simplex virus type 1

Explanation

This test may be requested as HSV 1 by DFA or HSV 1 by immunofluorescence. HSV 1 is primarily responsible for oral lesions frequently referred to as fever blisters or cold sores. Infectious agent antigen detection by immunofluorescence includes direct and indirect fluorescent antibody technique and involves using monoclonal antibodies and immunofluorescence microscopy. Cellular material must be obtained from the site for immunofluorescence to be an effective diagnostic technique.

87285

87285 Infectious agent antigen detection by immunofluorescent technique; Treponema pallidum

Explanation

The spirochete Treponema pallidum is the causative agent of syphilis. Infectious agent antigen detection by immunofluorescence includes direct and indirect fluorescent antibody technique and involves using monoclonal antibodies and immunofluorescence microscopy. Cellular material must be obtained from the site for immunofluorescence to be an effective diagnostic technique.

87320

87320 Infectious agent antigen detection by enzyme immunoassay technique, qualitative or semiquantitative, multiple-step method; Chlamydia trachomatis

Explanation

This test may be requested as Chlamydia trachomatis or C. trachomatis by enzyme immunoassay (EIA). C. trachomatis is a frequently occurring sexually transmitted disease. It may cause nonspecific urethritis or pelvic inflammatory disease (PID), although it is frequently asymptomatic in women. Another serotype also causes conjunctivitis. Enzyme immunoassay refers to a technique that utilizes a chemical bond between an enzyme and an antigen or antibody as a label to identify specific chemical or infectious agents. Special reagents and equipment are required for C. trachomatis EIA. Sensitivity of EIA is approximately 75 to 85 percent.

87340

87340 Infectious agent antigen detection by enzyme immunoassay technique, qualitative or semiquantitative, multiple-step method; hepatitis B surface antigen (HBsAg)

Explanation

This test may be requested as HBsAg by enzyme immunoassay (EIA). Hepatitis B is a retrovirus that can cause persistent infection leading to cirrhosis and hepatocellular carcinoma. HBsAg is a lipoprotein that coats the surface of the hepatitis B virus. Blood specimen is serum. This test may be requested as HBsAg by enzyme immunoassay (EIA) confirmation. This assay is performed only when a specimen is repeatedly reactive for Hepatitis B surface antigen. Elevated HBsAg levels beyond 6 months may indicate a chronic carrier (i.e., chronic hepatitis). The HBsAg neutralization test is performed to identify false positives. False positives on a standard HBsAg test will not neutralize with anti-HBs in the confirmatory assay. Hepatitis B is a retrovirus that can cause persistent infection leading to cirrhosis and hepatocellular carcinoma. HBsAg is a lipoprotein that coats the surface of the hepatitis B virus. Blood specimen is serum.

87350

87350 Infectious agent antigen detection by enzyme immunoassay technique, qualitative or semiquantitative, multiple-step method; hepatitis Be antigen (HBeAg)

Explanation

This test may be requested as HBeAg by enzyme immunoassay (EIA). Hepatitis B is a retrovirus that can cause persistent infection leading to cirrhosis and hepatocellular carcinoma. HBeAg is normally tested only on individuals who are chronically HBsAg positive. Blood specimen is serum.

87380

87380 Infectious agent antigen detection by enzyme immunoassay technique, qualitative or semiquantitative, multiple-step method; hepatitis, delta agent

Explanation

This test may be requested as hepatitis delta agent (HDAg) by enzyme immunoassay (EIA). Hepatitis delta agent is normally tested only on individuals who are chronically HBsAg positive or have an exacerbation of their hepatitis as HDAg requires the presence of HBsAg to become an infectious virus. Blood specimen is serum.

87389

87389 Infectious agent antigen detection by enzyme immunoassay technique, qualitative or semiquantitative, multiple-step method; HIV-1 antigen(s), with HIV-1 and HIV-2 antibodies, single result

Explanation

This test may be requested as human immunodeficiency virus type 1 (HIV-1) and type 2 (HIV-2) by EIA. HIV-1 is the causative agent of acquired immunodeficiency syndrome (AIDS). HIV-2 is a retrovirus closely related to simian AIDS and was found initially in West African nations and Portugal, but cases have been reported in the United States

since 1987. Blood specimen is obtained by venipuncture. Enzyme immunoassay refers to a technique that utilizes a chemical bond between an enzyme and an antigen or antibody as a label to identify specific chemical or infectious agents. If EIA is positive, it is repeated. Two out of three tests must be positive before the test is reported as positive. All positive EIA tests are confirmed with an additional test using a different technique, usually Western blot, which is reported separately.

87390

87390 Infectious agent antigen detection by enzyme immunoassay technique, qualitative or semiquantitative, multiple-step method; HIV-1

Explanation

This test may be requested as human immunodeficiency virus Type 1 (HIV-1) by EIA. HIV-1 is the causative agent of acquired immunodeficiency syndrome (AIDS). Blood specimen is obtained by venipuncture. Enzyme immunoassay refers to a technique that utilizes a chemical bond between an enzyme and an antigen or antibody as a label to identify specific chemical or infectious agents. If EIA is positive, it is repeated. Two out of three tests must be positive before the test is reported as positive. All positive EIA tests are confirmed with an additional test using a different technique, usually Western blot, which is reported separately.

87391

87391 Infectious agent antigen detection by enzyme immunoassay technique, qualitative or semiquantitative, multiple-step method; HIV-2

Explanation

This test may be requested as human immunodeficiency virus Type 2 (HIV-2) by EIA. HIV-2 is a retrovirus closely related to simian AIDS and found initially in West African nations and Portugal, but with cases also being reported in the United States since 1987. Blood specimen is serum. If EIA is positive, it is repeated. Two out of three tests must be positive before the test is reported as positive. All positive EIA tests are confirmed with an additional test using a different technique, usually Western blot, which is reported separately.

87480

87480 Infectious agent detection by nucleic acid (DNA or RNA); Candida species, direct probe technique

Explanation

This test is used to diagnosis an infection by any species of Candida, but usually C. albicans. This test would normally be performed to diagnosis systemic (invasive) candidiasis. Blood is serum. The specimen is treated to isolate nucleic acid (DNA, RNA). Nucleic acid is analyzed using direct probe technique.

87481

87481 Infectious agent detection by nucleic acid (DNA or RNA); Candida species, amplified probe technique

Explanation

This test is used to diagnosis an infection by any species of Candida, but usually C. albicans. This test would normally be performed to diagnosis systemic (invasive) candidiasis. Blood is serum. The specimen is treated to isolate the nucleic acid (DNA, RNA) and eliminate substances that inhibit amplification. The nucleic acid is amplified using specific primers for Candida sequences.

87482

87482 Infectious agent detection by nucleic acid (DNA or RNA); Candida species, quantification

Explanation

This test is used to diagnosis an infection by any species of Candida, but usually C. albicans. This test would normally be performed to diagnosis systemic (invasive) candidiasis. Blood is serum. The specimen is treated to isolate the nucleic acid (DNA, RNA). This code reports quantification only and is used primarily to assess extent of disease or disease progression.

87490

87490 Infectious agent detection by nucleic acid (DNA or RNA); Chlamydia trachomatis, direct probe technique

Explanation

This test may be requested as Chlamydia trachomatis or C. trachomatis by direct DNA probe. C. trachomatis is a frequently occurring sexually transmitted disease. It may cause nonspecific urethritis or pelvic inflammatory disease (PID), although it is frequently asymptomatic in women. Another serotype also causes conjunctivitis. The specimen is treated to isolate the DNA using direct probe.

87491

87491 Infectious agent detection by nucleic acid (DNA or RNA); Chlamydia trachomatis, amplified probe technique

Explanation

This test may be requested as Chlamydia trachomatis or C. trachomatis by polymerase chain reaction. C. trachomatis is a frequently occurring sexually transmitted disease. It may cause nonspecific urethritis or pelvic inflammatory disease (PID), although it is frequently asymptomatic in women. Another serotype also causes conjunctivitis. The DNA is amplified using a technique such as polymerase chain reaction (PCR).

87492

87492 Infectious agent detection by nucleic acid (DNA or RNA); Chlamydia trachomatis, quantification

Explanation

This test may be requested as Chlamydia trachomatis or C. trachomatis DNA quantification. C. trachomatis is a frequently occurring sexually transmitted disease. It may cause nonspecific urethritis or pelvic inflammatory disease (PID), although it is frequently asymptomatic in women. Another serotype also causes conjunctivitis. This code reports quantification only.

87493

87493 Infectious agent detection by nucleic acid (DNA or RNA); Clostridium difficile, toxin gene(s), amplified probe technique

Explanation

This code reports infectious agent detection by nucleic acid (DNA, RNA) amplified probe for clostridium difficile toxin B (tcdB). This test is used to diagnose patients whose symptoms include persistent non-bloody diarrhea, decreased appetite, abdominal discomfort, and elevated temperature following antibiotic therapy. Nucleic acid detection, also referred to as molecular pathology, is a rapidly developing diagnostic technique that is especially useful in identifying microorganisms that require tedious isolation and incubation and/or those which cannot be cultured. Another advantage of molecular methods is that they are able to detect infectious agents at much lower levels than required using other techniques. Amplified probe involves isolating and identifying the infectious agent DNA or RNA. This involves cell lysis and extraction of the DNA using phenol or chloroform. The nucleic acids are amplified using one of several techniques. Polymerase chain reaction (PCR) is the most frequently used amplification technique.

87501-87503

87501 Infectious agent detection by nucleic acid (DNA or RNA); influenza virus, reverse transcription and amplified probe technique, each type or subtype

87502 influenza virus, for multiple types or sub-types, multiplex reverse transcription and amplified probe technique, first 2 types or sub-types

87503 influenza virus, for multiple types or sub-types, multiplex reverse transcription and amplified probe technique, each additional influenza virus type or sub-type beyond 2 (List separately in addition to code for primary procedure)

Explanation

These codes report influenza virus infectious agent detection by nucleic acid (DNA or RNA) using reverse transcription and amplified probe technique. Nucleic acid detection, also referred to as molecular pathology, is a rapidly developing diagnostic technique that is especially useful in identifying microorganisms that require tedious isolation and incubation and/or those that cannot be cultured, and nucleic acid amplification tests are among the most sensitive and specific influenza tests. Specimen may be nasal, nasopharyngeal, or oropharyngeal swab; nasal or endotracheal aspirate; bronchoalveolar lavage (BAL); or pleural fluid. Testing for the influenza virus by amplified probe requires a molecular method referred to as reverse transcription polymerase chain reaction (RT-PCR). Report 87501 for each type or subtype and 87502 for the first two types or subtypes when testing for multiple types/subtypes. A separately reportable code (87503) is reported for each additional type or subtype beyond two.

87515

87515 Infectious agent detection by nucleic acid (DNA or RNA); hepatitis B virus, direct probe technique

Explanation

This test may be requested as HBV DNA direct probe. Hepatitis B is a retrovirus that can cause persistent infection leading to cirrhosis and hepatocellular carcinoma. Molecular (DNA) tests are useful in identifying potentially infectious individuals as well as chronic progression of the disease. Blood specimen is serum. A liver biopsy is required for analysis of liver tissue and is reported separately. The specimen is treated to isolate the DNA using direct probe.

87516

87516 Infectious agent detection by nucleic acid (DNA or RNA); hepatitis B virus, amplified probe technique

Explanation

This test may be requested as HBV DNA by polymerase chain reaction (PCR). Hepatitis B is a retrovirus that can cause persistent infection leading to cirrhosis and hepatocellular carcinoma. Molecular (DNA) tests are useful in identifying potentially infectious individuals as well as chronic progression of the disease. Blood specimen is serum. A liver biopsy is required for analysis of liver tissue and is reported separately The DNA is amplified using a technique such as polymerase chain reaction (PCR).

87517

87517 Infectious agent detection by nucleic acid (DNA or RNA); hepatitis B virus, quantification

Explanation

This test may be requested as HBV DNA quantification. Hepatitis B is a retrovirus that can cause persistent infection leading to cirrhosis and hepatocellular carcinoma. Blood specimen is serum. A liver biopsy is required for analysis of liver tissue and is reported separately. Quantification is used primarily to monitor response to therapy in chronic hepatitis B. This code reports quantification only.

87520

87520 Infectious agent detection by nucleic acid (DNA or RNA); hepatitis C, direct probe technique

Explanation

This test may be requested as HCV RNA direct probe. Hepatitis C is also referred to as non-A non-B (NANB) hepatitis. Blood specimen is serum. A liver biopsy is required for analysis of liver tissue and is reported separately. The specimen is treated to isolate the RNA using direct probe. This test is used primarily by research facilities.

87521-87522

87521 Infectious agent detection by nucleic acid (DNA or RNA); hepatitis C, reverse transcription and amplified probe technique

87522 hepatitis C, reverse transcription and quantification

Explanation

Hepatitis C is also referred to as non-A non-B (NANB) hepatitis. Blood specimen is plasma or serum. This test is used to detect infectious agents using the organism's DNA/RNA. In reverse transcription, the RNA from the organism is mapped to a single strand DNA allowing it to replicate. Report 87521 when the testing includes an amplified probe technique or reverse transcription polymerase chain reaction (RT-PCR) in which the reversely transcribed DNA is repeatedly duplicated (amplified) and detected using various methods. This test is used primarily by research facilities. Report 87522 if quantification of the RNA/DNA to monitor the effects of treatment is all that is performed.

Coding Tips

These codes have been revised for 2013 in the official CPT description.

87528

87528 Infectious agent detection by nucleic acid (DNA or RNA); Herpes simplex virus, direct probe technique

Explanation

This test may be requested as HSV by direct DNA probe. Herpes simplex may be classified as HSV type 1 (HSV 1) or HSV type 2 (HSV 2). HSV 1 is primarily responsible for oral lesions frequently referred to as

Appendix

fever blisters or cold sores. HSV 2 is a sexually transmitted disease with lesions occurring primarily in the genitourinary tract. Lesion swab/scrapings are obtained. CSF is obtained by spinal puncture. Blood specimen is serum. The specimen is treated to isolate the DNA using direct probe. Detection and typing (HSV1, HSV2) by direct DNA probe is superior to culture methods.

87529

87529 Infectious agent detection by nucleic acid (DNA or RNA); Herpes simplex virus, amplified probe technique

Explanation

This test may be requested as HSV by amplified DNA probe. Herpes simplex may be classified as HSV type 1 (HSV 1) or HSV type 2 (HSV 2). HSV 1 is primarily responsible for oral lesions frequently referred to as fever blisters or cold sores. HSV 2 is a sexually transmitted disease with lesions occurring primarily in the genitourinary tract. Lesion swab/scrapings are obtained. CSF is obtained by spinal puncture. Blood specimen is serum. The DNA is amplified using a technique such as polymerase chain reaction (PCR). Detection and typing (HSV 1, HSV 2) by amplified DNA probe is superior to culture methods.

87530

87530 Infectious agent detection by nucleic acid (DNA or RNA); Herpes simplex virus, quantification

Explanation

This test may be requested as HSV quantification by molecular technique. Herpes simplex may be classified as HSV type 1 (HSV 1) or HSV type 2 (HSV 2). HSV 1 is primarily responsible for oral lesions frequently referred to as fever blisters or cold sores. HSV 2 is a sexually transmitted disease with lesions occurring primarily in the genitourinary tract. Lesion swab/scrapings are obtained. CSF is obtained by spinal puncture. Blood specimen is serum. This code reports quantification only.

87531

87531 Infectious agent detection by nucleic acid (DNA or RNA); Herpes virus-6, direct probe technique

Explanation

This test may be requested as HHV-6 direct DNA probe. Human herpes virus-6 is most commonly associated with roseola in children, but also causes pneumonitis, encephalitis, and hepatitis in immunosuppressed individuals. Sputum is obtained by deep coughing or by separately reportable aerosol induced technique. Respiratory fluids may also be obtained endoscopically using bronchial alveolar lavage and reported separately. CSF is obtained by spinal puncture and reported separately. Blood specimen is serum. Liver tissue is obtained by biopsy, also reported separately. The

cells are lysed and DNA is extracted. HHV-6 DNA is identified by direct probe.

87532

87532 Infectious agent detection by nucleic acid (DNA or RNA); Herpes virus-6, amplified probe technique

Explanation

This test may be requested as HHV-6 amplified DNA probe. Human herpes virus-6 is most commonly associated with roseola in children, but also causes pneumonitis, encephalitis, and hepatitis in immunosuppressed individuals. Sputum is obtained by deep coughing or by separately reportable aerosol induced technique. Respiratory fluids may also be obtained endoscopically using bronchial alveolar lavage and reported separately. CSF is obtained by spinal puncture, which is reported separately. Blood specimen is serum. Liver tissue is obtained by biopsy, also reported separately. The cells are lysed and DNA is extracted. HHV-6 DNA is amplified using specific primers.

87533

87533 Infectious agent detection by nucleic acid (DNA or RNA); Herpes virus-6, quantification

Explanation

This test may be requested as HHV-6 quantification using nucleic acid technique. Human herpes virus-6 is most commonly associated with roseola in children, but also causes pneumonitis, encephalitis, and hepatitis in immunosuppressed individuals. Sputum is obtained by deep coughing or by separately reportable aerosol induced technique. Respiratory fluids may also be obtained endoscopically using bronchial alveolar lavage, which is reported separately. CSF is obtained by spinal puncture and reported separately. Blood specimen is serum. Liver tissue is obtained by biopsy, also reported separately. The cells are lysed and DNA is extracted. This code reports quantification only.

87534

87534 Infectious agent detection by nucleic acid (DNA or RNA); HIV-1, direct probe technique

Explanation

This test may be requested as human immunodeficiency virus Type 1 (HIV-1) by direct nucleic acid (DNA, RNA) probe. HIV is the causative agent of acquired immunodeficiency syndrome (AIDS). Blood specimen is serum. A random urine sample is obtained. Tissue is obtained by separately reportable biopsy procedure. The specimen is treated to isolate the DNA using direct probe.

87535-87536

87535 Infectious agent detection by nucleic acid (DNA or RNA); HIV-1, reverse transcription and amplified probe technique

87536 HIV-1, reverse transcription and quantification

Explanation

HIV is the causative agent of acquired immunodeficiency syndrome (AIDS). Specimen is serum. This test is used to detect infectious agents using the organism's DNA/RNA. In reverse transcription, the RNA from the organism is mapped to a single strand DNA allowing it to replicate. Report 87535 when the testing includes an amplified probe technique or reverse transcription polymerase chain reaction (RT-PCR) in which the reversely transcribed DNA is repeatedly duplicated (amplified) and detected using various methods. This test is used primarily by research facilities. Report 87536 if quantification of the RNA/DNA is all that is performed to monitor the effects of treatment.

Coding Tips

These codes have been revised for 2013 in the official CPT description.

87537

87537 Infectious agent detection by nucleic acid (DNA or RNA); HIV-2, direct probe technique

Explanation

This test may be requested as human immunodeficiency virus Type 2 (HIV-2) by EIA. HIV-2 is a retrovirus closely related to simian AIDS and found initially in West African nations and Portugal, but with cases also being reported in the United States since 1987. Blood specimen is serum. The specimen is treated to isolate the DNA using direct probe.

87538-87539

87538 Infectious agent detection by nucleic acid (DNA or RNA); HIV-2, reverse transcription and amplified probe technique

87539 HIV-2, reverse transcription and quantification

Explanation

This test may be requested as human immunodeficiency virus Type 2 (HIV-2). HIV-2 is a retrovirus closely related to simian AIDS and found initially in West African nations and Portugal, but with cases also being reported in the United States since 1987. Blood specimen is serum. This test is used to detect infectious agents using the organism's DNA/RNA. In reverse transcription, the RNA from the organism is mapped to a single strand DNA allowing it to replicate. Report 87538 when the testing includes an amplified probe technique

Appendix

or reverse transcription polymerase chain reaction (RT-PCR) in which the reversely transcribed DNA is repeatedly duplicated (amplified) and detected using various methods. This test is used primarily by research facilities. Report 87539 if quantification of the DNA is all that is performed to monitor the effects of treatment.

Coding Tips

These codes have been revised for 2013 in the official CPT description.

87590

87590 Infectious agent detection by nucleic acid (DNA or RNA); Neisseria gonorrhoeae, direct probe technique

Explanation

This test may be requested as gonorrhea direct DNA probe, gonorrhea molecular probe assay, or DNA detection of gonorrhea. Neisseria gonorrhea is one of the most common sexually transmitted infections. Molecular (nucleic acid probe) techniques offer rapid, accurate identification of Neisseria gonorrhea. While a cervical or urethral swab is preferred, molecular techniques are sensitive enough to detect the organism in urine also. Neisseria gonorrhea can be detected by DNA, RNA, or rRNA probes.

87591

87591 Infectious agent detection by nucleic acid (DNA or RNA); Neisseria gonorrhoeae, amplified probe technique

Explanation

This test may be requested as gonorrhea amplified DNA probe, gonorrhea molecular probe assay, or DNA detection of gonorrhea. Neisseria gonorrhea is one of the most common sexually transmitted infections. Molecular (nucleic acid probe) techniques offer rapid, accurate identification of Neisseria gonorrhea. While a cervical or urethral swab is preferred, molecular techniques are sensitive enough to detect the organism in urine also. Neisseria gonorrhea can be detected by DNA or rRNA probes. Amplification can be performed using a number of techniques. Polymerase chain reaction (PCR) and ligase chain reaction (LCR) detect gonorrhea DNA. An assay is also available which detects gonorrhea ribosomal RNA (rRNA)

87592

87592 Infectious agent detection by nucleic acid (DNA or RNA); Neisseria gonorrhoeae, quantification

Explanation

This test may be requested as gonorrhea nucleic acid quantification. Neisseria gonorrhea is one of the most common sexually transmitted infections. Molecular (nucleic acid probe) techniques offer rapid, accurate identification of Neisseria gonorrhea. While a cervical or urethral swab is preferred,

molecular techniques are sensitive enough to detect the organism in urine also. Neisseria gonorrhea can be detected by DNA or rRNA probes. This code reports quantification only.

87620

87620 Infectious agent detection by nucleic acid (DNA or RNA); papillomavirus, human, direct probe technique

Explanation

This test may be requested as human papillomavirus (HPV) direct DNA probe. Human papillomaviruses are a genus of viruses that causes warts (benign neoplasms of skin and mucous membranes). There are at least 58 known types. HPV is commonly associated with both plantar and genital warts. HPV infection of the cervix is of particular concern as it may be associated with cervical cancer. The specimen is probed with commercially available DNA probes for specific HPV types. DNA probes are specific for HPV types 6, 11, 16, 18, 31, 33, and 35.

87621

87621 Infectious agent detection by nucleic acid (DNA or RNA); papillomavirus, human, amplified probe technique

Explanation

This test may be requested as human papillomavirus (HPV) amplified DNA probe. Human papillomaviruses are a genus of viruses that causes warts (benign neoplasms of skin and mucous membranes). There are at least 58 known types. HPV is commonly associated with both plantar and genital warts. HPV infection of the cervix is of particular concern as it may be associated with cervical cancer. The specimen is amplified by polymerase chain reaction (PCR) and probed for specific HPV types. DNA probes are only able to detect a limited number of HPV types, including types 6, 11, 16, 18, 31, 33, and 35.

87622

87622 Infectious agent detection by nucleic acid (DNA or RNA); papillomavirus, human, quantification

Explanation

This test may be requested as human papillomavirus (HPV) amplified DNA probe. Human papillomaviruses are a genus of viruses that causes warts (benign neoplasms of skin and mucous membranes). There are at least 58 known types. HPV is commonly associated with both plantar and genital warts. HPV infection of the cervix is of particular concern as it may be associated with cervical cancer. The specimen is treated to encourage attachment of HPV DNA to filters. This code reports quantification only.

87660

87660 Infectious agent detection by nucleic acid (DNA or RNA); Trichomonas vaginalis, direct probe technique

Explanation

A microbiology test for trichomonas vaginalis, by direct probe technique, may be requested as trichomonas vaginalis direct DNA probe, molecular probe assay, or DNA detection of trichomonas vaginalis. Direct probe is a method to detect DNA of a target microorganism. This technique uses DNA probes that hybridize to whole chromosomes or specific target sequences for detection. The target DNA in the sample is fixed onto a slide and denatured from double-stranded DNA to single-stranded DNA. The target DNA is hybridized with that of the probe, reassociating into double-stranded nucleic acid. The unbound DNA is removed and the remaining DNA is counterstained and placed under fluoroscopy to visualize the hybridized probe attached to the target material.

87810

87810 Infectious agent antigen detection by immunoassay with direct optical observation; Chlamydia trachomatis

Explanation

This test may be requested as an optical immunoassay for Chlamydia trachomatis. C. trachomatis is a frequently occurring sexually transmitted disease. It may cause nonspecific urethritis or pelvic inflammatory disease (PID), although it is frequently asymptomatic in women. Another serotype also causes conjunctivitis. This test reports antigen detection using a competitive protein-binding assay, where an antigen binds to an antibody, which is fixed to a reflecting surface. This change in reflection can be observed directly as a color change.

87850

87850 Infectious agent antigen detection by immunoassay with direct optical observation; Neisseria gonorrhoeae

Explanation

This test may be requested as an optical immunoassay for Neisseria gonorrhea. N. Gonorrhea is one of the most common sexually transmitted infections. This test reports detection using a competitive protein-binding assay where an antigen binds to an antibody, which is fixed to a reflecting surface. This change in reflection can be observed directly as a color change.

Appendix

88104-88106

88104 Cytopathology, fluids, washings or brushings, except cervical or vaginal; smears with interpretation

88106 simple filter method with interpretation

Explanation

These tests have many different names, depending on the type of specimen obtained for analysis (e.g., bronchial cytology, esophageal cytology, etc.). Specimen is obtained by separately reportable washing or brushing procedure. Code 88104 reports cytopathology evaluation of smear specimens, including alcohol fixed, Papanicolaou, direct smear with 95 percent ethanol, or liquid fixative. Report 88106 for a simple filter method only.

88108

88108 Cytopathology, concentration technique, smears and interpretation (eg, Saccomanno technique)

Explanation

Cytopathology, concentration technique, (e.g., Saccomanno, cytocentrifugation, and cytospins) may be done on many different types of specimen samples like bronchial, cervicovaginal, and conjunctival brushings, nipple discharge, sputum, and gastrointestinal epithelial cell specimens. Cellular smear preparations (cervicovaginal, conjunctival, bronchial brushings, nipple discharge) are immediately fixated in 95 percent ethanol or pap fixative to eliminate drying. GI, urologic, and sputum samples are collected with a Saccomanno fixative added. Following preparation, the sample is centrifuged to yield a pellet at the bottom of the tube and overlying supernatant. The clear fluid supernatant is decanted completely and the pellet is used to make direct smears of the concentrated sample for cytopathology and cell counts. Cytocentrifugation, cytospins, smears and interpretations are then preformed.

88112

88112 Cytopathology, selective cellular enhancement technique with interpretation (eg, liquid based slide preparation method), except cervical or vaginal

Explanation

Selective cellular enhancement for cytopathology, such as liquid based slide preparation method, is reported when both concentration and enrichment of cytology specimens is done beyond a concentration technique alone reported with 88108 (e.g., Saccomanno, cytocentrifugation, and cytospins). Enhancement technologies allow not only for concentration of the diagnostic material, but also for removing of background debris on complicated specimens that cannot be evaluated with typical concentration techniques alone (see

88108). One liquid based slide preparation method uses a filtration system with a disposable filter, support, and means of drawing fluid where cells are caught within a large enough area to provide a high-quality, high-yield monolayer slide that has good quantity, distribution, and clarity for diagnostic purposes. When a sample is prepared using enhanced cytopathology, the slide preparation is examined and compared to previous studies. Report this for any specimen except cervical or vaginal.

88130

88130 Sex chromatin identification; Barr bodies

Explanation

This screening test will identify the presence or lack of sex chromatin. Specimen collection is by buccal mucosa scraping, Specimen should be chemically preserved with a fixative such as 95 percent ethanol. Method is by smear and microscopy. Examination of cells obtained by amniocentesis for the presence or absence of sex chromatin is a technique used to determine the infant's sex prior to birth.

88141

88141 Cytopathology, cervical or vaginal (any reporting system), requiring interpretation by physician

Explanation

This test is for the interpretation by a physician of a Papanicolaou (Pap) smear. This code is used in addition to the code for the technical service.

88142-88143

88142 Cytopathology, cervical or vaginal (any reporting system), collected in preservative fluid, automated thin layer preparation; manual screening under physician supervision

88143 with manual screening and rescreening under physician supervision

Explanation

These tests may be identified by the name "thin prep." Specimen collection is by cervical or endocervical scraping or aspiration of vaginal fluid. The physician obtaining the specimen places the specimen in a preservative suspension. At the laboratory, special instruments take the cells in the preservative suspension and "plate-out" a monolayer for screening-the careful review of the specimen for abnormal cells. Report 88142 for manual screening done under physician supervision and 88143 for manual screening followed by manual rescreening, done under physician supervision. System of reporting may be Bethesda or non-Bethesda.

88147-88148

88147 Cytopathology smears, cervical or vaginal; screening by automated system under physician supervision

88148 screening by automated system with manual rescreening under physician supervision

Explanation

These tests may be identified as a cervical smear, Pap smear, or vaginal cytology. Specimen collection is by cervical or endocervical scraping or aspiration of vaginal fluid. Method is microscopy examination of a spray or liquid fixated smear. Code 88147 should be used to report smears screened by automated system under physician supervision, while 88148 reports automated screening with manual rescreening under physician supervision. System of reporting may be Bethesda or non-Bethesda.

88150-88154

88150 Cytopathology, slides, cervical or vaginal; manual screening under physician supervision

88152 with manual screening and computer-assisted rescreening under physician supervision

88153 with manual screening and rescreening under physician supervision

88154 with manual screening and computer-assisted rescreening using cell selection and review under physician supervision

Explanation

These tests may also be identified as a cervical smear, Pap smear, or vaginal cytology. The specimen are cells collected by scraping or brushing the cervix or endocervix, or aspiration of vaginal fluid. The specimen is then smeared onto a slide and chemically treated with a preservative. These codes should be reported when any system other than the Bethesda System of evaluating and describing cervical/vaginal cytopathology slides is used. Code selection is based on the screening process used, with manual screening under physician supervision being reported with 88150, manual screening and computer-assisted rescreening under physician supervision with 88152, manual screening and rescreening under physician supervision with 88153, manual screening and computer-assisted rescreening using cell selection and review under physician supervision with 88154.

Coding Companion for Ob/Gyn

© 2012 OptumInsight, Inc.

88155

88155 Cytopathology, slides, cervical or vaginal, definitive hormonal evaluation (eg, maturation index, karyopyknotic index, estrogenic index) (List separately in addition to code[s] for other technical and interpretation services)

Explanation

This test may also be identified as the maturation index, cytologic estrogen effect, karyopyknotic index, or estrogenic index. Specimen collection is by tongue depressor or wooden spatula of the lateral vaginal wall. Method is microscopy examination of a spray or liquid fixated smear. The test may be used to determine the balance of estrogen and progesterone of the vaginal squamous epithelium.

88160-88162

88160 Cytopathology, smears, any other source; screening and interpretation
88161 preparation, screening and interpretation
88162 extended study involving over 5 slides and/or multiple stains

Explanation

Specimen collection is by separately reportable percutaneous needle biopsy. Methods include microscopy examination of smears or a centrifuge specimen. These codes report the pathology examination portion of the procedure only. Code 88160 reports screening and interpretation only. Code 88161 reports preparation, screening and interpretation. Code 88162 reports an extended study involving more than five slides and/or multiple stains.

88164-88167

88164 Cytopathology, slides, cervical or vaginal (the Bethesda System); manual screening under physician supervision
88165 with manual screening and rescreening under physician supervision
88166 with manual screening and computer-assisted rescreening under physician supervision
88167 with manual screening and computer-assisted rescreening using cell selection and review under physician supervision

Explanation

These tests may be identified as a cervical smear, Pap smear, or vaginal cytology. Specimen collection is by scraping or brushing the cervix or endocervix, or aspiration of vaginal fluid. Method is microscopy examination of a spray or liquid coated smear. These codes should be reported when the Bethesda System of evaluating and describing cervical/vaginal cytopathology slides is used. Code selection is based on the screening process used, with manual screening under physician supervision being reported with 88164, manual screening and rescreening under physician supervision with 88165, manual screening and computer-assisted rescreening under physician supervision with 88166, manual screening and computer-assisted rescreening using cell selection and review under physician supervision with 88167.

88172-88173 (88177)

88172 Cytopathology, evaluation of fine needle aspirate; immediate cytohistologic study to determine adequacy for diagnosis, first evaluation episode, each site
88173 interpretation and report
88177 immediate cytohistologic study to determine adequacy for diagnosis, each separate additional evaluation episode, same site (List separately in addition to code for primary procedure)

Explanation

Following fine needle aspiration (a procedure in which fluid or tissue is extracted using a long slender needle), the aspirated cells are often immediately examined microscopically by a physician in order to determine that diagnostic material is present. A preliminary diagnostic assessment may be rendered at that time in order to avoid a repeat operative procedure. Report 88172 for the first evaluation episode (a complete set of cytologic material submitted for evaluation, regardless of the number of needle passes or prepared slides) of each site and 88177 for each separate additional evaluation episode of the same site. Code 88173 reports the final interpretation and report from each anatomic site, regardless of the number of evaluation episodes or needle passes performed during the aspiration procedure.

88174-88175

88174 Cytopathology, cervical or vaginal (any reporting system), collected in preservative fluid, automated thin layer preparation; screening by automated system, under physician supervision
88175 with screening by automated system and manual rescreening or review, under physician supervision

Explanation

These tests may be identified by the brand name ThinPrep. Specimen collection is by cervical or endocervical scraping or aspiration of vaginal fluid. Report 88174 for automated screening done under physician supervision and 88175 when automated screening is followed by manual rescreening or review under physician supervision.

88267

88267 Chromosome analysis, amniotic fluid or chorionic villus, count 15 cells, 1 karyotype, with banding

Explanation

This is a prenatal technique used to analyze chromosomes from cells of extracted amniotic fluid or chorionic villus for possible genetic abnormalities that can be detected during embryonic development. The code includes a 15-cell count, one karyotype, with banding. Karyotype is the full chromosome set that genetically defines an individual. Banding refers to the appearance of stripes on stained paired bundles of chromosomes. This test would normally use more traditional techniques, such as direct microscopic analysis of cells arrested in metaphase with Giemsa or quinacrine banding techniques.

88269

88269 Chromosome analysis, in situ for amniotic fluid cells, count cells from 6-12 colonies, 1 karyotype, with banding

Explanation

This is a prenatal technique used to analyze intact chromosomes within the cells of amniotic fluid for possible genetic abnormalities that can be detected during embryonic development. The code includes a cell count from six to 12 colonies, one karyotype, with banding. Karyotype is the full chromosome set that genetically defines an individual. Banding refers to the appearance of stripes on stained paired bundles of chromosomes. By studying the occurrence of different DNA bands in the population, one can calculate the probability of two DNA samples matching one another. Any number of methods may be used, including polymerase chain reaction (PCR), restriction fragment length polymorphism (RFLP), and Northern or Southern blot.

88302

88302 Level II - Surgical pathology, gross and microscopic examination

Explanation

This examination may be ordered as a gross and microscopic pathology exam or a gross and microscopic tissue exam. The exam may not be specifically ordered ahead of time; rather, the tissue is harvested in the course of a surgery and sent for routine lab evaluation. Tissue is submitted in a container labeled with the tissue source, preoperative diagnosis, and patient identification information. Specimens from separate sites must be submitted in separate containers, each labeled with the tissue source. This procedure is used to describe examination of tissues presumed normal. It includes both a gross and microscopic examination with the microscopic exam mainly to confirm the tissue is free of disease. Examples of its use might include tissues from a fallopian tube or vas deferens performed in the course of sterilization procedures, newborn foreskin following circumcision, hernia sac, hydrocele sac, etc.

88304-88309

88304 Level III - Surgical pathology, gross and microscopic examination

88305 Level IV - Surgical pathology, gross and microscopic examination

88307 Level V - Surgical pathology, gross and microscopic examination

88309 Level VI - Surgical pathology, gross and microscopic examination

Explanation

These examinations would be ordered as a gross and microscopic pathology exam or a gross and microscopic tissue exam. Tissue is submitted in a container labeled with the tissue source, preoperative diagnosis, and patient identification information. Specimens from separate sites must be submitted in separate containers, each labeled with the tissue source. Codes 88304-88309 describe levels of service for specimens requiring additional levels of work due to a presumed presence of disease. Code 88304 describes the lowest level of complexity for diseased or abnormal tissue with each subsequent code (88305, 88307, and 88309) describing in ascending order higher levels of complexity and physician work. Specific types of disease and tissue sites are listed for each code in the CPT(r) description.

88360

88360 Morphometric analysis, tumor immunohistochemistry (eg, Her-2/neu, estrogen receptor/progesterone receptor), quantitative or semiquantitative, each antibody; manual

Explanation

Morphometric analysis may also be referred to as histomorphometry. A quantitative or semiquantitative test is done for tumor immunohistochemistry, such as the Her-2/neu receptor. The HER-2/neu protein is a cell surface growth factor receptor expressed on the cytoplasmic membrane of some epithelial cells. This protein regulates normal cell growth and division. An increased number of HER-2/neu genes in the cell nucleus causes over expression of the HER-2/neu oncoprotein, which in turn produces growth signals leading to cell transformation and cancer development. Microthin sections of the fixed, paraffin-embedded tissue are mounted on glass slides. Antigen retrieval with citrate buffers or microwaving is done to inhibit peroxidase activity and background staining. Immunostaining is done by adding a dilution containing the primary antibody to the receptor protein and incubating. Counterstaining with secondary antibodies is done

to visualize antibody location. Further analysis is done to determine the histologic organization of the tumor and measure its structure, form, and composition, quantitatively or semiquantitatively, manually. This codes is reported once for each antibody used to test for a specific protein receptor, such as Her-2/neu, estrogen, or progesterone receptor.

88361

88361 Morphometric analysis, tumor immunohistochemistry (eg, Her-2/neu, estrogen receptor/progesterone receptor), quantitative or semiquantitative, each antibody; using computer-assisted technology

Explanation

Morphometric analysis may also be referred to as histomorphometry. A quantitative or semiquantitative test is done for tumor immunohistochemistry, such as the Her-2/neu receptor. The HER-2/neu protein is a cell surface growth factor receptor expressed on the cytoplasmic membrane of some epithelial cells. This protein regulates normal cell growth and division. An increased number of HER-2/neu genes in the cell nucleus causes over expression of the HER-2/neu oncoprotein, which in turn produces growth signals leading to cell transformation and cancer development. Microthin sections of the fixed, paraffin-embedded tissue are mounted on glass slides. Antigen retrieval with citrate buffers or microwaving is done to inhibit peroxidase activity and background staining. Immunostaining is done by adding a dilution containing the primary antibody to the receptor protein and incubating. Counterstaining with secondary antibodies is done to visualize antibody location. Further analysis is done to determine the histologic organization of the tumor and measure its structure, form, and composition, quantitatively or semiquantitatively, using computer-assisted technology. This code is reported once for each antibody used to test for a specific protein receptor, such as Her-2/neu, estrogen, or progesterone receptor.

89250-89251

89250 Culture of oocyte(s)/embryo(s), less than 4 days;

89251 with co-culture of oocyte(s)/embryos

Explanation

Eggs (oocytes) are aspirated transvaginally using ultrasound guidance in a separately reportable procedure. Eggs or previously fertilized embryos are kept in an incubator in a Petri dish culture for less than four days in 89250. Code 89251 is reserved for those instances when co-culture techniques over and above those normally required are performed.

89253

89253 Assisted embryo hatching, microtechniques (any method)

Explanation

Assisted embryo hatching is performed in selected cases on the day of embryo transfer. A pipette is placed on one side of the embryo to keep it from moving. A very delicate, hollow needle called a hatching needle is placed on the other side of the embryo. An acidic solution is expelled from the needle against the outer shell (zona pellucida) of the embryo. The acidic solution digests a small area of the outer shell. The embryo is washed and replaced in the culture solution in the incubator.

89254

89254 Oocyte identification from follicular fluid

Explanation

Because the egg (oocyte) is microscopic, only the follicle (fluid filled structure surrounding the egg) can be seen during the ultrasound-guided retrieval. Upon aspiration of the follicle, specially trained personnel use a microscope to search for the oocyte-cumulus complex, which includes the egg and surrounding cumulus cells from the ovary. This is accomplished by pouring the collected fluid into flat dishes and using a microscope to search for eggs.

89255

89255 Preparation of embryo for transfer (any method)

Explanation

After the embryos have been cultured for two to six days, three to four healthy embryos are selected for transfer. Selected embryos are loaded into a transfer catheter. In a separately reportable procedure, the catheter is placed in the cervical canal and the embryos are transferred into the uterine cavity.

89257

89257 Sperm identification from aspiration (other than seminal fluid)

Explanation

A separately reportable testicular biopsy with aspiration is performed to obtain sperm. This may be required in cases where azoospermia is due to suspected obstruction to the spermatic ducts or in instances where the patient has had a failed reversal of a vasectomy. This procedure reports microscopic examination of aspirated fluid for the presence of sperm. If sperm are identified, further evaluation services may be performed and would be reported separately.

89258

89258 Cryopreservation; embryo(s)

© 2012 OptumInsight, Inc.

Appendix

Explanation

Embryos not required for current uterine transfer are frozen using a process referred to as cryopreservation. Pre-implantation embryo preservation is a relatively new procedure as compared to sperm preservation (see 89259), but more than two-thirds of the embryos survive the cryopreservation process and can be preserved for an indefinite period of time.

89259

89259 Cryopreservation; sperm

Explanation

A cryoprotectant, usually glycerol or Dimethyl Sulfoxide (DMSO), is mixed with the semen to reduce damage to sperm during the freezing process. The semen specimen is placed in a vial and frozen in liquid nitrogen at -196 C. This halts all biologic and metabolic processes allowing the sperm to be preserved for many years.

89260

89260 Sperm isolation; simple prep (eg, sperm wash and swim-up) for insemination or diagnosis with semen analysis

Explanation

Prior to insemination or further diagnostic studies, the sperm go through a spinning and washing process in a series of solutions. The purpose of this is to separate sperm from seminal fluids, allowing the sperm to go through a process referred to as capacitation. Capacitation is an invisible change mature spermatozoa must undergo to acquire accelerated movement, allowing them to navigate through the uterus and fallopian tube. In addition, this procedure checks the ability of the sperm to swim in a forward progressive fashion. This procedure includes a semen analysis (count, motility, volume and differential).

89261

89261 Sperm isolation; complex prep (eg, Percoll gradient, albumin gradient) for insemination or diagnosis with semen analysis

Explanation

Prior to insemination or further diagnostic studies, the sperm go through a spinning and washing process in a series of solutions. The purpose of this is to separate sperm from seminal fluids, allowing the sperm to go through a process referred to as capacitation. Capacitation is an invisible change mature spermatozoa must undergo to acquire accelerated movement, allowing them to navigate through the uterus and fallopian tube. This complex prep includes a Percoll gradient and albumin gradient. This procedure includes a semen analysis (count, motility, volume and differential).

89264

89264 Sperm identification from testis tissue, fresh or cryopreserved

Explanation

A separately reportable testicular biopsy is performed to obtain sperm. A small amount of testicular tissue is taken for microscopic evaluation for the presence of sperm. This test is used only when no other means is available of obtaining a sperm sample because of the possibility of causing further testicular damage.

89268

89268 Insemination of oocytes

Explanation

Insemination requires a sperm cell to be introduced to an egg (oocyte) for fertilization procedures. The sperm is prepared through a washing method, which separates the sperm cells from the seminal fluid. The washing filters out white blood cells, prostaglandins, and other debris, as well as cells with less motility, to provide the highest concentration of viable sperm. Once the concentrated spermatozoa have been prepared, they are placed in a culture medium with the eggs. If injection is required for fertilization, the protective coating of cells is removed from the egg and the sperm cell is directly injected.

89272

89272 Extended culture of oocyte(s)/embryo(s), 4-7 days

Explanation

Culture of eggs (oocytes) or embryos usually occurs for 48 to 72 hours. This code describes an extended period of time for the cells to incubate in a culture medium, which will improve the identification of the most viable embryos. It is sometimes necessary to wait up to five days for the embryo to become a blastocyte before implantation due to high risk of multiple gestation or repeated IVF failures.

89280-89281

89280 Assisted oocyte fertilization, microtechnique; less than or equal to 10 oocytes

89281 greater than 10 oocytes

Explanation

Assisted oocyte fertilization is done with microtechnique. A single sperm is injected into the egg (oocyte) to enable fertilization when sperm counts are very low or when sperm are non-motile. It requires micromanipulation of the sperm, which is also referred to as microtechnique. The usual method involves intracytoplasmic sperm injection (ICSI). Using ICSI technique, the mature egg is held in place with a holding pipette. A very delicate, sharp, hollow needle is used to immobilize and pick up a single sperm. This needle is inserted through the egg's outer shell (zona pellucida) into the cytoplasm of the egg. The sperm is injected into the cytoplasm and the needle removed. The eggs are checked the next day for evidence of fertilization. Report 89280 for 10 oocytes or less and 89281 for more than 10 oocytes.

89290-89291

89290 Biopsy, oocyte polar body or embryo blastomere, microtechnique (for pre-implantation genetic diagnosis); less than or equal to 5 embryos

89291 greater than 5 embryos

Explanation

Biopsy of an egg (oocyte) polar body or embryo blastomere (an embryo with six to eight cells) is indicated for patients who carry genetic disorders such as Sickle cell anemia, hemophilia, Fragile X syndrome, and others, and for those experiencing difficulty with a successful IVF or ICSI. The process of a biopsy includes inserting a microneedle into a fertilized egg to extract polar bodies of the oocyte, or to extract a single cell from a six to eight cell embryo. Screenings are performed through the process of FISH (fluorescent in-situ hybridization) and PCR (polymerase chain reaction). During FISH, a small amount of DNA is analyzed through staining of fluorochromes. PCR is able to detect gene-sequences or single genes, which may have abnormal mutations. Report 89290 for a biopsy of five or less embryos and 89291 for six or more embryos.

89300-89322

89300 Semen analysis; presence and/or motility of sperm including Huhner test (post coital)

89310 motility and count (not including Huhner test)

89320 volume, count, motility, and differential

89321 sperm presence and motility of sperm, if performed

89322 volume, count, motility, and differential using strict morphologic criteria (eg, Kruger)

Explanation

Semen analysis is generally performed in specialized infertility/andrology laboratories. Sexual activity culminating in ejaculation should be avoided for a minimum of 48 hours prior to testing. In 89300, a post coital specimen is obtained using a cervical swab. The test is timed to coincide with ovulation. Semen is tested for the presence (quantity) and/or motility of sperm. In 89310-89322, semen is collected using a condom-like seminal fluid collection device or by masturbation into a sterile container. In 89310, only sperm movement (motility) and number (concentration or count that measures how many million sperm are in each milliliter of fluid) are performed. Code 89320 reports a semen analysis that includes measurement of the ejaculate's volume, number, structure (shape) of sperm, sperm movement (motility), and direction of movement (forward motility). In addition, fluid thickness, acidity, and sugar content may be evaluated. Code 89321 tests only for the presence (quantity) and/or motility of sperm. In 89322, a detailed evaluation of the shape (morphology) is performed utilizing specially stained slides and microscopic examination of the sperm under high power magnification. In order to be considered normal, the sperm must meet a strict set of criteria regarding the shape and size of the head, mid-piece, and tail. A Kruger test is helpful in determining which reproductive techniques and methodologies may be most appropriate and successful. Tests reported with 89300-89322 may be accomplished using a variety of methods including semen function tests and computer-assisted sperm morphology/motility studies.

89325

89325 Sperm antibodies

Explanation

This procedure tests for antisperm antibodies in both the male and female. Semen and cervical mucus are placed together in a medium. Antisperm antibodies bind with the sperm inhibiting movement and their ability to fertilize. The sperm will appear clumped together on microscopic examination.

89329

89329 Sperm evaluation; hamster penetration test

Explanation

This test is also called sperm penetration assay (SPA) or hamster zona free ovum (HZFO) and tests the ability of the sperm to penetrate a hamster egg, which has been stripped of the zona pellucida (outer membrane). The patient should abstain from sexual activity culminating in ejaculation for a minimum of 48 hours. Semen is collected postcoitus using a condom-like seminal fluid collection device or by masturbation into a sterile container. Upon receiving the specimen in the laboratory, the sperm is washed and placed in a culture medium along with a single hamster egg. It is examined periodically using phase contrast microscopy. The test measures the ability of sperm to capacitate (invisible change which allows sperm to navigate rapidly forward), acrosome react (structural change fusing the outer membrane of the acrosome with the plasma membrane of the sperm head freeing enzymes in the acrosome which facilitate entry into the ovum), and fuse with the ovum.

89330

89330 Sperm evaluation; cervical mucus penetration test, with or without spinnbarkeit test

Explanation

Sperm mucus interaction is assessed in vitro. Human or bovine ovulatory mucus is placed in a capillary tube. Sperm penetration is measured over a period of 90 minutes. Sperm progression measures which sperm have progressed the farthest down the tube. Patient sperm penetration can be compared with fertile sperm specimens using in vitro methods.

89331

89331 Sperm evaluation, for retrograde ejaculation, urine (sperm concentration, motility, and morphology, as indicated)

Explanation

Retrograde ejaculation, in which the seminal fluid travels backward into the bladder following ejaculation, is often seen in patients with diabetes, or in men following transurethral surgery at or near the bladder neck, dissection of the retroperitoneal lymph nodes, or spinal cord injuries. The patient may present with low semen volume, motility (movement), and sperm concentration (count). In a urinalysis performed immediately after ejaculation, the specimen is examined under the microscope for the presence of sperm. If detected, the specimen is further processed to evaluate the concentration, motility, and morphology (shape).

89342-89346

89342 Storage (per year); embryo(s)
89343   sperm/semen
89344   reproductive tissue, testicular/ovarian
89346   oocyte(s)

Explanation

These codes report the long-term maintenance of preserved reproductive tissue samples and fertilized embryos in an appropriate storage facility per year. Report 89342 for embryo(s), 89343 for sperm/semen, 89344 for testicular or ovarian tissue, and 89346 for oocyte(s).

89352-89356

89352 Thawing of cryopreserved; embryo(s)
89353   sperm/semen, each aliquot
89354   reproductive tissue, testicular/ovarian
89356   oocytes, each aliquot

Explanation

Thawing of cryopreserved tissue requires thawing in different substances for set lengths of time so as to maintain the integrity of the specimen and prevent damage by thawing too quickly. The cryovial is removed from the liquid nitrogen and placed at room temperature until ice crystals have dissolved. A waterbath is prepared at the desired temperature in which the specimen is placed. After the water bath, each specimen is placed in a series of solutions to complete the thawing process. Report 89352 for embryos, 89353 for sperm/semen, 89354 for reproductive testicular/ovarian tissue, and 89356 for oocytes.

90281

90281 Immune globulin (Ig), human, for intramuscular use

Explanation

This code identifies the immune globulin (Ig), human, for intramuscular use. An immune globulin is a passive immunization agent obtained from donated, pooled human plasma. Passive immunity is achieved for a short period as the antibodies received through the immune globulin are circulated through the body. The recipient's immune system is not stimulated to build its own antibodies. Report this code with the appropriate administration code.

90283

90283 Immune globulin (IgIV), human, for intravenous use

Explanation

This code identifies the immune globulin (IgIV), human, for intravenous administration. An immune globulin is a passive immunization agent obtained from donated, pooled human plasma. Passive immunity is achieved for a short period as the antibodies received through the immune globulin are circulated through the body. The recipient's immune system is not stimulated to build its own antibodies. Report this code with the appropriate administration code.

90284

90284 Immune globulin (SCIg), human, for use in subcutaneous infusions, 100 mg, each

Explanation

This code identifies the human immune globulin for use in subcutaneous infusions (SCIg). An immune globulin is a passive immunization agent obtained from donated pooled human plasma. Passive immunity is achieved for a short period as the antibodies received through the immune globulin are circulated through the body. The recipient's immune system is not stimulated to build its own antibodies. Some patients have insufficient venous access or adverse reactions to intravenous treatments, making them unsuitable candidates for traditional IVIg therapy. Controlled doses of immune globulin are administered over a period of several hours through a small needle placed just under the skin. Report this code with the appropriate administration code.

90393

90393 Vaccinia immune globulin, human, for intramuscular use

Explanation

This code identifies the vaccinia immune globulin, human, for intramuscular use. This immune globulin is a passive immunization agent that gives protection against vaccinia and is obtained from donated, pooled human plasma. The vaccinia virus causes cutaneous and systemic reactions occurring as a complication of smallpox vaccination. Passive immunity is achieved for a short period as the antibodies received through the immune globulin are circulated through the body. The recipient's immune system is not stimulated to build its own antibodies. Report this code with the appropriate administration code.

90460-90461

90460 Immunization administration through 18 years of age via any route of administration, with counseling by physician or other qualified health care professional; first or only component of each vaccine or toxoid administered

90461 each additional vaccine or toxoid component administered (List separately in addition to code for primary procedure)

Explanation

The physician or other qualified health care professional instructs the patient or family on the benefits and risks related to the vaccine or toxoid. The physician counsels the patient or family regarding signs and symptoms of adverse effects and when to seek medical attention for any adverse effects. A physician, nurse, or medical assistant administers an immunization by any route to the patient. It may be a single vaccine or a combination vaccine/toxoid in one immunization administration (e.g., diphtheria, pertussis, and tetanus toxoids are in a single DPT immunization). Report 90460 for the first vaccine/toxoid component. Report 90461 for each additional component. These codes report immunization administration to patients 18 years of age or younger.

90471-90472

90471 Immunization administration (includes percutaneous, intradermal, subcutaneous, or intramuscular injections); 1 vaccine (single or combination vaccine/toxoid)

90472 each additional vaccine (single or combination vaccine/toxoid) (List separately in addition to code for primary procedure)

Explanation

A physician, nurse, or medical assistant administers an injectable (percutaneous, intradermal, subcutaneous, or intramuscular) immunization to the patient. It may be a single vaccine or a combination vaccine/toxoid in one immunization administration (e.g., diphtheria, pertussis, and tetanus toxoids are in a single DPT immunization). Report 90471 for one vaccine and 90472 for each additional vaccine (single or combination vaccine/toxoid).

90473-90474

90473 Immunization administration by intranasal or oral route; 1 vaccine (single or combination vaccine/toxoid)

90474 each additional vaccine (single or combination vaccine/toxoid) (List separately in addition to code for primary procedure)

Explanation

A physician, nurse, or medical assistant administers an immunization to a patient via an intranasal (e.g., nasal spray) or an oral route (e.g., a liquid that is swallowed). It may be a single vaccine or a combination vaccine/toxoid in one immunization administration (e.g., adenovirus, Rotavirus, typhoid, poliovirus). Report these codes with the appropriate administration code.

90645

90645 Hemophilus influenza b vaccine (Hib), HbOC conjugate (4 dose schedule), for intramuscular use

Explanation

A vaccine produces active immunization by inducing the immune system to build its own antibodies against specific microorganisms/viruses. The body retains memory of the antibody production pattern for long-term protection. The Hemophilus influenza b vaccine (Hib), HbOC conjugate, is prepared for intramuscular use, in a 4-dose schedule, to immunize a patient against influenza, caused by the bacteria species of the same name, Haemophilus influenzae. Report this code with the appropriate administration code.

90646

90646 Hemophilus influenza b vaccine (Hib), PRP-D conjugate, for booster use only, intramuscular use

Explanation

A vaccine produces active immunization by inducing the immune system to build its own antibodies against specific microorganisms/viruses. The body retains memory of the antibody production pattern for long-term protection. The Hemophilus influenza b vaccine (Hib), PRP-D conjugate, is prepared for intramuscular use, booster only, to immunize a patient against influenza, caused by the bacteria species of the same name, Haemophilus influenzae. Report this code with the appropriate administration code.

90647

90647 Hemophilus influenza b vaccine (Hib), PRP-OMP conjugate (3 dose schedule), for intramuscular use

Explanation

A vaccine produces active immunization by inducing the immune system to build its own antibodies against specific microorganisms/viruses. The body retains memory of the antibody production pattern for long-term protection. A Hemophilus influenza b vaccine (Hib), PRP-OMP conjugate, is prepared for intramuscular use, in a 3-dose schedule, to immunize a patient against influenza, caused by the bacteria species of the same name, Haemophilus influenzae. Report this code with the appropriate administration code.

90648

90648 Hemophilus influenza b vaccine (Hib), PRP-T conjugate (4 dose schedule), for intramuscular use

Explanation

A vaccine produces active immunization by inducing the immune system to build its own antibodies against specific microorganisms/viruses. The body retains memory of the antibody production pattern for long-term protection. A Hemophilus influenza b vaccine (Hib), PRP-T conjugate, is prepared for intramuscular use, in a 4-dose schedule, to immunize a patient against influenza, caused by the bacteria species of the same name, Haemophilus influenzae. Report this code with the appropriate administration code.

90649-90650

90649 Human Papilloma virus (HPV) vaccine, types 6, 11, 16, 18 (quadrivalent), 3 dose schedule, for intramuscular use

90650 Human Papilloma virus (HPV) vaccine, types 16, 18, bivalent, 3 dose schedule, for intramuscular use

Explanation

A vaccine produces active immunization by inducing the immune system to manufacture its own antibodies against specific microorganisms/viruses. The body retains memory of the antibody production pattern for long-term protection. A human papilloma virus (HPV) vaccine is prepared in a three-dose schedule for intramuscular use. The vaccine may be bivalent (types 16 and 18) or quadrivalent (types 6, 11, 16, and 18). The vaccine immunizes a patient against HPV or assists in producing an immune reaction to the E6 and E7 viral proteins to prevent or destroy the growth of abnormal or cancerous cells. Report the bivalent vaccine with 90650 and the quadrivalent vaccine with 90649. Report these codes with the appropriate administration code.

90653

90653 Influenza vaccine, inactivated, subunit, adjuvanted, for intramuscular use

Appendix

Explanation

A vaccine produces active immunization by inducing the immune system to build its own antibodies against specific microorganisms/viruses. The body retains memory of the antibody production pattern for long-term protection. An inactive virus suspension of the prevalent strains of influenza, with added adjuvant, is prepared for intramuscular injection. Report this code in addition to the appropriate administration code.

Coding Tips

This code is new for 2013.

90654

90654 Influenza virus vaccine, split virus, preservative-free, for intradermal use

Explanation

A vaccine produces active immunization by inducing the immune system to build its own antibodies against specific microorganisms/viruses. The body retains memory of the antibody production pattern for long-term protection. A split virus suspension of the prevalent strains of influenza is prepared for intradermal injection. Report this code in addition to the appropriate administration code.

90655-90656

90655 Influenza virus vaccine, trivalent, split virus, preservative free, when administered to children 6-35 months of age, for intramuscular use

90656 Influenza virus vaccine, trivalent, split virus, preservative free, when administered to individuals 3 years and older, for intramuscular use

Explanation

These codes report the supply of the vaccine only. A vaccine produces active immunization by inducing the immune system to build its own antibodies against specific microorganisms/viruses. The body retains memory of the antibody production pattern for long-term protection. A split virus suspension of three (two influenza A and one influenza B) of the most prevalent strains of influenza is prepared for intramuscular injection. Report 90655 for a preservative free, split virus influenza vaccine to be administered to children 6 to 35 months of age and 90656 if the vaccine is administered to individuals 3 years of age or older. Report these codes with the appropriate administration code.

Coding Tips

These codes have been revised for 2013 in the official CPT description.

90657-90658

90657 Influenza virus vaccine, trivalent, split virus, when administered to children 6-35 months of age, for intramuscular use

90658 Influenza virus vaccine, trivalent, split virus, when administered to individuals 3 years of age and older, for intramuscular use

Explanation

These codes report the supply of the vaccine only. A vaccine produces active immunization by inducing the immune system to build its own antibodies against specific microorganisms/viruses. The body retains memory of the antibody production pattern for long-term protection. A split virus suspension of three (two influenza A and one influenza B) of the most prevalent strains of influenza is prepared for intramuscular use. Report 90657 for the vaccine supply when administered to children ages 6 to 35 months and 90658 for vaccines administered to individuals 3 years of age or older. The vaccine induces active immunity to the highly contagious infection of the respiratory tract caused by a myxovirus and transmitted by airborne droplet infection. Report these codes with the appropriate administration code.

Coding Tips

These codes have been revised for 2013 in the official CPT description.

90660 (90672)

90660 Influenza virus vaccine, trivalent, live, for intranasal use

90672 Influenza virus vaccine, quadrivalent, live, for intranasal use

Explanation

A vaccine produces active immunization by inducing the immune system to build its own antibodies against specific microorganisms/viruses. The body retains memory of the antibody production pattern for long-term protection. A suspension of the prevalent strains of influenza virus is prepared for intranasal use. This live vaccination contains the actual pathogen that has been weakened. Report these codes with the appropriate administration code. Report 90660 when the vaccine contains three strains. Report 90672 if the vaccine is comprised of four strains.

Coding Tips

Code 90660 has been revised for 2013 in the official CPT description. Code 90672 is new for 2013. It is a resequenced code and will not display in numeric order.

90664-90668

90664 Influenza virus vaccine, pandemic formulation, live, for intranasal use

90666 Influenza virus vaccine, pandemic formulation, split virus, preservative free, for intramuscular use

90667 Influenza virus vaccine, pandemic formulation, split virus, adjuvanted, for intramuscular use

90668 Influenza virus vaccine, pandemic formulation, split virus, for intramuscular use

Explanation

These codes report pandemic formulations of the influenza virus vaccine. An influenza pandemic is a large-scale eruption of disease that takes place when a new influenza virus emerges in the human population, spreading easily between individuals and resulting in serious illness. A pandemic can rapidly travel across a whole region, a continent, or the world. Unlike seasonal influenza, individuals have little immunity to this virus. A suspension of the prevalent strain of pandemic influenza virus is prepared for intranasal use in 90664; this live vaccination contains the actual pathogen. Subvirion (split virus) vaccines do not contain the entire virus; rather, they contain purified portions. Split virus vaccines are believed to cause fewer adverse effects in children and young adults, while maintaining its ability to stimulate an immune response (immunogenicity) comparable to that of whole virus preparations. Due to their decreased rates of side effects, only split virus preparations are recommended for children younger than 13 years of age. A suspension of the prevalent strain of pandemic influenza virus is prepared for intramuscular use; 90668 reports the split virus vaccine, 90666 reports the preservative-free version, and 90667 reports the adjuvanted version. These codes identify the vaccine products only and must be reported in addition to the appropriate immunization administration codes.

90685-90688

90685 Influenza virus vaccine, quadrivalent, split virus, preservative free, when administered to children 6-35 months of age, for intramuscular use

90686 Influenza virus vaccine, quadrivalent, split virus, preservative free, when administered to individuals 3 years of age and older, for intramuscular use

90687 Influenza virus vaccine, quadrivalent, split virus, when administered to children 6-35 months of age, for intramuscular use

90688 Influenza virus vaccine, quadrivalent, split virus, when administered to individuals 3 years of age and older, for intramuscular use

Explanation

These codes report the supply of the vaccine only. A vaccine produces active immunization by inducing the immune system to build its own antibodies against specific microorganisms/viruses. The body retains memory of the antibody production pattern for long-term protection. A split virus suspension of four (two influenza A and two influenza B) of the most prevalent strains of influenza is prepared for intramuscular injection. Report 90685 for a preservative free, split virus influenza vaccine to be administered to children 6 to 35 months of age and 90686 if the vaccine is administered to individuals 3 years of age or older. Report 90687 for the vaccine supply when administered to children ages 6 to 35 months and 90688 for vaccines administered to individuals 3 years of age or older. The vaccine induces active immunity to the highly contagious infection of the respiratory tract caused by a myxovirus and transmitted by airborne droplet infection. Report these codes with the appropriate administration code.

Coding Tips

These codes are new for 2013.

90703

90703   Tetanus toxoid adsorbed, for intramuscular use

Explanation

This code reports supply of the toxoid only. A toxoid stimulates the body's own immune system to produce specific antitoxin antibodies that destroy the toxins secreted by bacteria. This provides immunity that is effective and long lasting. Code 90702 reports toxoids against diphtheria and tetanus (DT), adsorbed for intramuscular use, for administration to individuals younger than age seven. Report this code with the appropriate administration code.

90704-90706

90704   Mumps virus vaccine, live, for subcutaneous use

90705   Measles virus vaccine, live, for subcutaneous use

90706   Rubella virus vaccine, live, for subcutaneous use

Explanation

A vaccine produces active immunization by inducing the immune system to build its own antibodies against specific microorganisms/viruses. The body retains memory of these antibody production patterns for long-term protection. These codes all report a live vaccine for subcutaneous use. Code 90704 is for a mumps virus vaccine, 90705 reports a measles vaccine, and 90706 is for rubella. A live vaccine contains the actual pathogen. Report these codes with the appropriate administration code.

90707-90708

90707   Measles, mumps and rubella virus vaccine (MMR), live, for subcutaneous use

90708   Measles and rubella virus vaccine, live, for subcutaneous use

Explanation

A vaccine produces active immunization by inducing the immune system to build its own antibodies against specific microorganisms/viruses. The body retains memory of these antibody production patterns for long-term protection. Code 90707 reports the combined measles, mumps, and rubella (MMR) vaccine, live, for subcutaneous use. Code 90708 reports the measles and rubella virus vaccine, live, for subcutaneous use. A live vaccine contains the actual pathogens. Report these codes with the appropriate administration code.

90710

90710   Measles, mumps, rubella, and varicella vaccine (MMRV), live, for subcutaneous use

Explanation

A vaccine produces active immunization by inducing the immune system to build its own antibodies against specific microorganisms/viruses. The body retains memory of these antibody production patterns for long-term protection. This vaccine combines measles, mumps, rubella, and varicella (MMRV) for subcutaneous use. This live vaccine contains the actual pathogens. Report this code with the appropriate administration code.

90712

90712   Poliovirus vaccine, (any type[s]) (OPV), live, for oral use

Explanation

A vaccine produces active immunization by inducing the immune system to build its own antibodies against specific microorganisms/viruses. The body retains memory of these antibody production patterns for long-term protection. This code describes the poliovirus vaccine, (OPV) (any type), for oral use. This live vaccine contains the actual pathogen. Report this code with the appropriate administration code.

90713

90713   Poliovirus vaccine, inactivated (IPV), for subcutaneous or intramuscular use

Explanation

A vaccine produces active immunization by inducing the immune system to manufacture its own antibodies against specific microorganisms/viruses. The body retains memory of these antibody production patterns for long-term protection. This code describes the inactivated poliovirus vaccine (IPV) for subcutaneous or intramuscular use. Report this code with the appropriate administration code.

90714

90714   Tetanus and diphtheria toxoids (Td) adsorbed, preservative free, when administered to individuals 7 years or older, for intramuscular use

Explanation

This code reports supply of the toxoid only. A toxoid stimulates the body's own immune system to produce specific antitoxin antibodies that destroy the toxins secreted by bacteria. This provides immunity that is effective and long lasting. This code reports the immunization supply of tetanus and diphtheria toxoids (Td), adsorbed, preservative free, for intramuscular administration to patients seven years of age or older. Report this code with the appropriate administration code.

90715

90715   Tetanus, diphtheria toxoids and acellular pertussis vaccine (Tdap), when administered to individuals 7 years or older, for intramuscular use

Explanation

This code reports the vaccine/toxoid product supply only. A toxoid stimulates the body's own immune system to produce specific antitoxin antibodies that destroy the toxins secreted by bacteria. This provides immunity that is effective and long lasting. A vaccine produces active immunization by inducing the immune system to build its own antibodies against specific microorganisms/viruses. The body retains memory of these antibody production patterns for long-term protection. This code reports the immunization supply of tetanus, diphtheria toxoids, and acellular pertussis (synthetic form) vaccine (DTaP) for intramuscular administration to patients 7 years of age or older. Report this code with the appropriate administration code.

90716

90716   Varicella virus vaccine, live, for subcutaneous use

Explanation

A vaccine produces active immunization by inducing the immune system to build its own antibodies against specific microorganisms/viruses. The body retains memory of these antibody production patterns for long-term protection. This code describes a live varicella virus vaccine for subcutaneous use. This vaccine contains the actual pathogen. Report this code with the appropriate administration code.

90717

90717   Yellow fever vaccine, live, for subcutaneous use

Appendix

Explanation

A vaccine produces active immunization by inducing the immune system to build its own antibodies against specific microorganisms/viruses. The body retains memory of these antibody production patterns for long-term protection. This code reports the live vaccine against yellow fever for subcutaneous use. A live vaccine contains the actual pathogen. Report this code with the appropriate administration code.

90719

90719 Diphtheria toxoid, for intramuscular use

Explanation

This code reports supply of a toxoid only. A toxoid stimulates the body's own immune system to produce specific antitoxin antibodies that destroy the toxins secreted by bacteria. This provides active immunity that is effective and long lasting. Code 90719 reports a diphtheria toxoid alone for intramuscular use. Report this code with the appropriate administration code.

90720

90720 Diphtheria, tetanus toxoids, and whole cell pertussis vaccine and Hemophilus influenza B vaccine (DTP-Hib), for intramuscular use

Explanation

A toxoid stimulates the body's own immune system to produce specific antitoxin antibodies that destroy the toxins secreted by bacteria. This provides immunity that is effective and long lasting. A vaccine produces active immunization by inducing the immune system to build its own antibodies against specific microorganisms/viruses. The body retains memory of these antibody production patterns for long-term protection. Code 90720 describes a vaccine combining diphtheria and tetanus toxoids, whole cell pertussis vaccine, and Hemophilus influenza B vaccine, (DTP-Hib), for intramuscular use. Report this code with the appropriate administration code.

90721

90721 Diphtheria, tetanus toxoids, and acellular pertussis vaccine and Hemophilus influenza B vaccine (DtaP-Hib), for intramuscular use

Explanation

A toxoid stimulates the body's own immune system to produce specific antitoxin antibodies that destroy the toxins secreted by bacteria. This provides immunity that is effective and long lasting. A vaccine produces active immunization by inducing the immune system to build its own antibodies against specific microorganisms/viruses. The body retains memory of these antibody production patterns for long-term protection. Code 90721 reports a combination vaccine/toxoid of diphtheria and tetanus toxoids, acellular pertussis vaccine, and Hemophilus influenza B vaccine for intramuscular

use (DtaP-Hib). Report this code with the appropriate administration code.

90725

90725 Cholera vaccine for injectable use

Explanation

A vaccine produces active immunization by inducing the immune system to build its own antibodies against specific microorganisms/viruses. The body retains memory of these antibody production patterns for long-term protection. This code reports the supply of a cholera vaccine prepared for injectable use. Report this code with the appropriate administration code.

90727

90727 Plague vaccine, for intramuscular use

Explanation

A vaccine produces active immunization by inducing the immune system to build its own antibodies against specific microorganisms/viruses. The body retains memory of these antibody production patterns for long-term protection. This code reports the supply of a vaccine against plague for intramuscular use. Report this code with the appropriate administration code.

90732

90732 Pneumococcal polysaccharide vaccine, 23-valent, adult or immunosuppressed patient dosage, when administered to individuals 2 years or older, for subcutaneous or intramuscular use

Explanation

This code reports supply of a vaccine only. A vaccine produces active immunization by inducing the immune system to build its own antibodies against specific microorganisms/viruses. The body retains memory of these antibody production patterns for long-term protection. This code reports a pneumococcal polysaccharide vaccine, 23-valent, adult or immunosuppressed patient dosage, for subcutaneous or intramuscular administration to patients 2 years of age or older. Report this code with the appropriate administration code.

90733

90733 Meningococcal polysaccharide vaccine (any group(s)), for subcutaneous use

Explanation

A vaccine produces active immunization by inducing the immune system to build its own antibodies against specific microorganisms/viruses. The body retains memory of these antibody production patterns for long-term protection. This code reports a meningococcal polysaccharide vaccine (any group), for subcutaneous use. Report this code with the appropriate administration code.

90735

90735 Japanese encephalitis virus vaccine, for subcutaneous use

Explanation

A vaccine produces active immunization by inducing the immune system to build its own antibodies against specific microorganisms/viruses. The body retains memory of these antibody production patterns for long-term protection. This code describes a Japanese encephalitis virus vaccine for subcutaneous use. Report this code with the appropriate administration code.

90736

90736 Zoster (shingles) vaccine, live, for subcutaneous injection

Explanation

A vaccine produces active immunization by inducing the immune system to manufacture its own antibodies against specific microorganisms/viruses. The body retains memory of these antibody production patterns for long-term protection. This code reports a live herpes zoster (shingles) vaccine for subcutaneous injection. Shingles is a reactivation of the herpes zoster virus that causes chickenpox. The virus persists in a dormant state and may reactivate with certain conditions or advancing age that cause or is associated with immune system compromise. This vaccine prevents herpes zoster and postherpetic neuralgia as a result of the dormant virus in sensory nerve cells. Report this code with the appropriate administration code.

90739-90747

90739 Hepatitis B vaccine, adult dosage (2 dose schedule), for intramuscular use

90740 Hepatitis B vaccine, dialysis or immunosuppressed patient dosage (3 dose schedule), for intramuscular use

90743 Hepatitis B vaccine, adolescent (2 dose schedule), for intramuscular use

90744 Hepatitis B vaccine, pediatric/adolescent dosage (3 dose schedule), for intramuscular use

90746 Hepatitis B vaccine, adult dosage (3 dose schedule), for intramuscular use

90747 Hepatitis B vaccine, dialysis or immunosuppressed patient dosage (4 dose schedule), for intramuscular use

Explanation

A vaccine produces active immunization by inducing the immune system to build its own antibodies against specific microorganisms/viruses. The body retains memory of these antibody production patterns for long-term protection. These codes are used to report the supply of a hepatitis B vaccine for intramuscular use, prepared in various dosages. Report 90739 for an adult two-dose schedule;

90740 for a three-dose schedule for a dialysis or immunosuppressed patient; 90743 for an adolescent two-dose schedule; 90744 for a pediatric/adolescent three-dose schedule; 90746 for an adult three-dose schedule; and 90747 for a four-dose schedule for a dialysis or immunosuppressed patient. Report these codes with the appropriate administration code.

Coding Tips

Code 90739 is new for 2013. Code 90746 has been revised for 2013 in the official CPT description.

90748

90748 Hepatitis B and Hemophilus influenza b vaccine (HepB-Hib), for intramuscular use

Explanation

A vaccine produces active immunization by inducing the immune system to build its own antibodies against specific microorganisms/viruses. The body retains memory of these antibody production patterns for long-term protection. This code describes a combined hepatitis B and Hemophilus influenza B (HepB-Hib)) vaccine for intramuscular use. Report this code with the appropriate administration code.

92950

92950 Cardiopulmonary resuscitation (eg, in cardiac arrest)

Explanation

Cardiopulmonary arrest occurs when the patient's heart and lungs suddenly stop. In a clinical setting, cardiopulmonary resuscitation, the attempt at restarting the heart and lungs, is usually directed by a physician or another health care provider who is certified in Advanced Cardiac Life Support (ACLS). The patient's lungs are ventilated by mouth-to-mouth breathing or by a bag and mask. The patient's circulation is assisted using external chest compression. An electronic defibrillator may be used to shock the heart into restarting. Medications used to restart the heart include epinephrine and lidocaine.

93975

93975 Duplex scan of arterial inflow and venous outflow of abdominal, pelvic, scrotal contents and/or retroperitoneal organs; complete study

Explanation

The physician or assistant performs a Duplex ultrasound scan, which is a combination of real-time and Doppler studies, of the arteries and veins in the abdominal, pelvic, or genitorectal areas to evaluate vascular blood flow in relation to blockage. This code applies to a complete bilateral evaluation.

93976

93976 Duplex scan of arterial inflow and venous outflow of abdominal, pelvic, scrotal contents and/or retroperitoneal organs; limited study

Explanation

The physician or assistant performs a Duplex ultrasound scan, which is a combination of real-time and Doppler studies, of the arteries and veins in the abdominal, pelvic, or genitorectal areas to evaluate vascular blood flow in relation to blockage. This code applies to a limited evaluation.

96040

96040 Medical genetics and genetic counseling services, each 30 minutes face-to-face with patient/family

Explanation

The trained genetic counselor meets with an individual, couple, or family to investigate family genetic history and assess the risks associated with genetic defects in offspring. This code covers 30 minutes of face-to-face counseling, review of medical data, or data collection (interviews).

96360-96361

96360 Intravenous infusion, hydration; initial, 31 minutes to 1 hour
96361 each additional hour (List separately in addition to code for primary procedure)

Explanation

A physician or an assistant under direct physician supervision infuses a hydration solution (prepackaged fluid and electrolytes) for 31 minutes to one hour through an intravenous catheter inserted by needle into a patient's vein or by infusion through an existing indwelling intravascular access catheter or port. Report 96361 for each additional hour beyond the first hour. Intravenous infusion for hydration lasting 30 minutes or less is not reported.

96365-96368

96365 Intravenous infusion, for therapy, prophylaxis, or diagnosis (specify substance or drug); initial, up to 1 hour
96366 each additional hour (List separately in addition to code for primary procedure)
96367 additional sequential infusion of a new drug/substance, up to 1 hour (List separately in addition to code for primary procedure)
96368 concurrent infusion (List separately in addition to code for primary procedure)

Explanation

A physician or an assistant under direct physician supervision injects or infuses a therapeutic, prophylactic (preventive), or diagnostic medication other than chemotherapy or other highly complex drugs or biologic agents via intravenous route. Infusions are administered through an intravenous catheter inserted by needle into a patient's vein or by injection or infusion through an existing indwelling intravascular access catheter or port. Report 96365 for the initial hour and 96366 for each additional hour. Report 96367 for each additional sequential infusion of a different substance or drug, up to one hour, and 96368 for each concurrent infusion of substances other than chemotherapy or other highly complex drugs or biologic agents.

96369-96371

96369 Subcutaneous infusion for therapy or prophylaxis (specify substance or drug); initial, up to 1 hour, including pump set-up and establishment of subcutaneous infusion site(s)
96370 each additional hour (List separately in addition to code for primary procedure)
96371 additional pump set-up with establishment of new subcutaneous infusion site(s) (List separately in addition to code for primary procedure)

Explanation

A physician or an assistant under direct physician supervision infuses a therapeutic or prophylactic (preventive) medication other than chemotherapy or other highly complex drug or biologic agent via a subcutaneous route. Indications for subcutaneous infusion may include coma, dysphagia, nausea/vomiting, intestinal obstruction, malabsorption, or extreme weakness. Infusions are administered through a needle inserted beneath the skin; common infusion sites include the upper arm, shoulder, abdomen, and thigh. Report 96369 for infusions lasting longer than 15 minutes and up to one hour. This code includes pump set-up and the establishment of subcutaneous infusion sites. Report 96370 for each additional hour and 96371 for an additional pump set-up with the establishment of new subcutaneous infusion sites. Codes 96369 and 96371 should be reported only once per encounter.

Appendix

96372-96376

96372 Therapeutic, prophylactic, or diagnostic injection (specify substance or drug); subcutaneous or intramuscular
96373 intra-arterial
96374 intravenous push, single or initial substance/drug
96375 each additional sequential intravenous push of a new substance/drug (List separately in addition to code for primary procedure)
96376 each additional sequential intravenous push of the same substance/drug provided in a facility (List separately in addition to code for primary procedure)

Explanation

The physician or an assistant under direct physician supervision administers a therapeutic, prophylactic, or diagnostic substance by subcutaneous or intramuscular injection (96372), intra-arterial injection (96373), or by push into an intravenous catheter or intravascular access device (96374 for a single or initial substance, 96375 for each additional sequential IV push of a new substance, and 96376 for each additional sequential IV push of the same substance after 30 minutes have elapsed). The push technique involves an infusion of less than 15 minutes. Code 96376 may be reported only by facilities.

97597-97598

97597 Debridement (eg, high pressure waterjet with/without suction, sharp selective debridement with scissors, scalpel and forceps), open wound, (eg, fibrin, devitalized epidermis and/or dermis, exudate, debris, biofilm), including topical application(s), wound assessment, use of a whirlpool, when performed and instruction(s) for ongoing care, per session, total wound(s) surface area; first 20 sq cm or less
97598 each additional 20 sq cm, or part thereof (List separately in addition to code for primary procedure)

Explanation

A health care provider performs wound care management by using selective debridement techniques to remove devitalized or necrotic tissue from an open wound. Selective techniques are those in which the provider has complete control over which tissue is removed and which is left behind, and include high-pressure waterjet with or without suction and sharp debridement using scissors, a scalpel, or forceps. Wound assessment, topical applications, instructions regarding ongoing care of the wound, and the possible use of a whirlpool for treatment are included in these codes. Report 97597 for a total wound surface area less than or equal to 20 sq cm and 97598 for each additional 20 sq cm or part thereof.

97602

97602 Removal of devitalized tissue from wound(s), non-selective debridement, without anesthesia (eg, wet-to-moist dressings, enzymatic, abrasion), including topical application(s), wound assessment, and instruction(s) for ongoing care, per session

Explanation

The health care provider performs wound care management to promote healing using non-selective debridement techniques to remove devitalized tissue. Non-selective debridement techniques are those in which both necrotic and healthy tissue are removed. Non-selective techniques, sometimes referred to as mechanical debridement, include wet-to-moist dressings, enzymatic chemicals, autolytic debridement, and abrasion. Wet-to-moist debridement involves allowing a dressing to proceed from wet to moist, and manually removing the dressing, which removes both the necrotic and healthy tissue. Chemical enzymes are fast acting products that produce slough of necrotic tissue. Autolytic debridement is accomplished using occlusive or semi-occlusive dressings that keep wound fluid in contact with the necrotic tissue. Types of dressing applications used in autolytic debridement include hydrocolloids, hydrogels, and transparent films. Abrasion involves scraping the wound surface with a tongue blade or similar blunt instrument.

97605-97606

97605 Negative pressure wound therapy (eg, vacuum assisted drainage collection), including topical application(s), wound assessment, and instruction(s) for ongoing care, per session; total wound(s) surface area less than or equal to 50 square centimeters
97606 total wound(s) surface area greater than 50 square centimeters

Explanation

The health care provider performs negative pressure wound therapy (NPWT) with vacuum assisted drainage collection to promote healing of a chronic non-healing wound, including diabetic or pressure (decubitus) ulcer. This procedure includes topical applications to the wound, wound assessment, and patient or caregiver instruction related to on-going care per session. Negative pressure wound therapy uses controlled application of subatmospheric pressure to a wound. The subatmospheric pressure is generated using an electrical pump. The electrical pump conveys intermittent or continuous subatmospheric pressure through connecting tubing to a specialized wound dressing. The specialized wound dressing includes a porous foam dressing that covers the wound surface and an airtight adhesive dressing that seals the wound and contains the subatmospheric pressure at the wound site. Negative pressure wound therapy promotes healing by increasing local vascularity and oxygenation of the wound bed, evacuating wound fluid thereby reducing edema, and removing exudates and bacteria. Drainage from the wound is collected in a canister. Report 97605 for a wound(s) with a total surface area less than or equal to 50 sq. cm. Report 97606 for a wound(s) with a total surface area greater than 50 sq. cm.

97802-97804

97802 Medical nutrition therapy; initial assessment and intervention, individual, face-to-face with the patient, each 15 minutes
97803 re-assessment and intervention, individual, face-to-face with the patient, each 15 minutes
97804 group (2 or more individual(s)), each 30 minutes

Explanation

A dietetic professional provides medical nutrition therapy assessment or re-assessment and intervention in a face-to-face or group patient setting. After nutritional screening identifies patients at risk, preventive or therapeutic dietary therapy is initiated to induce a positive result in the role nutrition plays in improving health outcomes. Report 97802 for the initial assessment and intervention face-to-face with an individual patient for each 15 minutes of medical nutrition therapy. Report 97803 for re-assessment and intervention with an individual patient for each 15 minutes of medical nutrition therapy. Report 97804 for group medical nutrition therapy provided for two or more individuals, each 30 minutes.

98925-98929

98925 Osteopathic manipulative treatment (OMT); 1-2 body regions involved
98926 3-4 body regions involved
98927 5-6 body regions involved
98928 7-8 body regions involved
98929 9-10 body regions involved

Explanation

The physician uses these codes to report osteopathic manipulation, unique manual treatments that are used to treat somatic dysfunction and related disorders. Several techniques exist. Body regions included are head, cervical thoracic, lumbar, sacral, pelvic, extremities, rib cage, abdomen, and viscera. Report 98925 if one to two body regions are involved; 98926 if three to four body regions are involved; 98927 if five to six body regions are involved; 98928 if seven to eight body regions are involved; and 98929 if nine body regions are involved.

Coding Companion for Ob/Gyn

© 2012 OptumInsight, Inc.

Appendix

98966-98968

98966 Telephone assessment and management service provided by a qualified nonphysician health care professional to an established patient, parent, or guardian not originating from a related assessment and management service provided within the previous 7 days nor leading to an assessment and management service or procedure within the next 24 hours or soonest available appointment; 5-10 minutes of medical discussion

98967 11-20 minutes of medical discussion

98968 21-30 minutes of medical discussion

Explanation

A qualified health care professional (nonphysician) provides telephone assessment and management services to a patient in a non-face-to-face encounter. These episodes of care may be initiated by an established patient or by the patient's guardian. These codes are not reported if the telephone service results in a decision to see the patient within 24 hours or at the next available urgent visit appointment; instead, the phone encounter is regarded as part of the pre-service work of the subsequent face-to-face encounter. These codes are also not reported if the telephone call is in reference to a service performed and reported by the qualified health care professional that occurred within the past seven days or within the postoperative period of a previously completed procedure. This applies both to unsolicited patient follow-up or that requested by the health care professional. Report 98966 for telephone services requiring five to 10 minutes of medical discussion, 98967 for telephone services requiring 11 to 20 minutes of medical discussion, and 98968 for telephone services requiring 21 to 30 minutes of medical discussion. Do not report 98966-98968 if these codes have been reported within the previous seven days.

98969

98969 Online assessment and management service provided by a qualified nonphysician health care professional to an established patient or guardian, not originating from a related assessment and management service provided within the previous 7 days, using the Internet or similar electronic communications network

Explanation

On-line medical assessment and management services are provided to an established patient or guardian in response to a patient's on-line inquiry utilizing Internet resources in a non-face-to-face encounter. Services must be provided by a qualified health care professional (nonphysician). In order for these services to be reportable, the health care professional must provide a personal, timely response to the inquiry and the encounter must be permanently stored via electronic means or hard copy. A reportable service includes all communication related to the on-line encounter, such as phone calls, provision of prescriptions, and orders for laboratory services. This code is not reported if the on-line evaluation is in reference to a service performed and reported by the same health care professional within the past seven days or within the postoperative period of a previously completed procedure. Rather, the on-line service is considered to be part of the previous service or procedure. This applies both to unsolicited patient follow-up or that requested by the health care professional. Report 98969 only once for the same episode of care during a seven-day period.

Coding Tips

This code has been revised for 2013 in the official CPT description.

99000

99000 Handling and/or conveyance of specimen for transfer from the office to a laboratory

Explanation

This code is adjunct to basic services rendered. This code is reported for the handling and/or conveyance of a specimen from the provider's office to a laboratory.

Coding Tips

This code has been revised for 2013 in the official CPT description.

99001

99001 Handling and/or conveyance of specimen for transfer from the patient in other than an office to a laboratory (distance may be indicated)

Explanation

This code is adjunct to basic services rendered. This code is reported for the handling and/or conveyance of a specimen from the patient in a location other than the provider's office to the laboratory.

Coding Tips

This code has been revised for 2013 in the official CPT description.

99026-99027

99026 Hospital mandated on call service; in-hospital, each hour

99027 out-of-hospital, each hour

Explanation

The code reports the time for hospital mandated on call service provided by the physician. This code does not include prolonged physician attendance time for standby services or the time spent performing other reportable procedures or services. Report 99026 for each hour of hospital mandated on call service spent in the hospital and 99027 for each hour of hospital mandated on call service spent outside the hospital.

99050

99050 Services provided in the office at times other than regularly scheduled office hours, or days when the office is normally closed (eg, holidays, Saturday or Sunday), in addition to basic service

Explanation

This code is adjunct to basic services rendered. The physician reports this code to indicate services after posted office hours in addition to basic services.

99051

99051 Service(s) provided in the office during regularly scheduled evening, weekend, or holiday office hours, in addition to basic service

Explanation

This code is adjunct to basic services rendered. The physician reports this code to indicate services provided during posted evening, weekend, or holiday office hours in addition to basic services.

99053

99053 Service(s) provided between 10:00 PM and 8:00 AM at 24-hour facility, in addition to basic service

Explanation

This code is adjunct to basic services rendered. The physician reports this code to indicate services provided between 10 p.m. and 8 a.m. at a 24-hour facility in addition to basic services.

99056

99056 Service(s) typically provided in the office, provided out of the office at request of patient, in addition to basic service

Explanation

This code is adjunct to basic services rendered. The physician reports this code to indicate services typically provided in the office that are provided in a different location at the request of a patient.

99058

99058 Service(s) provided on an emergency basis in the office, which disrupts other scheduled office services, in addition to basic service

Explanation

This code is adjunct to basic services rendered. The physician reports this code to indicate services

Appendix

provided in the office on an emergency basis that disrupt other scheduled office services.

99060

99060 Service(s) provided on an emergency basis, out of the office, which disrupts other scheduled office services, in addition to basic service

Explanation

This code is adjunct to basic services rendered. The physician reports this code to indicate services provided on an emergency basis in a location other than the physician's office that disrupt other scheduled office services.

99143-99145

99143 Moderate sedation services (other than those services described by codes 00100-01999) provided by the same physician or other qualified health care professional performing the diagnostic or therapeutic service that the sedation supports, requiring the presence of an independent trained observer to assist in the monitoring of the patient's level of consciousness and physiological status; younger than 5 years of age, first 30 minutes intra-service time

99144 age 5 years or older, first 30 minutes intra-service time

99145 each additional 15 minutes intra-service time (List separately in addition to code for primary service)

Explanation

A physician or other trained health care provider administers medication that allows a decreased level of consciousness but does not put the patient completely asleep inducing a state called moderate (conscious) sedation. This allows the patient to breathe without assistance and respond to commands. This is used for less invasive procedures and/or as a second medication for pain. This code reports sedation services provided by the same provider performing the primary procedure with the assistance of an independently trained health care professional to assist in monitoring the patient. Report 99143 for the first 30 minutes of intra-service time for sedation services rendered to a patient younger than 5 years of age. Report 99144 for the first 30 minutes of intra-service time for sedation services rendered to a patient age 5 years of age or older. Report 99145 for each additional 15 minutes of service.

Coding Tips

These codes have been revised for 2013 in the official CPT description.

99148-99150

99148 Moderate sedation services (other than those services described by codes 00100-01999), provided by a physician or other qualified health care professional other than the health care professional performing the diagnostic or therapeutic service that the sedation supports; younger than 5 years of age, first 30 minutes intra-service time

99149 age 5 years or older, first 30 minutes intra-service time

99150 each additional 15 minutes intra-service time (List separately in addition to code for primary service)

Explanation

A physician or trained health care provider administers medication that allows a decreased level of consciousness but does not put the patient completely asleep, inducing a state called moderate (conscious) sedation. This allows the patient to breathe without assistance and respond to commands. This is used for less invasive procedures and/or as a second medication for pain. These codes report services provided by a qualified provider other than the health care provider performing the diagnostic or therapeutic service that the sedation supports. These codes are only reported for encounters in a facility setting (i.e., hospital, ASC, SNF) rather than an office or nonfacility setting. Report 99148 for the first 30 minutes of intra-service time for sedation services rendered to a patient younger than 5 years of age. Report 99149 for the first 30 minutes of intra-service time for sedation services rendered to a patient age 5 years of age or older. Report 99150 for each additional 15 minutes of service.

Coding Tips

These codes have been revised for 2013 in the official CPT description.

99601-99602

99601 Home infusion/specialty drug administration, per visit (up to 2 hours);

99602 each additional hour (List separately in addition to code for primary procedure)

Explanation

A home health professional visits the patient at home to perform the infusion of a specialty drug per a physician's order. The home health provider brings the supplies and medication required and administers and oversees the infusion. Each infusion takes up to two hours per visit for 99601. Report 99602 for each additional hour.

0058T-0059T

0058T Cryopreservation; reproductive tissue, ovarian

0059T oocyte(s)

Explanation

Cryopreservation is a technique of freezing and maintaining cells at extremely low temperatures to preserve the genetic and metabolic properties of the cell. The ovarian tissue or oocyte specimens are first preserved in a cryoprotectant solution to reduce cellular damage and the tissue is placed in storage vials. The sample is gradually frozen in liquid nitrogen. Cryopreserved samples are stored at temperatures of -80 to -196 degrees centigrade. The amount of cells being frozen, the source and amount of protective solution used, and the cooling technique may vary. Cryopreservation of ovarian reproductive tissue is reported with 0058T and oocyte(s) with 0059T.

0071T-0072T

0071T Focused ultrasound ablation of uterine leiomyomata, including MR guidance; total leiomyomata volume less than 200 cc of tissue

0072T total leiomyomata volume greater or equal to 200 cc of tissue

Explanation

Focused ultrasound ablation is a noninvasive surgical technique that uses thermal ablation to destroy uterine leiomyomata. In focused ultrasound ablation the ultrasound beam penetrates through soft tissues causing localized high temperatures for a few seconds at the targeted site, in this case the uterine leiomyomata. This produces thermocoagulation and necrosis of the uterine leiomyomata without damage to overlaying and surrounding tissues. Magnetic resonance (MR) guidance is used in conjunction with focused ultrasound ablation to provide more precise target definition. Since certain MR parameters are also temperature sensitive, MR guidance also allows estimation of optimal thermal doses to the uterine leiomyomata and detection of relatively small temperature elevations in surrounding tissues thereby preventing any irreversible damage to surrounding tissues. Report 0071T for total leiomyomata tissue volume less than 200 cc. Report 0072T for leiomyomata tissue volume equal to or greater than 200 cc.

Evaluation and Management

This section provides an overview of evaluation and management (E/M) services, tables that identify the documentation elements associated with each code, and the federal documentation guidelines with emphasis on the 1997 exam guidelines. This set of guidelines represent the most complete discussion of the elements of the currently accepted versions. The 1997 version identifies both general multi-system physical examinations and single-system examinations, but providers may also use the original 1995 version of the E/M guidelines; both are currently supported by the Centers for Medicare and Medicaid Services (CMS) for audit purposes.

Although some of the most commonly used codes by physicians of all specialties, the E/M service codes are among the least understood. These codes, introduced in the 1992 CPT® manual, were designed to increase accuracy and consistency of use in the reporting of levels of non-procedural encounters. This was accomplished by defining the E/M codes based on the degree that certain common elements are addressed or performed and reflected in the medical documentation.

The Office of the Inspector General (OIG) Work Plan for physicians consistently lists these codes as an area of continued investigative review. This is primarily because Medicare payments for these services total approximately $32 billion per year and are responsible for close to half of Medicare payments for physician services.

The levels of E/M services define the wide variations in skill, effort, and time and are required for preventing and/or diagnosing and treating illness or injury, and promoting optimal health. These codes are intended to represent physician work, and because much of this work involves the amount of training, experience, expertise, and knowledge that a provider may bring to bear on a given patient presentation, the true indications of the level of this work may be difficult to recognize without some explanation.

At first glance, selecting an E/M code may appear to be difficult, but the system of coding clinical visits may be mastered once the requirements for code selection are learned and used.

Providers

The AMA advises coders that while a particular service or procedure may be assigned to a specific section, the service or procedure itself is not limited to use only by that specialty group (see paragraphs 2 and 3 under "Instructions for Use of the CPT Codebook" on page x of the CPT Book). Additionally, the procedures and services listed throughout the book are for use by any qualified physician or other qualified health care professional or entity (e.g., hospitals, laboratories, or home health agencies).

The use of the phrase "physician or other qualified health care professional" (OQHCP) was adopted to identify a health care provider other than a physician. This type of provider is further described in CPT as an individual "qualified by education, training, licensure/regulation (when applicable), and facility privileging (when applicable)" State licensure guidelines determine the scope of practice and a qualified health care professional must practice within these guidelines, even if more restrictive than the CPT

guidelines. The qualified health care professional may report services independently or under incident-to guidelines. The professionals within this definition are separate from "clinical staff" and are able to practice independently. CPT defines clinical staff as "a person who works under the supervision of a physician or other qualified health care professional and who is allowed, by law, regulation, and facility policy to perform or assist in the performance of a specified professional service, but who does not individually report that professional service." Keep in mind that there may be other policies or guidance that can affect who may report a specific service.

Types of E/M Services

When approaching E/M, the first choice that a provider must make is what type of code to use. The following tables outline the E/M codes for different levels of care for:

- Office or other outpatient services—new patient
- Office or other outpatient services—established patient
- Hospital observation services—initial care, subsequent, and discharge
- Hospital inpatient services—initial care, subsequent, and discharge
- Observation or inpatient care (including admission and discharge services)
- Consultations—office or other outpatient
- Consultations—inpatient

The specifics of the code components that determine code selection are listed in the table and discussed in the next section. Before a level of service is decided upon, the correct type of service is identified.

Office or other outpatient services are E/M services provided in the physician or other qualified health care provider's office, the outpatient area, or other ambulatory facility. Until the patient is admitted to a health care facility, he/she is considered to be an outpatient.

A new patient is a patient who has not received any face-to-face professional services from the physician or other qualified health care provider within the past three years. An established patient is a patient who has received face-to-face professional services from the physician or other qualified health care provider within the past three years. In the case of group practices, if a physician or other qualified health care provider of the exact same specialty or subspecialty has seen the patient within three years, the patient is considered established.

If a physician or other qualified health care provider is on call or covering for another physician or other qualified health care provider, the patient's encounter is classified as it would have been by the physician or other qualified health care provider who is not available. Thus, a locum tenens physician or other qualified health care provider who sees a patient on behalf of the patient's attending physician or other qualified health care provider may not bill a new

© 2012 OptumInsight, Inc.

patient code unless the attending physician or other qualified health care provider has not seen the patient for any problem within three years.

Hospital observation services are E/M services provided to patients who are designated or admitted as "observation status" in a hospital.

Codes 99218-99220 are used to indicate initial observation care. These codes include the initiation of the observation status, supervision of patient care including writing orders, and the performance of periodic reassessments. These codes are used only by the provider "admitting" the patient for observation.

Codes 99234-99236 are used to indicate evaluation and management services to a patient who is admitted to and discharged from observation status or hospital inpatient on the same day. If the patient is admitted as an inpatient from observation on the same day, use the appropriate level of Initial Hospital Care (99221-99223).

Code 99217 indicates discharge from observation status. It includes the final physical examination of the patient, instructions, and preparation of the discharge records. It should not be used when admission and discharge are on the same date of service. As mentioned above, report codes 99234-99236 to appropriately describe same day observation services.

If a patient is in observation longer than one day, subsequent observation care codes 99224-99226 should be reported. If the patient is discharged on the second day, observation discharge code 99217 should be reported. If the patient status is changed to inpatient on a subsequent date, the appropriate inpatient code, 99221-99233, should be reported.

Initial hospital care is defined as E/M services provided during the first hospital inpatient encounter with the patient by the admitting provider. (If a physician other than the admitting physician performs the initial inpatient encounter, refer to consultations or subsequent hospital care in the CPT book.) Subsequent hospital care includes all follow-up encounters with the patient by all physicians or other qualified health care providers.

A consultation is the provision of a physician or other qualified health care provider's opinion or advice about a patient for a specific problem at the request of another physician or other appropriate source. CPT also states that a consultation may be performed when a physician or other qualified health care provider is determining whether to accept the transfer of patient care at the request of another physician or appropriate source. An office or other outpatient consultation is a consultation provided in the consultant's office, in the emergency department, or in an outpatient or other ambulatory facility including hospital observation services, home services, domiciliary, rest home, or custodial care. An inpatient consultation is a consultation provided in the hospital or partial hospital nursing facility setting. Report only one inpatient consultation by a consultant for each admission to the hospital or nursing facility.

If a consultant participates in the patient's management after the opinion or advice is provided, use codes for subsequent hospital or observation care or for office or other outpatient services (established patient), as appropriate.

CMS adopted new policies regarding the use of consultation codes beginning in 2010. Under these guidelines the inpatient and office/outpatient consultation codes contained in the CPT manual will not be a covered service for CMS. However, Medicare will cover telehealth consultations when reported with the appropriate HCPCS Level II G code.

Additional changes regarding inpatient services were initiated in 2010 by CMS. All outpatient services will be reported using the appropriate new or established evaluation and management (E/M) codes. Inpatient services for the first initial encounter should be reported by the physician providing the service using initial hospital care codes 99221–99223, and subsequent inpatient care codes 99231–99233. As there may only be one admitting physician, CMS has added HCPCS Level II modifier AI, Principal physician of record, which may be appended to the initial hospital care code by the attending physician or other qualified health care provider.

Note: The E/M codes were revised for 2013 to indicate that the majority of these services may be provided by a physician or other qualified health care professional. Unless otherwise indicated, the E/M services may be provided by the physician or other qualified health care professional.

Coding Companion for OB/GYN

Office or Other Outpatient Services—New Patient

E/M Code	History[1]	Exam[1]	Medical Decision Making[1]	Problem Severity	Coordination of Care; Counseling	Time Spent Face-to-Face (avg.)
99201	Problem-focused	Problem-focused	Straight-forward	Minor or self-limited	Consistent with problem(s) and patient's needs	10 min.
99202	Expanded problem-focused	Expanded problem-focused	Straight-forward	Low to moderate	Consistent with problem(s) and patient's needs	20 min.
99203	Detailed	Detailed	Low complexity	Moderate	Consistent with problem(s) and patient's needs	30 min.
99204	Comprehensive	Comprehensive	Moderate complexity	Moderate to high	Consistent with problem(s) and patient's needs	45 min.
99205	Comprehensive	Comprehensive	High complexity	Moderate to high	Consistent with problem(s) and patient's needs	60 min.

1 Key component. For new patients, all three components (history, exam, and medical decision making) are crucial for selecting the correct code.

Office or Other Outpatient Services—Established Patient[1]

E/M Code	History[2]	Exam[2]	Medical Decision Making[2]	Problem Severity	Coordination of Care; Counseling	Time Spent Face-to-Face (avg.)
99211	—	—	Physician supervision, but presence not required	Minimal	Consistent with problem(s) and patient's needs	5 min.
99212	Problem-focused	Problem-focused	Straight-forward	Minor or self-limited	Consistent with problem(s) and patient's needs	10 min.
99213	Expanded problem-focused	Expanded problem-focused	Low complexity	Low to moderate	Consistent with problem(s) and patient's needs	15 min.
99214	Detailed	Detailed	Moderate complexity	Moderate to high	Consistent with problem(s) and patient's needs	25 min.
99215	Comprehensive	Comprehensive	High complexity	Moderate to high	Consistent with problem(s) and patient's needs	40 min.

1 Includes follow-up, periodic reevaluation, and evaluation and management of new problems.
2 Key component. For established patients, at least two of the three components (history, exam, and medical decision making) are needed to select the correct code.

Hospital Observation Services

E/M Code	History[1]	Exam[1]	Medical Decision Making[1]	Problem Severity	Coordination of Care; Counseling	Time Spent Bedside and on Unit/Floor (avg.)
99217	Observation care discharge day management					
99218	Detailed or comprehensive	Detailed or comprehensive	Straight-forward or low complexity	Low	Consistent with problem(s) and patient's needs	30 min.
99219	Comprehensive	Comprehensive	Moderate complexity	Moderate	Consistent with problem(s) and patient's needs	50 min.
99220	Comprehensive	Comprehensive	High complexity	High	Consistent with problem(s) and patient's needs	70 min.

1 Key component. All three components (history, exam, and medical decision making) are crucial for selecting the correct code.

© 2012 OptumInsight, Inc.

Subsequent Hospital Observation Services[1]

E/M Code[2]	History[3]	Exam[3]	Medical Decision Making[3]	Problem Severity	Coordination of Care; Counseling	Time Spent Bedside and on Unit/Floor (avg.)
99224	Problem-focused interval	Problem-focused	Straight-forward or low complexity	Stable, recovering, or improving	Consistent with problem(s) and patient's needs	15 min.
99225	Expanded problem-focused interval	Expanded problem-focused	Moderate complexity	Inadequate response to treatment; minor complications	Consistent with problem(s) and patient's needs	25 min.
99226	Detailed interval	Detailed	High complexity	Unstable; significant new problem or significant complication	Consistent with problem(s) and patient's needs	35 min.

1 All subsequent levels of service include reviewing the medical record, diagnostic studies, and changes in the patient's status, such as history, physical condition, and response to treatment since the last assessment.
2 These codes are resequenced in CPT and printed following codes 99217-99220.
3 Key component. For subsequent care, at least two of the three components (history, exam, and medical decision making) are needed to select the correct code.

Hospital Inpatient Services—Initial Care[1]

E/M Code	History[2]	Exam[2]	Medical Decision Making[2]	Problem Severity	Coordination of Care; Counseling	Time Spent Bedside and on Unit/Floor (avg.)
99221	Detailed or comprehensive	Detailed or comprehensive	Straight-forward or low complexity	Low	Consistent with problem(s) and patient's needs	30 min.
99222	Comprehensive	Comprehensive	Moderate complexity	Moderate	Consistent with problem(s) and patient's needs	50 min.
99223	Comprehensive	Comprehensive	High complexity	High	Consistent with problem(s) and patient's needs	70 min.

1 The admitting physician should append modifier AI, Principal physician of record, for Medicare patients
2 Key component. For initial care, all three components (history, exam, and medical decision making) are crucial for selecting the correct code.

Hospital Inpatient Services—Subsequent Care[1]

E/M Code	History[2]	Exam[2]	Medical Decision Making[2]	Problem Severity	Coordination of Care; Counseling	Time Spent Bedside and on Unit/Floor (avg.)
99231	Problem-focused interval	Problem-focused	Straight-forward or low complexity	Stable, recovering or Improving	Consistent with problem(s) and patient's needs	15 min.
99232	Expanded problem-focused interval	Expanded problem-focused	Moderate complexity	Inadequate response to treatment; minor complications	Consistent with problem(s) and patient's needs	25 min.
99233	Detailed interval	Detailed	High complexity	Unstable; significant new problem or significant complication	Consistent with problem(s) and patient's needs	35 min.
99238	Hospital discharge day management					30 min. or less
99239	Hospital discharge day management					> 30 min.

1 All subsequent levels of service include reviewing the medical record, diagnostic studies, and changes in the patient's status, such as history, physical condition, and response to treatment since the last assessment.
2 Key component. For subsequent care, at least two of the three components (history, exam, and medical decision making) are needed to select the correct code.

Coding Companion for OB/GYN

Observation or Inpatient Care Services (Including Admission and Discharge Services)

E/M Code	History[1]	Exam[1]	Medical Decision Making[1]	Problem Severity	Coordination of Care; Counseling	Time[2]
99234	Detailed or comprehensive	Detailed or comprehensive	Straight-forward or low complexity	Low	Consistent with problem(s) and patient's needs	N/A
99235	Comprehensive	Comprehensive	Moderate	Moderate	Consistent with problem(s) and patient's needs	N/A
99236	Comprehensive	Comprehensive	High	High	Consistent with problem(s) and patient's needs	N/A

1 Key component. All three components (history, exam, and medical decision making) are crucial for selecting the correct code.
2 Typical times have not been established for this category of services.

Consultations—Office or Other Outpatient

E/M Code	History[1]	Exam[1]	Medical Decision Making[1]	Problem Severity	Coordination of Care; Counseling	Time Spent Face-to-Face (avg.)
99241	Problem-focused	Problem-focused	Straight-forward	Minor or self-limited	Consistent with problem(s) and patient's needs	15 min.
99242	Expanded problem-focused	Expanded problem-focused	Straight-forward	Low	Consistent with problem(s) and patient's needs	30 min.
99243	Detailed	Detailed	Low complexity	Moderate	Consistent with problem(s) and patient's needs	40 min.
99244	Comprehensive	Comprehensive	Moderate complexity	Moderate to high	Consistent with problem(s) and patient's needs	60 min.
99245	Comprehensive	Comprehensive	High complexity	Moderate to high	Consistent with problem(s) and patient's needs	80 min.

1 Key component. For office or other outpatient consultations, all three components (history, exam, and medical decision making) are crucial for selecting the correct code.

Consultations—Inpatient[1]

E/M Code	History[2]	Exam[2]	Medical Decision Making[2]	Problem Severity	Coordination of Care; Counseling	Time Spent Bedside and on Unit/Floor (avg.)
99251	Problem-focused	Problem-focused	Straight-forward	Minor or self-limited	Consistent with problem(s) and patient's needs	20 min.
99252	Expanded problem-focused	Expanded problem-focused	Straight-forward	Low	Consistent with problem(s) and patient's needs	40 min.
99253	Detailed	Detailed	Low complexity	Moderate	Consistent with problem(s) and patient's needs	55 min.
99254	Comprehensive	Comprehensive	Moderate complexity	Moderate to high	Consistent with problem(s) and patient's needs	80 min.
99255	Comprehensive	Comprehensive	High complexity	Moderate to high	Consistent with problem(s) and patient's needs	110 min.

1 These codes are used for hospital inpatients, residents of nursing facilities or patients in a partial hospital setting.
2 Key component. For initial inpatient consultations, all three components (history, exam, and medical decision making) are crucial for selecting the correct code.

© 2012 OptumInsight, Inc.

Emergency Department Services, New or Established Patient

E/M Code	History[1]	Exam[1]	Medical Decision Making[1]	Problem Severity[3]	Coordination of Care; Counseling	Time Spent[2] Face-to-Face (avg.)
99281	Problem-focused	Problem-focused	Straight-forward	Minor or self-limited	Consistent with problem(s) and patient's needs	N/A
99282	Expanded problem-focused	Expanded problem-focused	Low complexity	Low to moderate	Consistent with problem(s) and patient's needs	N/A
99283	Expanded problem-focused	Expanded problem-focused	Moderate complexity	Moderate	Consistent with problem(s) and patient's needs	N/A
99284	Detailed	Detailed	Moderate complexity	High; requires urgent evaluation	Consistent with problem(s) and patient's needs	N/A
99285	Comprehensive	Comprehensive	High complexity	High; poses immediate/ significant threat to life or physiologic function	Consistent with problem(s) and patient's needs	N/A
99288[4]			High complexity			N/A

1 Key component. For emergency department services, all three components (history, exam, and medical decision making) are crucial for selecting the correct code and must be adequately documented in the medical record to substantiate the level of service reported.

2 Typical times have not been established for this category of services.

3 NOTE: The severity of the patient's problem, while taken into consideration when evaluating and treating the patient, does not automatically determine the level of E/M service unless the medical record documentation reflects the severity of the patient's illness, injury, or condition in the details of the history, physical examination, and medical decision making process. Federal auditors will "downcode" the level of E/M service despite the nature of the patient's problem when the documentation does not support the E/M code reported.

4 Code 99288 is used to report two-way communication with emergency medical services personnel in the field.

Critical Care

E/M Code	Patient Status	Physician Attendance	Time[1]
99291	Critically ill or critically injured	Constant	First 30–74 minutes
99292	Critically ill or critically injured	Constant	Each additional 30 minutes beyond the first 74 minutes

1 Per the guidelines for time in *CPT 2012,* "A unit of time is attained when the mid-point is passed. For example, an hour is attained when 31 minutes have elapsed (more than midway between zero and 60 minutes)."

Nursing Facility Services—Initial Nursing Facility Care[1]

E/M Code	History[1]	Exam[1]	Medical Decision Making[1]	Problem Severity	Coordination of Care; Counseling
99304	Detailed or comprehensive	Detailed or comprehensive	Straight-forward or low complexity	Low	25 min.
99305	Comprehensive	Comprehensive	Moderate complexity	Moderate	35 min.
99306	Comprehensive	Comprehensive	High complexity	High	45 min.

1 These services must be performed by the physician. See CPT Corrections Document – CPT 2013 page 2.

2 Key component. For new patients, all three components (history, exam, and medical decision making) are crucial for selecting the correct code.

Nursing Facility Services—Subsequent Nursing Facility Care

E/M Code	History[1]	Exam[1]	Medical Decision Making[2]	Problem Severity	Coordination of Care; Counseling
99307	Problem-focused interval	Problem-focused	Straight-forward	Stable, recovering or improving	10 min.
99308	Expanded problem-focused interval	Expanded problem-focused	Low complexity	Responding inadequately or has developed a minor complication	15 min.
99309	Detailed interval	Detailed	Moderate complexity	Significant complication or a significant new problem	25 min.
99310	Comprehensive interval	Comprehensive	High complexity	Developed a significant new problem requiring immediate attention	35 min.

1 Key component. For established patients, at least two of the three components (history, exam, and medical decision making) are needed for selecting the correct code.

Nursing Facility Discharge and Annual Assessment

E/M Code	History[1]	Exam[1]	Medical Decision Making[1]	Problem Severity	Time Spent Bedside and on Unit/Floor (avg.)
99315	Nursing facility discharge day management				30 min. or less
99316	Nursing facility discharge day management				more than 30 min.
99318	Detailed interval	Comprehensive	Low to moderate complexity	Stable, recovering or improving	30 min.

1 Key component. For annual nursing facility assessment, all three components (history, exam, and medical decision making) are crucial for selecting the correct code.

Domiciliary, Rest Home (e.g., Boarding Home) or Custodial Care Services—New Patient

E/M Code	History[1]	Exam[1]	Medical Decision Making[1]	Problem Severity	Coordination of Care; Counseling	Time Spent Face-to-Face (avg.)
99324	Problem-focused	Problem-focused	Straight-forward	Low	Consistent with problem(s) and patient's needs	20 min.
99325	Expanded problem-focused	Expanded problem-focused	Low complexity	Moderate	Consistent with problem(s) and patient's needs	30 min.
99326	Detailed	Detailed	Moderate complexity	Moderate to high	Consistent with problem(s) and patient's needs	45 min.
99327	Comprehensive	Comprehensive	Moderate complexity	High	Consistent with problem(s) and patient's needs	60 min.
99328	Comprehensive	Comprehensive	High complexity	Unstable or developed a new problem requiring immediate physician attention	Consistent with problem(s) and patient's needs	75 min.

1 Key component. For new patients, all three components (history, exam, and medical decision making) are crucial for selecting the correct code and must be adequately documented in the medical record to substantiate the level of service reported.

© 2012 OptumInsight, Inc.

Domiciliary, Rest Home (e.g., Boarding Home) or Custodial Care Services— Established Patient

E/M Code	History[1]	Exam[1]	Medical Decision Making[1]	Problem Severity	Coordination of Care; Counseling	Time Spent Face-to-Face (avg.)
99334	Problem-focused interval	Problem-focused	Straight-forward	Minor or self-limited	Consistent with problem(s) and patient's needs	15 min.
99335	Expanded problem-focused interval	Expanded problem-focused	Low complexity	Low to moderate	Consistent with problem(s) and patient's needs	25 min.
99336	Detailed interval	Detailed	Moderate complexity	Moderate to high	Consistent with problem(s) and patient's needs	40 min.
99337	Comprehensive interval	Comprehensive	Moderate to high complexity	Moderate to high	Consistent with problem(s) and patient's needs	60 min.

1 Key component. For established patients, at least two of the three components (history, exam, and medical decision making) are needed for selecting the correct code.

Domiciliary, Rest Home (e.g., Assisted Living Facility), or Home Care Plan Oversight Services

E/M Code	Intent of Service	Presence of Patient	Time
99339	Individual physician supervision of a patient (patient not present) in home, domiciliary or rest home (e.g., assisted living facility) requiring complex and multidisciplinary care modalities involving regular physician development and/or revision of care plans, review of subsequent reports of patient status, review of related laboratory and other studies, communication (including telephone calls) for purposes of assessment or care decisions with health care professional(s), family member(s), surrogate decision maker(s) (e.g., legal guardian) and/or key caregiver(s) involved in patient's care, integration of new information into the medical treatment plan and/or adjustment of medical therapy, within a calendar month	Patient not present	15–29 min.
99340	Same as 99339	Patient not present	30 min. or more

Home Services—New Patient

E/M Code	History[1]	Exam[1]	Medical Decision Making[1]	Problem Severity	Coordination of Care; Counseling	Time Spent Face-to-Face (avg.)
99341	Problem-focused	Problem-focused	Straight-forward complexity	Low	Consistent with problem(s) and patient's needs	20 min.
99342	Expanded problem-focused	Expanded problem-focused	Low complexity	Moderate	Consistent with problem(s) and patient's needs	30 min.
99343	Detailed	Detailed	Moderate complexity	Moderate to high	Consistent with problem(s) and patient's needs	45 min.
99344	Comprehensive	Comprehensive	Moderate complexity	High	Consistent with problem(s) and patient's needs	60 min.
99345	Comprehensive	Comprehensive	High complexity	Usually the patient has developed a significant new problem requiring immediate physician attention	Consistent with problem(s) and patient's needs	75 min.

1 Key component. For new patients, all three components (history, exam, and medical decision making) are crucial for selecting the correct code and must be adequately documented in the medical record to substantiate the level of service reported.

Home Services—Established Patient

E/M Code	History[1]	Exam[1]	Medical Decision Making[1]	Problem Severity	Coordination of Care; Counseling	Time Spent Face-to-Face (avg.)
99347	Problem-focused interval	Problem-focused	Straight-forward	Minor or self-limited	Consistent with problem(s) and patient's needs	15 min.
99348	Expanded problem-focused interval	Expanded problem-focused	Low complexity	Low to moderate	Consistent with problem(s) and patient's needs	25 min.
99349	Detailed interval	Detailed	Moderate complexity	Moderate to high	Consistent with problem(s) and patient's needs	40 min.
99350	Comprehensive interval	Comprehensive	Moderate to high complexity	Moderate to high Usually the patient has developed a significant new problem requiring immediate physician attention	Consistent with problem(s) and patient's needs	60 min.

1 Key component. For established patients, at least two of the three components (history, exam, and medical decision making) are needed to select the correct code and must be adequately documented in the medical record to substantiate the level of service reported.

Newborn Care Services

E/M Code	Patient Status	Type of Visit
99460	Normal newborn	Inpatient initial inpatient hospital or birthing center per day
99461	Normal newborn	Inpatient initial treatment not in hospital or birthing center per day
99462	Normal newborn	Inpatient subsequent per day
99463	Normal newborn	Inpatient initial inpatient and discharge in hospital or birthing center per day
99464	Unstable newborn	Attendance at delivery
99465	High-risk newborn at delivery	Resuscitation, ventilation, and cardiac treatment

Neonatal and Pediatric Interfacility Transportation

E/M Code	Patient Status	Type of Visit
99466	Critically ill or injured infant or young child, to 24 months	Face-to-face transportation from one facility to another, initial 30-74 minutes
99467	Critically ill or injured infant or young child, to 24 months	Face-to-face transportation from one facility to another, each additional 30 minutes
99485	Critically ill or injured infant or young child, to 24 months	Supervision of patient transport from one facility to another, initial 30 minutes
99486	Critically ill or injured infant or young child, to 24 months	Supervision of patient transport from one facility to another, each additional 30 minutes

Inpatient Neonatal and Pediatric Critical Care

E/M Code	Patient Status	Type of Visit
99468	Critically ill neonate, aged 28 days or less	Inpatient initial per day
99469	Critically ill neonate, aged 28 days or less	Inpatient subsequent per day
99471	Critically ill infant or young child, aged 29 days to 24 months	Inpatient initial per day
99472	Critically ill infant or young child, aged 29 days to 24 months	Inpatient subsequent per day
99475	Critically ill infant or young child, 2 to 5 years	Inpatient initial per day
99476	Critically ill infant or young child, 2 to 5 years	Inpatient subsequent per day

Initial and Continuing Intensive Care Services

E/M Code	Patient Status	Type of Visit
99477	Neonate, aged 28 days or less	Inpatient initial per day
99478	Infant with present body weight of less than 1500 grams, no longer critically ill	Inpatient subsequent per day
99479	Infant with present body weight of 1501-2500 grams, no longer critically ill	Inpatient subsequent per day
99480	Infant with present body weight of 2501-5000 grams, no longer critically ill	Inpatient subsequent per day

Levels of E/M Services

Confusion may be experienced when first approaching E/M due to the way that each description of a code component or element seems to have another layer of description beneath. The three key components—history, exam, and decision making—are each comprised of elements that combine to create varying levels of that component.

For example, an expanded problem-focused history includes the chief complaint, a brief history of the present illness, and a system review focusing on the patient's problems. The level of exam is not made up of different elements but rather distinguished by the extent of exam across body areas or organ systems.

The single largest source of confusion are the "labels" or names applied to the varying degrees of history, exam, and decision-making. Terms such as expanded problem-focused, detailed, and comprehensive are somewhat meaningless unless they are defined. The lack of definition in CPT guidelines relative to these terms is precisely what caused the first set of federal guidelines to be developed in 1995 and again in 1997.

Documentation Guidelines for Evaluation and Management Services

Both versions of the federal guidelines go well beyond CPT guidelines in defining specific code requirements. The current version of the CPT guidelines does not explain the number of history of present illness (HPI) elements or the specific number of organ systems or body areas to be examined as they are in the federal guidelines. Adherence to some version of the guidelines is required when billing E/M to federal payers, but at this time, the CPT guidelines do not incorporate this level of detail into the code definitions. Although that could be interpreted to mean that non-governmental payers have a lesser documentation standard, it is best to adopt one set of the federal versions for all payer types for both consistency and ease of use.

The 1997 guidelines supply a great amount of detail relative to history and exam and will give the provider clear direction to following documentation elements. With that stated, the 1995 guidelines are equally valid and place a lesser documentation burden on the provider in regards to the physical exam.

The 1995 guidelines ask only for a notation of "normal" on systems with normal findings. The only narrative required is for abnormal findings. The 1997 version calls for much greater detail, or an "elemental" or "bullet-point" approach to organ systems, although a notation of normal is sufficient when addressing the elements within a system. The 1997 version works well in a template or electronic health record (EHR) format for recording E/M services.

The 1997 version did produce the single system specialty exam guidelines. When reviewing the complete guidelines listed below, note the differences between exam requirements in the 1995 and 1997 versions.

A Comparison of 1995 and 1997 Exam Guidelines

There are four types of exams indicated in the levels of E/M codes. Although the descriptors or labels are the same under 1995 and 1997 guidelines, the degree of detail required is different. The remaining content on this topic references the 1997 general multi-system speciality examination, at the end of this chapter.

The levels under each set of guidelines are:

1995 Exam Guidelines:

Problem focused:	One body area or system
Expanded problem focused:	Two to seven body areas or organ systems
Detailed:	Two to seven body areas or organ systems
Comprehensive:	Eight or more organ systems or a complete single-system examination

1997 Exam Guidelines:

Problem-focused:	Perform and document examination of one to five bullet point elements in one or more organ systems/body areas from the general multi-system examination
OR	
	Perform or document examination of one to five bullet point elements from one of the 10 single-organ-system examinations, shaded or unshaded boxes
Expanded problem-focused:	Perform and document examination of at least six bullet point elements in one or more organ systems from the general multi-system examination
OR	

Perform and document examination of at least six bullet point elements from one of the 10 single-organ-system examinations, shaded or unshaded boxes

Detailed:	Perform and document examination of at least six organ systems or body areas, including at least two bullet point elements for each organ system or body area from the general multi-system examination
OR	
	Perform and document examination of at least 12 bullet point elements in two or more organ systems or body areas from the general multisystem examination
OR	
	Perform and document examination of at least 12 bullet elements from one of the single-organ-system examinations, shaded or unshaded boxes
Comprehensive:	Perform and document examination of at least nine organ systems or body areas, with all bullet elements for each organ system or body area (unless specific instructions are expected to limit examination content with at least two bullet elements for each organ system or body area) from the general multi-system examination
OR	
	Perform and document examination of all bullet point elements from one of the 10 single-organ system examinations with documentation of every element in shaded boxes and at least one element in each unshaded box from the single-organ-system examination.

The Documentation Guidelines

The following guidelines were developed jointly by the American Medical Association (AMA) and the Centers for Medicare and Medicaid Services (CMS). Their mutual goal was to provide physicians and claims reviewers with advice about preparing or reviewing documentation for Evaluation and Management (E/M) services.

I. Introduction

What is Documentation and Why Is It Important?

Medical record documentation is required to record pertinent facts, findings, and observations about an individual's health history, including past and present illnesses, examinations, tests, treatments, and outcomes. The medical record chronologically documents the care of the patient and is an important element contributing to high quality care. The medical record facilitates:

- The ability of the physician and other health care professionals to evaluate and plan the patient's immediate treatment and to monitor his/her health care over time
- Communication and continuity of care among physicians and other health care professionals involved in the patient's care
- Accurate and timely claims review and payment
- Appropriate utilization review and quality of care evaluations
- Collection of data that may be useful for research and education

An appropriately documented medical record can reduce many of the problems associated with claims processing and may serve as a legal document to verify the care provided, if necessary.

What Do Payers Want and Why?

Because payers have a contractual obligation to enrollees, they may require reasonable documentation that services are consistent with the insurance coverage provided. They may request information to validate:

- The site of service
- The medical necessity and appropriateness of the diagnostic and/or therapeutic services provided
- Services provided have been accurately reported

II. General Principles of Medical Record Documentation

The principles of documentation listed below are applicable to all types of medical and surgical services in all settings. For Evaluation and Management (E/M) services, the nature and amount of physician work and documentation varies by type of service, place of service, and the patient's status. The general principles listed below may be modified to account for these variable circumstances in providing E/M services.

- The medical record should be complete and legible
- The documentation of each patient encounter should include:
  - A reason for the encounter and relevant history, physical examination findings, and prior diagnostic test results
  - Assessment, clinical impression, or diagnosis
  - Plan for care
  - Date and legible identity of the practitioner
- If not documented, the rationale for ordering diagnostic and other ancillary services should be easily inferred
- Past and present diagnoses should be accessible to the treating and/or consulting physician
- Appropriate health risk factors should be identified
- The patient's progress, response to, and changes in treatment and revision of diagnosis should be documented

© 2012 OptumInsight, Inc.

- The CPT and ICD-9-CM codes reported on the health insurance claim form or billing statement should be supported by the documentation in the medical record

III. Documentation of E/M Services 1995 and 1997

The following information provides definitions and documentation guidelines for the three key components of E/M services and for visits that consist predominately of counseling or coordination of care. The three key components—history, examination, and medical decision making—appear in the descriptors for office and other outpatient services, hospital observation services, hospital inpatient services, consultations, emergency department services, nursing facility services, domiciliary care services, and home services. While some of the text of the CPT guidelines has been repeated in this document, the reader should refer to CMS or CPT for the complete descriptors for E/M services and instructions for selecting a level of service. Documentation guidelines are identified by the symbol DG.

The descriptors for the levels of E/M services recognize seven components that are used in defining the levels of E/M services. These components are:

- History
- Examination
- Medical decision making
- Counseling
- Coordination of care
- Nature of presenting problem
- Time

The first three of these components (i.e., history, examination, and medical decision making) are the key components in selecting the level of E/M services. In the case of visits that consist predominately of counseling or coordination of care, time is the key or controlling factor to qualify for a particular level of E/M service.

Because the level of E/M service is dependent on two or three key components, performance and documentation of one component (e.g., examination) at the highest level does not necessarily mean that the encounter in its entirety qualifies for the highest level of E/M service.

These Documentation Guidelines for E/M services reflect the needs of the typical adult population. For certain groups of patients, the recorded information may vary slightly from that described here. Specifically, the medical records of infants, children, adolescents, and pregnant women may have additional or modified information, as appropriate, recorded in each history and examination area.

As an example, newborn records may include under history of the present illness (HPI) the details of the mother's pregnancy and the infant's status at birth; social history will focus on family structure; and family history will focus on congenital anomalies and hereditary disorders in the family. In addition, the content of a pediatric examination will vary with the age and development of the child. Although not specifically defined in these documentation guidelines, these patient group variations on history and examination are appropriate.

A. Documentation of History

The levels of E/M services are based on four types of history (Problem Focused, Expanded Problem Focused, Detailed, and Comprehensive). Each type of history includes some or all of the following elements:

- Chief complaint (CC)
- History of present illness (HPI)
- Review of systems (ROS)
- Past, family, and/or social history (PFSH)

The extent of history of present illness, review of systems, and past, family, and/or social history that is obtained and documented is dependent upon clinical judgment and the nature of the presenting problem.

The chart below shows the progression of the elements required for each type of history. To qualify for a given type of history all three elements in the table must be met. (A chief complaint is indicated at all levels.)

- DG: The CC, ROS, and PFSH may be listed as separate elements of history or they may be included in the description of the history of present illness

- DG: A ROS and/or a PFSH obtained during an earlier encounter does not need to be re-recorded if there is evidence that the physician reviewed and updated the previous information. This may occur when a physician updates his/her own record or in an institutional setting or group practice where many physicians use a common record. The review and update may be documented by:

  - Describing any new ROS and/or PFSH information or noting there has been no change in the information

  - Noting the date and location of the earlier ROS and/or PFSH

- DG: The ROS and/or PFSH may be recorded by ancillary staff or on a form completed by the patient. To document that the physician reviewed the information, there must be a notation supplementing or confirming the information recorded by others

- DG: If the physician is unable to obtain a history from the patient or other source, the record should describe the patient's condition or other circumstance that precludes obtaining a history

Definitions and specific documentation guidelines for each of the elements of history are listed below.

Chief Complaint (CC)

The CC is a concise statement describing the symptom, problem, condition, diagnosis, physician recommended return, or other factor that is the reason for the encounter, usually stated in the patient's words.

- DG: The medical record should clearly reflect the chief complaint

History of Present Illness	Review of systems (ROS)	PFSH	Type of History
Brief	N/A	N/A	Problem-focused
Brief	Problem Pertinent	N/A	Expanded Problem-Focused
Extended	Extended	Pertinent	Detailed
Extended	Complete	Complete	Comprehensive

History of Present Illness (HPI)

The HPI is a chronological description of the development of the patient's present illness from the first sign and/or symptom or from the previous encounter to the present. It includes the following elements:

- Location
- Quality
- Severity
- Duration
- Timing
- Context
- Modifying factors
- Associated signs and symptoms

Brief and extended HPIs are distinguished by the amount of detail needed to accurately characterize the clinical problem.

A brief HPI consists of one to three elements of the HPI.

- DG: The medical record should describe one to three elements of the present illness (HPI)

An extended HPI consists of at least four elements of the HPI or the status of at least three chronic or inactive conditions.

- DG: The medical record should describe at least four elements of the present illness (HPI) or for 1997 only the status of at least three chronic or inactive conditions

Review of Systems (ROS)

A ROS is an inventory of body systems obtained through a series of questions seeking to identify signs and/or symptoms that the patient may be experiencing or has experienced. For purposes of ROS, the following systems are recognized:

- Constitutional symptoms (e.g., fever, weight loss)
- Eyes
- Ears, nose, mouth, throat
- Cardiovascular
- Respiratory
- Gastrointestinal
- Genitourinary
- Musculoskeletal
- Integumentary (skin and/or breast)
- Neurological
- Psychiatric
- Endocrine
- Hematologic/lymphatic
- Allergic/immunologic

A problem pertinent ROS inquires about the system directly related to the problem identified in the HPI.

- DG: The patient's positive responses and pertinent negatives for the system related to the problem should be documented

An extended ROS inquires about the system directly related to the problem identified in the HPI and a limited number of additional systems.

- DG: The patient's positive responses and pertinent negatives for two to nine systems should be documented

A complete ROS inquires about the system directly related to the problem identified in the HPI plus all additional body systems.

- DG: At least 10 organ systems must be reviewed. Those systems with positive or pertinent negative responses must be individually documented. For the remaining systems, a notation indicating all other systems are negative is permissible. In the absence of such a notation, at least 10 systems must be individually documented

Past, Family, and/or Social History (PFSH)

The PFSH consists of a review of three areas:

- Past history (the patient's past experiences with illnesses, operations, injuries, and treatment)
- Family history (a review of medical events in the patient's family, including diseases that may be hereditary or place the patient at risk)
- Social history (an age appropriate review of past and current activities)

For certain categories of E/M services that include only an interval history, it is not necessary to record information about the PFSH. Those categories are subsequent hospital care, follow-up inpatient consultations, and subsequent nursing facility care.

A pertinent PFSH is a review of the history area directly related to the problem identified in the HPI.

- DG: At least one specific item from any of the three history areas must be documented for a pertinent PFSH

A complete PFSH is a review of two or all three of the PFSH history areas, depending on the category of the E/M service. A review of all three history areas is required for services that by their nature include a comprehensive assessment or reassessment of the patient. A review of two of the three history areas is sufficient for other services.

- DG: A least one specific item from two of the three history areas must be documented for a complete PFSH for the

© 2012 OptumInsight, Inc.

following categories of E/M services: office or other outpatient services, established patient; emergency department; domiciliary care, established patient; and home care, established patient

- DG: At least one specific item from each of the three history areas must be documented for a complete PFSH for the following categories of E/M services: office or other outpatient services, new patient; hospital observation services; hospital inpatient services, initial care; consultations; comprehensive nursing facility assessments; domiciliary care, new patient; and home care, new patient

B. Documentation of Examination 1997 Guidelines

The levels of E/M services are based on four types of examination:

- Problem Focused: A limited examination of the affected body area or organ system

- Expanded Problem Focused: A limited examination of the affected body area or organ system and any other symptomatic or related body area or organ system

- Detailed: An extended examination of the affected body area or organ system and any other symptomatic or related body area or organ system

- Comprehensive: A general multi-system examination or complete examination of a single organ system and other symptomatic or related body area or organ system

These types of examinations have been defined for general multi-system and the following single organ systems:

- Cardiovascular
- Ears, nose, mouth, and throat
- Eyes
- Genitourinary (Female)
- Genitourinary (Male)
- Hematologic/lymphatic/immunologic
- Musculoskeletal
- Neurological
- Psychiatric
- Respiratory
- Skin

Any physician regardless of specialty may perform a general multi-system examination or any of the single organ system examinations. The type (general multi-system or single organ system) and content of examination are selected by the examining physician and are based upon clinical judgment, the patient's history, and the nature of the presenting problem.

The content and documentation requirements for each type and level of examination are summarized below and described in detail in a table found later on in this document. In the table, organ systems and body areas recognized by CPT for purposes of describing examinations are shown in the left column. The content, or individual elements, of the examination pertaining to that body area or organ system are identified by bullets (•) in the right column.

Parenthetical examples "(e.g., ...)," have been used for clarification and to provide guidance regarding documentation. Documentation for each element must satisfy any numeric requirements (such as "Measurement of any three of the following seven...") included in the description of the element. Elements with multiple components but with no specific numeric requirement (such as "Examination of liver and spleen") require documentation of at least one component. It is possible for a given examination to be expanded beyond what is defined here. When that occurs, findings related to the additional systems and/or areas should be documented.

- DG: Specific abnormal and relevant negative findings from the examination of the affected or symptomatic body area or organ system should be documented. A notation of "abnormal" without elaboration is insufficient

- DG: Abnormal or unexpected findings from the examination of any asymptomatic body area or organ system should be described

- DG: A brief statement or notation indicating "negative" or "normal" is sufficient to document normal findings related to an unaffected areas or asymptomatic organ system

General Multi-System Examinations

General multi-system examinations are described in detail later in this document. To qualify for a given level of multi-system examination, the following content and documentation requirements should be met:

- Problem Focused Examination: It should include performance and documentation of one to five elements identified by a bullet (•) in one or more organ systems or body areas

- Expanded Problem Focused Examination: It should include performance and documentation of at least six elements identified by a bullet (•) in one or more organ systems or body areas

- Detailed Examination: It should include at least six organ systems or body areas. For each system/area selected, performance and documentation of at least two elements identified by a bullet (•) is expected. Alternatively, a detailed examination may include performance and documentation of at least 12 elements identified by a bullet (•) in two or more organ systems or body areas

- Comprehensive Examination: It should include at least nine organ systems or body areas. For each system/area selected, all elements of the examination identified by a bullet (•) should be performed, unless specific directions limit the content of the examination. For each area/system, documentation of at least two elements identified by a bullet (•) is expected

Single Organ System Examinations

The single organ system examinations recognized by CMS include eyes; ears, nose, mouth, and throat; cardiovascular; respiratory; genitourinary (male and female); musculoskeletal; neurologic; hematologic, lymphatic, and immunologic; skin; and psychiatric. Note that for each specific single organ examination type, the performance and documentation of the stated number of elements, identified by a bullet (•) should be included, whether in a box with a shaded or unshaded border. The following content and documentation requirements must be met to qualify for a given level:

- Problem Focused Examination: one to five elements
- Expanded Problem Focused Examination: at least six elements
- Detailed Examination: at least 12 elements (other than eye and psychiatric examinations)
- Comprehensive Examination: all elements (Documentation of every element in a box with a shaded border and at least one element in a box with an unshaded border is expected)

Content and Documentation Requirements

General Multisystem Examination 1997

System/Body Area	Elements of Examination
Constitutional	■ Measurement of any three of the following seven vital signs: 1) sitting or standing blood pressure, 2) supine blood pressure, 3) pulse rate and regularity, 4) respiration, 5) temperature, 6) height, 7) weight (May be measured and recorded by ancillary staff). ■ General appearance of patient (e.g., development, nutrition, body habitus, deformities attention to grooming)
Eyes	■ Inspection of conjunctivae and lids ■ Examination of pupils and irises (e.g., reaction to light and accommodation, size and symmetry) ■ Ophthalmoscopic examination of optic discs (e.g., size, C/D ratio, appearance) and posterior segments (e.g., vessel changes, exudates, hemorrhages)
Ears, nose, mouth, and throat	■ External inspection of ears and nose (e.g., overall appearance, scars, lesions, masses) ■ Otoscopic examination of external auditory canals and tympanic membranes ■ Assessment of hearing (e.g., whispered voice, finger rub, tuning fork) ■ Inspection of nasal mucosa, septum and turbinates ■ Inspection of lips, teeth and gums ■ Examination of oropharynx: oral mucosa, salivary glands, hard and soft palates, tongue, tonsils and posterior pharynx
Neck	■ Examination of neck (e.g., masses, overall appearance, symmetry, tracheal position, crepitus) ■ Examination of thyroid (e.g., enlargement, tenderness, mass)
Respiratory	■ Assessment of respiratory effort (e.g., intercostal retractions, use of accessory muscles, diaphragmatic movement) ■ Percussion of chest (e.g., dullness, flatness, hyperresonance) ■ Palpation of chest (e.g., tactile fremitus) ■ Auscultation of lungs (e.g., breath sounds, adventitious sounds, rubs)
Cardiovascular	■ Palpation of heart (e.g., location, size, thrills) ■ Auscultation of heart with notation of abnormal sounds and murmurs ■ Examination of: — carotid arteries (e.g., pulse amplitude, bruits) — abdominal aorta (e.g., size, bruits) — femoral arteries (e.g., pulse amplitude, bruits) — pedal pulses (e.g., pulse amplitude) — extremities for edema and/or varicosities
Chest (Breasts)	■ Inspection of breasts (e.g., symmetry, nipple discharge) ■ Palpation of breasts and axillae (e.g., masses or lumps, tenderness)
Gastrointestinal (Abdomen)	■ Examination of abdomen with notation of presence of masses or tenderness ■ Examination of liver and spleen ■ Examination for presence or absence of hernia ■ Examination (when indicated) of anus, perineum and rectum, including sphincter tone, presence of hemorrhoids, rectal masses ■ Obtain stool sample for occult blood test when indicated
Genitourinary	**Male:** ■ Examination of the scrotal contents (e.g., hydrocele, spermatocele, tenderness of cord, testicular mass) ■ Examination of the penis ■ Digital rectal examination of prostate gland (e.g., size, symmetry, nodularity tenderness) **Female:** ■ Pelvic examination (with or without specimen collection for smears and cultures), including: — examination of external genitalia (e.g., general appearance, hair distribution, lesions) and vagina (e.g., general appearance, estrogen effect, discharge, lesions, pelvic support, cystocele, rectocele) — examination of urethra (e.g., masses, tenderness, scarring) — examination of bladder (e.g., fullness, masses, tenderness) ■ Cervix (e.g., general appearance, lesions, discharge) ■ Uterus (e.g., size, contour, position, mobility, tenderness, consistency, descent or support) ■ Adnexa/parametria (e.g., masses, tenderness)

© 2012 OptumInsight, Inc.

System/Body Area	Elements of Examination
Lymphatic	Palpation of lymph nodes in **two or more** areas: ■ Neck ■ Groin ■ Axillae ■ Other
Musculoskeletal	■ Examination of gait and station *(if circled, add to total at bottom of column to the left) ■ Inspection and/or palpation of digits and nails (e.g., clubbing, cyanosis, inflammatory conditions, petechiae, ischemia, infections, nodes) *(if circled, add to total at bottom of column to the left) Examination of joints, bones and muscles of **one or more of the following six** areas: 1) head and neck; 2) spine, ribs, and pelvis; 3) right upper extremity; 4) left upper extremity; 5) right lower extremity; and 6) left lower extremity. The examination of a given area includes: ■ Inspection and/or palpation with notation of presence of any misalignment, asymmetry, crepitation, defects, tenderness, masses, effusions ■ Assessment of range of motion with notation of any pain, crepitation or contracture ■ Assessment of stability with notation of any dislocation (luxation), subluxation, or laxity ■ Assessment of muscle strength and tone (e.g., flaccid, cog wheel, spastic) with notation of any atrophy or abnormal movements
Skin	■ Inspection of skin and subcutaneous tissue (e.g., rashes, lesions, ulcers) ■ Palpation of skin and subcutaneous tissue (e.g., induration, subcutaneous nodules, tightening)
Neurologic	■ Test cranial nerves with notation of any deficits ■ Examination of deep tendon reflexes with notation of pathological reflexes (e.g., Babinski) ■ Examination of sensation (e.g., by touch, pin, vibration, proprioception)
Psychiatric	■ Description of patient's judgment and insight ■ Brief assessment of mental status including: — Orientation to time, place and person — Recent and remote memory — Mood and affect (e.g., depression, anxiety, agitation)

Content and Documentation Requirements

Level of exam	Perform and document
Problem focused	**One to five** elements identified by a bullet.
Expanded problem focused	**At least six** elements identified by a bullet.
Detailed	**At least 12** elements identified by a bullet, whether in a box with a shaded or unshaded border
Comprehensive	Performance of **all** elements identified by a bullet; whether in a box or with a shaded or unshaded box. Documentation of every element in each with a shaded border and at least one element in a box with un shaded border is expected

C. Documentation of the Complexity of Medical Decision Making 1995 and 1997

The levels of E/M services recognize four types of medical decision-making (straightforward, low complexity, moderate complexity, and high complexity). Medical decision-making refers to the complexity of establishing a diagnosis and/or selecting a management option as measured by:

• The number of possible diagnoses and/or the number of management options that must be considered

• The amount and/or complexity of medical records, diagnostic tests, and/or other information that must be obtained, reviewed, and analyzed

• The risk of significant complications, morbidity, and/or mortality, as well as comorbidities, associated with the patient's presenting problem, the diagnostic procedure, and/or the possible management options

The following chart shows the progression of the elements required for each level of medical decision-making. To qualify for a given type of decision-making, two of the three elements in the table must be either met or exceeded.

Number of Diagnoses or Management Option	Amount and/or Complexity of Data to be Reviewed	Risk of Complications and/or Morbidity or Mortality	Type of Decision Making
Minimal	Minimal or None	Minimal	Straightforward
Limited	Limited	Low	Low Complexity
Multiple	Moderate	Moderate	Moderate Complexity
Extensive	Extensive	High	High Complexity

Each of the elements of medical decision-making is described below.

Number of Diagnoses or Management Options
The number of possible diagnoses and/or the number of management options that must be considered is based on the number and types of problems addressed during the encounter, the complexity of establishing a diagnosis, and the management decisions that are made by the physician.

Generally, decision making with respect to a diagnosed problem is easier than that for an identified but undiagnosed problem. The number and type of diagnostic tests employed may be an indicator of the number of possible diagnoses. Problems that are improving or resolving are less complex than those that are worsening or failing to change as expected. The need to seek advice from others is another indicator of complexity of diagnostic or management problems.

- DG: For each encounter, an assessment, clinical impression, or diagnosis should be documented. It may be explicitly stated or implied in documented decisions regarding management plans and/or further evaluation

  - For a presenting problem with an established diagnosis, the record should reflect whether the problem is: a) improved, well controlled, resolving, or resolved; or b) inadequately controlled, worsening, or failing to change as expected

  - For a presenting problem without an established diagnosis, the assessment or clinical impression may be stated in the form of a differential diagnosis or as a "possible," "probable," or "rule-out" (R/O) diagnosis

- DG: The initiation of, or changes in, treatment should be documented. Treatment includes a wide range of management options including patient instructions, nursing instructions, therapies, and medications

- DG: If referrals are made, consultations requested, or advice sought, the record should indicate to whom or where the referral or consultation is made or from whom the advice is requested

Amount and/or Complexity of Data to be Reviewed
The amount and complexity of data to be reviewed is based on the types of diagnostic testing ordered or reviewed. A decision to obtain and review old medical records and/or obtain history from sources other than the patient increases the amount and complexity of data to be reviewed.

Discussion of contradictory or unexpected test results with the physician who performed or interpreted the test is an indication of the complexity of data being reviewed. On occasion, the physician who ordered a test may personally review the image, tracing, or specimen to supplement information from the physician who prepared the test report or interpretation; this is another indication of the complexity of data being reviewed.

- DG: If a diagnostic service (test or procedure) is ordered, planned, scheduled, or performed at the time of the E/M encounter, the type of service (e.g., lab or x-ray) should be documented

- DG: The review of lab, radiology, and/or other diagnostic tests should be documented. A simple notation such as WBC elevated" or "chest x-ray unremarkable" is acceptable. Alternatively, the review may be documented by initialing and dating the report containing the test results

- DG: A decision to obtain old records or a decision to obtain additional history from the family, caretaker, or other source to supplement that obtained from the patient should be documented

- DG: Relevant findings from the review of old records and/or the receipt of additional history from the family, caretaker, or other source to supplement that obtained from the patient should be documented. If there is no relevant information beyond that already obtained, that fact should be documented. A notation of "old records reviewed" or "additional history obtained from family" without elaboration is insufficient

- DG: The results of discussion of laboratory, radiology, or other diagnostic tests with the physician who performed or interpreted the study should be documented

- DG: The direct visualization and independent interpretation of an image, tracing, or specimen previously or subsequently interpreted by another physician should be documented

Risk of Significant Complications, Morbidity, and/or Mortality
The risk of significant complications, morbidity, and/or mortality is based on the risks associated with the presenting problem, the diagnostic procedure, and the possible management options.

- DG: Comorbidities/underlying disease or other factors that increase the complexity of medical decision making by increasing the risk of complications, morbidity, and/or mortality should be documented

- DG: If a surgical or invasive diagnostic procedure is ordered, planned, or scheduled at the time of the E/M encounter, the type of procedure (e.g., laparoscopy) should be documented

- DG: If a surgical or invasive diagnostic procedure is performed at the time of the E/M encounter, the specific procedure should be documented

- DG: The referral for or decision to perform a surgical or invasive diagnostic procedure on an urgent basis should be documented or implied

The following Table of Risk may be used to help determine whether the risk of significant complications, morbidity, and/or mortality is minimal, low, moderate, or high. Because the determination of risk

is complex and not readily quantifiable, the table includes common clinical examples rather than absolute measures of risk. The assessment of risk of the presenting problem is based on the risk related to the disease process anticipated between the present encounter and the next one. The assessment of risk of selecting diagnostic procedures and management options is based on the risk during and immediately following any procedures or treatment. The highest level of risk in any one category (presenting problem, diagnostic procedure, or management options) determines the overall risk.

Table of Risk.

Level of Risk	Presenting Problem(s)	Diagnostic Procedure(s) Ordered	Management Options Selected
Minimal	One self-limited or minor problem (e.g., cold, insect bite, tinea corporis)	Laboratory test requiring veinpuncture Chest x-rays EKG/EEG Urinalysis Ultrasound (e.g., echocardiography) KOH prep	Rest Gargles Elastic bandages Superficial dressings
Low	Two or more self-limited or minor problems One stable chronic illness (e.g., well controlled hypertension, non-insulin dependent diabetes, cataract, BPH) Acute, uncomplicated illness or injury (e.g., cystitis, allergic rhinitis, simple sprain)	Physiologic tests not under stress (e.g., pulmonary function tests) Non-cardiovascular imaging studies with contrast (e.g., barium enema) Superficial needle biopsies Clinical laboratory tests requiring arterial puncture Skin biopsies	Over-the-counter drugs Minor surgery with no identified risk factors Physical therapy Occupational therapy IV fluids without additives
Moderate	One or more chronic illnesses with mild exacerbation, progression or side effects of treatment Two or more stable chronic illnesses Undiagnosed new problem with uncertain prognosis (e.g., lump in breast) Acute illness with systemic symptoms (e.g., pyelonephritis, pneumonitis, colitis) Acute complicated injury (e.g., head injury with brief loss of consciousness)	Physiologic tests not under stress (e.g., cardiac stress test, fetal contraction stress test) Diagnostic endoscopies with no identified risk factors Deep needle or incisional biopsy Cardiovascular imaging studies with contrast and no identified risk factors (e.g., arteriogram, cardiac catheterization) Obtain fluid from body cavity (e.g., lumbar puncture, thoracentesis, culdocentesis)	Minor surgery with identified risk factors Effective major surgery (open, percutaneous or endoscopic) with no identified risk factors Prescription drug management Therapeutic nuclear medicine IV fluids with additives Closed treatment of fracture or dislocation without manipulation
High	One or more chronic illnesses with severe exacerbation, progression or side effects of treatment Acute/chronic illnesses that may pose a threat to life or bodily function (e.g., multiple trauma, acute MI, pulmonary embolus, severe respiratory distress, progressive severe rheumatoid arthritis, psychiatric illness with potential threat to self or others, peritonitis, acute renal failure An abrupt change in neurologic status (e.g., seizure, TIA, weakness or sensory loss)	Cardiovascular imaging studies with contrast with identified risk factors Cardiac electrophysiological tests Diagnostic endoscopies with identified risk factors Discography	Elective major surgery (open, percutaneous or endoscopic) with identified risk factors Emergency major surgery (open, percutaneous or endoscopic) Parenteral controlled substances Drug therapy requiring intensive monitoring for toxicity Decision not to resuscitate or to de-escalate care because of poor prognosis

D. Documentation of an Encounter Dominated by Counseling or Coordination of Care

In the case where counseling and/or coordination of care dominates (more than 50 percent) the physician/patient and/or family encounter (face-to-face time in the office or other outpatient setting or floor-unit time in the hospital or nursing facility), time is considered the key or controlling factor to qualify for a particular level of E/M service.

• DG: If the physician elects to report the level of service based on counseling and/or coordination of care, the total length of time of the encounter (face-to-face or floor time, as appropriate) should be documented and the record should describe the counseling and/or activities to coordinate care

Obstetrics and Gynecology Specifics

Each provider specialty has differences that typically lie in the approach and are likely to revolve around the physical exam.

There are 11 types of exams specified in the 1997 guidelines. Some of these exams will work better for some specialties than others. Not all specialists will find that the organ-system exam related to their specialty is the most practical. Find below suggestions related to the most problematic E/M audit areas: history and exam.

Many suggestions may pertain to the higher levels of service, new patient or consult levels four and five, or level four and five established patients. This is not an effort to steer a provider toward the use of those codes, but rather recognition that this is where the more demanding documentation elements reside.

Hospital admissions require comprehensive histories and exams at the two higher levels of admits. This is where documentation deficiencies most often occur. All admits for levels two and three require a complete (10) ROS. This area probably yields more deficiencies than any other. Hospitals generally require a complete "H & P." Under current guidelines, the history element can be met by indicating "all other ROS negative" after reviewing problem-pertinent systems, as well as any positive systems.

For subsequent hospital visits, the exam is often not very substantial (the patient just having had a complete H & P on admission). It is best to use the general system-level approach.

Physical Exam Section

For Ob/Gyn, the 1995 multi-system exam guidelines may be somewhat easier to document for follow-up patients, but, for this specialty, the 1997 single system exam stays very close to the normal exam elements for Ob/Gyn in particular. For Ob/Gyn, the comprehensive exam requires that 19 individual elements be addressed. This is one of the more lenient single-system exams, not because of the number of elements but because they are grouped logically within the organ systems pertinent to this specialty. For new patients and consults, the 1997 approach may work very well. A Genitourinary template can be easily created and may be of benefit for ease of documentation.

Evaluation and Management

CPT only © 2012 American Medical Association. All Rights Reserved.

Coding Companion for OB/GYN

© 2012 OptumInsight, Inc.

Evaluation and Management — 417

System/Body Area	Elements of Examination
Constitutional	■ Measurement of **any three of the following seven** vital signs: 1) sitting or standing blood pressure, 2) supine blood pressure, 3) pulse rate and regularity, 4) respiration, 5) temperature, 6) height, 7) weight (May be measured and recorded by ancillary staff). ■ General appearance of patient (e.g., development, nutrition, body habitus, deformities, attention to grooming)
Head and face	
Eyes	
Ears, nose, mouth and throat	
Neck	■ Examination of neck (e.g., masses, overall appearance, symmetry, tracheal position, crepitus) ■ Examination of thyroid (e.g., enlargement, tenderness, mass)
Respiratory	■ Assessment of respiratory effort (e.g., intercostal retractions, use of accessory muscles, diaphragmatic movements) ■ Auscultation of lungs (e.g., breath sounds, adventitious sounds, rubs)
Cardiovascular	■ Auscultation of heart with notation of abnormal sounds and murmurs ■ Examination of peripheral vascular system by observation (e.g., swelling, varicosities and palpation (e.g., pulses, temperature, edema, tenderness)
Chest (Breasts)	[See Genitourinary (female)]
Gastrointestinal (Abdomen)	■ Examination of abdomen with notation of presence of masses or tenderness ■ Examination for presence or absence of hernia ■ Examination of liver and spleen ■ Obtain stool sample for occult blood test when indicated
Genitourinary	**Male:** ■ Inspection of anus and perineum ■ Examination (with or without specimen collection for smears and cultures) of genitalia including: — scrotum (e.g., lesions, cysts, rashes) — epididymides (e.g., size, symmetry, masses) — testes (e.g., size, symmetry, masses) — urethral meatus (e.g., size, location, lesions, discharge) — penis (e.g., lesions, presence or absence of foreskin, foreskin retractability, plaque, masses, scarring deformities) ■ Digital rectal examination including: — prostate gland (e.g., size, symmetry, nodularity, tenderness) — seminal vesicles (e.g., symmetry, tenderness, masses, enlargement — sphincter tone, presence of hemorrhoids, rectal masses **Female:** ■ Includes **at least seven of the following eleven** elements identified by bullets: ■ Inspection and palpation of breasts (e.g., masses or lumps, tenderness, symmetry, nipple discharge) ■ Digital rectal examination including sphincter tone, presence of hemorrhoids, rectal masses ■ Pelvic examination (with or without specimen collection for smears and cultures), including — external genitalia (e.g., general appearance, hair distribution, lesions) — urethral meatus (e.g., size, location, lesions, prolapse) — urethra (e.g., masses, tenderness, scarring) — bladder (e.g., fullness, masses, tenderness) — vagina (e.g., general appearance, estrogen effect, discharge, lesions, pelvic support, cystocele, rectocele) — cervix (e.g., general appearance, lesions, discharge) — uterus (e.g., size, contour, position, mobility, tenderness, consistency, descent or support) — adnexa/parametria (e.g., masses, tenderness, organomegaly, nodularity) — anus and perineum
Lymphatic	■ Palpation of lymph nodes in neck, axillae, groin and/or other location
Musculoskeletal	
Extremities	
Skin	■ Inspection and/or palpation of skin and subcutaneous tissue (e.g., rashes, lesions, ulcers)
Neurological/ psychiatric	Brief assessment of mental status including: — orientation to time, place and person and — mood and affect (e.g., depression, anxiety, agitation)

Content and Documentation Requirements

Level of exam	Perform and document
Problem focused	**One to five** elements identified by a bullet.
Expanded problem focused	**At least six** elements identified by a bullet.
Detailed	**At least 12** elements identified by a bullet, whether in a box with a shaded or unshaded border
Comprehensive	Performance of **all** elements identified by a bullet; whether in a box or with a shaded or unshaded box. Documentation of every element in each with a shaded border and at least one element in a box with un shaded border is expected

© 2012 OptumInsight, Inc.

Index

CPT Index

CPT Index

CFTR, 81220-81223
Change
Catheter
  With Contrast, 75984
Fetal Position
  by Manipulation, 59412
Chemiluminescent Assay, 82397
Chemistry Tests
Organ or Disease Oriented Panel
  Electrolyte, 80051
  General Health Panel, 80050
  Lipid Panel, 80061
  Obstetric Panel, 80055
Chemosurgery
Destruction
  Malignant Lesion, 17270-17276
Chest
Ultrasound, 76604
X-ray, 71010, 71020
Chest Wall
Reconstruction, 49904
Chicken Pox (Varicella)
Immunization, 90716
Chlamydia
Antibody, 86631-86632
Antigen Detection
  Direct
    Optical Observation, 87810
  Direct Fluorescent, 87270
  Enzyme Immunoassay, 87320
  Nucleic Acid, 87490-87492
  Culture, 87110
Chloramphenicol, 82415
Chloride
Blood, 82435
Urine, 82436
CHOL, 82465, 83718-83721
Cholecalciferol
Blood Serum Level 25 Hydroxy,
  82306
I, 25 Dyhydroxy, 82652
Cholera Vaccine
Injectable, 90725
Cholesterol
Measurement, 83721
Serum, 82465
Testing, 83718-83719
Choline Esterase I, 82013
Choriogonadotropin, 80414, 84702-84703
Stimulation, 80414-80415
Chorionic Gonadotropin, 80414, 84702-84704
Stimulation, 80414-80415
Chorionic Growth Hormone, 83632
Chorionic Villi, 59015
Chorionic Villus
Biopsy, 59015
Chromatography
Column
  Mass Spectrometry, 82541-82544
Gas–Liquid or HPLC, 82486, 82491-82492
Paper, 82487-82488
Thin–Layer, 82489
Chromium, 82495
Chromosome Analysis
Amniotic Fluid, 88267-88269
Chorionic Villus, 88267
Pregnancy Associated Plasma Protein A, 84163
Chromotubation
Oviduct, 58350
Cl, 82435-82436
Clitoroplasty
for Intersex State, 56805
Clostridium Difficile Toxin
Amplified Probe Technique, 87493
Closure, 12001-12007, 12020-12047, 13100-13102, 13131-13133, 13160
Fistula
  Rectovaginal, 57305-57308
  Urethrovaginal, 57310-57311
  Vesicouterine, 51920-51925
  Vesicovaginal, 51900, 57320-57330
Rectovaginal Fistula, 57300-57308

Closure—*continued*
Skin
  Abdomen
    Complex, 13100-13102
    Intermediate, 12031-12037
    Layered, 12031-12037
    Simple, 12001-12007
    Superficial, 12001-12007
  Breast
    Complex, 13100-13102
    Intermediate, 12031-12037
    Layered, 12031-12037
    Simple, 12001-12007
    Superficial, 12001-12007
  Buttock
    Complex, 13100-13102
    Intermediate, 12031-12037
    Layered, 12031-12037
    Simple, 12001-12007
    Superficial, 12001-12007
  External
    Genitalia
      Intermediate, 12041-12047
      Layered, 12041-12047
      Simple, 12001-12007
      Superficial, 12001-12007
  Genitalia
    Complex, 13131-13133
    External
      Intermediate, 12041-12047
      Layered, 12041-12047
      Simple, 12001-12007
      Superficial, 12001-12007
  Trunk
    Complex, 13100-13102
    Intermediate, 12031-12037
    Layered, 12031-12037
    Simple, 12001-12007
    Superficial, 12001-12007
  Vagina, 57120
CMG (Cystometrogram), 51725-51729
Coagulation
Factor III, 85730-85732
Factor IV, 82310
Cocaine
Screen, 82486
Coccyx
X-ray, 72220
Codeine Screen, 82486
Coffey Operation
Uterus, Repair, Suspension, 58400
  with Presacral Sympathectomy, 58410
Collection and Processing
Specimen
  Capillary, 36416
  Vein, 36415
  Washings
    Abdomen, 49320
    Peritoneal, 58943, 58960
Colpectomy
Partial, 57106
Total, 57110
with Hysterectomy, 58275
  with Repair of Enterocele, 58280
Colpo–Urethrocystopexy, 58152, 58267, 58293
  Marshall–Marchetti–Krantz procedure, 58152, 58267, 58293
  Pereyra Procedure, 58267, 58293
Colpocentesis, 57020
Colpocleisis, 57120
Colpoperineorrhaphy, 57210
Colpopexy, 57280
Extra–peritoneal, 57282
Intraperitoneal, 57283
Laparoscopic, 57425
Open, 57280
Colporrhaphy
Anterior, 57240, 57289
  with Insertion of Mesh, 57267
  with Insertion of Prosthesis, 57267
Anteroposterior, 57260-57265
  with Enterocele Repair, 57265
  with Insertion of Mesh, 57267
  with Insertion of Prosthesis, 57267

Colporrhaphy—*continued*
Manchester, 58400
Nonobstetrical, 57200
Posterior, 57250
  with Insertion of Mesh, 57267
  with Insertion of Prosthesis, 57267
Colposcopy
Biopsy, 56821, 57421, 57454-57455, 57460
  Endometrial, 58110
Cervix, 57421, 57452-57461
Exploration, 57452
Loop Electrode Biopsy, 57460
Loop Electrode Conization, 57461
Vagina, 57420-57421
Vulva, 56820
  Biopsy, 56821
Colpotomy
Drainage
  Abscess, 57010
Exploration, 57000
Column Chromatography/Mass Spectrometry, 82541-82544
Combined Vaccine, 90710
Comparative Analysis Using STR Markers, 81265-81266
Complement
Fixation Test, 86171
Complete Blood Count, 85025-85027
Computed Tomography (CT Scan)
Guidance
  Cyst Aspiration, 77012
  Needle Biopsy, 77012
with Contrast
  Abdomen, 74160, 74175
  Pelvis, 72191, 72193
without Contrast
  Abdomen, 74150
  Pelvis, 72192
without Contrast, followed by Contrast
  Abdomen, 74170
  Pelvis, 72194
Computer
Aided Detection
  Mammography
    Diagnostic, 77051
    Screening, 77052
COMVAX, 90748
Concentration of Specimen, 87015
Condyloma
Destruction
  Anal, 46900-46922
  Vagina, 57061-57065
  Vulva, 56501-56515
Confirmation
Drug, 80102
Conization
Cervix, 57461, 57520-57522
Construction
Vagina
  with Graft, 57292
  without Graft, 57291
Contraception
Cervical Cap
  Fitting, 57170
Diaphragm
  Fitting, 57170
Intrauterine Device (IUD)
  Insertion, 58300
  Removal, 58301
Contraceptive Capsules, Implantable
Insertion, 11981
Removal, 11976
Coombs Test, 86880
Cordocentesis, 59012
Corpus Uteri, 58100-58285
Cortisol, 80418, 82530
Total, 82533
Cotte Operation, 58400-58410
  Repair, Uterus, Suspension, 58400-58410
CPR (Cardiopulmonary Resuscitation), 92950
CR, 82565-82575
Creatinine
Blood, 82565

Creatinine—*continued*
Clearance, 82575
Other Source, 82570
Urine, 82570-82575
Creation
Catheter Exit Site, 49436
CRIT, 85013
Cryofixation
Embryo, 89258
Sperm, 89259
Thawing
  Embryo, 89352
  Oocytes, 89353
  Reproductive Tissue, 89354
  Sperm, 89356
Cryopreservation
Embryo, 89258
Oocyte, 0059T
Sperm, 89259
Testes
  Embryo, 89352
  Oocytes, 89353
  Reproductive Tissue, 89354
  Sperm, 89356
Thawing
  Embryo, 89352
  Oocytes, 89353
  Reproductive Tissue, 89354
  Sperm, 89356
Cryosurgery, 17270-17276
Cervix, 57511
Lesion
  Anus, 46916
  Vagina, 57061-57065
  Vulva, 56501-56515
CS, 99143-99150
CSF, 86325
CST, 59020
CT Scan
Angiography
  Abdomen and Pelvis, 74174
Drainage, 75989
Guidance
  Needle Biopsy, 77012
  Parenchymal Tissue Ablation, 77013
  Tissue Ablation, 77013
  Visceral Tissue Ablation, 77013
with Contrast
  Abdomen, 74160, 74175
    and Pelvis, 74177
  Pelvis, 72191, 72193
    and Abdomen, 74177
without Contrast
  Abdomen, 74150
    and Pelvis, 74176
  Pelvis, 72192
    and Abdomen, 74176
without Contrast, followed by Contrast
  Abdomen, 74170
    and Pelvis, 74178
  Pelvis, 72194
    and Abdomen, 74178
Culdocentesis, 57020
Culdoplasty
McCall, 57283
Culdoscopy, 57452
Culdotomy, 57000
Culture
Acid Fast Bacilli, 87116
Bacteria
  Additional Methods, 87077
  Aerobic, 87040-87070
  Anaerobic, 87075-87076
  Blood, 87040
  Feces, 87045-87046
  Other, 87070-87071
  Screening, 87081
  Urine, 87086-87088
Chlamydia, 87110
Fertilized Oocyte
  for In Vitro Fertilization, 89250
  Assisted Microtechnique, 89280-89281
  with Co–Culture of Embryo, 89251

Culture—*continued*
Fungus
Blood, 87103
Identification, 87106
Other, 87102
Skin, 87101
Mycobacteria, 87116-87118
Oocyte/Embryo
Extended Culture, 89272
for In Vitro Fertilization, 89250
with Co-Culture of Embryo, 89251
Pathogen
by Kit, 87084
Stool, 87045-87046
Tubercle Bacilli, 87116
Typing, 87140-87147, 87158
Culture, 87140-87147, 87158
Yeast, 87106
Curettage
Cervix
Endocervical, 57454, 57456, 57505
Hydatidiform Mole, 59870
Postpartum, 59160
Curettement
Skin Lesion, 17270
CVS, 59015
CXR, 71010, 71020
CYP2C19, 81225
CYP2C9, 81227
CYP2D6, 81226
Cyst
Abdomen
Destruction, 49203-49205
Excision, 49203-49205
Bartholin's Gland
Excision, 56740
Repair, 56440
Breast
Incision and Drainage, 19020
Puncture Aspiration, 19000-19001
Excision
Pilonidal, 11770-11772
Incision and Drainage, 10060-10061
Pilonidal, 10080-10081
Puncture Aspiration, 10160
Ovarian
Excision, 58925
Incision and Drainage, 58800-58805
Pilonidal
Excision, 11770-11772
Incision and Drainage, 10080-10081
Retroperitoneum
Destruction, 49203-49205
Excision, 49203-49205
Skin
Puncture Aspiration, 10160
Vaginal
Excision, 57135
Cystatin C, 82610
Cystectomy
Ovarian
Laparoscopic, 58661
Open, 58925
Cystic Fibrosis Transmembrane Conductance Regulator Gene Analysis, 81220-81223
Cystometrogram, 51725-51729
Cystoscopy, 52000
Cystostomy
with Fulguration, 51020
with Insertion
Radioactive Material, 51020
Cystotomy
with Destruction Intravesical Lesion, 51030
with Fulguration, 51020
with Insertion
Radioactive Material, 51020
Urethral Catheter, 51045
Cystourethropexy, 51840-51841
Cystourethroscopy, 52000, 53500
Cytochrome Gene Analysis, 81225-81227

Cytogenomic Constitutional Microarray Analysis, 81228-81229
Cytomegalovirus
Antigen Detection
Direct Fluorescence, 87271
Cytopathology
Cervical or Vaginal
Requiring Interpretation by Physician, 88141
Thin Layer Prep, 88142-88143, 88174-88175
Concentration Technique, 88108
Evaluation, 88172-88173, 88177
Immediate Cytohistologic Study, 88172, 88177
Fine Needle Aspirate, 88172-88173, 88177
Fluids, Washings, Brushings, 88104-88108
Other Source, 88160-88162
Selective Cellular Enhancement Technique, 88112
Smears
Cervical or Vaginal, 88141-88155, 88164-88167, 88174-88175
Other Source, 88160-88162
Cytotoxic Screen
Lymphocyte, 86805-86806

D

D and C (Dilation and Curettage), 59840
D and E (Dilation and Evacuation), 59841-59851
Dark Field Examination, 87164-87166
Debridement
Muscle
Infected, 11004-11006
Necrotizing Soft Tissue, 11004-11008
Skin
Subcutaneous Tissue
Infected, 11004-11006
Wound
Non–Selective, 97602
Selective, 97597-97598
Debulking Procedure
Ovary
Pelvis, 58952-58954
DECAVAC, 90714
Dehiscence
Suture
Abdominal Wall
Skin and Subcutaneous Tissue
Complex, 13160
Complicated, 13160
Extensive, 13160
Skin and Subcutaneous Tissue
Simple, 12020
with Packing, 12021
Superficial, 12020
with Packing, 12021
Wound
Abdominal Wall
Skin and Subcutaneous Tissue
Complex, 13160
Complicated, 13160
Extensive, 13160
Skin and Subcutaneous Tissue
Simple, 12020
with Packing, 12021
Superficial, 12020
with Packing, 12021
Dehydroepiandrosterone, 82626
Dehydroepiandrosterone–Sulfate, 82627
Deoxycorticosterone, 82633
Desoxycorticosterone, 82633
Destruction
Bladder, 51020
Condyloma
Anal, 46900-46922

Destruction—*continued*
Condyloma—*continued*
Vagina, 57061-57065
Vulva, 56501-56515
Cyst
Abdomen, 49203-49205
Retroperitoneal, 49203-49205
Endometrial Ablation, 58356
Endometriomas
Abdomen, 49203-49205
Retroperitoneal, 49203-49205
Hemorrhoids
Thermal, 46930
Lesion
Anus, 46900-46917
Bladder, 51030
Nerve
Superior Hypogastric Plexus, 64681
Skin
Malignant, 17270-17276
Urethra, 53265
Vagina
Extensive, 57065
Simple, 57061
Vulva
Extensive, 56515
Simple, 56501
Nerve, 64681
Polyp
Urethra, 53260
Skene's Gland, 53270
Skin Lesion
Malignant, 17270-17276
Tumor
Abdomen, 49203-49205
Mesentery, 49203-49205
Peritoneum, 49203-49205
Retroperitoneal, 49203-49205
Urethra
Prolapse, 53275
Device
Contraceptive, Intrauterine
Insertion, 58300
Removal, 58301
Intrauterine
Insertion, 58300
Removal, 58301
DHEA (Dehydroepiandrosterone), 82626
DHEAS, 82627
Diaphragm
Vagina
Fitting, 57170
Diaphragm Contraception, 57170
Differential Count
White Blood Cell Count, 85007, 85009
Dihydrocodeinone Screen, 82486
Dihydromorphinone, 82486
Dihydroxyvitamin D, 82652
Dilation
Cervix
Canal, 57800
Stump, 57558
Curettage, 57558
Urethra
General, 53665
Suppository and/or Instillation, 53660-53661
Vagina, 57400
Dilation and Curettage
Cervical Stump, 57558
Cervix, 57558, 57800
Corpus Uteri, 58120
Hysteroscopy, 58558
Induced Abortion, 59840
with Amniotic Injections, 59851
with Vaginal Suppositories, 59856
Postpartum, 59160
Dilation and Evacuation, 59841
with Amniotic Injections, 59851
Diphtheria
Immunization, 90714-90715, 90719-90721
Doppler Echocardiography, 76827-76828

Doppler Scan
Fetal
Middle Cerebral Artery, 76821
Umbilical Artery, 76820
Double-J Stent
Cystourethroscopy, 52000
Drainage
Abdomen
Abdominal Fluid, 49082-49083
Paracentesis, 49082-49083
Peritoneal, 49020
Peritoneal Lavage, 49084
Peritonitis, Localized, 49020
Wall
Skin and Subcutaneous Tissue, 10060-10061
Complicated, 10061
Multiple, 10061
Simple, 10060
Single, 10060
Abscess
Abdomen
Peritoneal
Open, 49020
Percutaneous, 49021
Peritonitis, localized, 49020
Skin and Subcutaneous Tissue
Complicated, 10061
Multiple, 10061
Simple, 10060
Single, 10060
Bartholin's Gland
Incision and Drainage, 56420
Breast
Incision and Drainage, 19020
Contrast Injection
with X-ray, 75989
Hematoma
Vagina, 57022-57023
Ovary
Incision and Drainage
Abdominal Approach, 58822
Percutaneous, 58823
Vaginal Approach, 58820
Paraurethral Gland
Incision and Drainage, 53060
Pelvic
Percutaneous, 58823
Pelvis
Incision and Drainage
Percutaneous, 58823
Pericolic
Percutaneous, 58823
Perineum
Incision and Drainage, 56405
Peritoneum, 49020
Open, 49020
Percutaneous, 49021
Skene's Gland
Incision and Drainage, 53060
Skin
Incision and Drainage
Complicated, 10061
Multiple, 10061
Simple, 10060
Single, 10060
Puncture Aspiration, 10160
Vagina
Incision and Drainage, 57010
Vulva
Incision and Drainage, 56405
X-ray, 75989
Amniotic Fluid
Diagnostic Aspiration, 59000
Therapeutic Aspiration, 59001
Cyst
Breast, 19000-19001
Fetal Fluid, 59074
Hematoma
Vagina, 57022-57023
Skin, 10060-10180
Drug
Confirmation, 80102
Infusion, 96365-96371
Screening, 80100-80101
Tissue Preparation, 80103

Exploration—*continued*
 Pelvis, 49320
 Peritoneum
  Endoscopic, 49320
 Vagina, 57000
  Endoscopic Endocervical, 57452
External Cephalic Version, 59412

F

Factor
 Blood Coagulation
  III, 85730-85732
  IV, 82310
 Hyperglycemic-Glycogenolytic, 82943
 Sulfation, 84305
Fallopian Tube
 Anastomosis, 58750
 Catheterization, 58345, 74742
 Destruction
  Endoscopy, 58670
 Ectopic Pregnancy, 59121
  with Salpingectomy and/or Oophorectomy, 59120
 Excision, 58700-58720
 Ligation, 58600-58611
 Lysis
  Adhesions, 58740
 Occlusion, 58615
  Endoscopy, 58671
 Placement
  Implant for Occlusion, 58565
 Repair, 58752
  Anastomosis, 58750
  Creation of Stoma, 58770
 Tumor
  Resection, 58950, 58952-58956
 X-ray, 74742
FANCC, 81242
Fanconi Anemia
 Complementation Group C Gene Analysis, 81242
Farr Test, 82784-82785
Fe, 83540
Fern Test
 Smear and Stain, Wet Mount, 87210
Ferric Chloride
 Urine, 81005
Ferritin
 Blood or Urine, 82728
Fertility Test
 Semen Analysis, 89300-89322
 Sperm Evaluation
  Cervical Mucus Penetration Test, 89330
  Hamster Penetration, 89329
Fertilization
 Oocytes (Eggs)
  In Vitro, 89250-89251
   Assisted (Microtechnique), 89280-89281
   with Co-Culture of Embryo, 89251
Fetal Biophysical Profile, 76818-76819
Fetal Contraction Stress Test, 59020
Fetal Hemoglobin, 83030-83033, 85460-85461
Fetal Lung Maturity Assessment, Lecithin Sphingomyelin Ratio, 83661
Fetal Non-Stress Test, 59025
 Ultrasound, 76818
Fetal Procedure
 Amnioinfusion, 59070
 Cord Occlusion, 59072
 Fluid Drainage, 59074
 Shunt Placement, 59076
Fetal Testing
 Amniotic Fluid Lung Maturity, 83661, 83663-83664
 Biophysical Profile, 76818-76819
 Lung Maturity, 83661, 83663-83664

Fetal Testing—*continued*
 Heart, 76825-76826
  Doppler
   Complete, 76827
   Follow-up or Repeat Study, 76828
 Hemoglobin, 83030-83033, 85460-85461
 Scalp Blood Sampling, 59020
 Ultrasound, 76801-76828
  Heart, 76825
  Middle Cerebral Artery, 76821
  Umbilical Artery, 76820
Fibrinolysis
 Plasminogen, 85420-85421
 Plasminogen Activator, 85415
Fibroadenoma
 Excision, 19120-19126
Fibroids Tumor of Uterus
 Excision
  Abdominal Approach, 58140
  Vaginal Approach, 58145
Fibronectin, Fetal, 82731
Fimbrioplasty, 58760
 Laparoscopic, 58672
Fine Needle Aspiration
 Evaluation, 88172-88173, 88177
Finger
 Collection of Blood, 36415-36416
Fistula
 Rectovaginal
  Abdominal Approach, 57305
  Transperineal Approach, 57308
  with Concomitant Colostomy, 57307
  Transperineal Approach, 57308
 Urethrovaginal, 57310
  with Bulbocavernosus Transplant, 57311
 Vesicouterine
  Closure, 51920-51925
 Vesicovaginal
  Closure, 51900
  Transvesical and Vaginal Approach, 57330
  Vaginal Approach, 57320
Fitting
 Cervical Cap, 57170
 Diaphragm, 57170
Fixation (Device)
 Sacrospinous Ligament
  Vaginal Prolapse, 57282
Flu Vaccines, 90645-90660
FLUARIX, 90656
Fluid Collection
 Incision and Drainage
  Skin, 10140
Fluid Drainage
 Abdomen, 49082-49084
FluMist, 90660
Fluorescent Antibody, 86255-86256
Fluoroscopy
 Drain Abscess, 75989
 Hourly, 76001
 Needle Biopsy, 77002
Fluvirin, 90656, 90658
Fluzone, 90655-90658
FMR1, 81243-81244
Foam Stability Test, 83662.
Folic Acid, 82746
 RBC, 82747
Follicle Stimulating Hormone (FSH), 80418, 80426, 83001
Foreign Body
 Removal
  Hysteroscopy, 58562
  Peritoneum, 49402
  Subcutaneous, 10120-10121
  Uterus, 58562
  Vagina, 57415
Forensic Exam
 Phosphatase, Acid, 84061
Fragile-X
 Mental Retardation 1 Gene Analysis, 81243-81244
FSH, 83001
 with Additional Tests, 80418, 80426

FT-4, 84439
FTI, 84439
Fulguration
 Bladder, 51020
Fungal Wet Prep, 87220
Fungus
 Culture
  Blood, 87103
  Identification, 87106
  Other, 87102
  Skin, 87101
 Tissue Exam, 87220
Furuncle
 Incision and Drainage, 10060-10061

G

G6PC, 81250
Galactogram, 77053-77054
 Injection, 19030
Gamete Intrafallopian Transfer (GIFT), 58976
Gamete Transfer
 In Vitro Fertilization, 58976
Gammaglobulin
 Blood, 82784-82787
Gap Junction Protein Gene Analysis, 81252-81254
GARDASIL, 90649
GBA, 81251
Gel Diffusion, 86331
Gene
 Analysis
  APC, 81201-81203
  ASPA, 81200
  BCKDHB, 81205
  BLM, 81209
  BRCA1, 81214-81215
  BRCA1, BRCA2, 81211-81213
  BRCA2, 81216-81217
  Comparative Analysis Using Short Tandem Repeat (STR) Markers, 81265-81266
  CTR, 81220-81223
  CYP1C19, 81225
  CYP2C9, 81227
  CYP2D6, 81226
  Cytogenomic Constitutional Microarray Analysis, 81228-81229
  FANCC, 81242
  FMR1, 81243-81244
  G6PC, 81250
  GBA, 81251
  GJB2, 81252-81254
  HBA1/HBA2, 81257
  HEXA, 81255
  HFE, 81256
  HLA
   High Resolution
    Class I and II Typing, 81378
    Class I Typing, 81379-81381
    Class II Typing, 81382-81383
   IKBKAP, 81260
   Low Resolution
    Class I and II Typing, 81370-81371
    Class I Typing, 81372-81374
    Class II Typing, 81375-81377
  MCOLN1, 81290
  MECP2, 81302-81304
  MTHFR, 81291
  SNRPN/UBE3A, 81331
  UGT1A1, 81350
  VKORC1, 81355
Genitalia
 Tissue Transfer, Adjacent, 14040-14041
Gentamicin, 80170
 Assay, 80170
GH, 83003
GHb, 83036

GIFT, 58976
GJB2 Gene Analysis, 81252-81254
GLC, 82486
Globulin
 Antihuman, 86880-86885
 Immune, 90281-90284, 90384-90386, 90393
 Sex Hormone Binding, 84270
Globulin, Rh Immune, 90384-90386
Globulin, Thyroxine-Binding, 84442
Glucagon, 82943
 Tolerance Test, 82946
Glucose, 80434
 Blood Test, 82947-82950, 82962
 Body Fluid, 82945
 Tolerance Test, 82951-82952
  with Tolbutamide, 82953
Glucose-6-Phosphatase, Catalytic Subunit Gene Analysis, 81250
Glucose-6-Phosphate
 Dehydrogenase, 82955-82960
Glucosidase
 Beta Acid Gene Analysis, 81251
Glucuronide Androstanediol, 82154
Glutamate Pyruvate Transaminase, 84460
Glutamic Alanine Transaminase, 84460
Glutamic Aspartic Transaminase, 84450
Glycohemoglobin, 83036
Gonadotropin
 Chorionic, 84702-84703
 FSH, 83001
 ICSH, 83002
 LH, 83002
Gonadotropin Panel, 80426
Growth Hormone, 83003
 Human, 80418
GTT, 82951-82952

H

HAA (Hepatitis Associated Antigen), 87340, 87350-87380, 87515-87522
HAAb (Antibody, Hepatitis), 86708-86709
Hamster Penetration Test, 89329
Handling
 Specimen, 99000-99001
Haptoglobin, 83010
Harvesting
 Eggs for In Vitro Fertilization, 58970
HBA1/HBA2, 81257
HBcAb, 86704-86705
HBeAb, 86707
HBeAg, 87350
HBsAb, 86706
HBsAg (Hepatitis B Surface Antigen), 87340
HCG, 84702-84704
Hct, 85013-85014
HDL (High Density Lipoprotein), 83718
Heart
 Resuscitation, 92950
Heel
 Collection of Blood, 36415-36416
Hematoma
 Incision and Drainage
  Skin, 10140
 Puncture Aspiration, 10160
 Skin
  Incision and Drainage, 10140
  Puncture Aspiration, 10160
 Vagina
  Incision and Drainage, 57022-57023
Hemochromatosis Gene Analysis, 81256
Hemoglobin
 A1C, 83036
 Analysis
  O2 Affinity, 82820
  Chromatography, 83021
  Electrophoresis, 83020
 Fetal, 83030-83033, 85460-85461

Coding Companion for OB/GYN

Implant—continued
Hormone Pellet, 11980
Mesh
Vaginal Repair, 57267
Ovum, 58976
Tubouterine, 58752
In Vitro Fertilization
Biopsy Oocyte, 89290-89291
Culture Oocyte, 89250-89251
Extended, 89272
Embryo Hatching, 89253
Fertilize Oocyte, 89250
Microtechnique, 89280-89281
Identify Oocyte, 89254
Insemination of Oocyte, 89268
Prepare Embryo, 89255, 89352
Retrieve Oocyte, 58970
Transfer Embryo, 58974-58976
Transfer Gamete, 58976
Incision
Abdomen, 49000
Exploration, 58960
Bladder
Catheterization, 51045
with Destruction, 51020-51030
with Radiotracer, 51020
Hemorrhoid
External, 46083
Hymenotomy, 56442
Skin, 10060-10180
Uterus
Remove Lesion, 59100
Vagina
Exploration, 57000
Incision and Drainage
Abdomen
Fluid, 49082-49083
Abscess
Abdomen, Abdominal
Percutaneous, 49021
Peritoneal, 49020
Peritonitis, Localized, 49020
Skin and Subcutaneous Tissue
Complicated, 10061
Multiple, 10061
Simple, 10060
Single, 10060
Bartholin's Gland, 56420
Breast, 19020
Ovary, 58820-58822
Abdominal Approach, 58822
Vaginal Approach, 58820
Paraurethral Gland, 53060
Perineum, 56405
Peritoneum
Open, 49020
Percutaneous, 49021
Skene's Gland, 53060
Skin, 10060-10061
Vagina, 57010-57020
Vulva, 56405
Bulla
Skin
Puncture Aspiration, 10160
Cyst
Ovarian, 58800-58805
Skin, 10060-10061
Pilonidal, 10080-10081
Puncture Aspiration, 10160
Fluid Collection
Skin, 10140
Foreign Body
Skin, 10120-10121
Furuncle, 10060-10061
Hematoma
Skin, 10140
Puncture Aspiration, 10160
Vagina, 57022-57023
Pilonidal Cyst, 10080-10081
Seroma
Skin, 10140
Vagina, 57020
Wound Infection
Skin, 10180
Inclusion Bodies
Fluid, 88106
Smear, 87207, 87210

Incomplete
Abortion, 59812
Induced
Abortion
by Dilation and Curettage, 59840
by Dilation and Evacuation, 59841
by Saline, 59850-59851
by Vaginal Suppositories, 59855-59856
with Hysterotomy, 59100, 59852, 59857
Infection
Drainage
Postoperative Wound, 10180
Immunoassay, 86317-86318
Infectious Agent Detection
Antigen Detection
Direct Fluorescence
Chlamydia Trachomatis, 87270
Cytomegalovirus, 87271
Treponema Pallidum, 87285
Enzyme Immunoassay
Chlamydia Trachomatis, 87320
Hepatitis B Surface Antigen (HBsAg), 87340
Hepatitis Be Antigen (HBeAg), 87350
Hepatitis, Delta Agent, 87380
HIV-1, 87390
HIV-2, 87391
Multiple Step Method, 87320, 87340, 87350-87380, 87389-87391
Immunofluorescence, 87274
Herpes Simplex, 87274
Concentration, 87015
Detection
by Immunoassay
Chlamydia Trachomatis, 87810
Neisseria Gonorrhoeae, 87850
with Direct Optical Observation, 87810-87850
by Nucleic Acid
Candida Species, 87480-87482
Chlamydia Trachomatis, 87490-87492
Hepatitis B Virus, 87515-87517
Hepatitis C, 87520-87522
Herpes Simplex Virus, 87528-87530
Herpes Virus-6, 87531-87533
HIV-1, 87534-87536
HIV-2, 87537-87539
Influenza, 87501-87503
Neisseria Gonorrhoeae, 87590-87592
Papillomavirus, Human, 87620-87622
Trichomonas Vaginalis, 87660
Influenza B Vaccine, 90645-90648, 90720-90721, 90748
Influenza Vaccine, 90645-90648, 90653-90660, 90664-90668, 90672, 90685-90688, 90720-90721, 90748
Influenza Virus
Antibody
Vaccine, 90657-90660
Infusion
Amnion, Transabdominal, 59072
Hydration, 96360-96361
Intra-Arterial
Diagnostic, Prophylactic, Diagnostic, 96373
IV
Diagnostic, Prophylactic, Therapeutic, 96365-96368
Hydration, 96360-96361
Subcutaneous, 96369-96371

Infusion—continued
Therapy
Home Infusion Procedures, 99601-99602
Intravenous, 96360-96368
Inhibitor
of Kappa Light Polypeptide Gene Enhancer in B-Cells, Kinase Complex-Associated Protein Gene Analysis, 81260
Injection
Anesthetic
Sympathetic Nerves, 64517
Breast
Radiologic, 19030
Hemorrhoids
Sclerosing Solution, 46500
Hydration, 96360-96361
Intra-amniotic, 59850-59852
Intra-arterial, 96373
Intramuscular, 96372
Intravenous, 96365-96368
Diagnostic, 96365-96368
Mammary Ductogram
Galactogram, 19030
Radiologic
Breast, 19030
Subcutaneous, 96369-96371
Insemination
Artificial, 58321-58322, 89268
Insertion
Catheter
Abdomen, 49324, 49435
Bladder, 51045, 51701-51703
Breast
for Interstitial Radioelement Application, 19296-19298
Pelvic Organs and/or Genitalia, 55920
Suprapubic, 51102
Urethra, 51701-51703
Venous, 36415-36416
Cervical Dilator, 59200
Drug Delivery Implant, 11981, 11983
Heyman Capsule
Uterus
for Brachytherapy, 58346
Intrauterine Device (IUD), 58300
Laminaria, 59200
Mesh
Pelvic Floor, 57267
Needle
Pelvic Organs and/or Genitalia, 55920
Oviduct
Chromotubation, 58350
Hydrotubation, 58350
Ovoid
Vagina
for Brachytherapy, 57155
Packing
Vagina, 57180
Pessary
Vagina, 57160
Prostaglandin, 59200
Prosthesis
Pelvic Floor, 57267
Radiation Afterloading Apparatus, 57156
Radioactive Material
Bladder, 51020
Interstitial Brachytherapy, 77776-77778
Intracavitary Brachytherapy, 77761-77762
Stent
Bladder, 51045
Tandem
Uterus
for Brachytherapy, 57155
Urethral
Catheter, 51701-51703
Suppository, 53660-53661
Insulin, 80434

Integumentary System
Breast
Excision, 19100-19103, 19120-19126
Incision, 19000-19030
Metallic Localization Clip Placement, 19295
Preoperative Placement of Needle Localization, 19290-19291
Debridement, 11004-11006
Destruction
Malignant Lesion, 17270-17276
Drainage, 10060-10180
Excision
Benign Lesion, 11420-11426
Debridement, 11004-11006
Malignant Lesion, 11620-11626
Graft, 14040-14041
Tissue Transfer or Rearrangement, 14040-14041
Incision, 10060-10180
Introduction
Drug Delivery Implant, 11981, 11983
Removal
Drug Delivery Implant, 11982-11983
Repair
Adjacent Tissue Transfer Rearrangement, 14040-14041
Complex, 13100-13102, 13131-13133, 13160
Intermediate, 12031-12047
Simple, 12001-12007, 12020-12021
Internet E/M Service
Nonphysician, 98969
Intersex State
Clitoroplasty, 56805
Vaginoplasty, 57335
Intestine(s)
Lysis of Adhesions
Laparoscopic, 44180
Intestines, Small
Repair
Enterocele
Abdominal Approach, 57270
Vaginal Approach, 57268
Intradermal Influenza Virus Vaccine, 90654
Intramuscular Injection, 96372
Intrauterine
Contraceptive Device (IUD)
Insertion, 58300
Removal, 58301
Insemination, 58322
Intrauterine Synechiae
Lysis, 58559
Intravenous Therapy, 96360-96368, 96374-96376
Introduction
Breast
Metallic Localization Clip Placement, 19295
Preoperative Placement, Needle, 19290-19291
Contraceptive Capsules
Implantable, 11981
Drug Delivery Implant, 11981, 11983
IPOL, 90713
IPV, 90713
Iron, 83540
Iron Binding Capacity, 83550
Irrigation
Vagina, 57150
Irving Sterilization
Ligation, Fallopian Tube, Oviduct, 58600-58611, 58670
ISG Immunization, 90281-90283
Isolation
Sperm, 89260-89261
IUD, 58300-58301
Insertion, 58300
Removal, 58301
IUI (Intrauterine Insemination), 58322

© 2012 OptumInsight, Inc.

IV, 96365-96368, 96374-96376
  Hydration, 96360-96361
IV Infusion Therapy, 96365-96368
  Hydration, 96360-96361
IV Injection, 96374-96376
IVF (In Vitro Fertilization), 58970-58976, 89250-89255
Ivy Bleeding Time, 85002

J

Japanese Encephalitis Virus Vaccine, 90735
JE-VAX, 90735
Jones and Cantarow Test
  Clearance, Urea Nitrogen, 84545

K

K+, 84132
Kala Azar Smear, 87207
Keitzer Test, 51727, 51729
Kelly Urethral Plication, 57220
Kleihauer–Betke Test, 85460
Kloramfenikol, 82415
KOH
  Hair, Nails, Tissue, Examination for Fungi, 87220

L

L/S, 83661
L/S Ratio
  Amniotic Fluid, 83661
Labial Adhesions
  Lysis, 56441
Lactate, 83605
Lactic Acid, 83605
Lactic Dehydrogenase, 83615-83625
Lactogen, Human Placental, 83632
Laminaria
  Insertion, 59200
Laparoscopy
  Abdominal, 49320-49322, 49324-49327
    Surgical, 49321-49322, 49324-49326
  Aspiration, 49322
  Biopsy, 49321
    Ovary, 49321
  Bladder
    Repair
      Sling Procedure, 51992
      Urethral Suspension, 51990
  Destruction
    Lesion, 58662
  Diagnostic, 49320
  Ectopic Pregnancy, 59150
    with Salpingectomy and/or Oophorectomy, 59151
  Enterolysis, 44180
  Fimbrioplasty, 58672
  Graft Revision
    Vaginal, 57426
  Hysterectomy, 58541-58554, 58570-58573
    Radical, 58548
    Total, 58570-58573
  In Vitro Fertilization, 58976
    Retrieve Oocyte, 58970
    Transfer Embryo, 58974
    Transfer Gamete, 58976
  Incontinence Repair, 51990-51992
  Lysis of Adhesions, 58660
  Lysis of Intestinal Adhesions, 44180
  Omentopexy, 49326
  Ovary
    Biopsy, 49321
  Oviduct Surgery, 58670-58671
  Pelvis, 49320
  Placement Interstitial Device, 49327
  Removal
    Fallopian Tubes, 58661
    Leiomyomata, 58545-58546
    Ovaries, 58661

Laparoscopy—continued
  Salpingostomy, 58673
  Surgical, 44180, 49321-49322, 49324-49327, 51992, 57425, 58545-58546, 58552, 58554
  Urethral Suspension, 51990
  Vaginal Hysterectomy, 58550-58554
  Vaginal Suspension, 57425
Laparotomy
  Exploration, 49000-49002, 58960
  Hemorrhage Control, 49002
  Second Look, 58960
  Staging, 58960
  with Biopsy, 49000
Laparotomy, Exploratory, 49000-49002
Laroyenne Operation
  Vagina, Abscess, Incision and Drainage, 57010
Laser Surgery
  Anal, 46917
  Lesion
    Skin, 17270-17276
Laser Treatment, 17270-17276
Latzko Procedure
  Colpocleisis, 57120
LAV Antibodies, 86689, 86701-86703
LAV-2, 86702-86703
Lavage
  Peritoneal, 49084
LD (Lactic Dehydrogenase), 83615
LDH, 83615-83625
LDL, 83721
Lead, 83655
Lecithin–Sphingomyelin Ratio, 83661
LEEP Procedure, 57460
LeFort Procedure
  Vagina, 57120
Leiomyomata
  Embolization, 37210
  Removal, 58140, 58545-58546, 58561
Lesion
  Anal
    Destruction, 46900-46917
    Excision, 46922
  Bladder
    Destruction, 51030
  Breast
    Excision, 19120-19126
  Excision, 59100
    Urethra, 53265
  Pelvis
    Destruction, 58662
  Skin
    Destruction
      Malignant, 17270-17276
    Excision
      Benign, 11420-11426
      Malignant, 11620-11626
  Vagina
    Destruction, 57061-57065
  Vulva
    Destruction
      Extensive, 56515
      Simple, 56501
Leukoagglutinins, 86021
Leukocyte
  Antibody, 86021
Leukocyte Count, 85032, 85048
LH (Luteinizing Hormone), 80418, 80426, 83002
Ligation
  Fallopian Tube
    Oviduct, 58600-58611, 58670
  Hemorrhoids, 46221
  Oviducts, 59100
Lipoprotein
  Blood, 83718-83721
  LDL, 83721
Localization
  Nodule Radiographic, Breast, 77032
LRH (Luteinizing Releasing Hormone), 83727
LSD (Lysergic Acid Diethylamide), 80100-80104
LUSCS, 59514-59515, 59618-59622
LUSS (Liver Ultrasound Scan), 76705

Luteinizing Hormone (LH), 80418, 80426, 83002
Luteinizing Release Factor, 83727
Luteotropic Hormone, 80418, 84146
Luteotropin, 80418, 84146
Luteotropin Placental, 83632
Lutrepulse Injection, 11980
Lymph Node(s)
  Excision
    Abdominal, 38747
    Inguinofemoral, 38760-38765
    Limited, for Staging
      Para–Aortic, 38562
      Pelvic, 38562
    Pelvic, 38770
    Retroperitoneal Transabdominal, 38780
  Removal
    Abdominal, 38747
    Inguinofemoral, 38760-38765
    Pelvic, 38747, 38770
    Retroperitoneal Transabdominal, 38780
Lymphadenectomy
  Abdominal, 38747
  Bilateral Inguinofemoral, 56632, 56637
  Bilateral Pelvic
    Total, 57531, 58210
  Diaphragmatic Assessment, 58960
  Inguinofemoral, 38760-38765
  Inguinofemoral, Iliac and Pelvic, 56640
  Limited Para–Aortic, Resection of Ovarian Malignancy, 58951
  Limited Pelvic, 58954
  Limited, for Staging
    Para–Aortic, 38562
    Pelvic, 38562
  Malignancy, 58951, 58954
  Para-Aortic, 58958
  Pelvic, 58958
  Peripancreatic, 38747
  Portal, 38747
  Radical
    Groin Area, 38760-38765
    Pelvic, 58548
  Retroperitoneal Transabdominal, 38780
  Unilateral Inguinofemoral, 56631, 56634
Lymphocyte
  Toxicity Assay, 86805-86806
Lymphocytotoxicity, 86805-86806
Lysergic Acid Diethylamide, 80102-80103
Lysergide, 80102-80103
Lysis
  Adhesions
    Fallopian Tube, 58740
    Labial, 56441
    Ovary, 58740
    Oviduct, 58740
    Ureter, 50722
    Urethra, 53500
    Uterus, 58559
  Labial
    Adhesions, 56441

M

Machado Test
  Complement, Fixation Test, 86171
MacLean–De Wesselow Test
  Clearance, Urea Nitrogen, 84540-84545
Madlener Operation, 58600
Magnesium, 83735
Magnetic Resonance Angiography (MRA)
  Abdomen, 74185
  Pelvis, 72198
Malaria Smear, 87207
Maltose
  Tolerance Test, 82951-82952
Mammary Abscess, 19020

Mammary Duct
  X-ray with Contrast, 77053-77054
Mammary Ductogram
  Injection, 19030
  Radiologic Supervision and Interpretation, 77053-77054
Mammary Stimulating Hormone, 80418, 84146
Mammogram
  Breast
    Localization Nodule, 77032
  Screening, 77057
  with Computer-Aided Detection, 77051-77052
Mammography
  Diagnostic, 77055-77056
    with Computer–aided Detection, 77051
  Screening, 77057
    with Computer–aided Detection, 77052
  with Computer-Aided Detection, 77051-77052
Mammotropic Hormone, Pituitary, 80418, 84146
Mammotropic Hormone, Placental, 83632
Mammotropin, 80418, 84146
Manchester Colporrhaphy, 58400
Mandated Services
  Hospital, on call, 99026-99027
Manipulation
  Osteopathic, 98925-98929
Marcellation Operation
  Hysterectomy, Vaginal, 58260-58270, 58550
Marshall–Marchetti–Krantz Procedure, 51840-51841, 58152, 58267, 58293
Marsupialization
  Bartholin's Gland Cyst, 56440
  Cyst
    Bartholin's Gland, 56440
    Urethral Diverticulum, 53240
Mass Spectrometry and Tandem Mass Spectrometry
  Analyte
    Qualitative, 83788
    Quantitative, 83789
Mastotomy, 19020
Maternity Care and Delivery, 59400-59871
MBC, 87181-87190
McCall Culdoplasty, 57283
McDonald Operation, 57700
McIndoe Procedure, 57291
MCOLN1, 81290
MEA (Microwave Endometrial Ablation, 58563
Measles Immunization, 90705, 90707, 90710
Measles Vaccine, 90705, 90708-90710
Measles, German
  Vaccine, 90706-90710
Measles, Mumps, Rubella Vaccine, 90707
MECP2, 81302-81304
Medical Genetics
  Counseling, 96040
Medical Nutrition Therapy, 97802-97804
Meningococcal Vaccine
  Polysaccharide, Any Groups, 90733
Menomune, 90733
MERUVAX, 90706
Mesh
  Insertion
    Pelvic Floor, 57267
  Removal
    Abdominal Infected, 11008
Mesh Implantation
  Vagina, 57267
Methemalbumin, 83857
Methyl CpG Binding Protein 2 Gene Analysis, 81302-81304
Metroplasty, 58540
Mg, 83735

Pregnanediol, 84135
Pregnanetriol, 84138
Pregnenolone, 84140
Prenatal Procedure
  Amnioinfusion
    Transabdominal, 59070
  Drainage
    Fluid, 59074
  Occlusion
    Umbilical Cord, 59072
  Shunt, 59076
Prenatal Testing
  Amniocentesis, 59000
    with Amniotic Fluid Reduction, 59001
  Chorionic Villus Sampling, 59015
  Cordocentesis, 59012
  Fetal Blood Sample, 59030
  Fetal Monitoring, 59050
    Interpretation Only, 59051
  Non-Stress Test, Fetal, 59025, 99500
  Oxytocin Stress Test, 59020
  Stress Test
    Oxytocin, 59020
  Ultrasound, 76801-76817
    Fetal Biophysical Profile, 76818-76819
    Fetal Heart, 76825
Preparation
  for Transfer
    Embryo, 89255
  Thawing
    Embryo
      Cryopreserved, 89352
    Oocytes
      Cryopreserved, 89356
    Reproductive Tissue
      Cryopreserved, 89354
    Sperm
      Cryopreserved, 89353
Procalcitonin (PCT), 84145
Profibrinolysin, 85420-85421
Progesterone, 84144
Progesterone Receptors, 84234
Progestin Receptors, 84234
Prolactin, 80418, 84146
Prolapse
  Urethra, 53275
Pronuclear Stage Tube Transfer (PROST), 58976
PROST (Pronuclear Stage Tube Transfer), 58976
Prostaglandin, 84150
  Insertion, 59200
Prosthesis
  Vagina
    Insertion, 57267
Protein
  A, Plasma (PAPP-A), 84163
  Other Source, 84157
  Serum, 84155
  Total, 84155-84157
  Urine, 84156
    by Dipstick, 81000-81003
Prothrombin
  Time, 85610-85611
Prothrombinase
  Partial Time, 85730-85732
Protime, 85610-85611
Protoporphyrin, 84202-84203
Provitamin A, 84590
PT, 85610-85611, 97597-97606
Pteroylglutamic Acid, 82746-82747
PTT, 85730-85732
PUBS (Percutaneous Umbilical Blood Sampling), 59012
Pudendal Nerve
  Injection
    Anesthetic, 64430
Puncture Aspiration
  Abscess
    Skin, 10160
  Bulla, 10160
  Cyst
    Breast, 19000-19001
    Skin, 10160

Puncture Aspiration—continued
  Hematoma, 10160
  PV, 90712-90713

Q

Quick Test
  Prothrombin Time, 85610-85611

R

Radical Vaginal Hysterectomy, 58285
Radical Vulvectomy, 56630-56640
Radioelement
  Application, 77761-77778
    with Ultrasound, 76965
Radioelement Substance
  Catheter Placement
    Breast, 19296-19298
    Pelvic Organs or Genitalia, 55920
  Needle Placement
    Pelvic Organs and Genitalia, 55920
Radioimmunosorbent Test
  Gammaglobulin, Blood, 82784-82785
Radiological Marker
  Preoperative Placement
    Excision of Breast Lesion, 19125-19126
Radiotherapy
  Afterloading
    Catheter Insertion, 19296-19298
Rapid Plasma Reagin Test, 86592-86593
Raz Procedure, 51845
RBC, 85007, 85014, 85041, 85651-85652, 86850-86870
RBC ab, 86850-86870
Receptor
  Estrogen, 84233
  Progesterone, 84234
  Progestin, 84234
Receptor Assay
  Endocrine, 84235
  Estrogen, 84233
  Non-Hormone, 84238
  Progesterone, 84234
RECOMBIVAX HB, 90740-90746
Reconstruction
  Abdominal Wall
    Ometal Flap, 49905
  Chest Wall
    Omental Flap, 49905
  Fallopian Tube, 58673, 58750-58752, 58770
  Oviduct
    Fimbrioplasty, 58760
  Urethra, 53430
    Hypospadias
      Suture to Bladder, 51840-51841
  Uterus, 58540
  Wound Repair, 13100-13102, 13131-13133, 13160
Rectocele
  Repair, 45560
Rectum
  Repair
    Rectocele, 45560
Red Blood Cell (RBC)
  Antibody, 86850-86870
  Count, 85032-85041
  Hematocrit, 85014
  Morphology, 85007
  Platelet Estimation, 85007
  Sedimentation Rate
    Automated, 85652
    Manual, 85651
Red Blood Cell ab, 86850-86870
Reductase, Lactic Cytochrome, 83615-83625
Reduction
  Pregnancy
    Multifetal, 59866
Rehydration, 96360-96361

Reimplantation
  Ovary, 58825
Reinsertion
  Drug Delivery Implant, 11983
Relative Density
  Body Fluid, 84315
Remodeling
  Bladder/Urethra, 53860
Removal
  Bladder, 51597
  Cerclage
    Cervix, 59871
  Contraceptive Capsules, 11976
  Drug Delivery Implant, 11982-11983
  Fallopian Tube
    Laparoscopy, 58661
      with Hysterectomy, 58542, 58544, 58548
  Foreign Bodies
    Hysteroscopy, 58562
    Peritoneum, 49402
    Subcutaneous, 10120-10121
    Uterus, 58562
    Vagina, 57415
  Implant
    Contraceptive Capsules, 11976
  Intrauterine Device (IUD), 58301
  Leiomyomata, 58545-58546, 58561
  Lymph Nodes
    Abdominal, 38747
    Inguinofemoral, 38760-38765
    Pelvic, 38770
    Retroperitoneal Transabdominal, 38780
  Mesh
    Abdominal Wall, 11008
  Ovaries
    Laparoscopy, 58661
      with Hysterectomy, 58542, 58544, 58548
  Prosthesis
    Abdominal Wall, 11008
  Sling
    Vagina, 57287
  Tissue
    Vaginal, Partial, 57107
  Vagina
    Partial
      Tissue, 57106
      Wall, 57107, 57110-57111
      with Nodes, 57109
Repair
  Bladder
    Fistula, 51900-51925
    Neck, 51845
  Cervix
    Cerclage, 57700
      Abdominal, 59320-59325
    Suture, 57720
    Vaginal Approach, 57720
  Cyst
    Bartholin's Gland, 56440
  Cystocele, 57240
  Enterocele
    Hysterectomy, 58263, 58270, 58292, 58294
    Vaginal Approach, 57268
    with Colporrhaphy, 57265
  Episiotomy, 59300
  Fallopian Tube, 58752
    Anastomosis, 58750
    Create Stoma, 58770
  Fistula
    Rectovaginal, 57308
  Intestines
    Enterocele
      Abdominal Approach, 57270
      Vaginal Approach, 57268
  Introitus, Vagina, 56800
  Laceration, Skin
    Abdomen
      Complex, 13100-13102
      Intermediate, 12031-12037
      Layered, 12031-12037
      Simple, 12001-12007
      Superficial, 12001-12007
    Breast
      Complex, 13100-13102

Repair—continued
  Laceration, Skin—continued
    Breast—continued
      Intermediate, 12031-12037
      Layered, 12031-12037
      Simple, 12001-12007
      Superficial, 12001-12007
    Buttock
      Complex, 13100-13102
      Intermediate, 12031-12037
      Layered, 12031-12037
      Simple, 12001-12007
      Superficial, 12001-12007
    External
      Genitalia
        Complex/Intermediate, 12041-12047
        Layered, 12041-12047
        Simple, 12001-12007
        Superficial, 12041-12047
    Genitalia
      Complex, 13131-13133
      External
        Complex/Intermediate, 12041-12047
        Layered, 12041-12047
        Simple, 12001-12007
        Superficial, 12041-12047
    Trunk
      Complex, 13100-13102
      Intermediate, 12031-12037
      Layered, 12031-12037
      Simple, 12001-12007
      Superficial, 12001-12007
  Microsurgery, 69990
  Oviduct, 58752
    Create Stoma, 58770
  Paravaginal Defect, 57284-57285, 57423
  Pelvic Floor
    with Prosthesis, 57267
  Perineum, 56810
  Rectocele, 45560, 57250
  Rectovaginal Fistula, 57308
  Rectum
    Rectocele, 45560, 57250
  Simple, Integumentary System, 12001-12007, 12020-12021
  Skin
    Wound
      Complex, 13100-13102, 13131-13133, 13160
      Intermediate, 12031-12047
      Simple, 12020-12021
  Ureter
    Lysis Adhesions, 50722
  Urethra
    Diverticulum, 53240
    Urethrocele, 57230
    Wound, 53502
  Urethral Sphincter, 57220
  Uterus
    Anomaly, 58540
    Fistula, 51920-51925
    Rupture, 58520, 59350
    Suspension, 58400-58410
      Presacral Sympathectomy, 58410
  Vagina
    Anterior, 57240, 57289
      with Insertion of Mesh, 57267
      with Insertion of Prosthesis, 57267
    Cystocele, 57240, 57260
    Enterocele, 57265
    Episiotomy, 59300
    Fistula, 51900
      Rectovaginal, 57300-57307
      Transvesical and Vaginal Approach, 57330
      Urethrovaginal, 57310-57311
      Vesicovaginal, 57320-57330
    Hysterectomy, 58267, 58293
    Incontinence, 57288
    Pereyra Procedure, 57289
    Postpartum, 57200
    Prolapse, 57282, 57284
    Rectocele, 57250-57260

Coding Companion for OB/GYN

© 2012 OptumInsight, Inc.

Toxoplasma
Antibody, 86777-86778
Trachelectomy, 57530
Radical, 57531
Trachelorrhaphy, 57720
Transaminase
Glutamic Oxaloacetic, 84450
Glutamic Pyruvic, 84460
Transfer
Adjacent Tissue, 14040-14041
Blastocyst, 58974-58976
Cryopreserved, 89352
Gamete Intrafallopian, 58976
Tubal Embyo Stage, 58974
Transferase
Aspartate Amino, 84450
Glutamic Oxaloacetic, 84450
Transfusion
Blood
Fetal, 36460
Transposition
Ovary, 58825
Transurethral
Radiofrequency Micro-Remodeling
Female Bladder, 53860
Treatment, Tocolytic, 59412
Treponema Pallidum
Antibody, 86780
Antigen Detection
Direct Fluorescent Antibody,
87285
Triacylglycerol, 84478
Trichomonas Vaginalis
Antigen Detection
Nucleic Acid, 87660
Triglycerides, 84478
TriHIBt, 90721
Triiodothyronine
Free, 84481
Resin Uptake, 84479
Reverse, 84482
Total, 84480
True, 84480
Trophoblastic Tumor GTT, 59100,
59870
Trypanosomiases, 86171
Trypanosomiasis, 86171
TSA, 86316
TSH, 80418, 84443
TSI, 84445
TT-3, 84480
TT-4, 84436
Tubal Embryo Stage Transfer, 58976
Tubal Ligation, 58600
Laparoscopic, 58670
Postpartum, 58605
with Cesarean Section, 58611
Tubal Pregnancy, 59121
with Salpingectomy and/or Oopho-
rectomy, 59120
Tubectomy, 58700-58720
Tubercle Bacilli
Culture, 87116
Tuberculosis
Culture, 87116
Tudor Rabbit Ear
Urethra, Repair
Diverticulum, 53240
Sphincter, 57220
Urethrocele, 57230
Wound, 53502
Tumor
Abdomen
Destruction
Excision, 49203-49205
Breast
Excision, 19120-19126
Destruction
Abdomen, 49203-49205
Fallopian Tube
Resection, 58950, 58952-58956
Immunoassay for Antigen, 86294,
86316
CA 125, 86304
CA 15–3, 86300
CA 19–9, 86301

Tumor—continued
Ovary
Resection, 58950, 58952-58954
Peritoneum
Resection, 58950-58956
Retroperitoneal
Destruction
Excision, 49203-49205
Uterus
Excision, 58140-58145
Vagina
Excision, 57135
TVCB (Transvaginal Chorionic Villus
Biopsy), 59015
TVH (Total Vaginal Hysterectomy),
58262-58263, 58285, 58291-
58292
TVS (Transvaginal Sonography),
76817, 76830
Tylectomy, 19120-19126
Typing
Blood, 86900-86901, 86906
HLA, 81370-81383
Tissue, 81370-81383
Tyrosine, 84510
Tzanck Smear, 88160-88161

U

Uchida Procedure
Tubal Ligation, 58600
UCX (Urine Culture), 87086-87088
UDP Glucuronosyltransferase
1 Family, Polypeptide A1 Gene
Analysis, 81350
UFE, 37210
UFR, 51736-51741
UGT1A1, 81350
Ultrasound
Abdomen, 76700-76705
Ablation
Uterine Leiomyomata, 0071T-
0072T
Artery
Middle Cerebral, 76821
Umbilical, 76820
Breast, 76645
Chest, 76604
Drainage
Abscess, 75989
Fetus, 76818-76819
Follow–Up, 76970
Guidance
Amniocentesis, 59001, 76946
Amnioinfusion, 59070
Chorionic Villus Sampling, 76945
Drainage
Fetal Fluid, 59074
Endometrial Ablation, 58356
Fetal Cordocentesis, 76941
Fetal Transfusion, 76941
Needle Biopsy, 76942
Occlusion
Umbilical Cord, 59072
Ova Retrieval, 76948
Radiation Therapy, 76950
Radioelement, 76965
Shunt Placement
Fetal, 59076
Thoracentesis, 76942
Heart
Fetal, 76825
Hysterosonography, 76831
Intraoperative, 76998
Pelvis, 76856-76857
Pregnant Uterus, 76801-76817
Sonohysterography, 76831
Umbilical Artery, 76820
Uterus
Tumor Ablation, 0071T-0072T
Vagina, 76830
Umbilical
Artery Ultrasound, 76820
Umbilical Cord
Occlusion, 59072

UPP (Urethral Pressure Profile),
51727, 51729
Urea Nitrogen, 84525
Blood, 84520-84525
Clearance, 84545
Quantitative, 84520
Semiquantitative, 84525
Urine, 84540
Urecholine Supersensitivity Test
Cystometrogram, 51725-51726
Ureter
Lysis
Adhesions, 50722
Repair
Lysis of Adhesions, 50722
Ureterolysis
for Ovarian Vein Syndrome, 50722
Urethra
Adhesions
Lysis, 53500
Dilation
General, 53665
Suppository and/or Instillation,
53660-53661
Diverticulum
Endoscopy, 52000
Excision, 53230
Marsupialization, 53240
Repair, 53240
Endoscopy, 52000
Excision
Diverticulum, 53230
Incision and Drainage, 53060
Insertion
Catheter, 51701-51703
Lesion
Destruction, 53265
Excision, 53260
Lysis
Adhesions, 53500
Paraurethral Gland
Incision and Drainage, 53060
Polyp
Destruction, 53260
Excision, 53260
Pressure Profile Studies, 51727,
51729
Prolapse
Destruction, 53275
Excision, 53275
Repair, 53275
Reconstruction, 53430
Repair
Diverticulum, 53240
Sphincter, 57220
Urethrocele, 57230
Wound, 53502
Skene's Gland
Incision and Drainage, 53060
Suture
to Bladder, 51840-51841
Wound, 53502
Urethral
Diverticulum Marsupialization,
53240
Pressure Profile, 51727, 51729
Urethral Diverticulum
Marsupialization, 53240
Urethral Pressure Profile, 51727,
51729
Urethrocele
Repair, 57230-57240
Urethrocystopexy, 51840-51841
Urethropexy, 51840-51841
Urethroplasty
Reconstruction
Female Urethra, 53430
Urethrorrhaphy, 53502
Urethroscopy, 52000
Urinalysis, 81000-81050
Automated, 81001, 81003
Glass Test, 81020
Microalbumin, 82043-82044
Microscopic, 81015
Pregnancy Test, 81025
Qualitative, 81005

Urinalysis—continued
Routine, 81002
Screen, 81007
Semiquantitative, 81005
Volume Measurement, 81050
without Microscopy, 81002
Urine
Albumin, 82042-82044
Blood, 81000-81005
Colony Count, 87086
Pregnancy Test, 81025
Tests, 81000-81050
Urine Sensitivity Test, 87181-87190
Urodynamic Tests
Cystometrogram, 51725-51729
Uroflowmetry, 51736-51741
Voiding Pressure Studies
Bladder, 51728-51729
Uroflowmetry, 51736-51741
Urothromboplastin
Partial Time, 85730-85732
Uterine
Adhesion
Lysis, 58559
Hemorrhage
Postpartum, 59160
Uterus
Ablation
Endometrium, 58353-58356
Tumor
Ultrasound Focused, 0071T-
0072T
Biopsy
Endometrium, 58100
Endoscopy, 58558
Catheterization
X–ray, 58340
Chromotubation, 58350
Curettage, 58356
Postpartum, 59160
Dilation and Curettage, 58120
Postpartum, 59160
Ectopic Pregnancy
Interstitial
Partial Resection Uterus,
59136
Total Hysterectomy, 59135
Embolization
Fibroid, 37210
Endoscopy
Endometrial Ablation, 58563
Exploration, 58555
Surgery, 58558-58565
Treatment, 58558-58565
Excision
Laparoscopic, 58550
Total, 58570-58573
with Removal of Ovaries,
58552, 58554
Partial, 58180
Radical
Laparoscopic, 58548
Open, 58210, 58285
Removal of Tubes and/or Ovaries,
58262-58263, 58291-
58293, 58552, 58554
Sonohysterography, 76831
Total, 58150-58152, 58200,
58953-58956
Vaginal, 58260-58270, 58290-
58294, 58550-58554
with Colpectomy, 58275-
58280
with Colpo–Urethrocystopexy,
58267
with Repair of Enterocele,
58270, 58294
Hemorrhage
Postpartum, 59160
Hydatidiform Mole
Excision, 59100
Hydrotubation, 58350
Hysterosalpingography, 74740
Hysterosonography, 76831
Incision
Removal of Lesion, 59100

terus—*continued*
  Insertion
    Heyman Capsule
      for Brachytherapy, 58346
    Intrauterine Device, 58300
    Tandem
      for Brachytherapy, 57155
  Lesion
    Excision, 58545-58546, 59100
  Reconstruction, 58540
  Removal
    Intrauterine Device (IUD), 58301
  Repair
    Fistula, 51920-51925
    Rupture, 58520, 59350
    Suspension, 58400
      with Presacral Sympathec-
        tomy, 58410
  Sonohysterography, 76831
  Suture
    Rupture, 59350
  Tumor
    Ablation
      Ultrasound Focused, 0071T-
        0072T
    Embolization, 37210
    Excision
      Abdominal Approach, 58140,
        58146
      Vaginal Approach, 58145
  X-ray with Contrast, 74740

V

-Y Operation, Bladder, Neck, 51845
-Y Plasty
  Skin, Adjacent Tissue Transfer,
    14040-14041
accines
  Chicken Pox, 90716
  Cholera Injectable, 90725
  Diphtheria Toxoid, 90719
  Diphtheria, Tetanus, Acellular Per-
    tussis and Hemophilus Influ-
    enza B (Hib) (DtaP-Hib), 90721
  Diphtheria, Tetanus, and Acellular
    Pertussis, (Tdap), 90715
  Diphtheria, Tetanus, Whole Cell Per-
    tussis and Hemophilus Influ-
    enza B (DTP-Hib), 90720
  Encephalitis, Japanese, 90735
  Hemophilus Influenza B, 90645-
    90648
  Hepatitis B, 90739-90747
  Hepatitis B and Hemophilus Influ-
    enza B (HepB-Hib), 90748
  Human Papilloma Virus (HPV),
    90649-90650
  Influenza, 90653-90660, 90664-
    90668, 90672, 90685-90688
  Measles, 90705
  Measles and Rubella, 90708
  Measles, Mumps and Rubella (MMR),
    90707
  Measles, Mumps, Rubella and Vari-
    cella (MMRV), 90710
  Meningococcal, 90733
  Mumps, 90704
  Plague, 90727
  Pneumococcal, 90732
  Poliovirus, Inactivated
    Intramuscular, 90713
    Subcutaneous, 90713
  Poliovirus, Live
    Oral, 90712
  Rubella, 90706
  Tetanus and Diphtheria, 90714
  Tetanus Toxoid, 90703
  Tetanus, Diphtheria and Acellular
    Pertussis (Tdap), 90715
  Tetanus, Diphtheria, and Acellular
    Pertussis (TdaP), 90715
  Varicella (Chicken Pox), 90716
  Yellow Fever, 90717
  Zoster, 90736

Vagina
  Abscess
    Incision and Drainage, 57010
  Biopsy
    Colposcopy, 57421
    Endocervical, 57454
    Extensive, 57105
    Simple, 57100
  Closure, 57120
  Colposcopy, 57420-57421, 57455-
    57456, 57461
  Construction
    with Graft, 57292
    without Graft, 57291
  Cyst
    Excision, 57135
  Dilation, 57400
  Endocervical
    Biopsy, 57454
    Exploration, 57452
  Excision
    Closure, 57120
    Complete
      with Removal of Paravaginal
        Tissue, 57111
      with Removal of Paravaginal
        Tissue with Lymphade-
        nectomy, 57112
      with Removal of Vaginal Wall,
        57110
    Partial
      with Removal of Paravaginal
        Tissue, 57107
      with Removal of Paravaginal
        Tissue with Lymphade-
        nectomy, 57109
      with Removal of Vaginal Wall,
        57106
    Total, 57110
      with Hysterectomy, 58275-
        58280
      with Repair of Enterocele,
        58280
  Exploration
    Endocervical, 57452
    Incision, 57000
  Hematoma
    Incision and Drainage, 57022-
      57023
  Hemorrhage, 57180
  Hysterectomy, 58290, 58550-58554
  Incision and Drainage, 57020
  Insertion
    Ovoid
      for Brachytherapy, 57155
    Packing for Bleeding, 57180
    Pessary, 57160
  Irrigation, 57150
  Lesion
    Destruction, 57061-57065
      Extensive, 57065
      Simple, 57061
  Prolapse
    Sacrospinous Ligament Fixation,
      57282
  Removal
    Foreign Body, 57415
    Prosthetic Graft, 57295-57296
    Sling
      Stress Incontinence, 57287
    Tissue, Partial, 57106
    Wall, Partial, 57107
  Repair, 56800
    Cystocele, 57240, 57260
      Combined Anteroposterior,
        57260-57265
      Posterior, 57240
    Enterocele, 57265
    Fistula, 51900
      Rectovaginal, 57300-57308
      Transvesical and Vaginal
        Approach, 57330
      Urethrovaginal, 57310-57311
      Vesicovaginal, 51900, 57320-
        57330
    Hysterectomy, 58267, 58293
    Incontinence, 57288
    Obstetric, 59300

Vagina—*continued*
  Repair—*continued*
    Paravaginal Defect, 57284
    Pereyra Procedure, 57289
    Prolapse, 57282, 57284
    Prosthesis Insertion, 57267
    Rectocele
      Combined Anteroposterior,
        57260-57265
      Posterior, 57250
    Suspension, 57280-57283
      Laparoscopic, 57425
    Urethra Sphincter, 57220
    Wound, 57200-57210
      Colpoperineorrhaphy, 57210
      Colporrhaphy, 57200
  Revision
    Prosthetic Graft, 57295-57296,
      57426
    Sling
      Stress Incontinence, 57287
  Septum
    Excision, 57130
  Suspension, 57280-57283
    Laparoscopic, 57425
  Suture
    Cystocele, 57240, 57260
    Enterocele, 57265
    Fistula, 51900, 57300-57330
    Rectocele, 57250-57260
    Wound, 57200-57210
  Tumor
    Excision, 57135
  Ultrasound, 76830
  X-ray with Contrast, 74775
Vaginal Delivery, 59400, 59610-59614
  After Previous Cesarean Section,
    59610-59612
  Attempted, 59618-59622
  Antepartum Care Only, 59425-
    59426
  Attempted, 59618-59622
  Cesarean Delivery After Attempted
    Delivery Only, 59620
    with Postpartum Care, 59622
  Delivery After Previous Vaginal Deliv-
    ery Only
    with Postpartum Care, 59614
  Delivery Only, 59409
  External Cephalic Version, 59412
  Placenta, 59414
  Postpartum Care only, 59410
  Routine Care, 59400
Vaginal Smear, 88141-88155, 88164-
  88167, 88174-88175
Vaginal Suppositories
  Induced Abortion, 59855
    with Dilation and Curettage,
      59856
    with Hysterotomy, 59857
Vaginal Tissue
  Removal, Partial, 57106
Vaginal Wall
  Removal, Partial, 57107
Vaginectomy
  Partial, 57109
    with Nodes, 57109
Vaginoplasty
  Intersex State, 57335
Vaginorrhaphy, 57200
Vaginoscopy
  Biopsy, 57454
  Exploration, 57452
Vaginotomy, 57000-57010
Valentine's Test
  Urinalysis, Glass Test, 81020
Van Den Bergh Test, 82247-82248
Vancomycin
  Assay, 80202
Varicella (Chicken Pox)
  Immunization, 90710, 90716
VARIVAX, 90716
Vascular Studies
  Artery Studies
    Middle Cerebral Artery, Fetal,
      76821
    Umbilical Artery, Fetal, 76820

Vascular Studies—*continued*
  Visceral Studies, 93975-93976
VBAC, 59610-59614
VDRL, 86592-86593
Venereal Disease Research Labora-
  tory (VDRL), 86592-86593
Venipuncture
  Routine, 36415
Version, Cephalic
  External, of Fetus, 59412
Very Low Density Lipoprotein, 83719
Vesication
  Puncture Aspiration, 10160
Vesicourethropexy, 51840-51841
Vesicovaginal Fistula
  Closure
    Abdominal Approach, 51900
    Transvesical/Vaginal Approach,
      57330
    Vaginal Approach, 57320
Villus, Chorionic
  Biopsy, 59015
Viral
  AIDS, 87390
  Human Immunodeficiency
    Antibody, 86701-86703
    Antigen, 87390-87391, 87534-
      87539
    Confirmation Test, 86689
  Influenza
    Vaccine, 90657-90660
  Salivary Gland
    Cytomegalovirus
      Antigen Detection, 87271
Viscosities, Blood, 85810
    Epoxide Reductase Complex,
      Subunit 1 Gene Analysis,
      81355
  Not Otherwise Specified, 84591
VKORC1, 81355
VLDL, 83719
Voiding
  Pressure Studies
    Bladder, 51728-51729
VP, 51728-51729
Vulva
  Abscess
    Incision and Drainage, 56405
  Colposcopy., 56820
  Biopsy, 56821
  Excision
    Complete, 56625, 56633-56640
    Partial, 56620, 56630-56632
    Radical, 56630-56631, 56633-
      56640
      Complete, 56633-56640
      Partial, 56630-56632
    Simple
      Complete, 56625
      Partial, 56620
  Lesion
    Destruction, 56501-56515
  Perineum
    Biopsy, 56605-56606
    Incision and Drainage, 56405
  Repair
    Obstetric, 59300
Vulvectomy
  Complete, 56625, 56633-56640
  Partial, 56620, 56630-56632
  Radical, 56630-56640
    Complete
      with Bilateral Inguinofemoral
        Lymphadenectomy,
        56637
      with Inguinofemoral, Iliac, and
        Pelvic Lymphadenec-
        tomy, 56640
      with Unilateral Inguinofemo-
        ral Lymphadenectomy,
        56634
    Partial, 56630-56632
    Simple
      Complete, 56625
      Partial, 56620